SEX FROM PLATO TO PAGLIA

Advisory Board

David Archard
University of Lancaster

Martha Cornog

John Corvino
Wayne State University

Joseph A. Diorio
Unitec, New Zealand

Ann Garry
California State University, Los Angeles

Christine E. Gudorf
Florida International University

Sarah Hoffman
University of Saskatchewan

Richard T. Hull
State University of New York at Buffalo (Emeritus)

Edward Johnson
University of New Orleans

John Kleinig
John Jay College of Criminal Justice

Timothy F. Murphy
University of Illinois College of Medicine at Chicago

James Lindemann Nelson
Michigan State University

Igor Primoratz
Hebrew University of Jerusalem

J. Martin Stafford

Robert M. Stewart
California State University, Chico

Edward Collins Vacek, S.J.
Weston Jesuit School of Theology

Alan Wertheimer
University of Vermont

SEX FROM PLATO TO PAGLIA
A PHILOSOPHICAL ENCYCLOPEDIA

VOLUME 2: M–Z

Edited by
ALAN SOBLE

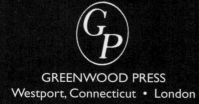

GREENWOOD PRESS
Westport, Connecticut • London

Library of Congress Cataloging-in-Publication Data

Sex from Plato to Paglia : a philosophical encyclopedia / edited by Alan Soble.
    p. cm.
   Includes bibliographical references and index.
    ISBN 0–313–32686–X (set : alk. paper)—ISBN 0–313–33424–2 (v. 1 : alk. paper)—
ISBN 0–313–33425–0 (v. 2 : alk. paper)
    1. Sex—History—Encyclopedias. 2. Sex—Philosophy—Encyclopedias. I. Soble,
Alan.
  HQ12.S423   2006
   306.7'03—dc22   2005019218

British Library Cataloguing in Publication Data is available.

Library of Congress Catalog Card Number: 2005019218
ISBN: 0–313–32686–X (set)
      0–313–33424–2 (vol. 1)
      0–313–33425–0 (vol. 2)

First published in 2006

Greenwood Press, 88 Post Road West, Westport, CT 06881
An imprint of Greenwood Publishing Group, Inc.
www.greenwood.com

Printed in the United States of America

The paper used in this book complies with the
Permanent Paper Standard issued by the National
Information Standards Organization (Z39.48–1984).

10 9 8 7 6 5 4 3 2 1

For Rachel Soble

Pinball Wizard

Marital continence is so much more difficult than continence outside marriage, because the spouses grow accustomed to intercourse.... Once they begin to have sexual intercourse as a habit, and a constant inclination is created, a mutual need for intercourse comes into being.

Karol Wojtyła (Pope John Paul II)

[R]estricting sex to a single partner ... reduce[s] its overall frequency. Marriage translates a maximum of opportunity into a minimum of desire by continually allowing the release of sexual tension before an ample amount of erotic passion can accumulate.... Thus marriage seems almost intentionally designed to make sex boring.

Murray Davis

CONTENTS

PREFACE

In early 2002, with the encouragement and guidance of Lawrence C. Becker (and, later, Charlotte B. Becker, also an experienced encyclopedist), I undertook this project to assemble an encyclopedia devoted exclusively to a relatively new and quickly growing area in philosophy, the *philosophy of sex*.

The result, *Sex from Plato to Paglia: A Philosophical Encyclopedia*, is a reference tool and resource book directed to undergraduate and graduate students in philosophy, theology, gender studies, psychology, sexology, and the arts and humanities in general, as well as to high school, college, and university teachers (of philosophy of sex courses, and others) and professional researchers and writers, whether independent or affiliated with or housed in an educational institution or think tank. The entries have, with only a few exceptions, been written in such a way that students, faculty persons, and writers in other areas, including the natural and social sciences and the professions, will profit from perusing the encyclopedia, if only out of curiosity. They might be pleasantly surprised and discover that philosophical discussions of sexuality deserve greater attention. The general goal of the encyclopedia is to educate its readers in the fundamental questions, approaches, insights, and conclusions in the continuing and expanding field of the philosophical study of human sexuality and, in the process, to be not only instructive but also thought-provoking and occasionally entertaining.

CONTENT

The encyclopedia is eclectic. It contains entries written in diverse philosophical styles and from various perspectives. Analytic, continental, religious, secular, solemn, curious, liberal, conservative, and feminist pieces cover a wide range of themes in the philosophy of sex, from "Abortion" to "Wojtyła, Karol." The final catalog of contributors and entries is mostly the result of the conscious deliberations of several human brains, but—as editors of large projects and presidents are bound to know—serendipity, too, played a role. Not every possible topic has been covered, but the included entries pick up some of the slack. For example, the intersection of medicine and sex is explored in, among others, these entries: "Diseases, Sexually Transmitted," "Ethics, Professional Codes of," "Intersexuality," "Money, John," "Paraphilia," and "Reproductive Technology."

Sex from Plato to Paglia is composed of 153 entries that break down into these three types: figures, topics/concepts, and history/schools of thought. Fifty entries discuss people who have said something philosophically noteworthy (or more) about sexuality. Most are deceased, from Plato (427–347 BCE) and Aristotle (384–322 BCE) to Michel Foucault (1926–1984), Jacques Lacan (1901–1981), and Robert Rimmer (1917–2001). Eleven, including Albert Ellis (1913–   ), John Money (1921–   ), and Irving Singer (1925–   ), are still alive. Purists will be sure to register the fact that the encyclopedia violates its own title by including entries on figures, topics, and schools that antedate Plato (pre-Platonic philosophy of sex, both Occidental and Oriental); also, some included figures, topics, or history/schools (or a piece of same) fall within a hair space to a decade after the publication of Camille Paglia's (1947–) *Sexual Personae* (1990), *Sex, Art, and American Culture* (1992), and *Vamps and Tramps* (1994) (post-Paglian philosophy of sex, both Philadelphian and Opelousan). Philosophers and librarians will also have discriminating opinions about this conundrum—whether the entry "Freudian Left, The" (and others) should be included among figures instead of schools of thought (as the editor did). About 60 entries cover topics or concepts such as abstinence, bestiality, flirting, jealousy, objectification, seduction, and rape, and about 40 entries cover history/schools of thought, such as Catholicism, existentialism, Islam, Jainism, and poststructuralism. Here, too, whether something is a topic or more precisely a school of thought could be puzzling, for example, the entries "Consequentialism," "Nudism," and "Pedophilia." The editor used the following criteria: If the word ended with "ism," or if the word's first letter could, in some context (other than at the beginning of a sentence) exist without too much strain in the upper case, the term was a *good candidate* for the "schools of thought" category. These tests work well for "consequentialism" and "nudism." The editor is not yet convinced that "pedophilia" as a "school of behavior" that has (for some writers) an underlying philosophy—as nudism is both a practice and a philosophy—is properly something other than a topic, despite ancient Greek philosophical pederasty and the more recent exertions of the North American Man-Boy Love Association. Nor are "Heterosexism" and "Sadomasochism" counted as schools of thought, despite the "ism."

STATISTICS

The entries range in length from slightly over 700 words (e.g., "Mead, Margaret") to a hundred or so words over 6,000 (e.g., "Activity, Sexual," "Arts, Sex and the," "Catholicism, History of," "Judaism, History of," and "Masturbation"), including the entry's "References." The average length is roughly 3,500 words per entry. The 153 entries were written by 103 contributors, with 33 contributors writing more than one entry. If we discount the loquacious volume editor's 8 entries, J. Martin Stafford led the pack with 5 entries. Joseph A. Diorio, Christine E. Gudorf, Edward Johnson, and Carol V. Quinn wrote 4 each. Four entries were written by teams of two scholars: Peter B. Anderson and Cindy Struckman-Johnson coauthored "Coercion (by Sexually Aggressive Women)"; Charles M. Culver and Bernard Gert wrote "Paraphilia"; and Jan Steutel and Ben Spiecker cranked out both "Disability" and "Incest."

Most of the authors are philosophers or trained in philosophy. Scholars from other fields also contributed, primarily religious studies and theology, and a handful came from political science, psychology, history, and sociology. Most are inhabitants of the United States, but 21 are from other countries: Canada (4), Finland (4), the United Kingdom (4), Australia (3), Israel (2), Netherlands (2), Denmark (1) and New Zealand (1). American contributors come from 28 states and from Guam (2) and the District of Columbia (2). California (11) beat its nearest competitors, Florida and New York, by 3.

The members of the encyclopedia's advisory board dutifully performed their administrative tasks, which included proposing figures, topics, and schools to be covered in the encyclopedia; suggesting and refining the entry descriptions and thereby the content of the entries; nominating candidate contributors for the entries; volunteering to write entries; reviewing some of the manuscripts; offering general advice about various matters; and providing occasional support and solace to the volume editor. The volume editor takes responsibility, and welcomes both the praise and the blame, for having edited, as editors are wont to do, all the entries.

FORMAT

The entries are arranged alphabetically by title, which was selected by the editor. If the entry is on an individual, his or her birth and death dates (or, in the case of living subjects, only the birth date) are supplied, attached to the title in parentheses. The text of the entry is followed immediately by a "See also" section listing other entries (chosen by the editor) that extend, elaborate, or provide details about the content of the entry. Each entry concludes with two bibliographies. The first, "References," contains works that are referred to or mentioned in the entry's text. The second, "Additional Reading," lists works that are relevant to the content of the entry but not referred to in the text of the entry. The "Additional Reading" items are, to resort to a well-known way of expressing it, "Suggestions for Further Reading." Immediately following "References" is the name of the contributor(s), whose affiliation(s) can be found in the "Editors and Contributors" section at the back of the book.

In the text of the entry, words in boldface type (e.g., **abortion**) are cross-references to other entries in the encyclopedia. Throughout the book, blind entries provide alternative ways of looking up a topic; for instance, users who go to the *E* section to look up "Education" will find the cross-reference "Education, Sex. *See* Sex Education" to lead them to the entry they seek in the *S* section. The first time a deceased person is mentioned in an entry, his or her birth and death dates (the abbreviation "ca." is used to alert the reader to approximate dates) are inserted parenthetically. (Occasionally the year of birth of a still-living person is provided in the text, out of respect for our senior citizens, among whom the editor "self-identifies.") "BCE" and, in a few cases, "CE" are employed instead of "BC" and "AD" for life dates as well as dates of events, appearance of a particular piece of writing, and so on. In the absence of "BCE," assume the date referred to is "CE."

No entry contains any footnotes or endnotes, but the entries do contain in-text citations to material listed in their "References" bibliographies. In-text references are central to the encyclopedia's mission as a research resource, even if they might at times seem to clutter the text. For example, if the entry teaches the reader (and claims) that St. Augustine presented an ingenious but fallacious argument that evil things *cannot* exist, the reader will be told exactly where (in the *Confessions*) Augustine's argument can be located (§7.12), so that the reader is not compelled to page through the entire *book* to find it. The in-text references, then, are meant to make the encyclopedia user-helpful. However, although page references are usually supplied to material in *articles*, sometimes they are not, since in some cases articles are brief and it would not be difficult for readers to find the relevant passage that is paraphrased or discussed. For *quoted* passages, whether from a book or an article, an appropriate reference is given, so that the reader can find it. If a quoted passage contains italicized words, assume that the original was italicized unless advised otherwise.

Note, however, that the in-text references are not always to page numbers in a book or an article. Especially for famous works in the history of philosophy, which exist today in many editions and translations that are paginated differently, it is more convenient for the author and the reader that reference be made not to page number but to, say, chapter number and paragraph number, so that no matter what edition or translation of the work is available, the reader can find the passage that is quoted or referred to. For example, standard marginal numbers are used for anything written by Plato and Aristotle; book, chapter, and section numbers are used for the works of Augustine, Thomas Aquinas, David Hume, and others; "Akademie" numbers are sometimes used for the works of Immanuel Kant; paragraph numbers for G.W.F. Hegel's *Philosophy of Right*; "Remark" letters for Bernard Mandeville's *Fable of the Bees*; and so on. If reference is made to a particular book or article early in a paragraph, and no other, different material is referred to in that paragraph, then the reader should assume that any later in-text references in that paragraph (say, page numbers standing alone) are to that only-named particular book or article. Exceptions to these principles occur in the case of materials referred to that exist on the World Wide Web, which ordinarily have no page or marginal numbers. But these items are almost always brief and, in any event, the reader who accesses a Web page can use his or her browser's search function to find the passage. This procedure is efficient if one searches for a unique word or short string of words.

The "Additional Reading" bibliographies were compiled largely by the volume editor. Every entry, with two exceptions ("Manichaeism" and "Spencer, Herbert"), concludes with an "Additional Reading" list. Many philosophical articles and books on sexuality are valuable sources, yet not all could be discussed or mentioned in the individual entries. The "Additional Reading" lists are meant to alert readers who are interested in the breadth of the philosophical literature, and who wish to pursue matters of special concern more deeply, to this additional material. Also listed are more general philosophical treatises about issues, concepts, and figures that will help readers situate the philosophy of sex within the history of, and current debates in, philosophy. Further, important nonphilosophical articles and books on sexuality, from the humanities and the sciences (some of which are classics in their fields), are significant sources not only for those who wish to evaluate philosophical perspectives on sexuality in the broader context of general human knowledge but also for those who believe, as many scholars do, that knowledge of a wide variety of disciplines is essential to understanding and making progress in the philosophy of sex, which is, and is best approached as, an interdisciplinary field.

The "Additional Reading" bibliography does not include sources discussed, mentioned, or cited in an entry; all these items are listed only in an entry's "References" list. However, occasionally a few sources not referred to in an entry are nevertheless included in its "References" bibliography by virtue of their importance to the content of the entry. Further, an entry's "Additional Reading" list includes not only additional material but also—for the benefit of readers intent on tracking down a particular source or who do not have access to a specific item listed in the "References"—information about reprints and other editions of the sources contained in the "References." This information about reprints and alternative editions has the independent value of providing a historical record of writings in the philosophy of sex.

Readers may notice some repetition in the "References" and "Additional Reading" bibliographies. An item listed in the "References" of one entry may show up in another entry's "References" or in another entry's "Additional Reading." Some items appear in more than one "Additional Reading" list (and may or may not be listed in any entry's "References"). This repetition results from interconnections between the various topics and concepts in the philosophy of sex. It is not to be bemoaned. Rather, the repetition will usefully assist readers in locating relevant material for further research. The essay on the phenomenology of prostitution by Clelia Anderson and Yolanda Estes might be overlooked by readers interested in phenomenological approaches to sexuality, were the essay included only in the bibliographies of the "Prostitution" entry; or it might be missed by those interested in prostitution, were it listed only in the bibliographies of the "Phenomenology" entry. Similarly, Ermanno Bencivegna's "Kant's Sadism," Drucilla Cornell's *The Imaginary Domain: Abortion, Pornography, and Sexual Harassment*, and other "compound" items simply had to be listed several times. The editor suspects that any item listed once could, with justification, have been listed twice, but he wisely eschewed that route. The repetition that does exist will be helpful to those students and scholars—probably most—who read or browse selectively instead of reading universally, that is, digesting the entire encyclopedia.

The encyclopedia's editor is fully responsible for the final selection of the items included in each "Additional Reading" bibliography. The editor, however, received much assistance from the authors of the individual entries, who suggested many items to be included in their entry's "Additional Reading" list and who are therefore responsible (only) for the accuracy of the bibliographic information for the particular items they submitted toward this list. That an item is listed should not necessarily be taken as an endorsement of the book or article or as meaning that either the author of the entry or the editor thinks that the work has merit (although in many cases it does). That is, some items are listed for the sake of completeness and to provide another piece of the intricate historical record. Besides, philosophical tastes vary and change. That which is eminently vacuous in one decade might be eminently sagacious in the next. This could apply to all readers or even only to one reader, who might have "matured"—or "regressed"—as a scholar.

Had space allowed, brief annotations for each item listed could have further enhanced the usefulness of the "Additional Reading" bibliographies. For example, it is obvious why Laura Kipnis's essay "Adultery" is listed for the "Adultery" entry. (Even so, a few words about Kipnis's view of adultery would help the reader.) But its being included for the "Freudian Left" entry may be puzzling. It could be explained easily by appending: "Kipnis coins the term 'surplus monogamy,' deliberately fashioned after Marcuse." Alas, pressing space considerations, as well as time and energy requirements, placed severe limits on what could be accomplished. The reader is encouraged to trust the editor's judgment that good reason exists for the seemingly odd placement of some items. (In a few instances, where it was thought essential, an extremely brief annotation, surrounded by square brackets, has been inserted.)

The following principles were employed by the editor in structuring the items in the bibliographies:

- In the "Additional Reading" lists alone, and never in an entry's "References" bibliography, abbreviations for books are occasionally used, usually when an item has been reprinted in a popular (well-known or much-referred-to) anthology or collection of articles. These books are listed in the "Abbreviations" section found at the front of the book. Sometimes these items are referred to in the "References" as appearing in these collections; there abbreviations are not used, thereby usually (but not always; see the exception, below) signaling that the item's original or primary location of appearance was in fact the anthology itself and not, say, a journal (the item does not appear in the collection as a reprint). This might occur in the "Additional Reading" section of an entry as well, indicating again that the anthology is the original or main location of publication. An exception occurs when a contributor chose to refer in the text of the entry to a reprint of the article in a collection instead of to the original, sometimes on the grounds that the reprint would be more accessible to the reader and sometimes because only the reprint was accessible to the writer. When this happens, it will be made clear in the "Additional Reading" bibliography where the original location of publication, with its earlier date, is provided.

- If an article or essay by an author is included in a book entirely written by that author, the author's name appears only once, as the author of the essay, and not repeated later as author of the whole book. For example,

  Swiss, Charles E. "How to Play Pinball Like a Wizard." In *Games and Other Diversions: A Philosophical Exploration*. Bogalusa, La.: Cheeseworks Enterprises, 2004, 77–93.

  In this case, because no other author or editor is provided for *Games and Other Diversions*, the reader should assume that the whole work was authored by Swiss. That is, the formats "In his [or her] *Games . . .*" or "In Charles E. Swiss, *Games . . .*" are not employed. If someone else edited the book, or if the author of the article is in fact the editor of a (this) book that contains essays by other writers, then the editor's name, different or the same, is explicitly provided. In such a case, expect to see:

  Swiss, Charles E. "How to Play Pinball Like a Wizard." In Charles E. Swiss, ed., *Games and Other Diversions: A Philosophical Exploration*. Bogalusa, La.: Cheeseworks Enterprises, 2004, 77–93.

  Or if Swiss did not edit the book, it would appear as "In Lucy Butterworth, ed., *Games. . . .*"

- The goal (appreciably achieved but not always) was to supply thoroughly complete bibliographic information. For journal articles, this means full names of author(s); full title of essay; name(s) of translator(s), if any; journal name; volume; issue number (or quarter, season, month); year; and inclusive page numbers. For books, this means full names of all authors or editors ("et al." was used neither for books nor articles; it was deemed by the editor inappropriate for a reference book, which should provide a complete historical record); full name of book, including subtitle, if any; name(s) of translator(s), if any; name of the publisher; place of publication; and year of publication. For an item translated into English, its original date of publication (if available) in its original language is provided after the author's name. Sometimes a year date after the author's name indicates, instead, the year of the item's first edition in English, if a later edition is the one listed in the bibliography. Multiple dates indicate successive editions (for items in any language). And sometimes a year date after the author's name indicates, in particular for ancient texts and classic works, when (roughly) it was written and unleashed onto the world (*perhaps* published, if "published," a relatively modern concept, and grist for the social constructionist mill, even makes sense for these works). The context should successfully disclose what the year date refers to.

The encyclopedia contains other helpful sections. At the end of the front matter is a "Guide to Related Topics," which groups together under a single heading entries having a significant feature in common. A reader who wants to explore ancient thought about sex will find entries of that sort grouped under "Classical Philosophy." Other readers may want to focus on the entries grouped under "Continental Philosophy," "Feminism," "Sexology," and so on. There are twenty-two groupings, from "Analytic Philosophy" to "Theories of

Sexuality." Some entries are listed more than once. "Jealousy," for example, is placed under "Analytic Philosophy," "Ethics," and "Psychology" because the entry discusses in an analytic manner an emotion that has ethical implications.

At the end of the second volume are the "Selected General Bibliography," a section devoted to the authors of the entries and the members of the advisory board, and the indices. The "Selected General Bibliography" lists a number of anthologies and textbooks about the philosophy and theology of sex, works that along with those listed in "Abbreviations" in the first volume might well be said to complete the core literature in the field. This general bibliography also includes helpful treatises in general philosophy, important collections, books, and reference materials from other fields, and (segregated from the rest) the names of journals that exclusively publish studies about sexuality.

Readers curious about the authors of the entries and the members of the encyclopedia's advisory board will find professional and personal information about them in the next section. Their academic positions, affiliations, education, publications, and assorted biographical details were supplied by the persons themselves and only mildly edited by the volume editor. The encyclopedia closes with both a name index and a subject index.

ACKNOWLEDGMENTS

The editor owes some words of thanks to friends and colleagues. From among the contributors to this encyclopedia, these colleagues performed duties above and beyond sending me their entries more or less on time and more or less in good shape: Elizabeth Brake, Keith Burgess-Jackson, David Carr, Carol Steinberg Gould, Mane Hajdin, Raja Halwani, Jeffrey Hershfield, Berel Dov Lerner, Michael P. Levine, Ed Pluth, Lee C. Rice, Lance Byron Richey, and Celia Wolf-Devine. From among the members of the advisory board, these colleagues performed duties above and beyond those required by their burdensome administrative functions: Martha Cornog, Ann Garry, Sarah Hoffman, Richard T. Hull, Edward Johnson, J. Martin Stafford, Robert M. Stewart, and Edward Collins Vacek. From among the contemporary scholars whose work was addressed in entries in the encyclopedia, these writers were especially cooperative in providing generous, witty, or acerbic criticism: Vern L. Bullough, Albert Ellis, John Finnis ("Natural Law, New"), Gilbert Herdt, John Money, Camille Paglia, Roger Scruton, Irving Singer, and Robert C. Solomon ("Communication Model").

Other people who graciously replied to the editor's requests for help or offered it out of the blue include Dirk Baltzly, Steven Barbone, Charlotte Becker, Larry Becker, Aaron Ben-Ze'ev, Charles Bronstein, Ronna Burger, Judy Crane, Russell Dancy, Carrie Delorge, Lara Denis, Laura Drago, Forrai Gábor, Jancy Hoeffel, Rebecca Homiski, Noretta Koertge, Nan Levinson, Peggy Brinkman Matteliano, Elijah Millgram, Seiriol Morgan, Alan Pasch, Sylvia Walsh Perkins, Timothy Perper, Patricia Petersen, Heidi Ravven, Eric Reitan, Marga Ryersbach, Laurie Shrage, Rachel Soble, Edward Stein, Jim Stone, Rosemarie Tong, John Wagner, Yuko Yoshida, Michael Zeleny, and several "I-prefer-to-be-anonymous" reviewers of manuscripts.

To the staff of the Interlibrary Loan Department of the University of New Orleans, I express my gratitude for the stream of books and journal articles they secured for me over the last three years. Finally, a tip of the hat to the personnel at Café Roma (Jefferson Davis Parkway), Rue de la Course (S. Carrollton), the New Orleans East Donut Shoppe ("South Shore Grill"), the Metairie-Causeway Donut Shoppe ("Joe's Cafe"), Z'otz Coffeehouse (Oak Street), Brown's Donut Shop (Read Boulevard), 13 Monaghan (Marigny), Central Perk ("Not Central Park, but Close"), Community Coffee at Riverbend (deceased), Coffee Bean Cafe (a.k.a. "European Coffee House"), and the world-famous house of nunches, the Hoff Street Delicatessen—the only place that survived Katrina.

INTRODUCTION

Human sexuality and animal sexuality have been extensively studied by the natural and social sciences. Tens of thousands of books and hundreds of thousands of journal articles, plus a substantial number of excellent reference works (some of which are listed in the "Selected General Bibliography"), attest to the long history of the sexological sciences and to the continuing and irresistible interest among scholars in investigating the variety of sexual desires, sexual behaviors, sexual couplings, and sexual curiosities exhibited by both humans and other animals. This abundant research has seemingly covered every imaginable aspect of sex, from the microscopic to the social, from the mundane to the improbable, from the unspeakably, intimately personal to the public, the political, and the economic. And, of course, the poets, novelists, artists, sculptors, opera writers, musicians, photographers, filmmakers, choreographers, and even the architects and landscapers have illuminated, in their own distinctive, sometimes only implicit, ways the many forms and styles of sexuality. I would not be surprised were a congress of methodical and determined librarians and information historians to discover that of all the topics on which the human mind has pondered, sex is (nearly) the most frequently entertained and dissected.

Indeed, I have heard it said (but have never believed) that men—human males—think about sex once every six to ten seconds. Women, for their part—or so I have been instructed by several authoritative feminists—tend to dwell on food. (In a culture that connives women to be thin, a deliciously fattening but forbidden meal is often in the back of their salivating minds.) Now, what counts, exactly, as "thinking about sex" or "having a thought about sex" (or about food) deserves careful analysis, and this is the sort of thing that *philosophers* do, at least some of them. Consider the question seriously, for it is not far removed from, "What is a *sexual picture*?" and "What is an *obscene image*?"—incomparably difficult questions raised, discussed, and argued over both by philosophers of sex and law and by jurisprudentialists and legal scholars. *Sex from Plato to Paglia* focuses on a slice of all the human thought about sex, the philosophical slice, not the architectural slice nor the choreographical slice and, as such, has its own methods, its own ways of proceeding through the sexual maze, and its own sorts of results.

Moreover, the goals and content of an encyclopedia of the philosophy of sex must, at the beginning, be distinguished from the goals and content of what in popular culture often *passes as* philosophy of sex, by which I mean the stream of lectures and interviews, newspaper columns and books, audio- and videotapes, radio broadcasts, and television programs on sex: from Dr. Ruth's motherly or auntish advice to Dr. Phil's fatherly or uncleish advice, from Rabbi Boteach's fiery encyclicals to Jerry Springer's reconciliatory end-of-the-show monologues. There are differences between popularized philosophy of sex—to be sure, a good deal of it mentions *bona fide* philosophers like Plato (427–347 BCE), St. Augustine (354–430), and Sigmund Freud (1856–1939)—and technical, professional, scholarly, academic philosophy of sex, which also discusses the same catalog of figures.

The central difference may be that whereas pop-culture philosophizing promises a quick fix to ubiquitous problems (indeed, this is its appeal, and it *is* undeniably good for some things), hardcore philosophy promises absolutely no quick fixes at all. What professional philosophy of sex has to offer are "fixes," so to speak, but fixes that take a long time to achieve and require sustained mental attention and deliberation. This is *not* to insist, self-righteously, that (to employ Jeremy Bentham's [1748–1832] metaphor) poetry is always better than pushpin; nor is it to insist (to rely backhandedly on Socrates [469–399 BCE] and John Stuart Mill [1806–1873]) that the unexamined life has absolutely nothing at all going for it—recall the physically gorgeous and ignorantly blissful young heterosexual couple that Alvie (Woody Allen) unabashedly envies in *Annie Hall*. Simply put, philosophy of sex has something to offer to a different group of people, having different needs and interests, who hold a different vision of the valuable or fun life. My own favorites among the entries—an editor can also be a reader—in terms of their value and fun for me, not necessarily the ones that are objectively the best, include: "Augustine (Saint)"; "Descartes, René"; "Desire, Sexual"; "Existentialism"; "Fichte, Johann Gottlieb"; "Hegel, G.W.F."; "Hobbes, Thomas"; "Jealousy"; "Kierkegaard, Søren"; "Mandeville, Bernard"; "Paraphilia"; "Rousseau, Jean-Jacques"; and "Russell, Bertrand." Other readers, having their own equally eccentric standards of value and fun, will construct their own equally compelling lists of favorite entries.

The philosophy of sex provides instruction and practice in clarifying our thought processes, enabling us to progress from an ordinarily quite acceptable, everyday, and usually harmless sloppiness to greater precision in thinking and speaking. It will not offer any psychological consolation. Quite the contrary. Often what is revealed by deep and protracted philosophical thought is hardly the comfort or contentment one might have hoped for, and it is frequently unsettling and upsetting. For what philosophical thought about sexuality tends to reveal, even flaunt, is that the Human Condition cannot be reduced to easy formulas and platitudes, that our sexual existence—our yearnings, desires, motives, actions, and identities—is barely recognized by ourselves and much too complex to be neatly ordered, categorized, and comprehended the way accountants can immaculately sum things up with Power Point in black, white, and red.

For example, sexual jealousy can be painful and difficult to handle, often gaining the better of us. It is not to sell the humanities short by admitting that an attack of severe jealousy is best attended to by psychotherapy, tranquilizers, or several close friends and not by the philosophy of sex. But, again, this is *not* to say that professional, technical, or scholarly philosophy of sex must be arcane, boring, or irrelevant—as the term "academic" often means to those uninitiated to the world of letters. What the philosophy of sex can do will be valuable and interesting in its own right, in the right context. It will help us gain a glimmer of understanding of the existential significance of feeling jealous, inserting it into a larger picture of the meaning of life. It will illuminate how our feeling jealous links up with, even depends on, certain beliefs and attitudes that we possess, ideas we have willy-nilly or, instead, as the result of entrenched social patterns. It will also teach us how to think clearly about exactly what we are experiencing, so that we are able to distinguish jealousy from its various close relatives, such as envy, resentment, and insulted anger, and hence be in a better position to understand and communicate to others the quality and focus of our emotions.

The fear of loss is a ubiquitous human state, but that does not mean we must succumb to it blindly, without any intellectual appreciation of it at all. To take what is for some a less threatening example, consider the practice or phenomenon of "cybersex." Philosophical reflection on cybersex makes us reevaluate the notion of our having a discretely defined body. It forces us to rethink what it means to have "sexual contact" with another person and, derivatively, what forms adultery might, or might not, take in the technologically sophisticated twenty-first century. It also compels us to ask critically why we need or want "actual" or "real" embodied other people when engaging in sex, instead of being happily orgasmic with their virtual representations. The philosophical questions that arise here are in many ways similarly macabre to those that arise about cloning and are equally troublesome and no less pressing.

The philosophy of sex began, in the West, with the ancient Greek philosopher Plato (if not earlier, with Sappho [ca. 610–580 BCE], the pre-Socratics, and the Hebrews), and in the East with ancient religious teachings, including those of Hinduism and Buddhism. Like all subareas in philosophy (ethics, logic, epistemology, and so forth), the philosophy of sex has a history. In the West, for example, it proceeds from Plato to and through—to name just a few figures—Michel Montaigne (1533–1592), David Hume (1711–1776), Immanuel Kant (1724–1804), Søren Kierkegaard (1813–1855), Bertrand Russell (1872–1970), Jean-Paul Sartre (1905–1980), Michel Foucault (1926–1984), and Catharine MacKinnon (1946–). That is only *secular* philosophy of sex in the West; the history of the philosophy of sex also has an intertwining theological, religious path, from Plato, again, to and through St. Paul (5–64?), St. Augustine, St. Thomas Aquinas (1224/25–1274), Søren Kierkegaard, and a handful of twentieth-century popes.

It was in the twentieth century that the philosophy of sex blossomed (as did other areas in philosophy, for example, logic, the philosophy of language, and legal philosophy), partially as the result of Thomas Nagel's (1937–) pioneering essay "Sexual Perversion," published in the prestigious *Journal of Philosophy* in 1969. "Pioneering" and "prestigious" are used circumspectly, with both trepidation and reluctance, because by the twenty-first century it has become hackneyed, an entrenched professional cliché, to use precisely those words in recounting this revolutionary event. But revolutionary it was, in a genuine sense, for Nagel successfully applied the techniques of (stereotypically) cold analytic philosophy to a rich human phenomenon. Further, he also demonstrated that Anglo-American analytic philosophy had much to learn from the Continental (in this instance, the French) philosophical tradition. After the essay appeared, philosophers increasingly took sexual matters seriously, writing about sexuality unhysterically and without sermonizing, treating sex not as something especially delicate or especially dangerous but as another topic, among other topics of no more or no less importance, about which philosophical thought might fruitfully yield illumination.

There are already in print several reference works in the philosophy of sex. One is Igor Primoratz's *Human Sexuality* (1997), which reprints in a 500-page volume twenty-five of the most important journal articles in the philosophy of sex published during the final thirty years of the twentieth century. *Human Sexuality* is not only historically significant; it is also an indispensable resource for research. (Each article is reprinted as a facsimile, exactly as it appeared when first published, including original font, page numbers, etc.) But the volume is not encyclopedic, nor was it intended to be. Another is Alan Soble's *Sex, Love, and Friendship* (1997), which collects together, in 650 pages, sixty philosophical essays prepared for the Society for the Philosophy of Sex and Love in the period 1977–1992. Like Primoratz's volume, *Sex, Love, and Friendship* is a historically important record and a valuable resource for research but is not encyclopedic. A third is Earl E. Shelp's two-volume, 550-page *Sexuality and Medicine* (1987), whose twenty-eight essays are devoted to the special intersection of sexual ethics and biomedical science. Anyone who has more than a passing interest in the philosophy of sex should obtain copies of, or at least ensure having access to, these three works. The rationale behind *Sex from Plato to Paglia* is that while a great deal of interesting and important philosophical writing has been done on human sexuality, this material remained to be integrated and presented in such a way that a large amount of philosophical thought about sex is succinctly yet accurately and comprehensively summarized. Further, significant advances in the field needed to be distinctly noted and described, and additional lines of research, and questions and issues insufficiently explored or yet to be explored, brought to the attention of those feeling an itch to contribute to the development of the philosophy of sex.

ABBREVIATIONS

The abbreviations listed below are used throughout the entry bibliographies to designate frequently cited works.

HS   Primoratz, Igor, ed. *Human Sexuality*. Aldershot, U.K.: Ashgate, 1997.

P&S1   Baker, Robert B., and Frederick A. Elliston, eds. *Philosophy and Sex*, 1st ed. Buffalo, N.Y.: Prometheus, 1975.

P&S2   Baker, Robert B., and Frederick A. Elliston, eds. *Philosophy and Sex*, 2nd ed. Buffalo, N.Y.: Prometheus, 1984.

P&S3   Baker, Robert B., Kathleen J. Wininger, and Frederick A. Elliston, eds. *Philosophy and Sex*, 3rd ed. Amherst, N.Y.: Prometheus, 1998.

POS1   Soble, Alan, ed. *The Philosophy of Sex: Contemporary Readings*, 1st ed. Totowa, N.J.: Rowman and Littlefield, 1980.

POS2   Soble, Alan, ed. *The Philosophy of Sex: Contemporary Readings*, 2nd ed. Savage, Md.: Rowman and Littlefield, 1991.

POS3   Soble, Alan, ed. *The Philosophy of Sex: Contemporary Readings*, 3rd ed. Lanham, Md.: Rowman and Littlefield, 1997.

POS4   Soble, Alan, ed. *The Philosophy of Sex: Contemporary Readings*, 4th ed. Lanham, Md.: Rowman and Littlefield, 2002.

SLF   Soble, Alan, ed. *Sex, Love, and Friendship: Studies of the Society for the Philosophy of Sex and Love, 1977–1992*. Amsterdam, Holland: Rodopi, 1997.

STW   Stewart, Robert, ed. *Philosophical Perspectives on Sex and Love*. New York: Oxford University Press, 1995.

GUIDE TO RELATED TOPICS

Analytic Philosophy

Abstinence
Activity, Sexual
Adultery
Casual Sex
Completeness, Sexual
Consent
Desire, Sexual
Fantasy
Flirting
Friendship
Harassment, Sexual
Jealousy
Masturbation
Orientation, Sexual
Paraphilia
Perversion, Sexual
Philosophy of Sex, Overview of
Privacy
Seduction

Catholicism, Roman

Abortion
Abstinence
Animal Sexuality
Anscombe, G.E.M.
Augustine (Saint)
Bible, Sex and the
Catholicism, History of
Catholicism, Twentieth- and Twenty-First-
    Century
Completeness, Sexual
Contraception
Natural Law (New)
Paul (Saint)
Thomas Aquinas (Saint)
Wojtyła, Karol (Pope John Paul II)

Classical Philosophy

Aristotle
Augustine (Saint)
Gnosticism
Greek Sexuality and Philosophy, Ancient
Manichaeism
Paul (Saint)
Plato
Roman Sexuality and Philosophy, Ancient

Continental Philosophy

Bataille, Georges
Existentialism
Feminism, French
Fichte, Johann Gottlieb
Foucault, Michel
Freudian Left, The
Hegel, G.W.F.
Heidegger, Martin
Kant, Immanuel
Kierkegaard, Søren
Kolnai, Aurel
Lacan, Jacques
Leibniz, Gottfried
Levinas, Emmanuel
Marxism
Nietzsche, Friedrich
Phenomenology
Poststructuralism
Sade, Marquis de
Schopenhauer, Arthur
Spinoza, Baruch

Ethics

Abortion
Adultery

Existentialism

Feminism

Gay/Lesbian/Bisexual/Transgendered (GLBT)

Diseases, Sexually Transmitted
Dworkin, Andrea
Feminism, French
Feminism, Lesbian
Feminism, Men's
Foucault, Michel
Greek Sexuality and Philosophy, Ancient
Herdt, Gilbert
Heterosexism
Homosexuality, Ethics of
Homosexuality and Science
MacKinnon, Catharine
Marriage, Same-Sex
Mead, Margaret
Military, Sex and the
Orientation, Sexual
Philosophy of Sex, Teaching the
Queer Theory
Roman Sexuality and Philosophy,
   Ancient
Social Constructionism

History

African Philosophy
Beauty
Bible, Sex and the
Boswell, John
Bullough, Vern L.
Catholicism, History of
Catholicism, Twentieth- and Twenty-First-
   Century
Desire, Sexual
Ethics, Professional Codes of
Existentialism
Feminism, History of
Gnosticism
Greek Sexuality and Philosophy,
   Ancient
Incest
Judaism, History of
Judaism, Twentieth- and Twenty-First-
   Century
Love
Manichaeism
Marriage
Philosophy of Sex, Overview of
Poststructuralism
Protestantism, History of

Protestantism, Twentieth- and Twenty-
   First-Century
Psychology, Twentieth- and Twenty-First-
   Century
Roman Sexuality and Philosophy, Ancient
Sexology
Social Constructionism
Utopianism

Legal Philosophy

Arts, Sex and the
Bestiality
Consent
Disability
Diseases, Sexually Transmitted
Dworkin, Andrea
Harassment, Sexual
Humor
Law, Sex and the
Liberalism
MacKinnon, Catharine
Marriage, Same-Sex
Military, Sex and the
Nudism
Paglia, Camille
Pornography
Posner, Richard
Privacy
Prostitution
Rape
Rape, Acquaintance and Date
Sadomasochism
Sex Work

Liberalism

Consent
Consequentialism
Ellis, Albert
Ethics, Sexual
Feminism, Liberal
Hobbes, Thomas
Kant, Immanuel
Law, Sex and the
Liberalism
Nudism
Paglia, Camille
Pornography
Privacy

Prostitution
Rimmer, Robert
Russell, Bertrand
Sadomasochism
Seduction
Sex Work
Singer, Irving

Marxism

Ethics, Sexual
Existentialism
Freudian Left, The
Hegel, G.W.F.
Marxism

Medicine

Addiction, Sexual
Bestiality
Contraception
Disability
Diseases, Sexually Transmitted
Dysfunction, Sexual
Ellis, Albert
Ellis, Havelock
Ethics, Professional Codes of
Firestone, Shulamith
Freud, Sigmund
Genital Mutilation
Homosexuality and Science
Incest
Intersexuality
Money, John
Paraphilia
Pedophilia
Perversion, Sexual
Reproductive Technology
Sexology
Sherfey, Mary Jane

Modern Philosophy

Descartes, René
Hobbes, Thomas
Hume, David
Leibniz, Gottfried
Rousseau, Jean-Jacques
Spinoza, Baruch

Non-Western Philosophy

African Philosophy
Buddhism
Chinese Philosophy
Hinduism
Indian Erotology
Islam
Jainism
Tantrism

Philosophers (Secular)

Aristotle
Bataille, Georges
Boswell, John
Bullough, Vern L.
Descartes, René
Dworkin, Andrea
Ellis, Albert
Ellis, Havelock
Fichte, Johann Gottlieb
Firestone, Shulamith
Foucault, Michel
Freud, Sigmund
Hegel, G.W.F.
Heidegger, Martin
Herdt, Gilbert
Hobbes, Thomas
Hume, David
Kant, Immanuel
Kierkegaard, Søren
Kolnai, Aurel
Lacan, Jacques
Leibniz, Gottfried
Levinas, Emmanuel
MacKinnon, Catharine
Mandeville, Bernard
Mead, Margaret
Money, John
Nagel, Thomas
Nietzsche, Friedrich
Paglia, Camille
Plato
Posner, Richard
Rimmer, Robert
Rousseau, Jean-Jacques
Russell, Bertrand
Sacher-Masoch, Leopold von

Sade, Marquis de
Schopenhauer, Arthur
Scruton, Roger
Sherfey, Mary Jane
Singer, Irving
Spencer, Herbert
Spinoza, Baruch
Westermarck, Edward
Wittgenstein, Ludwig

Philosophers (Theological)

Anscombe, G.E.M.
Augustine (Saint)
Kierkegaard, Søren
Paul (Saint)
Thomas Aquinas (Saint)
Wojtyła, Karol (Pope John Paul II)

Politics

African Philosophy
Arts, Sex and the
Consequentialism
Disability
Diseases, Sexually Transmitted
Dworkin, Andrea
Ellis, Albert
Existentialism
Feminism, Men's
Firestone, Shulamith
Foucault, Michel
Freud, Sigmund
Freudian Left, The
Heterosexism
Law, Sex and the
Liberalism
MacKinnon, Catharine
Mandeville, Bernard
Marriage, Same-Sex
Marxism
Military, Sex and the
Natural Law (New)
Paglia, Camille
Pornography
Privacy
Prostitution
Queer Theory
Rape

Rape, Acquaintance and Date
Scruton, Roger
Sex Education
Sex Work
Sexology
Spencer, Herbert
Utopianism
Violence, Sexual
Wittgenstein, Ludwig

Psychology

Beauty
Completeness, Sexual
Ellis, Albert
Freud, Sigmund
Homosexuality and Science
Humor
Jealousy
Lacan, Jacques
Language
Nagel, Thomas
Plato
Psychology, Evolutionary
Psychology, Twentieth- and Twenty-First-
    Century
Sexology

Religion (Western, Non-Catholic)

Abstinence
Bible, Sex and the
Gnosticism
Islam
Judaism, History of
Judaism, Twentieth- and Twenty-First-
    Century
Manichaeism
Protestantism, History of
Protestantism, Twentieth- and Twenty-
    First-Century

Sexology

Bullough, Vern L.
Dysfunction, Sexual
Ellis, Albert
Ellis, Havelock

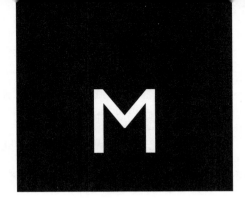

MACKINNON, CATHARINE (1946–). Catharine Alice MacKinnon is a feminist and legal activist whose work aims to theorize women's oppression independently of psychoanalysis, **Marxism**, and **liberalism** (Ring, 755). Born in Minnesota, MacKinnon attended Smith College, gained a law degree and a Ph.D. in political science from Yale University, and was appointed Elizabeth A. Long Professor of Law at the University of Michigan. She is well known for having established **sexual harassment** as a legally actionable form of sex discrimination, and she wrote, with **Andrea Dworkin** (1946–2005), an ordinance (MacKinnon, *Women's Lives*, 493n.22 [to 497]) that would have enabled women harmed by **pornography** to sue its producers in civil court. Considered in Minneapolis, Los Angeles County, and Massachusetts, and passed in Indianapolis in 1984, the ordinance was struck down as unconstitutional by U.S. federal courts (MacKinnon and Dworkin, 426–61; Downs, 95–143; Duggan et al., 130; Vadas, 94–100). A controversial figure, MacKinnon has been described as "the best philosophical mind since Aristotle" (Vadas, 96) and as the author of "the incoherent rants of a lunatic fringe" (Soble, *Pornography*, 178).

Sex and Gender. Sexuality is the keystone of MacKinnon's theory of women's oppression. "Sexuality is to feminism," she writes, "what work is to Marxism" (*Toward*, 3). While women's condition in patriarchy parallels that of workers in capitalism, MacKinnon believes that a class-based Marxist analysis cannot explain women's oppression, because it does not address the fundamentally social origins of the categories "men" and "women" (W. Brown, 79–81). MacKinnon believes these categories are not generated by nature but are produced by male power. Male power is the source, not the consequence, of gender differences: "[I]n life, 'woman' and 'man' are widely experienced as features of being, not constructs of perception, cultural interventions, or forced identities. Gender, in other words, is lived as ontology, not as epistemology" (*Toward*, 237). Ontology is what is real and, for MacKinnon, it is inherently inaccessible. Epistemology includes socially constructed beliefs about what is real and emerges out of the power structures of given societies. As a social constructionist, MacKinnon denies control over social organization to ontology or male/female biological differences (Allen, *Power*, 11–12). Epistemology controls the hierarchical definition of male/female categories.

Patriarchy has not misunderstood gender differences or applied them unjustly in assigning men and women to different social roles; patriarchy has *created* oppressive gender differences in the first place, by creating the categories "men" and "women" and by building dominance and subordination into their definitions (MacKinnon, *Feminism Unmodified*, 3; Allen, "Pornography," 513). "Men create the world," MacKinnon states, "from their own point of view, which then becomes the truth to be described. . . . *Power to create the world from one's own point of view is power in its male form*. The male epistemological stance, which corresponds to the world it creates, is objectivity" ("Feminism . . . Agenda," 537–38). Power predates epistemology. Regardless of how natural the hierarchical social structure of male and female categories appears to be, this structure is a social production that already reflects male power. The persons who originally occupied the male standpoint of objectivity had to have the power to impose it. While masculine power created gender and is exercised through it, this power itself could not depend on gender (Allen, "Pornography," 513). Male power generates the epistemology that constructs the sex/gender categories through which male power is exercised. Power makes gender, and gender serves power.

Gendering is a social process that makes people into women and men, and their resulting characteristics have nothing to do with their biology (MacKinnon, *Toward*, 46). For men, being gendered means power, control, assertiveness, aggression, strength, agency, and income, while for women it means subordination, vulnerability, weakness, passivity, and relative impoverishment (*Toward*, 110). "Women's situation," MacKinnon writes, "combines unequal pay with allocation to disrespected work, sexual targeting for rape, domestic battering, sexual abuse as children, and systematic sexual harassment; depersonalization, demeaned physical characteristics, use in denigrating entertainment, deprivation of reproductive control, and forced prostitution" ("From Practice to Theory," 15).

Gendering serves sexuality. The feminine gender stereotype makes women sexually attractive to men. "What defines women as such," MacKinnon writes, "is what turns men on" (*Toward*, 110). Gender and sexuality, like the categories "men" and "women," are "fundamentally social" (*Toward*, xiii). Sexuality, as socially constructed, requires gender difference: Without submissive women and aggressive men, sexuality would not be erotically arousing (*Feminism Unmodified*, 51). Inequality makes sex sexy (*Feminism Unmodified*, 7; *Toward*, 113). "Male dominance," she writes, "is sexual. Meaning: men in particular, if not men alone, sexualize hierarchy" (*Toward*, 127). For a sexual charge to be felt, even in same-sex relationships, one person must be gendered "male" and dominate the other. When a man is raped by another man, he is socially gendered female ("Desire and Power," 111–12). Equality and sexuality are opposed; the conjunction of force and sex is inescapable.

Society can sexualize anything: Sexuality is "whatever a given culture (even subculture) defines it as" ("Reply," 186). By sexualizing the gender stereotypes of weakness and strength, patriarchy makes sexuality oppressive for women. Women accept being sexual playthings for men. No force is apparent in this process unless the oppressed resist. When slaves see their status as natural, and labor without being forced, harmony apparently prevails. Similarly, when women willingly assume the feminine role and excite men—and themselves—through submissive behavior, no overt power is apparent. But since sexuality is gendered and unequal, force is always (at least implicitly) present. Willing women engaging in submissive sexuality undergo oppression.

Having theorized (male) sexuality as inherently aggressive, MacKinnon assimilates heterosexual intercourse to **rape** (*Feminism Unmodified*, 86). She denies that sexual relationships involve equal partners interacting out of affection or erotic arousal (168). Distinguishing rape from normal sex rests on the mistaken belief that normal sex is nonviolent, and rape, which is supposedly abnormal, unacceptably introduces violence into sex. Rape cannot be distinguished from normal sex in this way, however, because the essence of normal sex *is* violence (Rapaport, 133–34). MacKinnon charges that rape laws jail rapists for doing to women what nonrapists regularly do to them as a matter of course ("Feminism . . . Jurisprudence," 643).

Laws against rape presume that women should control their own **sexual activity** through a presumptive right to refuse (*Toward*, 174 ff.). MacKinnon notes, however, that "when sex is violent, women may have lost control over what is done to them, but absence of force does not ensure . . . control" (*Toward*, 178). Intercourse is rape with **consent**, and consent, even when overtly present, is suspect: Women may consent out of fear, or to avoid more force than already has been used, or because they, like men, have eroticized dominance (*Toward*, 177). Intercourse without force is conceptually impossible. "If there is no inequality, no violation, no dominance, no force, there is no sexual arousal" (*Feminism Unmodified*, 160).

Pornography. MacKinnon sees pornography as "the manufacture from skin and blood and ruined lives of a vicious product by vicious people" (Dworkin and MacKinnon, 25). In the production of pornography, women are "bound, battered, tortured, harassed, raped, and sometimes killed; or . . . 'merely' humiliated, molested, objectified and used" ("Pornography as Defamation," 796). Pornography is "a major way that gender hierarchy is enjoyed and practiced" (Dworkin and MacKinnon, 47). It shows men getting aroused by their domination of women, and women enjoying being dominated.

Pornography is a pervasive school for patriarchal sexuality. MacKinnon believes that pornography teaches men and women that sex is pleasurable and that sexual pleasure *means* inequality and violence. Pornography damages women through a general behavioral conditioning of arousal and orgasm to domination and submission (Dworkin and MacKinnon, 46; MacKinnon, "Pornography as Defamation," 802; Vadas, 96). Pornography *is* sex: It gives men erections through viewing the abuse of women, and it encourages them to abuse women—which also gives them erections and reinforces their abusive behavior. The primary impact of pornography is not cognitive but physiological and behavioral (Douglas, 183; McGowan, 157–58). Consumers of pornography become addicted and desensitized, needing increasingly violent images to obtain an erotic kick (MacKinnon, "Does Sexuality," 125). Increasingly violent pornography makes men increasingly violent: "[T]he more pornography men see, the more abusive and violent they want it to be; the more abusive and violent it becomes, the more they enjoy it, the more abusive and violent they become, and the less harm they see in it" (Dworkin and MacKinnon, 47).

Pornography precludes sexual equality by presenting women as inherently usable objects (MacKinnon, *Feminism Unmodified*, 178; B. Brown, 75; Scales, 364; Vadas, 96). Intending no hyperbole, MacKinnon calls the pornographic enforcement of this inequality "world war" against women. When men do to each other what they do regularly to women, it is called "war," but when they do it to women it is "everyday life" (MacKinnon, "State of Emergency," 7–8). MacKinnon argues that by normalizing **sexual violence** pornography leads men to believe that women want forced sex ("Pornography as Defamation," 799). This makes "it impossible for [men] to tell when sex is forced . . . that rape is rape" (Dworkin and MacKinnon, 47–48). In a claim developed more fully by her supporters (e.g., Langton), MacKinnon suggests that pornography disables women's ability to say no to sex.

MacKinnon concentrates on visual pornography. The camera demands that things actually be done to be shown (*Only Words*, 3–4; MacKinnon and Dworkin, 5). Since sex is supposed to be enjoyable, women in pornographic pictures and films are shown having fun. Pornography involves "buying and selling captive smiling women to make such pictures, *acting as if* they like it" (*Only Words*, 5; emphasis added). This enjoyment is a charade, but men see and believe only the smiles. Visual pornography apparently proves that women enjoy sexual abuse. Men see women in pornography not only enjoying what men do to them but playing at saying no in a flirtatious game of pseudorefusal in which they really mean yes (Bird, 6; West, 400). Since women have been objectified universally as sexual playthings, the presumption that they always want sex is generalized to real life: Women's refusals are silenced, and "no" is heard as "yes." Consider a tyrant who, while people slept, secretly implanted in their brains a meaning-scrambler that made the speeches of dissidents sound like government support. Dissidents could say anything, but the scramblers would make audiences hear pro-government propaganda. This would violate freedom of speech (West, 409–11). If pornography scrambled women's speech by making refusals of sexual advances sound like invitations, this would similarly violate women's speech rights.

MacKinnon draws broadly on J. L. Austin's (1911–1960) account of performative utterances, speech acts that do things as well as say things (*Only Words*, 21; Austin, *How to Do Things*; *Papers*, 233–52; Langton, 295–96). For MacKinnon, pornography is speech that acts. It does not merely express the view that women should not be listened to but actually silences them. In its oppressive impact on women, pornography is as much an action as saying "kill" to an attack dog or "shoot" to a firing squad (*Only Words*, 12, 37; Douglas, 183; Langton, 294–95; McGowan, 157). "Social inequality is substantially created and enforced—that is, *done*—through words and images . . . in which saying it is doing it" (*Only Words*, 13). As performative speech, pornography must be judged by what it does, as discriminatory action against women, not only in terms of what it says (Langton, 297; Palczewski, 7–10).

Austin distinguished what he called the locutionary, perlocutionary, and illocutionary forces of utterances (*How to Do Things*, 98–120). Saying "George Bush is a good president" has the locutionary force of expressing a factual proposition. It also has the variable perlocutionary force of generating agreement or disgust among hearers. "I nominate George Bush to be the Republican Party candidate for president in 2004," when uttered by a qualified speaker following the rules of the party's convention and spoken to delegates who grasp what she/he is doing, actually *makes* Bush a nominee and thereby creates a state of affairs (McGowan, 158). Austin called this doing-by-saying "illocution." Some illocutionary acts require a speaker to hold an authoritative position (Langton, 298–99, 314–15). Only a judge can sentence a convicted prisoner; only a military officer can order troops to attack. Other types of illocutionary acts, however, are or should be available to anyone: refusing to pick up a hitchhiker, ordering a dish in a restaurant, or refusing sexual advances. Some of MacKinnon's followers apply the concept of illocutionary speech directly to pornography, which they see as an oppressive form of speech that in itself silences the legitimate, sex-refusing illocutions of women. MacKinnon herself supports this link at most implicitly.

Rae Langton distinguishes three kinds of cases in which women's illocutionary refusals may be silenced. First, recognizing that they are relatively powerless, women may not refuse because they despair of being listened to; they go along, often out of fear, with whatever is demanded. Second, women may openly refuse, but men may disregard the "no" they hear and force sex on them against their will (Langton, 315; West, 398). Cases of this kind may constitute rape. In the third kind of case, women's refusals of sex simply are not heard *as* refusals at all. "Sex," MacKinnon says, "is what women are *for*" ("Feminism . . . Jurisprudence," 653). Women in pornography always want sex, despite pretending to resist, so when real-life women say no, they are assumed to mean yes. The illocutionary force of their refusals is disabled (Langton, 315–16; McGowan, 182; West, 399–403).

This disablement explains how men can misunderstand what their aggressive behavior means to women (MacKinnon, "Feminism . . . Jurisprudence," 652–53). If women say no, but men hear yes, then men can force sex upon women without thinking they are doing so. Pornography opens a gap between women's experience of being raped—she said no—and men's belief that they engaged in consensual sex—he heard yes. As MacKinnon states, "[A] woman is raped, but not by a rapist" ("Feminism . . . Jurisprudence," 654). This gap between saying and being heard involves what Austin called "uptake" (*How to Do Things*, 117; Bird, 2; Hornsby, 134). Some philosophers argue that uptake is essential for illocution; how could Bush be nominated if the convention delegates did not understand what the nominating speaker was intending to do? Others believe that illocutions can be performed effectively regardless of whether they are taken up by hearers (Bird, 7 ff.; Jacobson, 77–78).

MacKinnon apparently acknowledges that pornography has locutionary, perlocutionary, and illocutionary dimensions. But she has been interpreted as taking the latter to be the most important: "[P]ornography contains ideas. . . . But the way it works is not as a thought or through its ideas as such. . . . Its place in abuse requires understanding it more in active than in passive terms, as constructing and performative rather than as merely referential or connotative" (*Only Words*, 21; Langton, 293–95). To actually *do* the silencing of women, rather than just convince men not to listen to them or to take their refusals seriously, pornography seemingly must operate in the illocutionary rather than only the locutionary and perlocutionary domains. Cynthia Stark distinguishes what she calls the causal and the conceptual views of how pornography harms women in MacKinnon's work. Agreeing with MacKinnon that pornography has subordinating effects on women, Stark argues that MacKinnon goes beyond the widely accepted claim "that certain sexually explicit materials are causally related to various harms to women" and advances the additional "notion that pornography is itself an act of harm" (278). Stark calls this additional notion the conceptual view of pornography as an instance of harm-in-itself, and she identifies it as one of the original contributions of MacKinnon's work. While Stark rejects MacKinnon's claim that pornography *is* harm rather than a *cause* of harm, she explains that the conceptual view—implicitly for MacKinnon but explicitly in the work of Langton— entails seeing a significant part of the impact of pornography as illocutionary. The issue between these writers is not whether pornography disables the illocutionary speech of women, about which they agree, but whether it does this through its illocutionary force. Pornography's performative impact, whether illocutionary or perlocutionary, is directed in the first instance toward men. Pornography may convince men, through perlocution, to disregard what women say, but it may also—if it has illocutionary force—directly disable the illocutionary refusals of women by making men unable to hear them. Either way, pornography oppresses women through men.

This interpretation is problematic, because any illocutionary action of pornography on men is difficult to define in Austinian terms. When an authorized priest says, "I declare you man and wife," the two people involved are immediately married. Once the priest speaks, the people *are* married, and no one has to do or think anything else to make it so. For any silencing effects of pornography to be enacted, however, something beyond the pornographic saying would be needed. Illocutionary speech produces its effects "without any lapse of time" (Butler, 17). Once the saying is said, the doing is done. Pornography does not have this direct effect but must be mediated through the behaviors of its consumers.

MacKinnon states that consumers of pornography "are sexually habituated to [its] kick, a process that is largely unconscious and works as primitive conditioning" (*Only Words*, 16; see McGowan, 168–69; West, 412–13). Pornography therefore involves conditioning or behavioral modification (Schaeffer, 702). If so, it is not clear that pornography can be construed as being illocutionary, since conditioning works through the mediating and potentially variable processes of behavioral shaping. Behavior modification is not an instantaneous event but a process in which behavior is produced over time by environmental factors that operate both before and after the behaviors being shaped. According to B. F. Skinner (1904–1990), "[T]he environment not only prods or lashes, it selects. Its role is similar to that in natural selection, though on a very different time scale. . . . [W]e must take into account what the environment does to an organism not only before but after it responds. Behavior is shaped and maintained by its consequences" (18).

Behavior modification is an interactive process between organisms and environments. Illocutionary speech acts are not mediated through subsequent processes. Rather than the saying being the doing, with pornography the saying seems to be the start of processes that may lead to the doing. Thus, the more pornography is understood as behavioral conditioning, the less it looks like illocutionary speech. Caroline West's examples illustrate the point. In addition to the dictator who implants meaning-scramblers, she describes a pharmaceutical company that manufactures pills with the same effect as the scramblers (410, 414). The scramblers and the pills both could make men think that women who said no to sex meant yes. Making the scramblers or the pills, or installing or swallowing them, might violate women's speech rights, but doing these things is not to perform an illocutionary speech act (see Austin, *How to Do Things*, 113–14).

Further, to the extent that illocutions require authority, it is specifically the pornography that silences women, through men, only if pornography has, for the men at least, the requisite authority. Langton (312) thinks it does; Alan Soble ("Bad Apples," 370–77) disagrees. In MacKinnon's theoretical universe, however, the question of the authority of pornography is otiose. Of course pornography is authoritative. In the gendered hierarchy of patriarchy it is the master's voice. Pornography, writes MacKinnon, "is not at all divergent or unorthodox. It is the ruling ideology" (*Toward*, 205). Whether this reflects reality is another matter.

Even if it is not illocutionary, pornography is still perlocutionary speech. But pornography as perlocutionary is subject to greater variability; and because the uptake of its meaning by audiences will be more variable, invoking pornography as the global *explanans* for men's sexual behavior will be less successful. But looking at pornography *qua* perlocutionary material is at least consistent with MacKinnon's idea that pornography does not work cognitively but physiologically and behaviorally instead.

MacKinnon has been criticized for homogenizing pornography into an undifferentiated field of politically invincible common meaning (Butler, 73–74; Fraiman, 746). Soble argues that MacKinnon unjustifiably assumes that pornography always means the same thing to all men (*Pornography*, 38). Emphasizing pornography's ability to convey multiple meanings, he objects that MacKinnon pretends to know what goes on uniformly in all men's minds when they view pornography (125). He asserts that a picture of a woman exposing her bare bottom in itself means nothing, much less conveys a clear message of submission and vulnerability. According to Soble, "get her," "love her," and "be her" all are equally plausible interpretations of the message or meaning of such a picture, contrary to MacKinnon's claim that "get her" (rape her, dominate her) is its sole meaning (27–28). Judith Butler argues similarly that pornography, like all speech, is equivocal and its interpretation uncertain (87).

MacKinnon could reply that variability in the perlocutionary meaning of pornography is irrelevant, because for her pornography works primarily at the visceral level of genital responses: "[T]ry arguing with an orgasm sometime" (*Only Words*, 17). The message "get her," she says, "is addressed directly to the penis, delivered through an erection" (*Only Words*, 21). MacKinnon believes that listening to women's own accounts exposes pornography's impact on their lives in every context from everyday sexuality, in which "woman after woman used by consumers of pornography recount its causal role in her sexual violation by a man close to her," to extreme criminality in which "serial murderers use pornography to prepare and impel them to rape and kill" (MacKinnon and Dworkin, 5–6). If pornography is causally responsible for a great deal of harm done to women by men, it is plausible to conclude, perhaps by abduction, that "get her" *is* its meaning, even if men do not acknowledge or are not conscious of it.

MacKinnon's appeal here to listening to what women say about their experiences with and from pornography is not an unusual move among feminists. It goes along with another common feminist strategy, consciousness raising, both of which contribute to women's understanding of the world independently of the presumptively objective accounts provided by male knowledge. For MacKinnon, there is no independent epistemological position from which to see sexuality and pornography objectively, and what is called "objectivity" is the male outlook from the stance of power ("Points," 690; Rapaport, 127–28). It does not matter whether men agree with the emerging understanding. Consciousness raising is a political process that sifts through individual variations in experience, locating a platform for unified political resistance ("Feminism . . . Agenda," 535). Through consciousness raising, women reconstruct themselves from their own real experience: "[F]eminism makes its 'women' from the ground up, out of particularities, from practice" ("Points," 696). Even though she claims that women's experiences must be interpreted by them freely and collectively, MacKinnon has been criticized for assuming in advance what the content of that process will be (Grant, 78; Réaume, 473–74). To some, MacKinnon assumes the role of a feminist didactician, telling women how they really should understand their lives.

Pornography's depiction of sexuality does not reflect or distort any presocial or biological phenomena (MacKinnon, *Feminism Unmodified*, 148–49; "Reply," 186). Sex and pornography are not "imagery in some relation to a reality elsewhere constructed, . . . not a distortion, reflection, projection, expression, fantasy, representation, or symbol" (*Feminism Unmodified*, 149). Despite this **social constructionism**, MacKinnon frequently implies an extrasocial dimension to sexuality. She writes that "pornography . . . eroticizes hierarchy . . . sexualizes inequality . . . makes dominance and submission into sex" (*Feminism Unmodified*, 172). She does not explain where pornography gets the eroticism with which it eroticizes hierarchy or what constitutes the "sex" *into which* pornography makes dominance and submission. Is there implicitly an extrasocial sexuality on which pornography draws in carrying out its constructions?

The answer may reside in the male body: "[U]nder male dominance, whatever sexually arouses a man is sex" (*Feminism Unmodified*, 160). Pornography links violence to male arousal. Male dominance, however, does not create male arousal; but without arousal, there would be nothing sexualizing to link dominance *to*. Violence is not inherently sexual. It is made sexual by being linked to penile arousal. But why is *this* sexualizing? The male body must respond genitally to something for that something to be sexual. Penile arousal grounds sexualization, rooting sexuality in the body. As MacKinnon says, "[W]hatever it takes to make a penis shudder and stiffen . . . is what sexuality means culturally" (*Toward*, 137). If "whatever sexually arouses a man is sex," then to know what counts as sex, we first have to know what sexually arouses men. But how do we know, without circularity, what *sexual* arousal is? (See Diorio.)

Women's Sexuality. Erections eroticize. Since male power controls sexuality, women cannot eroticize or sexualize anything. Sexuality, for MacKinnon, is nothing more than women "being fucked," in both the physically literal and negatively figurative senses of the term. MacKinnon believes that women overwhelmingly would choose freedom from "being fucked" over greater freedom to engage in sexuality (*Toward*, 153–54). Because sexuality offers women no possible haven from oppression, for them to choose sexuality over freedom would be like slaves choosing forced labor over emancipation. Women and sexuality are antagonistic, and MacKinnon rejects any extrasocial sexual domain that could provide liberating erotic enjoyment (Nussbaum, 231).

Some of MacKinnon's feminist critics want to retrieve a positive sexual space within which women can assert independent erotic interests. MacKinnon paints such a gloomy picture of the subordinate, dominated, powerless position of women in patriarchy that we might wonder how any woman, including MacKinnon, could be successful at anything, let alone press for her own sexuality, a realm in which male force and control are, in her account, especially prodigious (see Valverde, 243). In particular, Drucilla Cornell objects that MacKinnon needlessly closes off sexuality as a domain within which women could contest oppression by pursuing nonoppressive pleasure (129). MacKinnon's absolute division between women's freedom and their oppression through sexuality denies women the opportunity to be "being[s] of the flesh" (114) and leaves them no potential to affirm an alternative form of desire (106). Women cannot become free by being cut off from their sexuality, because they need the physical intimacy of sexual caressing, kissing, and embracing (135–36).

The question whether there is any potentially independent women's sexuality outside patriarchy has been pursued by other feminist critics of MacKinnon, who argue that her theory makes sense only if it is based on some presocial concept of women and women's sexuality against which their oppression can be measured (indeed, against which their oppression can be said to exist). Denise Schaeffer claims that MacKinnon attacks the patriarchal construction of sex and gender precisely because it *distorts* women; MacKinnon "disputes the social meaning of womanhood not on the grounds that identity is inherently indeterminate but because there is something to 'woman' that is authentic and real" (704). Jeanne Schroeder argues similarly that "MacKinnon's message is not that women have been formed by society, it is that women have been *deformed*. There is some concept of an authentic woman external to our current society" (194); otherwise, it would make no sense to speak of women as "deformed" and "oppressed" or to know in which ways they are deformed and oppressed.

This sort of philosophical account of women (and men)—a philosophical anthropology—buttressed by the sciences, could create space for an undistorted and newly eroticized sexuality emerging from women's experience. These authors invoke a broadly liberal conception of a presocial women's identity that constitutes the respect-deserving entity oppressed by patriarchy. MacKinnon explicitly rejects any essentially liberal account of her work, however, just as she explicitly rejects liberalism itself, stating that she "analyze[s] women and men as socially and politically constituted throughout, an approach that neither reveals nor presupposes 'authentic' or 'arbitrary' beings but rather exposes thoroughly socially contingent ones" (" 'The Case,' " 710).

MacKinnon has sought to redefine **feminism** (as "unmodified") and in doing so stridently confronts patriarchy in terms of sexuality, gender, and the social definition of women. Her work has polarized debate both within and outside feminist circles. She offers a complex account of the role of sexuality in human life that, while profoundly unsettling to many writers, continues to draw serious philosophical attention.

See also Activity, Sexual; Dworkin, Andrea; Ethics, Sexual; Feminism, Lesbian; Feminism, Liberal; Freudian Left, The; Harassment, Sexual; Language; Liberalism; Marxism; Objectification, Sexual; Paglia, Camille; Personification, Sexual; Pornography; Privacy; Rape; Social Constructionism; Violence, Sexual

REFERENCES

Allen, Amy. "Pornography and Power." *Journal of Social Philosophy* 32:4 (2001), 512–31; Allen, Amy. *The Power of Feminist Theory: Domination, Resistance, and Solidarity.* Boulder, Colo.: Westview, 1999; Austin, J. L. (1962) *How to Do Things with Words*, 2nd ed. Ed. J. O. Urmson and Marina Sbisá. Cambridge, Mass.: Harvard University Press, 1975; Austin, J. L. (1961) *Philosophical Papers*, 2nd ed. Ed. J. O. Urmson and G. J. Warnock. London: Oxford University Press, 1970; Bird, Alexander. "Illocutionary Silencing." *Pacific Philosophical Quarterly* 83:1 (2002), 1–15; Brown, Beverley. "Pornography and Feminism: Is Law the Answer?" *Critical Quarterly* 34:2 (1992), 72–82; Brown, Wendy. *States of Injury: Power and Freedom in Late Modernity.* Princeton, N.J.: Princeton University Press, 1995; Butler, Judith. *Excitable Speech: A Politics of the Performative.* New York: Routledge, 1997; Cornell, Drucilla. *Transformations: Recollective Imagination and Sexual Difference.* New York: Routledge, 1993; Diorio, Joseph A. "Feminist-Constructionist Theories of Sexuality and the Definition of Sex Education." *Educational Philosophy and Theory* 21:2 (1989), 23–31; Douglas, Lawrence. "The Force of Words: Fish, Matsuda, MacKinnon, and the Theory of Discursive Violence." *Law and Society Review* 29:1 (1995), 169–90; Downs, Donald Alexander. *The New Politics of Pornography.* Chicago, Ill.: University of Chicago Press, 1989; Duggan, Nancy, Nan Hunter, and Carole S. Vance. "False Promises: Feminist Antipornography Legislation in the U.S." In Varda Burstyn, ed., *Women against Censorship.* Vancouver, Can.: Douglas and McIntyre, 1985, 130–51; Dworkin, Andrea, and Catharine A. MacKinnon. *Pornography and Civil Rights: A New Day for Women's Equality.* Minneapolis, Minn.: Organizing Against Pornography, 1988; Fraiman, Susan. "Catharine MacKinnon and the Feminist Porn Debates." *American Quarterly* 47:4 (1995), 743–49; Grant, Judith. *Fundamental Feminism: Contesting the Core Concepts of Feminist Theory.* New York: Routledge, 1993; Hornsby, Jennifer. "Disempowered Speech." *Philosophical Topics* 23:2 (1995), 127–47; Jacobson, Daniel. "Freedom of Speech Acts? A Response to Langton." *Philosophy and Public Affairs* 24:1 (1995), 64–79; Langton, Rae. "Speech Acts and Unspeakable Acts." *Philosophy and Public Affairs* 22:4 (1993), 293–330; MacKinnon, Catharine A. " 'The Case' Responds." *American Political Science Review* 95:3 (2001), 709–11; MacKinnon, Catharine A. "Desire and Power: A Feminist Perspective." In Cary Nelson and Lawrence Grossberg, eds., *Marxism and the Interpretation of Culture.* Urbana: University of Illinois Press, 1988, 105–21; MacKinnon, Catharine A. "Does Sexuality Have a History?" In Domna C. Stanton, ed., *Discourses of Sexuality: From Aristotle to AIDS.* Ann Arbor: University of Michigan Press, 1992, 117–36; MacKinnon, Catharine A. "Feminism, Marxism, Method, and the State: An Agenda for Theory." *Signs* 7:3 (1982), 515–44; MacKinnon, Catharine A. "Feminism, Marxism, Method, and the State: Toward Feminist Jurisprudence." *Signs* 8:4 (1983), 635–58; MacKinnon, Catharine A. *Feminism Unmodified: Discourses on Life and Law.* Cambridge, Mass.: Harvard University Press, 1987; MacKinnon, Catharine A. "From Practice to Theory, or What Is a White Woman Anyway?" *Yale Journal of Law and Feminism* 4:1 (1991), 13–22; MacKinnon, Catharine A. *Only Words.* Cambridge, Mass.: Harvard University Press, 1993; MacKinnon, Catharine A. "Points against Postmodernism." *Chicago-Kent Law Review* 75:3 (2000), 687–712; MacKinnon, Catharine A. "Pornography as Defamation and Discrimination." *Boston University Law Review* 71:5 (1991), 793–815; MacKinnon, Catharine A. "Reply to Miller, Acker and Barry, Johnson, West, and Gardiner." *Signs* 10 (Autumn 1984), 184–88; MacKinnon, Catharine A. *Sexual Harassment of Working Women: A Case of Sex Discrimination.* New Haven, Conn.: Yale University Press, 1979; MacKinnon, Catharine A. "State of Emergency." *Women's Review of Books* 19:6 (2002),

7–8; MacKinnon, Catharine A. *Toward a Feminist Theory of the State*. Cambridge, Mass.: Harvard University Press, 1989; MacKinnon, Catharine A. *Women's Lives, Men's Laws*. Cambridge, Mass.: Harvard University Press, 2005; MacKinnon, Catharine A., and Andrea Dworkin, eds. *In Harm's Way: The Pornography Civil Rights Hearings*. Cambridge, Mass.: Harvard University Press, 1997; McGowan, Mary Kate. "Conversational Exercitives and the Force of Pornography." *Philosophy and Public Affairs* 31:2 (2003), 155–89; Nussbaum, Martha C. "Objectification." In *Sex and Social Justice*. New York: Oxford University Press, 1999, 213–39; Palczewski, Catherine Helen. "Contesting Pornography: Terministic Catharsis and Definitional Argument." *Argumentation and Advocacy* 38 (Summer 2001), 1–17; Rapaport, Elizabeth. "Generalizing Gender: Reason and Essence in the Legal Thought of Catharine MacKinnon." In Louise Antony and Charlotte Witt, eds., *A Mind of One's Own: Feminist Essays on Reason and Objectivity*. Boulder, Colo.: Westview, 1993, 127–43; Réaume, Denise G. "The Social Construction of Women and the Possibility of Change: Unmodified Feminism Revisited." *Canadian Journal of Women and the Law* 5:2 (1992), 463–83; Ring, Jennifer. "Toward a Feminist Epistemology." *American Journal of Political Science* 31:4 (1987), 753–72; Scales, Ann. "Avoiding Constitutional Depression: Bad Attitudes and the Fate of Butler." *Canadian Journal of Women and the Law* 7:2 (1994), 349–92; Schaeffer, Denise. "Feminism and Liberalism Reconsidered: The Case of Catharine MacKinnon." *American Political Science Review* 95:3 (2001), 699–708; Schroeder, Jeanne L. "*Abduction from the Seraglio*: Feminist Methodologies and the Logic of Imagination." *Texas Law Review* 70:1 (1991), 109–210; Skinner, B. F. *Beyond Freedom and Dignity*. New York: Knopf, 1971; Soble, Alan. "Bad Apples: Feminist Politics and Feminist Scholarship." *Philosophy of the Social Sciences* 29:3 (1999), 354–88; Soble, Alan. *Pornography, Sex, and Feminism*. Amherst, N.Y.: Prometheus, 2002; Stark, Cynthia A. "Is Pornography an Action? The Causal vs. the Conceptual View of Pornography's Harm." *Social Theory and Practice* 23:2 (1997), 277–306; Vadas, Melinda. "The Pornography/Civil Rights Ordinance v. The BOG: And the Winner Is . . . ?" *Hypatia* 7:3 (1992), 94–109; Valverde, Mariana. "Beyond Gender Dangers and Private Pleasures: Theory and Ethics in the Sex Debates." *Feminist Studies* 15:2 (1989), 237–54; West, Caroline. "The Free Speech Argument against Pornography." *Canadian Journal of Philosophy* 33:3 (2003), 391–422.

Joseph A. Diorio

ADDITIONAL READING

Bartlett, Katharine T., and Rosanne Kennedy, eds. *Feminist Legal Theory: Readings in Law and Gender*. Boulder, Colo.: Westview, 1991, 370–403; Bernick, Susan E. "The Logic of the Development of Feminism; or, Is MacKinnon to Feminism as Parmenides Is to Greek Philosophy?" *Hypatia* 7:1 (1992), 1–15; Berns, Walter. "Dirty Words." *The Public Interest*, no. 114 (Winter 1994), 119–25; Chancer, Lynn S. "Feminist Offensives: *Defending Pornography* and the Splitting of Sex from Sexism." *Stanford Law Review* 48 (February 1996), 739–60; Colker, Ruth. "Feminism, Sexuality, and Authenticity." In Martha A. Fineman and Nancy S. Thomadsen, eds., *At the Boundaries of Law*. New York: Routledge, 1991, 135–47; Colker, Ruth. "Feminism, Sexuality, and Self: A Preliminary Inquiry into the Politics of Authenticity." *Boston University Law Review* 68:1 (1988), 217–64; De Lauretis, Teresa. "Eccentric Subjects: Feminist Theory and Historical Consciousness." *Feminist Studies* 16:1 (1990), 115–50; Douglass, Carol Ann. "What We're Trying to Save: Thoughts after Reading Catharine A. MacKinnon's *Feminism Unmodified* and Andrea Dworkin's *Intercourse*." *Off Our Backs* 17 (June 1987), 14–15; Dworkin, Ronald. "Is There a Right to Pornography?" *Oxford Journal of Legal Studies* 1:2 (1981), 177–212. Reprinted in Susan Dwyer, ed., *The Problem of Pornography*. Belmont, Calif.: Wadsworth, 1995, 77–90; Dworkin, Ronald. "Liberty and Pornography." *New York Review of Books* (21 October 1993), 12–15. Reprinted in Susan Dwyer, ed., *The Problem of Pornography*. Belmont, Calif.: Wadsworth, 1995, 113–21; Dworkin, Ronald. (1996) "MacKinnon's Words." In Hugh LaFollette, ed., *Ethics in Practice: An Anthology*, 2nd ed. Malden, Mass.: Blackwell, 2002, 356–63; Dworkin, Ronald. "Women and Pornography." *New York Review of Books* (21 October 1993), 36–42; [reply to letter] *New York Review of Books* (3 March 1994), 48–49; Emerson, Thomas

I. "Pornography and the First Amendment: A Reply to Professor MacKinnon." *Yale Law and Policy Review* 3 (Fall 1984), 130–43; Estlund, David M. "MacKinnon." [Reply to Catharine A. MacKinnon, "Pornography Left and Right" (q.v.)] In David M. Estlund and Martha C. Nussbaum, eds., *Sex, Preference, and Family: Essays on Law and Nature.* New York: Oxford University Press, 1997, 164–68; Estlund, David M. "The Visit and the Video: Publication and the Line between Sex and Speech." In David M. Estlund and Martha C. Nussbaum, eds., *Sex, Preference, and Family: Essays on Law and Nature.* New York: Oxford University Press, 1997, 126–47; Ferguson, Frances. "Pornography, the Theory." In *Pornography, the Theory: What Utilitarianism Did to Action.* Chicago, Ill.: University of Chicago Press, 2004, 34–56; Groenhout, Ruth E. "Essentialist Challenges to Liberal Feminism." *Social Theory and Practice* 28:1 (2002), 51–75; Harris, Angela P. "Race and Essentialism in Feminist Legal Theory." In Katharine T. Bartlett and Rosanne Kennedy, eds., *Feminist Legal Theory: Readings in Law and Gender.* Boulder, Colo.: Westview, 1991, 235–62; Haslanger, Sally. "On Being Objective and Being Objectified." In Louise Anthony and Charlotte Witt, eds., *A Mind of One's Own: Feminist Essays on Reason and Objectivity.* Boulder, Colo.: Westview, 1993, 85–125; Herman, Barbara. "Could It Be Worth Thinking about Kant on Sex and Marriage?" In Louise Antony and Charlotte Witt, eds., *A Mind of One's Own: Feminist Essays on Reason and Objectivity.* Boulder, Colo.: Westview, 1993, 49–67; Hornsby, Jennifer, and Rae Langton. "Free Speech and Illocution." *Legal Theory* 4:1 (1998), 21–37; Jackson, Emily. "The Problem with Pornography: A Critical Survey of the Current Debate." *Feminist Legal Studies* 3:1 (1995), 49–70; Jaggar, Alison M. Review of *Feminism Unmodified: Discourses on Life and Law*, by Catharine A. MacKinnon. *New York Times Book Review* (3 May 1987), 3, 51; Jeffreys, Sheila. *Anticlimax: A Feminist Perspective on the Sexual Revolution.* London: Women's Press, 1990. New York: New York University Press, 1991; Kennedy, Duncan. "Sexual Abuse, Sexy Dressing, and the Eroticization of Domination." In *Sexy Dressing Etc.* Cambridge, Mass.: Harvard University Press, 1993, 126–213; Laden, Anthony Simon. "Radical Liberals, Reasonable Feminists: Reason, Power, and Objectivity in MacKinnon and Rawls." *Journal of Political Philosophy* 11:2 (2003), 133–52; Landry, Donna. "Treating Him Like an Object: William Beatty Warner's 'Di(va)lution.'" In Linda Kauffman, ed., *Feminism and Institutions: Dialogues on Feminist Theory.* Cambridge, Mass.: Blackwell, 1989, 126–38; Langton, Rae. "Pornography, Speech Acts, and Silence." In Hugh LaFollette, ed., *Ethics in Practice: An Anthology.* Cambridge, Mass.: Blackwell, 1997, 338–49; Langton, Rae. "Subordination, Silence, and Pornography's Authority." In R. C. Post, ed., *Censorship and Silencing: Practices of Cultural Regulation.* Los Angeles, Calif.: Getty Research Institute, 1998, 261–83; Langton, Rae. "Whose Right? Ronald Dworkin, Women, and Pornographers." *Philosophy and Public Affairs* 19:4 (1990), 311–59. Reprinted in Susan Dwyer, ed., *The Problem of Pornography.* Belmont, Calif.: Wadsworth, 1995, 91–112; MacKinnon, Catharine A. "The Logic of Experience: Reflections on the Development of Sexual Harassment Law." *Georgetown Law Journal* 90:3 (2002), 813–33; MacKinnon, Catharine A. "Pornography Left and Right." [Review of *Sex and Reason*, by Richard A. Posner, and *Girls Lean Back Everywhere: The Law of Obscenity and the Assault on Genius*, by Edward de Grazia] *Harvard Civil Rights–Civil Liberties Law Review* 30 (Winter 1995), 143–68. Reprinted in David M. Estlund and Martha C. Nussbaum, eds., *Sex, Preference, and Family: Essays on Law and Nature.* New York: Oxford University Press, 1997, 102–25; MacKinnon, Catharine A. "Preface." In Jeffrey Moussaieff Masson, *A Dark Science: Women, Sexuality, and Psychiatry in the Nineteenth Century.* New York: Farrar, Straus and Giroux, 1986, xi–xxii. Reprinted as "Sex, Lies, and Psychotherapy," in *Women's Lives, Men's Laws.* Cambridge, Mass.: Harvard University Press, 2005, 251–58; MacKinnon, Catharine A. "Roe v. Wade: A Study in Male Ideology." In Jay L. Garfield and Patricia Hennessey, eds., *Abortion: Moral and Legal Perspectives.* Amherst: University of Massachusetts Press, 1984, 45–54; MacKinnon, Catharine A. *Sex Equality.* New York: Foundation Press, 2001; MacKinnon, Catharine A. "Sexuality, Pornography, and Method: 'Pleasure under Patriarchy.'" *Ethics* 99:2 (1989), 314–46; MacKinnon, Catharine A. "Vindication and Resistance: A Response to the Carnegie Mellon Study of Pornography in Cyberspace." *Georgetown Law Journal* 83:4 (1995), 1959–67; Mahoney, Martha R. "Whiteness and Women, in Practice and Theory: A Reply to Catharine MacKinnon." *Yale Journal of Law and Feminism* 5:2 (1993), 217–51; Mason-Grant, Joan. *Pornography Embodied: From Speech to Sexual Practice.*

Lanham, Md.: Rowman and Littlefield, 2004; Muehlenhard, Charlene L., and Lisa C. Hollabaugh. "Do Women Sometimes Say No When They Mean Yes? The Prevalence and Correlates of Women's Token Resistance to Sex." *Journal of Personality and Social Psychology* 54:5 (1988), 872–79; Nussbaum, Martha C. "Objectification." *Philosophy and Public Affairs* 24:4 (1995), 249–91. Reprinted in POS3 (283–321); POS4 (381–419). Reprinted, revised, in *Sex and Social Justice*. New York: Oxford University Press, 1999, 213–39; Parent, W. A. "A Second Look at Pornography and the Subordination of Women." *Journal of Philosophy* 87:4 (1990), 205–11; Pateman, Carole. "Sex and Power." [Review of *Feminism Unmodified*, by Catharine A. MacKinnon] *Ethics* 100:2 (1990), 398–407; Posner, Richard A. "Obsession." [Review of *Only Words*, by Catharine A. MacKinnon] *The New Republic* (18 October 1993), 31–36; Rimm, Marty. "Marketing Pornography on the Information Superhighway: A Survey of 917,410 Images, Descriptions, Short Stories, and Animations Downloaded 8.5 Million Times by Consumers in Over 2000 Cities in Forty Countries, Provinces, and Territories." *Georgetown Law Journal* 83 (1995), 1849–1934; Ring, Jennifer. "Saving Objectivity for Feminism: MacKinnon, Marx, and Other Possibilities." *Review of Politics* 49 (Fall 1987), 467–89; Roiphe, Katie. *The Morning After: Sex, Fear, and Feminism*. London: Hamish Hamilton, 1993; Rorty, Richard. "Feminism and Pragmatism." *Michigan Quarterly Review* 30:2 (1991), 231–58; Schroeder, Jeanne L. "Feminism Historicized: Medieval Misogynist Stereotypes in Contemporary Feminist Jurisprudence." *Iowa Law Review* 75 (1990), 1135–1217; Scruton, Roger. "Kiss Me, Cate." [Review of *Only Words*, by Catharine A. MacKinnon] *National Review* (1 November 1993), 61–62; Soble, Alan. "Pornography." In *Sexual Investigations*. New York: New York University Press, 1996, 214–49; Soble, Alan. "Pornography and the Social Sciences." *Social Epistemology* 2:2 (1988), 135–44. Reprinted in POS2 (317–31); POS4 (421–34); St. John, Maria. "How to Do Things with the *Starr Report*: Pornography, Performance, and the President's Penis." In Linda Williams, ed., *Porn Studies*. Durham, N.C.: Duke University Press, 2004, 27–49; Vadas, Melinda. "A First Look at the Pornography/Civil Rights Ordinance: Could Pornography Be the Subordination of Women?" *Journal of Philosophy* 84:9 (1987), 487–511; Warner, William Beatty. "Treating Me Like an Object: Reading Catharine MacKinnon's Feminism." In Linda Kauffman, ed., *Feminism and Institutions: Dialogues on Feminist Theory*. Cambridge, Mass.: Blackwell, 1989, 90–125; West, Caroline. "Pornography and Censorship." In Edward Zalta, ed., *Stanford Encyclopedia of Philosophy*. <plato.stanford.edu/entries/pornography-censorship/> [accessed 18 January 2005]; West, Robin. "Unwelcome Sex: Toward a Harm-Based Analysis." In Catharine MacKinnon and Reva Siegel, eds., *Directions in Sexual Harassment Law*. New Haven, Conn.: Yale University Press, 2004, 138–52.

MAIMONIDES. *See* Judaism, History of

MANDEVILLE, BERNARD (1670–1733).

Bernard Mandeville was born and educated in Holland but moved to London by the late 1690s. He lived there until the end of his life, working successfully as a doctor (specializing in nervous and gastric disorders) while at the same time acquiring some reputation, and later notoriety, for his books and pamphlets. Mandeville was a keen and perceptive student of human nature but was not systematic in setting out his views, some of which are mutually inconsistent. It is with good reason that the first book to be published in England about him for 250 years (by Hector Monro [1911–2001]) was called *The Ambivalence of Bernard Mandeville*.

Mandeville's treatment of human affairs is almost invariably colored by his conviction that men and women are clever animals governed by their passions, not by principles rooted in reason or spirituality. He applied this maxim to human sexuality and stood by it right up to the end of his life. This is evident from a comment in his last work *A Letter to*

Dion, published in 1732, only a few months before his death: "[W]ithout Lust, if you give it a softer Name, our Species could not be preserv'd, any more than that of Bulls or Goats" (21). Since sexual instincts are among our most powerful passions, it is not surprising that Mandeville examined them even in his early books.

In his first prose work, *The Virgin Unmask'd: or, Female Dialogues betwixt an Elderly Maiden Lady and her Niece* (1709), the interlocutors discuss such matters as modesty of dress, the artificiality of courtship, and the subjugation of women, both to their fathers before **marriage** and to their husbands thereafter. Mandeville believed that women's inferior status was socially determined rather than natural. He also thought that women's libidinous propensities were just as strong as men's, a thesis he substantially modified in *A Modest Defence of Publick Stews* (1724), where he lists four types of women, categorized in part by the different degrees of force with which they experience **sexual desire** (42–48). By discussing these issues, he was participating in a debate that flourished in the late seventeenth and early eighteenth centuries (see Cook, chap. 3).

By far the best known of Mandeville's books is *The Fable of the Bees*, which appeared in 1714. It includes a poem ("The Grumbling Hive, or Knaves turn'd Honest," first published in 1705) and twenty discursive remarks. His observations on **love** and lust occur in Remark N, which was added to the second edition (1723), the publication of which quickly rendered the book a subject of controversy and scandal. The introduction of human sexuality is somewhat gratuitous, as Remark N is initially about envy. Though interesting and provocative, his account of sex is seriously flawed by the tension, that Mandeville fails to address, between his concession that the good of society requires that "This Impulse of Nature" be carefully regulated and often suppressed and his castigation of the restrictive conventions and educative processes by which this end is achieved. (This problem later perplexed **Sigmund Freud** [1856–1939]; see *Civilization and Its Discontents*.) Mandeville does not explain why "the Peace and Happiness of the Civil Society" depend on stifling our sexual cravings. He denies that the refinements wrought by civilization are useful embellishments; they are, instead, accretions that warp a natural appetite and cause it to "degenerate from its honest Original and primitive Simplicity."

Like other sections of Part I of the *Fable*, Remark N contains unambiguous indications of Mandeville's conspiratorial account of the origin of morality and society: Politicians have labored to perpetrate a confidence trick on mankind by means of which they are civilized. The effect of this imposture on our sexual appetite affords a particularly striking instance of how one passion can be played off against another—a doctrine central to Mandeville's psychology and important in this instance as "Nature never fails to furnish us largely with this Passion, tho' she is often sparing to bestow upon us such a Portion of Reason and Reflection as is necessary to curb it" (*Publick Stews*, 7). By flattering our pride and instilling in us a sense of shame, "Artful Moralists" have induced us

> to encounter ourselves, and if not subdue, at least so to conceal and disguise our darling Passion, Lust, that we scarce know it when we meet with it in our own Breasts. . . . What we call Love then is not a Genuine, but an Adulterated Appetite, or rather a Compound, a heap of several contradictory Passions blended in one. As it is a product of Nature warp'd by Custom and Education, so the true Origin and first Motive of it . . . is stifled in well-bred People, and almost concealed from themselves. (*Fable*, Remark N)

The 1723 edition of the *Fable* met with a torrent of criticism from ethical rationalists and orthodox Christians, who believed that human beings, created in God's image, were inherently social and that morality was intuitively perceived and further reinforced by God's commandments. In a 1724 pamphlet, William Law (1686–1761) challenged Mandeville to specify the time when and place where society was established by political imposture (18–19). The sustained criticism of his conspiratorial thesis prompted Mandeville to move to a more evolutionary account. In the six dialogues constituting Part II of the *Fable*, published in 1729, there are clear intimations that moral and social institutions evolved in the light of experience. Had this insight been applied to his 1714 account of sexuality, it might have been more consistent and complete. However, it is not only human institutions that have evolved but human nature itself, a possibility that Mandeville, in common with many eighteenth-century thinkers, consistently denied. His failure in the *Fable* to appreciate the evolution of mankind from animals into sophisticated intellectual and social beings, and his stubborn and exclusive insistence on the animal part of our nature, explain the deficiencies in his account of sexuality. Although he did not say so, **David Hume**'s (1711–1776) account of sexual desire was probably a reaction against Mandeville (*A Treatise of Human Nature*, bk. II. ii.11). Still, Hume's account of the social conventions governing sexual relationships (III.ii.12) incorporates some of Mandeville's radical insights.

Mandeville's scant regard for consistency is exasperating. In *Publick Stews*, he offers an account of the incentive to marriage that is in sharp contrast to the account of sexual appetite found in the *Fable*.

> When a Man and a Woman select one another out of the whole Species, it is not merely for Propagation; nay, that is generally the least in their Thoughts: What they chiefly have in View, is to pass the remainder of their Lives happily together, to enjoy the soft Embraces and mutual Endearments of Love; to divide their Joys and Griefs; to share their Pleasures and Afflictions; and, in short, to make one another as happy as possible. . . . Now all these Enjoyments depend upon the mutual Affection of these two. (33–34)

The shift from sexual *appetite* to conjugal *affection* and the gulf alleged to exist between them are striking. It is almost as if he failed to perceive that they are connected.

Remark H of the *Fable* (1714 edition) includes Mandeville's first defense of **prostitution**, which makes it surprising that its publication attracted little attention and generated no recorded controversy on its first appearance. (It was the target of much invective nine years later.) His reason for advocating toleration is that "it is Wisdom in all Governments to bear with lesser Inconveniences to prevent greater. If Courtesans and Strumpets were to be prosecuted with as much Rigour as some silly People would have it, what Locks or Bars would be sufficient to preserve the Honour of our Wives and Daughters?" He proceeds to describe the brothels "conniv'd at," though not actually licensed, by the authorities in Amsterdam. In *Publick Stews*, Mandeville went farther, setting out detailed proposals for licensed and regulated brothels in all towns of any size (12–15). He once again maintained, against the received wisdom of his day, that easy access to prostitutes is necessary to preserve the chastity of decent women from the advances of lecherous men. He also believed that the provision of such facilities would forestall evils that thrived without regulation, most notably the transmission of venereal disease and the murder of illegitimate children born to prostitutes. However, some of his arguments are far from convincing. Not all premarital and extramarital relationships are prompted by lust that could as well be vented in a brothel, for in many cases both parties are prompted by genuine affection. Nor is it true that if men could procure the services of a prostitute for as little as half a crown (a tidy sum in Mandeville's time), they would desist from **masturbation**, a practice Mandeville believed was harmful (30–31) but one that would be more convenient and economical than recourse to a prostitute. *Publick Stews* is Mandeville's most extensive treatment of sexuality, incorporating discussion of matters physiological (recall that he was a doctor), psychological, sociological, and ethical. It is also the only work in which he openly professes a utilitarian morality.

A vigorous response to Mandeville's defense of prostitution can be found in Section VI of *An Enquiry whether a general Practice of Virtue tends to the Wealth or Poverty, Benefit or Disadvantage of a People*, a book published anonymously in 1725 and now attributed to George Bluet, about whom nothing is known. Bluet feared that if brothels were licensed by authority, the temptation to excess would be unrestrained. He disputed Mandeville's conviction that only the lower ranks of women would be recruited to work in them, believing that licensed brothels would render marriage less fashionable and that women of quality would be tempted into promiscuity and prostitution. Also, by making opportunities more readily available, brothels would increase promiscuity among people who would not otherwise be tempted. He also raised the possibility of brothels in which women could hire the services of men! Whereas Mandeville thought that wide-ranging sexual experience prior to marriage would temper men's unrealistic expectations of conjugal life and make them better husbands (*Publick Stews*, 35–37), Bluet believed that by promoting promiscuous sexual behavior before marriage, brothels would make marital fidelity less likely. Further, by fostering an ill opinion of the character of women, brothels would increase suspicion and **jealousy**. As marriage declined, human sexual relations would, he feared, become increasingly bestial.

See also Casual Sex; Consequentialism; Evolution; Freud, Sigmund; Hume, David; Love; Marriage; Masturbation; Prostitution; Russell, Bertrand; Westermarck, Edward

REFERENCES

Bluet, George. *An Enquiry whether a general Practice of Virtue tends to the Wealth or Poverty, Benefit or Disadvantage of a People*. London, 1725. Reprinted in J. Martin Stafford, ed., *Private Vices, Publick Benefits?—the Contemporary Reception of Bernard Mandeville*. Solihull, U.K.: Ismeron, 1997, 227–382; Cook, Richard I. *Bernard Mandeville*. Boston, Mass.: Twayne's English Authors Series No. 170, 1974; Freud, Sigmund. (1930) *Civilization and Its Discontents*. In *The Standard Edition of the Complete Psychological Works of Sigmund Freud*, vol. 21. Trans. James Strachey. London: Hogarth Press, 1953–1974, 57–145; Hume, David. (1739–1740) *A Treatise of Human Nature*. Ed. David Fate Norton and Mary J. Norton. Oxford, U.K.: Oxford University Press, 2000; Law, William. *Remarks upon a Late Book entitled, The Fable of the Bees*. London, 1724. Reprinted in J. Martin Stafford, ed., *Private Vices, Publick Benefits?—the Contemporary Reception of Bernard Mandeville*. Solihull, U.K.: Ismeron, 1997, 45–94; Mandeville, Bernard. (1714, 1723) *The Fable of the Bees*, 2 vols. Ed. F. B. Kaye. Oxford, U.K.: Clarendon Press, 1924; Mandeville, Bernard. *A Letter to Dion [Occasion'd by his* (George Berkeley's) *Book Call'd Alciphron, or The Minute Philosopher]*. London, 1732. Reprinted in J. Martin Stafford, ed., *Private Vices, Publick Benefits?—the Contemporary Reception of Bernard Mandeville*. Solihull, U.K.: Ismeron, 1997, 573–611; Mandeville, Bernard. *A Modest Defence of Publick Stews: or, An Essay on Whoring as it is now practis'd in these Kingdoms*. London, 1724. Reprinted, with an introduction by Richard I. Cook. Los Angeles, Calif.: Augustan Reprint Society, Publication No. 162, 1973. Reprinted, New York: AMS Press, 2000; Mandeville, Bernard. *The Virgin Unmask'd: or, Female Dialogues betwixt an Elderly Maiden Lady and her Niece*. London, 1709. Reprint, Delmar, N.Y.: Scholars' Facsimiles, 1975; Monro, Hector. *The Ambivalence of Bernard Mandeville*. Oxford, U.K.: Clarendon Press, 1975; Stafford, J. Martin, ed. *Private Vices, Publick Benefits?—the Contemporary Reception of Bernard Mandeville*. Solihull, U.K.: Ismeron, 1997.

J. Martin Stafford

ADDITIONAL READING

Cook, Richard I. "The Great Leviathan of Lechery: Mandeville's *Modest Defence of Publick Stews*." In Irwin Primer, ed., *Mandeville Studies*. The Hague, Holland: Martinus Nijhoff, 1975, 22–33; Freud, Sigmund. (1912) "Contributions to a Discussion on Masturbation." In *The Standard Edition of the Complete Psychological Works of Sigmund Freud*, vol. 12. Trans. James Strachey. London: Hogarth Press, 1953–1974, 243–54; Frey, Roger G. "Mandeville, Bernard." In Lawrence C. Becker and Charlotte B. Becker, eds., *Encyclopedia of Ethics*, 2nd ed., vol. 2. New York: Routledge, 2001, 1039–41; Goldsmith, M. M. *Private Vices, Public Benefits: Bernard Mandeville's Social and Political Thought*. Cambridge: Cambridge University Press, 1985; Mandeville, Bernard. (1714, 1723) *The Fable of the Bees, or Private Vices, Publick Benefits*, 2 vols. Ed. F. B. Kaye. Oxford, U.K.: Clarendon Press, 1924. Reprinted, Indianapolis, Ind.: Liberty Classics, 1988. Abridged edition: *The Fable of the Bees and Other Writings*. Ed. E. J. Hundert. Indianapolis, Ind.: Hackett, 1997; Stafford, J. Martin. "Mandeville's Contemporary Critics." *1650–1850: Ideas, Aesthetics, and Inquiries in the Early Modern Era* 7 (2002), 387–401; Vichert, Gordon S. "Bernard Mandeville's *The Virgin Unmask'd*." In Irwin Primer, ed., *Mandeville Studies*. The Hague, Holland: Martinus Nijhoff, 1975, 1–10.

MANICHAEISM. Manichaeism takes it name from its founder, Mani (216–276 CE). The religion spread quickly to the West, into the Roman Empire, and eastward into central Asia and as far as China. Though suffering from sporadic and sometimes intense persecutions, the movement had a renewal with the "Cathar heresy" in thirteenth-century France and continued into the seventeenth century, when Portuguese merchants reported finding Manichees in China.

For centuries our knowledge of the Manichaean religion came only from the writings of its Christian, Zoroastrian, and Muslim opponents. This changed with the European expeditions to Turfan in China (1896–1916) that resulted in the discovery of Manichaean texts in Chinese as well as in Persian and Old Turkish. In 1930 Carl Schmidt (1868–1938) came upon a collection of Manichaean works in Egypt that were written in Coptic. These date to about 400 CE and are much older than the Turfan finds. The most important is a work known as the *Kephalaia* ("principal doctrines") that purports to give the teachings Mani delivered to his disciples, often in response to their questions. In 1969 announcement was made of the first Greek Manichaean text to be recovered. Referred to today as the Cologne Mani Codex (see Cameron and Dewey), it dates to the fourth to fifth century. It contains an account of Mani's life and teachings. Additional, though mainly fragmentary, Manichaean texts have turned up in quantity among the papyrus manuscripts found (1991–1993) at Kellis in Egypt, where there was a Manichaean community from the late third to the late fourth century (Armstrong, 16–17).

Mani was born in southern Mesopotamia in the region of Seleucia-Ctesiphon, which was the capital of the Parthian Empire. His mother was reputed to have belonged to the royal family. His father Pattak was a major influence in his early religious formation. Pattak belonged to a sect that placed great emphasis on baptism, most likely the Elkesaites, a heretical Jewish Christian group (Lieu, *Mesopotamia*, 81–87). Besides regular ablutions, the group practiced a rigorous asceticism such as would later characterize Manichaeism. Mani had his first revelation when he was twelve. The being who appeared to him was his heavenly "twin," later identified as the "Comforter" or Holy "Spirit," in imitation of Christian terminology. From this time on Mani realized the errors and shortcomings of the Elkesaites and began making his objections known. The Cologne Mani Codex (73:8–16) colorfully describes Mani's situation: "For while he was still in that sect of the Baptists, he was like a lamb dwelling in a strange flock, or like a bird living with other birds of a different song" (translation by Cameron and Dewey, 59). When he was twenty-four years old, he left the group along with his father and two disciples.

Mani soon gathered more followers and began sending out missionaries to spread his message. He traveled to India, visiting the Indus Valley, where he had some success. By 242 he was back in Persia, where he gained some favor with Shapur I, king of the Sasanian Empire (242–273) that had recently replaced the Parthians. Some members of the royal family had converted to his religion. Shapur I's successor, Ohrmuzd I, continued this policy of toleration during his short rule (273–274). But when Bahram I came to the throne (274–277), he condemned (at the urging of Kartir, an influential Zoroastrian priest) Mani to a martyr's death in 276 and persecuted his followers.

Mani understood himself to be the final messenger of a truth that had been taught by a long line of teachers, including the Buddha, Zoroaster, and especially Jesus. Their teachings had been corrupted over time, but Mani now restored them to their original form. His goal, therefore, was to present to the world a universal religion that both embraced and supplanted all previous religions. At its core, Manichaeism is a Gnostic religion in that it emphasizes a fundamental struggle between good and evil, expressed in contrasting pairs (light/darkness, spirit/body). It is Mani's teaching that points the way for the individual to escape the present evil world. Figuring prominently in this teaching is his account of how humans came into their present predicament.

In the beginning, good and evil existed as eternally opposite and separate principles. The kingdom of light, ruled by the Father of Greatness, represents good. The kingdom of darkness is the location of evil and is ruled by the King of Darkness. Somehow darkness perceives the light and strives to conquer it. To counter this, the Father evokes the Great Spirit, also known as the Mother of Life, who then brings forth the Primal Man. Primal Man descends to do battle with the forces of evil but is overcome by them. As a result, that part of the light that Primal Man represents becomes intermingled with and trapped in darkness. Though this seems a tragedy, it actually sets the stage for the ultimate triumph of good over evil.

At this point more emanations from the light move the drama forward. The Living Spirit is called forth and defeats some of the rulers of darkness. From their bodies the Living Spirit creates ten heavens and eight earths. The Father of Greatness then evokes the Third Ambassador, who is associated with the sun, and his female counterpart, the Virgin of Light, who is associated with the moon. (Texts such as the *Kephalaia* also allow that the Virgin of Light is the female aspect of the Ambassador instead of a distinct separate being.) The Ambassador and the Virgin show their naked forms to the male and female rulers of darkness, and these demonic rulers respond by ejaculating semen or aborting embryos. From the semen come plants that represent a freeing of the particles of light formerly held prisoner by the rulers, and from the abortions come more demon forces of evil that are the source of animal life. Finally, one demonic pair, Saklas and Nebroel, have lustful intercourse and produce Adam and Eve. In Adam and Eve, especially, are found particles of light from the defeat of Primal Man but so, too, **sexual desire**, which keeps them imprisoned in the physical bodies of this world. Overcoming lustful desire thus becomes the key to the process of salvation. Helping in this endeavor is Jesus the Splendor. He approaches Adam in the Garden and reveals to him his true nature and how to be saved. He also calls forth the Mind of Light, who inspires the great religious thinkers that attempt to enlighten the human race by their teachings.

This account has many similarities with known Gnostic texts, especially in its use of the concept of emanations. However, evil is here eternally existent and not the result of a diminution of goodness as the emanations proceed ever farther from their perfect source, or of Sophia's self-willed action, as in the Gnostic teachings. Also, in Manichaeism there is less emphasis on male-female pairings among the emanations, though they do turn up at key points such as the Third Ambassador–Virgin of Light and Saklas-Nebroel. Of course, the Adam-Eve pair is also central to Mani's system. But questions arise about Eve. While the texts indicate that Adam and Eve are both born from the intercourse of Saklas and Nebroel, when it comes to matters of redemption the texts seem to address only Adam. Since Adam is created to regather the light lost when the Primal Man was defeated, Eve seems irrelevant. This is further born out by the fact that it is only to Adam that Jesus the Splendor appears. So is Eve even capable of salvation? A.V.W. Jackson, basing his thinking on **Saint Augustine**'s (354–430) *On the Morals of the Manichaeans* (388) and the *Fihrist* of the Muslim writer Al-Nadim (ca. 935–995), says, "In Adam the light predominates but Eve is wholly composed of darkness" (252n.137). But the matter is hardly settled.

The community that Mani founded consisted of two groups. The first was the Elect who lived a strictly ascetic way of life, studiously avoiding bringing harm to the particles of light trapped in the present world. The Elect abided by the "Three Seals" of the mouth, the hand, and the sexual organs, which entailed abstaining from eating meat, drinking wine, and telling lies and, above all, renouncing sexual intercourse. The reward for their efforts would be their return to the realm of light.

The Elect were supported in their endeavors by the Hearers, much as the Buddhist monks of the Sangha were supported by the laity. The Hearers provided food to the Elect, which was accepted with both a proclamation of innocence for any suffering its production may have caused and a prayer for the one who offered it. In contrast to the Elect, Hearers were allowed to marry, though producing offspring was, presumably, not encouraged (Jackson, 4). Still, Augustine in *On the Morals of the Manichaeans* (§65) charges that the Manichees are more approving of sexual intercourse than they are of procreation. For Augustine this necessarily means that they are opposed to the very reason for **marriage**. The Hearers were required to keep ten Commandments: "monogamy, the renunciation of fornication, lying, hypocrisy, idolatry, magic, the killing of animals, theft and any doubt of their religion, as well as the duty of the indefatigable care of the elect" (Rudolph, 341). Their fate was to be reborn again into this world, though if their deeds were worthy enough, perhaps reborn as one of the Elect.

The role of women in the Manichaean community has been variously assessed. According to Kurt Rudolph, "Women can attain the station of the elect but cannot take office" (340). More convincingly, J. Kevin Coyle notes that women Elect are depicted in frescoes at Kara-Kotscho in Chinese Turkestan and mentioned in Turfan fragments (81–82, n.11, n.13). Moreover, women Elect are specifically mentioned in a Greek papyrus probably sent by bishop Theonas of Alexandria (ca. 300) to warn his flock of the dangers of Manichaean teachings (see Lieu, *Mesopotamia*, 96–97). Women could even be missionaries: The *Life of Saint Porphyry* mentions a certain Julia who was one of the Elect and traveled from Antioch Gaza around the year 400 to spread the faith (see Lieu, *Mesopotamia*, 48). In addition, we have a fourth-century tombstone of an unknown woman who was one of the Elect and also likely a missionary (105). However, there is no conclusive proof that women were admitted to the highest levels of community leadership consisting of presbyters, bishops, and apostles (Coyle, 82).

While the characteristic attitude of the Manichees toward **sexual activity** was **abstinence,** here and there emerge reports of the ritual use of semen and menstrual discharge, for example, the dipping of a dried fig into semen collected from the wet dreams of men and the menstrual blood of women, a fig that was then eaten by Manichees in some sort of communion rite. While reports of such activities have long been discounted by scholars, they do receive some support from the Greek papyrus of Theonas of Alexandria. Toward the end he enjoins the faithful to beware of "those women whom they call 'elect' and whom they hold in honour, manifestly because they require their menstrual blood for the abominations of their madness" (translation by C. H. Roberts, quoted by Lieu, *Mesopotamia*, 96). Such practices were also reported about a Gnostic group called the Borborites; the similarity has led at least one expert on **Gnosticism** to propose that the Borborite practice "may actually have been influenced by the Manichees" (Layton, 200).

See also Abstinence; Augustine (Saint); Buddhism; Catholicism, History of; Chinese Philosophy; Gnosticism; Hinduism; Tantrism

REFERENCES

Armstrong, Steven A. "The First Generation of Manichaeans and Other Communities in the Egyptian Deserts: Methodology, the Available Evidence, and Conclusions." *Rose + Croix Journal* 1:1 (2004), 10–49; Augustine. (388) *On the Morals of the Manichaeans*. Trans. R. Strothert. In Philip Schaff, ed., *Nicene and Post-Nicene Fathers*. 1st series, vol. 4. Edinburgh, Scot.: T. and T. Clark, 1887, 69–89; BeDuhn, Jason. *The Manichaean Body in Discipline and Ritual*. Baltimore, Md.: Johns Hopkins University Press, 2000; Cameron, Ron, and Arthur Dewey. *The Cologne Mani Codex: "Concerning the Origin of His Body."* Texts and translations. Missoula, Mont.: Scholars Press, 1979; Clark, Elizabeth A. "Vitiated Seeds and Holy Vessels: Augustine's Manichean Past." In *Ascetic Piety and Women's Faith: Essays on Late Ancient Christianity*. Lewiston, N.Y.: Mellen Press, 1986, 291–349; and Karen L. King, ed., *Images of the Feminine in Gnosticism*. Philadelphia, Pa.: Fortress Press, 1988, 367–401; Coyle, J. Kevin. "Prolegomena to a Study of Women in Manichaeism." In P. Mirecki and J. BeDuhn, eds., *The Light and the Darkness: Studies in Manichaeism and Its World*. Leiden, Holland: Brill, 2001, 79–92; Gardner, Iain. *The Kephalaia of the Teacher: The Edited Coptic Manichaean Texts in Translation with Commentary*. Leiden, Holland: Brill, 1995; Gardner, Iain, and Samuel N. C. Lieu, eds. *Manichaean Texts from the Roman Empire*. New York: Cambridge University Press, 2004; Jackson, A. V. Williams. *Researches in Manichaeism with Special Reference to the Turfan Fragments*. New York: Columbia University Press, 1932; Layton, Bentley. *The Gnostic Scriptures: Ancient Wisdom for the New Age*. New York: Doubleday, 1987; Legge, F. (1897) *Western Manichaeism and the Turfan Discoveries*. Whitefish, Mont.: Kessinger, 2005; Lieu, Samuel N. C. *Manichaeism in Central Asia and China*. Leiden, Holland: Brill, 1998; Lieu, Samuel N. C. *Manichaeism in Mesopotamia and the Roman East*. Leiden, Holland: Brill, 1994; Lieu, Samuel N. C. *Manichaeism in the Later Roman Empire and Medieval China: A Historical Survey*. Dover, N.H.: Manchester University Press, 1985. 2nd ed., Tübingen, Ger.: Mohr, 1992; Rudolph, Kurt. (1980) *Gnosis: The Nature and History of Gnosticism*. San Francisco, Calif.: Harper and Row, 1987.

Erik W. Larson

MARCUSE, HERBERT. *See* Freudian Left, The

MARRIAGE. Philosophers have reflected on marriage since **Plato** (427–347 BCE) colored his dialogues with stories about Socrates's home life, and Confucianism recognized family relationships as the exemplar for all social institutions. Marriage is often an arrangement for expressing **love** and intimacy, but the philosophical understanding of these concepts varies widely (and they change even within the same marriage at different stages). Yet marriage has other dimensions, which makes thinking philosophically about it complex; it intersects with law, economics, ethnicity, culture, and systems of ethical and religious beliefs. The widespread role of marriage as a way to perpetuate religions, let alone its role as a mechanism for producing new generations and for taming or constraining the sexual impulse, guarantees ongoing philosophical argument and practical struggle over marriage's value (its individual and social advantages and disadvantages) and its structure (what form shall it take?).

The Ancient Greeks. When explaining in the *Crito* why he should not escape from prison to avoid death, Socrates (469–399 BCE) mentions various benefits he received from Athens, including that his very existence was provided for by laws supporting his parents' marriage (50d–51). In Plato's work on the best possible state, *Laws*, marriage regulations are among the first determined (bk. IV, 721). Men should marry between age thirty and thirty-five, women between sixteen and twenty. Anyone reaching thirty-five without marrying, perhaps for economic benefit, must pay a yearly fine and is deprived of honors extended to other elders. In marriage, humans naturally participate in immortality through reproduction, but celibacy is also a social vice. Thus early in philosophical reflection on marriage is a provocative idea that sounds strange to twentieth-century ears: Reproduction by citizens is a civic duty. The best citizens do not pursue marriage for their own pleasure; benefit to the state comes first. For Plato, community spirit would be fostered by marriages that disregard both class lines and intellectual differences (VI, 773). Marriage should also improve the characters of spouses and offspring. Marriage ceremonies should be economically modest and ensure that the spouses remain sober. Plato was concerned with the effect of alcohol on the unborn (VI, 775).

Marital incompatibility is addressed by the guardians of the laws and women delegated the responsibility of overseeing marriage. Both emphasize reconciliation. Plato's state does not allow no-fault divorce. It does recognize that irreconcilable differences may warrant divorce, but this does not absolve citizens of the duty to reproduce. Divorced couples with insufficient children are helped to find new partners (XI, 930a). Plato also expressed concern about the effects of single parenting on children and urged widowers not to expose children to a stepmother. Widows are advised to remain single if they have fulfilled their reproductive duty. Remarriage is always guided by family members and state-appointed marriage overseers. Marriage is a social matter arranged by family members (e.g., fathers) and guided by social workers, whose goal is to harmonize reproduction for the state's benefit and direct **sexual activity** rationally for the citizens' good. (For an illuminating account of arranged marriage, see Goode.) A father may not disown a son without approval from 50 percent of the family's adult members. The children of a female slave belong to her master; whether the father is a slave or free citizen is irrelevant. But the children of a master and his female slave and those of a mistress and her male slave are exiled (XI, 930d).

The *Laws'* conception of marriage as primarily a social tool is preserved from Plato's earlier dialogue, the utopian *Republic*, in which marriage serves as the means of population maintenance, and children are considered a social resource (V, 460–62). The best citizens are encouraged to mate with each other, and their children are reallocated to overseers capable of developing their innate talents. For the sake of a harmonious society, the *Laws* abandons this mating among the best and leaves the natural family intact. In the *Republic*, marriage is communal within the guardian class. In the *Laws* marriage is communal, too, in the weak sense that other family members and state agents participate in arranging marriage and divorce. Illegitimacy is handled by the death of the infant in the *Republic* (461a–c) and by exile in the *Laws* (XI, 930d–e). (For a comparison of the *Republic* and the *Laws*, see Bobonich.)

Erotic love is missing from both discussions of marriage. For Plato, **sexual desire** is natural but must be controlled and directed by law for social benefit. In the *Symposium*, he expresses the idea—the vehicle is Aristophanes's speech (190–92)—that love (*eros*) is a desire for the completion of a fragmented self through union with another person. Plato's own account of *eros*, perhaps voiced by Diotima (210b–e), involves passionate longing and a search not for another person but for absolute **beauty** and goodness. Plato, aware of *eros*'s power, deflects it in two ways. In the context of the personal life, desire is directed away from particular persons toward abstract values (Vlastos [1907–1991]). Those who merely desire physical beauty and do not "ascend" to higher beauty manage only to reproduce themselves physically. This love, and the heterosexual marriage with which it may be associated, has relatively little value for Plato. In the context of civil society, desire is directed to the formation of unions that will be beneficial. But decisions about marriage are not left to a couple "in love," a private, selfish, and dangerous unit.

Heterosexual marriage fares no better in **Aristotle**'s (384–322 BCE) philosophy. In the *Politics*, he agrees with Plato that reproduction, leaving behind an image of oneself, is a natural desire (1252a30). But the major reason for family is the satisfaction of men's everyday needs (1252b13). The family is not self-sufficient, so the community and the state develop naturally to minister to the family (1253a20). Facilitated by marriage, the family grooms citizens and fosters the good life through a division of labor. The male naturally rules over the female, like the rational rule the passionate (1254b15). Some possibility exists for love or **friendship** (*philia*) in the family between father and son. Yet Aristotle is not convinced that genuine *philia* between unequals is possible; children are always indebted to parents for the gift of life. (For similar Aristotelian uncertainty, see *Nicomachean Ethics*, bk. 8, 1158b12–b30.) If a family fosters human excellence, it will produce children equal in virtue to the father and hence worthy of love. Women, inferior by nature, cannot attain a level of human excellence worthy of male love.

Aristotle is wary of the effects of young fathers on children and reluctant to allow mating between men and women outside their prime. The preferred age at marriage for men is thirty-seven, when they are old enough to have acquired practical wisdom and are able to command respect from children. These men should marry and mate with nineteen-year-old females, guaranteeing that married life would correspond to the periods of male and female prime fertility (*Politics*, 1335a). Aristotle regarded **adultery** as disgraceful and urged penalties for the offending party. It serves as his example of an action for which there is no mean; there is no way to commit adultery at the right time, in the right place, with the right woman (*Nicomachean Ethics*, 1107a15). As an advocate of proper prenatal care, Aristotle urged pregnant women to eat properly, avoid stress, and take daily walks to the temples of the gods who watch over births (*Politics*, 1335a–b). The state has a serious interest in fostering the health and virtue of future citizens.

Christianity. Aristophanes's myth in the *Symposium* suggests that the single life is a fallen, defective state. Humans, having displeased Zeus, were separated into halves, which significantly reduces their power. Their lives are henceforth consumed by trying to repair themselves by melding with their other halves (selves) to form a couple, a whole. The Judeo-Christian tradition also provides details of the "Fall" but allows a more positive assessment of the single life. In the Old Testament, paradise was originally populated by a married couple, and so Christianity strongly encourages marriage and procreation as a contribution to the fulfillment of God's creation. At the same time, however, many Church patricians argued that remaining single was superior to marriage; celibacy, even though it encompassed childlessness, was the more holy state. The beginning of the debate was **Saint Paul**'s (5–64?) encouraging Christians to remain single, the best state, yet also giving them permission to marry (contrast 1 Cor. 7:1, 7:7–8, 7:27 with 7:6, 7:9, 7:28). For those who have strong sexual desires and cannot abstain, monogamous marriage is an acceptable option, one designed to quell or satisfy desire within reasonable and regulated bounds.

An optimistic Christian assessment of marriage is found in **Saint Augustine** (354–430). All humanity is tainted by original sin, even the conception, birth, and lives of infants. Augustine, in the *Confessions*, speaks of watching a naturally jealous baby (bk. 1, chap. 7). He also recounts his personal experiences of uncontrollable lust (2.1–2.3, 3.1) as a young man. To cure this (in Pauline manner), his parents—he thought, but they failed to do so—should have imposed order on his life by arranging marriage: "Then the stormy waves of my youth would have [been] broken" (2.2). When he finally did take a concubine (in the fashion of a long marriage), their relationship was still lusty (4.2). They had only one child. It is likely that Augustine (a Manichee at the time) and his concubine engaged in sex for reasons other than procreation and used rudimentary contraceptive methods. Much later, as a Catholic bishop, Augustine redeemed marriage, despite his view of the superiority of an **abstinence** that refuses to make concessions to original sin and that renounces personal satisfaction in the pursuit of spirituality. Among theologians his three goods of marriage are well known: reproduction, fidelity, and the sacramental bond (*Marriage and Concupiscence*, 1.11.10; 1.19.17; 1.23.21). This was part of his optimism.

For Augustine, the corruption of the flesh, concupiscence, is a consequence, not the cause, of the Fall. Augustine insisted that prelapsarian Adam and Eve "lived in a partnership of unalloyed felicity" and would have had sexual intercourse and reproduced in Eden (had they not fallen). But they would not have experienced concupiscence (*City of God*, 14.10; 14.26). Indeed, in contrast to Aristotle, Augustine "presented sexual intercourse [between prelapsarian Adam and Eve] as secondary to friendship. . . . Friendship, and not sexual desire, had set the pace of their relations" (Brown, 402). Eve was Adam's "only companion" (*City*, 14.11), a role as important as, if not more important than, her role as procreative partner (see Clark). Augustine—more optimism—hoped that postlapsarian marriages could attain this ideal of marital friendship.

The views of St. Jerome (330/347?–420) were less flattering to marriage. Jerome endorses a remark of the Stoic philosopher Sextus (second century), that a man who ardently desires his wife commits adultery (*Against Jovinianus*, I, 49; note, however, that similar sentiments can be found in Augustine [*Marriage and Concupiscence*, 1.17] and **Thomas Aquinas** [1224/25–1274; *Summa theologiae*, supp., ques. 49, art. 6]). Ardent love of another person for, say, its sexual pleasure is blasphemous; it elevates a human above God. Instead of coming to his wife as a lover he should come to her as a husband (I, 49). Jerome denied Augustine's view of the occurrence of sexual intercourse in Eden, claiming that Adam and Eve would have stayed virgins had there been no Fall (I, 16). Postlapsarian marriage may populate the earth, but the superior virginity populates heaven. Jerome (like Paul, 1 Cor. 7:40) advises widows to remain unmarried. Priests must be unmarried and abstain because sexuality distracts from study and prayer, and priests must be prepared to tend to their flocks. But if the number of people for whom celibacy is possible is insufficient for clerical needs, priests may marry. Jerome (again following Paul, 1 Cor. 7:32–33) observes that a married man is too occupied in attending to his spouse's needs, while unmarried men are free to attend to God (I, 35). Jerome looks positively on marriages dedicated to raising children who will remain virgins but fears that marriages based on sexual desire dissolve quickly as lust is satisfied.

One writer in the Christian tradition, Saint Thomas Aquinas, at least partially switches the emphasis from the sinful sexual tendencies of adults to the relationship between marriage and the good of children. To be sure, he agrees with Augustine that were Adam and Eve to have engaged in intercourse, lustful desires would have been absent (*Summa theologiae* Ia, ques. 98, art. 2)—yet their pleasure would have been greater than our postlapsarian pleasure (Ia, ques. 98, art. 2, reply 3). Further, Aquinas is well known for developing a Natural Law ethics that condemns as mortal sins all nonprocreative sexual activity, including **homosexuality**, heterosexual oral and anal sex, **masturbation**, and **bestiality** (IIa–IIae, ques. 154).

This same Natural Law philosophy allows Aquinas to argue that a female parent is not competent to raise children on her own: "[T]he fitness of human life requires man to stand by woman after the sexual act is done, and not to go off at once and form connections with anyone he meets, as is the way with fornicators." Aquinas here uses a broad sense of "procreation" when claiming that the purpose of sex is procreation. Children need both parents for a long time for procreation in the broad sense to be completed, until the time they can care for themselves and produce their own children. What they need from parents is more than material support; they also need the discipline and education that only the father can provide. This consideration suggests to Aquinas that monogamy is mandatory (a man cannot realistically spread his resources and energy beyond one family). It also suggests that marriage is lifelong, for the raising of children virtually never ends. But Aquinas argues for the indissolubility of marriage on other grounds as well: (1) Property, which is necessary for a child's survival even as an adult, can be conveyed from male parent to child only if he remains continually concerned for the child; (2) men significantly harm women materially and socially by leaving them after the blush is off the rose; and (3) divorce can lead to confusion of parentage. Aquinas expects that love and friendship will develop between the partners, creating a permanent commitment to each other, and this will make the question of divorce moot. (See *Summa contra gentiles*, par. 120–23.) Official Catholicism in the twenty-first century remains committed to the sinfulness of nonprocreative (and contracepted) sexuality, celibacy for those with religious vocations, and marriage's indissolubility.

When Paul wrote to the Corinthian converts, he answered questions about the religious significance of circumcision and the status of existent marriages between converts and unbelievers (see 1 Cor. 7). Religious involvement with the details of marriage, then, has long been motivated by considerations other than encouraging procreation and structuring the satisfaction of sexual desire. During the early medieval period spouses were often selected more by parents and families than by the choice and mutual **consent** of the betrothed. For guidance in marital planning, the participants in these affairs turned to priests (Flandrin, 126). Perhaps the Church increasingly preferred that marriages at least seem voluntary (see Ariès, "Love in Married Life"). Christianity also seemed to embrace the notion (adopted from the Romans) that love would often evolve between spouses after an arranged marriage, although Christians had their own special conception of love: the spiritual love of unconditional commitment that resembles the bind between Christ and the Church and Christ and humanity. This type of love, which **Immanuel Kant** (1724–1804) called "practical" (i.e., moral) love, as opposed to "pathological" passionate, romantic love (*Groundwork*, 67; *Lectures*, 163; see Schott, 111), can be promised and even commanded. Such a Christian deployment of love must of course be distinguished from the Romantic maneuver of incorporating love into marriage (see Letwin). That sort of love/marriage combination, unlike the Christian combination, makes divorce seem more natural, because passionate romance eventually declines or even dies (see Ariès, "Love").

Christian marriage was originally a private affair, the ceremony was performed by the groom's father in the home, and the marriage was dissoluble if it did not produce children (see Ariès, "Indissoluble Marriage"). The progeny stakes were high in the families of nobles, and the marriage ceremony included the blessing of the bed by the groom's father. Priests eventually took over this function, blessing the bed with holy water. But when no great amount of property and prestige were involved in a marriage, these and other devices to insure paternity were dispensed with. A lack of property in poorer families meant that not all children could marry and had to seek other sexual outlets. From the ninth century to the thirteenth the Church gradually developed the Augustinian idea that marriage was a sacrament. The aristocratic use of marriage to form an alliance between families; Paul's and Jerome's ascetic, sexless ideal marriage; social tolerance of concubines, informal marriage, and masturbation—all these were gradually rejected and replaced by consensual, indissoluble marriage whose ceremony was performed by a priest in a public place, the church. Of course, these marriages were to be not only lifelong but monogamous. The polygyny of the Old Testament found no space in the development of Christianity.

Polygamy. Polygamy comes in three varieties: polygyny, in which one man has a number of wives; polyandry, the marriage of one woman to several husbands; and communal marriage, in which roughly equal numbers of males and females form a union. In *Republic*, Plato endorsed communal marriage for the guardians. Later, **David Hume** (1711–1776), although he admitted that polygamy was a defensible family form, preferred monogamy. He valued friendship between the sexes (as in Aquinas) and thought that it would be more difficult to develop in polygamy. Hume also worried that the sheer number of children would make it difficult for fathers to have intimate, affectionate relationships with them (*Essays*, pt. 1, 19.69, 12–13). Modern feminist **Shulamith Firestone** proposed communal marriage in households where biological parents were released both from special rights over and responsibilities for offspring; this was seen as an important component in eliminating family chauvinism (230–36). Another defender of communal marriage, Alan Donagan, argues nonetheless that biological parents should practice temporary monogamy while attempting to conceive a child to assure paternity (101–3). Those causally and voluntarily responsible for the child's existence must be identified, because communal arrangements often dissolve, and (again, Aquinas) the child's right to be raised to be socially independent must be respected.

The views of **Arthur Schopenhauer** (1788–1860) on sexuality and marriage are intriguing. He sees the sexual impulse as the will of Nature working through what appears (wrongly) to the individual as a voluntary, personal choice. Whom we select to mate with is ultimately Nature's choice determining the composition of the next generation. Schopenhauer examines two types of monogamous union and finds fault with both: marriages for love and arranged marriages. The happiness in love marriages will be brief, because the spouses will be mismatched in many ways that the temporary madness of sexual attraction obscures. Yet these instinctual marriages are valuable in that the needs of the species are attained, albeit at the expense of individuals. More stable marriages are those arranged by parents for economic and other practical reasons. But they thwart the working of instinct and so have costs for both the species and the individual. The spouses forgo sexual gratification or must find it elsewhere (*World as Will*, vol. 2, 565–67). This creates **prostitution,** in which some women are "human sacrifices upon the altar of monogamy." The benefits of rational, arranged marriage to a relatively few women do not justify the suffering of so many other women ("Women," 86–88). So Schopenhauer favored polygamy. It increases reproductive access and marginalizes those males who should not reproduce. He commented favorably on polygamy among the Mormons. Polygamous societies provide for all women, while monogamous societies provide a decent life for only a select group of women. Further, a man whose wife is barren, has become too old, or suffers from chronic illness should be allowed to have another. Polygamy, on his view, benefits both women and men; it is a better alternative than divorce, prostitution, or illegitimacy ("Women," 85–88).

Even though Christianity forbids polygamy, other religions find it agreeable. One example is the Church of the Latter-day Saints (LDS). Like Augustine, LDS theologians believe that there was marriage in Eden between Adam and Eve; they also believe that there will be marriage again in heaven. The highest houses in heaven are open to those who practice polygamy on earth. The Utah Territory was the homeland of many Mormon polygamists, but Utah received statehood in 1896 only after its constitution made polygamy illegal (see Porter). There are still Mormons who practice this lifestyle. In 1991 the Joseph family from Utah, neither Mormon nor members of the LDS, received significant media attention when Elizabeth Joseph, an attorney, addressed the Utah chapter of the National Organization for Women (NOW). Mrs. Joseph was a plural wife—wife number seven, of nine— who argued that polygamy was good **feminism**. Like Schopenhauer, she argued that a woman does not want just any husband but the best husband she can find, even if he is a married man. She also argued that polygamy facilitates careers for women, provides excellent day care for children, removes the drudgery of daily domestic chores and the sexual marriage debt, and reintroduces into marriage special romantic nights with the husband. Men benefit as well: They enjoy sexual variety and engage in sexual relations with more willing partners; and they can spend more time with children, since several wives work outside the home. Subsequently, Utah NOW issued a statement that it neither condemns nor endorses polygamy.

Islam also has a favorable view of polygamy. The prophet Mohammed married four times in his fifties and sixties after the death of his first wife. Mohammed permitted a maximum of four wives but required that the husband be able to provide economically for all his wives and children. He must not exhibit any favoritism but love all his wives equally and spend the same time with each (Polygamy.com). Some predominantly Muslim countries have made polygamy illegal, and Egypt has given women the legal right to divorce men who take a second wife. One Islamic argument for polygamy is that it has always existed without regulation and continues to exist today in the officially monogamous West in the form of mistresses, prostitutes, and serial marriages. Islam also regards polygamy as justified when a woman is barren, because procreation is a religious duty. Muslims also think that this wife will find consolation in the children of the other wives. Polygamy is a superior alternative to prostitutes, mistresses, divorce, and the birth of illegitimate children who will lack proper parental care.

The views of Kant on sexuality and marriage contrast sharply with those favorable to polygamy. Augustine offered the uncontrollability of the sexual organs as a visible manifestation of the Fall; the genitals are in ongoing revolt against rational control and, in effect, against God (*City*, 14.16 ff.). Kant also sees sexual desire as an indication of human decadence. Sexual desire by its nature insults human dignity, treating that person who arouses it as an object, a mere source of pleasure, and hence violating the duty to respect persons as ends in themselves. Sexual desire in particular treats persons merely as things because it is directed primarily at body parts, especially the genitals (*Lectures*, 163–64). If sexual desire is by its nature decadent in this way, it would seem that humans should be celibate (a Pauline conclusion). However, Kant proposes marriage as the solution to this immorality of sexual desire (167). Although the right way to interpret these difficult passages in Kant is controversial, one possibility is that marriage fuses two persons into one (in a sense, they achieve Aristophanes's ideal state), and since the couple exists as one, there can be no question of using another merely as a means (Baker and Elliston, 1st ed., 18; 2nd ed., 26–27; 3rd ed., 31; contrast Herman). Kant argues specifically against polygamy, employing his idea that marriage involves a fusion of two into one. For in polygyny, in which one man is married to several wives, the man cannot achieve with any one wife the complete fusion that would make sexual relations permissible.

Other Contemporary Views. In the nineteenth century, Aquinas's embryonic idea of marital friendship and the sexual equality implicit in Kant's notion of marriage fueled (along with other influences, including the writings of Mary Wollstonecraft [1759–1797]) the feminist movement in the United States in the work of Margaret Fuller (1810–1850), a Transcendentalist and intimate of Ralph Waldo Emerson (1803–1882). Fuller, urging women to choose sexual abstinence over an unequal marriage, outlined four types of equal marriage. *Domestic partnership* required the equal economic rights and responsibilities associated with a family business. *Mutual idolatry* meant exclusive romantic and sexual love. *Intellectual companionship* was a marriage between educated equals who shared common interests, perhaps in art or politics. Fuller seems to have regarded the fourth type, *mutual pilgrimage*, as slightly superior to the others. Partners will prophesize to each other on their journey toward a common shrine; they have an interest in a common intellectual, religious, or political issue pursued together as partners, with the added commitment that change in direction will also be undertaken as a couple. Fuller may have lived this sort of life, serving as editor of *The Dial* and acting as a full partner in her eventual husband's political activities in Italy. We are not far from the union of John Stuart Mill (1806–1873) and Harriet Taylor (1807–1858), one consistent with the doctrines of *Subjection of Women*.

A provocative twentieth-century analysis of marriage was offered by philosopher **Bertrand Russell** (1872–1970). Russell expressed surprise at the lack of family feeling in the United States and forecast, in 1929, that the family in the States would become matriarchal. Russell advocated trial marriage of a year or two for young couples before they entered a more permanent marriage. Even marriage is essentially a trial period for Russell until children are born. Although he preferred that childless marriages be dissolved by mutual consent, Russell's only requirement for divorce was that the woman produce a medical affidavit that she was not pregnant (a proposal indicative of Russell's feminist leanings). Russell also advocated a form of open marriage. Marriage is an institution for family building and not particularly suited to romantic and sexual satisfaction over the long run. Russell saw extramarital affairs as a useful outlet for sexual desire, provided children did not result from such liaisons. (Similarly, Richard Taylor [1919–2003] did not think that legal marriage guarantees stability and commitment and was a staunch defender of extramarital affairs.) Russell's position on divorce when a marriage has already produced children was that divorce is permissible only when the children are at grave risk from the alcoholism, habitual crime, mental illness, or venereal disease of the adults. Russell specifically excludes adultery as a justification of divorce; **jealousy** is not tenable, and sexual outlets should be available outside the marriage to each partner in the marriage (221–39).

It is difficult not to be struck by the differences between ancient views of marriage and contemporary views. Although there are many exceptions to this pattern, marriage as conceived and practiced in the West has evolved from an ownership relation to an emotionally significant relationship between equal partners. Whether two (or more) people—even in the best of economic and social conditions—can be friends, marriage partners, lovers, and parents all at once (while permitting outside relationships) is, however, a question likely to puzzle us for quite some time.

See also Adultery; African Philosophy; Augustine (Saint); Bible, Sex and the; Catholicism, History of; Catholicism, Twentieth- and Twenty-First-Century; Chinese Philosophy; Ellis, Albert; Feminism, History of; Feminism, Liberal; Fichte, Johann Gottlieb; Friendship; Gnosticism; Greek Sexuality and Philosophy, Ancient; Islam; Judaism, History of; Love; Marriage, Same-Sex; Paul (Saint); Plato; Protestantism, History of; Rimmer, Robert; Roman Sexuality and Philosophy, Ancient; Rousseau, Jean-Jacques; Russell, Bertrand; Utopianism; Westermarck, Edward; Wojtyła, Karol (Pope John Paul II)

REFERENCES

Ariès, Philippe. "The Indissoluble Marriage." In Philippe Ariès and André Béjin, eds., *Western Sexuality: Practice and Precept in Past and Present Times*. Trans. Anthony Forster. New York: Blackwell, 1985, 140–57; Ariès, Philippe. "Love in Married Life." In Philippe Ariès and André Béjin, eds., *Western Sexuality: Practice and Precept in Past and Present Times*. Trans. Anthony Forster. New York: Blackwell, 1985, 130–39; Aristotle. (ca. 325 BCE?) *Nicomachean Ethics*. Trans. Terence Irwin. Indianapolis, Ind.: Hackett, 1985; Aristotle. (ca. 330 BCE?) *Politics*. Trans. Benjamin Jowett. In Richard McKeon, ed., *The Basic Works of Aristotle*. New York: Random House, 1941, 1127–1324; Augustine. (413–427) *The City of God*. Trans. Henry Bettenson. New York: Penguin Classics, 1984; Augustine. (397) *The Confessions*. Trans. Henry Chadwick. New York: Oxford University Press, 1991; Augustine. (418?–421) *On Marriage and Concupiscence*. Trans. Peter Holmes. In Marcus Dods, ed., *Works*, vol. 12. Edinburgh, Scot.: T. and T. Clark, 1874, 93–202; Baker, Robert B., and Frederick A. Elliston, eds. *Philosophy and Sex*, 1st ed. Buffalo, N.Y.: Prometheus, 1975. 2nd ed., 1984; Baker, Robert B., Kathleen J. Wininger, and Frederick A. Elliston, eds. *Philosophy and Sex*, 3rd ed. Amherst, N.Y.: Prometheus, 1998; Bobonich, Christopher. *Plato's Utopia Recast: His Later Ethics and Politics*. Oxford, U.K.: Clarendon Press, 2002; Brown, Peter. *The Body and Society: Men, Women, and Sexual Renunciation in Early Christianity*. New York: Columbia University Press, 1988; Clark, Elizabeth A. " 'Adam's Only Companion': Augustine and the Early Christian Debate on Marriage." *Recherches Augustiniennes* 21 (1986), 139–62; Donagan, Alan. *A Theory of Morality*. Chicago, Ill.: University of Chicago Press, 1977; Firestone, Shulamith. *The Dialectic of Sex: The Case for Feminist Revolution*. New York: Morrow, 1970; Flandrin, Jean-Louis. "Sex in Married Life in the Early Middle Ages: The Church's Teaching and Behavioral Reality." In Philippe Ariès and André Béjin, eds., *Western Sexuality: Practice and Precept in Past and Present Times*. Trans. Anthony Forster. New York: Blackwell, 1985, 114–29; Fuller, Margaret. "The Great Lawsuit." *The Dial* 4 (July 1843–1844), 1–47; Goode, William J. "The Theoretical Importance of Love." *American Sociological Review* 24:1 (1959), 38–47; Herman, Barbara. "Could It Be Worth Thinking About Kant on Sex and Marriage?" In Louise Antony and Charlotte Witt, eds., *A Mind of One's Own: Feminist Essays on Reason and Objectivity*. Boulder, Colo.: Westview, 1993, 49–67; Hume, David. (1742) *Essays, Moral, Political, and Literary*. Part I. Ed. Eugene F. Miller. Indianapolis, Ind.: Liberty Classics, 1985; Jerome. (393) *Against Jovinianus*. In *St. Jerome: Letters and Select Works*. Trans. W. H. Fremantle. *Select Library of Nicene and Post-Nicene Fathers*, ser. 2, vol. 6. Edinburgh, Scot.: 1892. Web site, Christian Classics Ethereal Library: <www.ccel.org/fathers2/NPNF2-06/Npnf2-06-10.htm#P6119_1832142> [accessed 27 September 2004]; Joseph, Elizabeth. "Polygamy Is Good Feminism." *New York Times* (23 May 1991), A31; Kant, Immanuel. (1785) *Groundwork of the Metaphysic of Morals*. Trans. H. J. Paton. New York: Harper Torchbooks, 1964; Kant, Immanuel. (ca. 1780) *Lectures on Ethics*. Trans. Louis Infield. New York: Harper Torchbooks, 1963; Letwin, Shirley Robin. "Romantic Love and Christianity." *Philosophy* 52 (1977), 131–45; Mill, John Stuart. (1869)

The Subjection of Women. In Alice Rossi, ed., *Essays on Sex Equality: John Stuart Mill and Harriet Taylor Mill.* Chicago, Ill.: University of Chicago Press, 1970, 123–242; Plato. *Crito* (ca. 390 BCE); *Laws* (ca. 355–347 BCE); *Symposium* (ca. 380 BCE); *Republic* (ca. 375–370 BCE). Trans. Benjamin Jowett. In *The Dialogues of Plato,* 2 vols. New York: Random House, 1937, vol. 1 (427–38), vol. 2 (407–788), vol. 1 (301–45), vol. 1 (591–879), respectively; Polygamy.com. (Web site) "Polygamy by Light of Life." <www.polygamy.com/Islam/Polygamy.htm> [accessed 27 September 2004]; Porter, Perry L. *A Chronology of Federal Legislation on Polygamy.* Perry Porter's Page (4 January 1998). <www.xmission.com/~plporter/lds/chron.htm> [accessed 27 September 2004]; Russell, Bertrand. (1929) *Marriage and Morals.* New York: Norton, 1970; Schopenhauer, Arthur. (1851) "On Women." In R. J. Hollingdale, ed., *Arthur Schopenhauer: Essays and Aphorisms.* New York: Penguin, 1970, 80–89; Schopenhauer, Arthur. (1818, 1844, 1859) *The World as Will and Representation,* 2 vols. Trans. Eric F. C. Payne. New York: Dover, 1969; Schott, Robin May. *Cognition and Eros: A Critique of the Kantian Paradigm.* University Park: Pennsylvania State University Press, 1993; Taylor, Richard. (1982) *Love Affairs: Marriage and Infidelity.* Amherst, N.Y.: Prometheus, 1997; Thomas Aquinas. (1258–1264) *On the Truth of the Catholic Faith. Summa contra gentiles. Book Three: Providence. Part II.* Trans. Vernon J. Bourke. Garden City, N.Y.: Image Books, 1956; Thomas Aquinas. (1265–1273) *Summa theologiae,* 60 vols. Cambridge, U.K.: Blackfriars, 1964–1976; Utah National Organization for Women. "No Stand on Polygamy." <www.now.org/press/08–97/utahnow.html> [accessed 27 September 2004]; Vlastos, Gregory. "The Individual as an Object of Love in Plato." In *Platonic Studies.* Princeton, N.J.: Princeton University Press, 1973, 3–34; Wollstonecraft, Mary. (1792) *A Vindication of the Rights of Women.* Buffalo, N.Y.: Prometheus, 1989.

Anthony J. Graybosch

ADDITIONAL READING

Abbey, Ruth. "Odd Bedfellows: Nietzsche and Mill on Marriage." *History of European Ideas* 23:2–4 (1997), 81–104; Allgeier, Elizabeth, and Wiederman, Michael. "Mate Selection." In Vern L. Bullough and Bonnie Bullough, eds., *Human Sexuality: An Encyclopedia.* New York: Garland, 1994, 386–90; Applbaum, Kalman D. "Marriage with the Proper Stranger: Arranged Marriage in Metropolitan Japan." *Ethnology* 34:1 (1995), 37–51; Ariès, Philippe, and André Béjin, eds. *Western Sexuality: Practice and Precept in Past and Present Times.* New York: Blackwell, 1985; Bayles, Michael D. "Marriage, Love, and Procreation." In Robert B. Baker and Frederick A. Elliston, eds., *Philosophy and Sex,* 1st ed. Buffalo, N.Y.: Prometheus, 1975, 190–206. Reprinted in P&S2 (130–45); P&S3 (116–29); Berger, Michael S. "Two Models of Medieval Jewish Marriage: A Preliminary Study." *Journal of Jewish Studies* 52:1 (2001), 59–84; Bornoff, Nicholas. *Pink Samurai: Love, Marriage, and Sex in Contemporary Japan.* New York: Pocket Books, 1991; Brake, Elizabeth. "Justice and Virtue in Kant's Account of Marriage." *Kantian Review* 9 (March 2005), 58–94; Brake, Elizabeth. "Love's Paradox: Making Sense of Hegel on Marriage." In Stella Stanford and Alison Stone, eds., *Hegel and Feminism, Women's Philosophy Review,* Special Issue no. 22 (Autumn 1999), 80–104; Brooke, Christopher. *The Medieval Idea of Marriage.* Oxford, U.K.: Oxford University Press, 1989; Brophy, Brigid. "The Immorality of Marriage." In *Don't Never Forget: Collected Views and Reviews.* London: Jonathan Cape, 1966, 22–27; Brown, Peter. *Augustine of Hippo.* Berkeley: University of California Press, 2000; Burch, Robert W. "The Commandability of Pathological Love." *Southwestern Journal of Philosophy* [*Philosophical Topics*] 3:3 (1972), 131–40. Reprinted in Alan Soble, ed., *Eros, Agape, and Philia: Readings in the Philosophy of Love.* New York: Paragon House, 1989, 245–53; Cicovacki, Predrag. "Can Love Resolve the Problem of Marriage?" In Thomas Magnell, ed., *Explorations of Value.* Amsterdam, Holland: Rodopi, 1997, 221–33; Coleman, Julie. *Love, Sex, and Marriage: A Historical Thesaurus.* Amsterdam, Holland: Rodopi, 1999; Cott, Nancy F. *Public Vows: A History of Marriage and the Nation.* Cambridge, Mass.: Harvard University Press, 2000; Denis, Lara. "From Friendship to Marriage: Revising Kant." *Philosophy and Phenomenological Research* 63:1 (2001), 1–28; Devlin, Patrick. (1963) "Morals and the Law of Marriage." In *The Enforcement of Morals.* Oxford, U.K.: Oxford University Press, 1965, 61–85; duBois, Page. "The Platonic

Appropriation of Reproduction." In Nancy Tuana, ed., *Feminist Interpretations of Plato*. University Park: Pennsylvania State University Press, 1994, 139–56. Taken from *Sowing the Body: Psychoanalysis and Ancient Representations of Women*. Chicago, Ill.: University of Chicago Press, 1988, 169–83; Engels, Frederick. (1884) "A Recently Discovered Case of Group Marriage." In *The Origin of the Family, Private Property, and the State*. Peking, China: Foreign Languages Press, 1978, 217–21; Ertman, Martha M. "Marriage as a Trade: Bridging the Private/Private Distinction." *Harvard Civil Rights–Civil Liberties Law Review* 36:1 (2001), 79–132; Falco, Maria J., ed. *Feminist Interpretations of Mary Wollstonecraft*. University Park: Pennsylvania State University Press, 1996; Fisher, Helen E. *Anatomy of Love: The Natural History of Monogamy, Adultery, and Divorce*. New York: Norton, 1992. *Anatomy of Love: A Natural History of Mating, Marriage, and Why We Stray*. New York: Ballantine, 1994; Foster, Michael Smith. *Annulment: The Wedding That Was. How the Church Can Declare a Marriage Null*. New York: Paulist Press, 1998; Fuller, Margaret. "The Great Lawsuit." *The Dial* 4 (July 1843–1844), 1–47. Reprinted in Eve Kornfeld, *Margaret Fuller: A Brief Biography with Documents*. New York: St. Martin's Press, 1996, 156–90; Geach, Mary. "Marriage: Arguing to a First Principle in Sexual Ethics." In Luke Gormally, ed., *Moral Truth and Moral Tradition: Essays in Honour of Peter Geach and Elizabeth Anscombe*. Dublin, Ire.: Four Courts Press, 1994, 177–93; George, Robert P., and Gerard V. Bradley. "Marriage and the Liberal Imagination." *Georgetown Law Journal* 84:2 (1995), 301–20; Goode, William J. "The Theoretical Importance of Love." *American Sociological Review* 24:1 (1959), 38–47. Reprinted in Ashley Montagu, ed., *The Practice of Love*. Englewood Cliffs, N.J.: Prentice-Hall, 1975, 120–35; Goode, William J., ed. *Readings on the Family and Society*. Englewood Cliffs, N.J.: Prentice-Hall, 1964; Gregory, Paul. "Against Couples." *Journal of Applied Philosophy* 1:2 (1984), 263–68; Himmelfarb, Gertrude. *Marriage and Morals among the Victorians*. New York: Knopf, 1986; Houlgate, Laurence D., ed. *Morals, Marriage, and Parenthood*. Belmont, Calif.: Wadsworth, 1999; Kant, Immanuel. (1762–1794) *Lectures on Ethics*. Trans. Peter Heath. Ed. Peter Heath and Jerome Schneewind. Cambridge: Cambridge University Press, 1997; Lawrence, D. H. *Phoenix II: Uncollected, Unpublished, and Other Prose Works*. New York: Viking, 1959; McEvoy, James. "Friendship within Marriage: A Philosophical Essay." In Luke Gormally, ed., *Moral Truth and Moral Tradition: Essays in Honour of Peter Geach and Elizabeth Anscombe*. Dublin, Ire.: Four Courts Press, 1994, 194–202; Mencken, H. L. "Marriage." In *In Defense of Women*. New York: Knopf, 1924, 65–122; Mendus, Susan. "Marital Faithfulness." *Philosophy* 59 (1984), 243–52. Reprinted in Alan Soble, ed., *Eros, Agape, and Philia: Readings in the Philosophy of Love*. New York: Paragon House, 1989, 235–44; P&S3 (130–38); Mohr, Richard D. "The Case for Gay Marriage." *Notre Dame Journal of Law, Ethics, and Public Policy* 9:1 (1995), 216–29. Reprinted in HS (231–55); P&S3 (190–211); Murstein, Bernard I. "Physical Attractiveness and Marital Choice." *Journal of Personality and Social Psychology* 22:1 (1972), 8–12; O'Driscoll, Lyla H. "On the Nature and Value of Marriage." In Mary Vetterling-Braggin, Frederick Elliston, and Jane English, eds., *Feminism and Philosophy*. Totowa, N.J.: Littlefield, Adams, 1977, 249–63; Okin, Susan Moller. "Plato." In *Women in Western Political Thought*. Princeton, N.J.: Princeton University Press, 1979, 15–50; Pagels, Elaine. *Adam, Eve, and the Serpent*. New York: Vintage, 1988; Palmer, David. "The Consolation of the Wedded." In Robert B. Baker and Frederick A. Elliston, eds., *Philosophy and Sex*, 1st ed. Buffalo, N.Y.: Prometheus, 1975, 178–89. Reprinted in P&S2 (119–29); Pateman, Carole. "Hegel, Marriage, and the Standpoint of Contract." In Patricia J. Mills, ed., *Feminist Interpretations of G.W.F. Hegel*. University Park: Pennsylvania State University Press, 1996, 209–23; Pius XI (Pope). "On Christian Marriage." *Catholic Mind* 29:2 (1931), 21–64; "Polygamy: Frequently Asked Questions." Absolom Industries. <www.absalom.com/mormon/polygamy/faq.htm> [accessed 27 September 2004]; Posner, Richard A., and Katharine B. Silbaugh. "Bigamy." In *A Guide to America's Sex Laws*. Chicago, Ill.: University of Chicago Press, 1996, 143–54; Rice, F. Philip. *Sexual Problems in Marriage*. Philadelphia, Pa.: Westminster, 1978; Rosenblum, Nancy L. "Democratic Sex: Reynolds v. U.S., Sexual Relations, and Community." In David M. Estlund and Martha C. Nussbaum, eds., *Sex, Preference, and Family: Essays on Law and Nature*. New York: Oxford University Press, 1997, 63–85; Shanley, Mary Lyndon. *Just Marriage*. Ed. Joshua Cohen and Deborah Chasman. New York: Oxford University Press, 2004;

Shanley, Mary Lyndon. "Marital Slavery and Friendship: John Stuart Mill's *The Subjection of Women*." *Political Theory* 9:2 (1981), 229–47; Singer, Irving. "Marriage: Same-Sex and Opposite-Sex." In *Sex: A Philosophical Primer*, expanded ed. Lanham, Md.: Rowman and Littlefield, 2004, ix–xxxii; Smart, Carol. *The Ties That Bind: Law, Marriage, and the Reproduction of Patriarchal Relations*. London: Routledge and Kegan Paul, 1974; Spurlock, John C. *Free Love: Marriage and Middle-Class Radicalism in America, 1825–1860*. New York: New York University Press, 1988; Taylor, Richard. *Love Affairs: Marriage and Infidelity*. Amherst, N.Y.: Prometheus, 1997. Previously published as *Having Love Affairs*. Buffalo, N.Y.: Prometheus, 1982, 1990; Taylor, Richard. "Why Marriage? The Tie That Binds Need Not Be Legal." *Free Inquiry* 23:3 (2003), 49–51; Teichman, Jenny. "Marriage." In *Illegitimacy: A Philosophical Examination*. Oxford, U.K.: Blackwell, 1982, 76–85; Trainor, Brian T. "The State, Marriage, and Divorce." *Journal of Applied Philosophy* 9:2 (1992), 135–48; Van Wagoner, Richard S. *Mormon Polygamy: A History*, 2nd ed. Salt Lake City, Utah: Signature Books, 1989; Vlastos, Gregory. "The Individual as an Object of Love in Plato." In *Platonic Studies*. Princeton, N.J.: Princeton University Press, 1973, 3–34. Reprinted in Alan Soble, ed., *Eros, Agape, and Philia: Readings in the Philosophy of Love*. New York: Paragon House, 1989, 96–124; Wellwood, John, ed. *Challenge of the Heart: Love, Sex, and Intimacy in Changing Times*. Boston, Mass.: Shambhala, 1985; Wilson, Holly. "Kant's Evolutionary Theory of Marriage." In Jane Kneller, ed., *Autonomy and Community*. Albany: State University of New York Press, 1998, 283–306.

MARRIAGE, SAME-SEX. Marriage is a *social institution* whose nature, value, symbolic meaning, and normative requirements are elaborated within particular religious communities and cultural traditions. Marriage is also a *legal status*; civil marriage consists of a set of special rights, benefits, and obligations, such as the right to give proxy **consent**, to inherit when a spouse dies without a will, to refuse to testify against one's spouse, and to receive Social Security survivor's benefits. The prospect of same-sex marriage raises questions about the cultural meaning of marriage, the significance of sexuality, gender roles, family, and marriage within different religious traditions, and the state's interest in promoting some relationships through marriage **law**. Fundamentalist and liberal Protestant sects, Catholicism, and Reformed and Orthodox **Judaism** have reached different conclusions about whether to celebrate or condemn same-sex unions within their faiths. The main focus of public debate, however, is *civil* marriage. Who is entitled to the special rights and benefits of legal marriage? Civil marriage for same-sex couples is already a reality in some parts of the world, including (in Europe) the Netherlands, Belgium, and Spain, and (in North America) Canada and, as of 2004, in the state of Massachusetts in the United States.

Traditionalism, Expansionism. The debate over same-sex civil marriage might best be characterized as a debate between traditionalists and expansionists. Traditionalists argue that the meaning of marriage should not be expanded to include same-sex couples. Expansionists argue that it should. Those forwarding traditionalist arguments face the difficult task of showing how legal bars to same-sex marriage are consistent with basic values of liberty, equality, and the disestablishment of religion. Those forwarding expansionist arguments face the task of addressing the central implication of their arguments, namely, that civil marriage should be extended to *any* private committed relationship between two or more adults, including adult incestuous and polygamous marriages.

One central bone of contention between traditionalists and expansionists is over what the essential nature of marriage is and thus which relationships can meaningfully be called marriages (Coolidge; Mohr; Wedgwood). Traditionalists cite the widespread and historically enduring cultural assumption that "marriage" refers only to relationships between a man and a woman. Expansionists typically reject the claim that "marriage" has one fixed definition, citing both cross-cultural variation in marriage forms and historical change in the institution of marriage within particular cultures (Cott, 9–23, 200–227; Eskridge, *The Case*, 15–50).

An equally central bone of contention is over which features of intimate relationships the state has an interest in promoting. Both traditionalists, as well as many expansionists, agree that the state has an interest in promoting stable long-term relationships that meet the individual's needs for companionship and emotional support. The state also has an interest in promoting the economic support of individuals within private relationships rather than their dependence on state resources. And the state has an interest in promoting those intimate relationships that provide stable environments for rearing children. Traditionalists, however, argue that only in relationships where both sexes are present can the state's interests be met. Only heterosexual couples form a reproductive unit, and thus the state's interest in promoting families is reasonably focused on heterosexual couples. Moreover, some also claim that social science research indicates that children fare less well in the absence of both a father and a mother. Drawing on views that originated in psychoanalytic theory of the 1950s and 1960s and stereotypes of gay male culture, some traditionalists also argue that both homosexual persons and same-sex relationships are deficient in important ways: Homosexual persons are promiscuous and incapable of true marital unity. As a result, same-sex relationships lack sexual fidelity and are unstable, thus failing to provide children with an adequate home environment.

Though some expansionists agree that the state's primary interest is in promoting long-term, committed, sexually monogamous relationships, no expansionist regards the requirement of different-sexed partners as relevant to the state's interests. Expansionists typically argue that the primary function of marriage is unitive, not reproductive. As evidence, they observe that marriage licenses are issued to sterile and elderly individuals as well as to those who plan to adopt or remain childless. Expansionists point to social science research indicating that children fare just as well with gay or lesbian parents as with heterosexual ones. Given the importance of child welfare, the state has an interest in promoting stable family environments without regard to the biological relatedness of parents to children.

"Traditionalism" and "expansionism" do not, however, name unified political views. Expansionist positions emerge from political liberalism's emphases on state neutrality and on equality. Traditionalist positions have their roots in both communitarianism and Natural Law theory. There is also a third party to these debates, marriage abolitionists, who for various reasons think that the state should get out of the marriage licensing business altogether. All told, the central arguments emerge from neutral **liberalism**, liberal egalitarianism, communitarianism, and **New Natural Law**.

Liberalism. Neutral liberalism is especially hospitable to individual and group pluralism, including pluralism about the meaning and value of marriage, because it assumes that the state should remain neutral with respect to conceptions of the good and should not favor any one particular ethical, religious, metaphysical, or epistemological doctrine. For neutral liberalism, the determination of the right—that is, the rules defining just social arrangements—is prior to the good, rather than dependent on any particular conception of the good. This basic principle of state neutrality entails that, in determining who may marry, the obligations of marriage, and conditions for divorce, the state should not appeal to particular ethical or religious views. It should appeal only to such neutral considerations as the constitutional values of liberty and equality and the conditions for the orderly pursuit of happiness and the reproduction of society over time. Current bars to same-sex marriage are largely premised on moral arguments that appeal to a particular ethical conception of intimate relationships (as monogamous, long-term, and reproductive) and a particular view about what kinds of **sexual activity** are valuable or valueless. Though perhaps broadly shared, such moral views do not provide an appropriate basis, so far as neutral liberalism is concerned, for setting public policy. Once moral and religious arguments are set aside in favor of politically neutral considerations, the case for restricting marriage exclusively to heterosexuals would seem to be substantially undercut. A strong commitment to accommodating pluralism seems to entail extending the right to marry to same-sex couples (Ball, 15–40). Whether it also entails extending that right to polygamous intimacies depends on whether women's equality can be sustained within polygamous relationships.

Some appeal to neutral liberalism to reach the quite different conclusion that the state should not recognize marriages at all. Given that the state must remain neutral with respect to the value of different kinds of relationships, it should not single out any relationship for special support (Vanderheiden). This is not to say that the state cannot have interests in promoting relationships that involve economic and other caretaking support, including the care and education of children. However, there are many relationships, some of which are also stable and long term, that have these characteristics. These include relationships between friends, adult siblings, cohabiting sexual intimates, extended family relationships, and poor individuals who pool economic resources. Since individuals may choose a plurality of relationships to satisfy their needs for **love** and affection, economic support, caretaking, and the production and education of children, it would be a violation of state neutrality to single out one of the multiplicity of relationships for special state protection. Some conclude, then, that civil marriage—the licensing of a particular form of relationship—should be abolished rather than expanded to include same-sex marriages. In its place there might instead be full freedom to contract whatever personal arrangements one pleases (Kymlicka).

While neutral liberalism grounds marriage arguments on the value of *liberty* to pursue one's own conception of the good, other liberal arguments appeal to an equally defining feature of liberalism: its commitment to the *equality* of individuals. Indeed, equality figures prominently in legal arguments for same-sex marriages. Vermont, for example, created a legal alternative to marriage for same-sex couples—civil unions—because Vermont's Common Benefits Clause declares that "government is, or ought to be, instituted for the common benefit, protection, and security of the people, nation, or community, and not for the particular emolument or advantage of any single person, family, or set of persons, who are a part only of that community." Three Canadian provinces extended marriage rights to same-sex couples on the basis of Canada's Charter of Rights and Freedoms, which declares, "Every individual . . . has the right to the equal protection and equal benefit of the law without discrimination."

Equality arguments may appeal either to gay and lesbian equality or to the equality of the sexes. Same-sex marriage bars deny to gays and lesbians the fundamental right to marry that heterosexual citizens enjoy, including heterosexual rapists, child molesters, and deadbeat dads (Eskridge, *The Case*, 123–52). The right to marry is, arguably, a central right of citizenship (Calhoun, 123–31; Gerstmann, 67–111; Kaplan). Since fitness to enter intimate relationships or to care for children is not a condition of heterosexuals' right to marry, same-sex marriage bars appear motivated primarily by animus toward gays and lesbians. In *Loving v. Virginia*, the Supreme Court invalidated laws barring interracial marriage because they were designed to preserve a racial caste system motivated by prejudice. Later, the U.S. Supreme Court ruled in *Romer v. Evans* that laws motivated by animus against gays and lesbians are unconstitutional, because "a bare . . . desire to harm a politically unpopular group cannot constitute a legitimate government interest."

The equality argument more commonly raised in court suits appeals to sex equality, not **sexual orientation** equality. It might appear that same-sex marriage bars treat the sexes alike because men and women are equally barred from marrying a same-sex partner. But the marriage bar prevents one sex from doing what the other can do, namely, marry a particular person. George can marry Sally, but Linda cannot marry Sally, and the only relevant difference between George and Linda is their sex (Koppelman; Strasser, 133–50). If sex is an impermissible basis for differential treatment of either men or women, then same-sex marriage bars are impermissible. The Hawaii Supreme Court took this route in *Baehr v. Lewin*, arguing that failure to issue marriage licenses to same-sex couples violated Hawaii's Equal Rights Amendment.

Same-sex marriage bars also are integrally connected with women's oppression (Eskridge *The Case*, 153–72; Hunter; Koppelman; Sunstein). Both sexism against women and **heterosexism** against gays and lesbians rest on the assumptions that masculinity is natural for males, femininity for females, that these gender roles are hierarchically ranked, and that it is reasonable to expect individual compliance with a person's "natural" gender role. Specifically, marital gender roles have played a significant role in women's oppression, as has the idea that women are naturally suited for some but not other social roles. The idea that there are separate husband and wife gender roles in marriage and that only a male-female couple is naturally equipped to enact them also underlies many arguments against same-sex marriage, especially those that insist that children need both a mother and a father. Because the same-sex marriage bar operates from the same assumptions that sustain women's oppression, some conclude that gay and lesbian marriage rights would promote women's equality.

An important strand of feminist thought, however, opposes same-sex marriage rights precisely because ending women's oppression matters (Card; Ettelbrick; Polikoff; Robson). In the 1980s, radical and lesbian feminists argued that the institution of marriage has always operated as a central support of patriarchy. The sexual division of labor within marriage makes women primarily responsible for unpaid labor in the home, often resulting in women's reduced investment in developing their own career assets and their increased economic dependence on men. Law and social practices have assumed a male-headship model of the family, instantiated most clearly in eighteenth- and nineteenth-century *coverture* laws that made husband and wife legally one person, endowing only the husband with civil and political rights. Within marriage women have had little protection against husbands' violence. Although marriage law has changed over time, women continue to be disadvantaged by marriage; this is perhaps most obvious in the dramatically different economic prospects of men and women after divorce. A realistic appraisal of the history of marriage suggests that marriage is an irredeemably sexist institution. Thus some conclude that eliminating women's oppression depends on abolishing civil marriage.

Although both liberal neutralism and liberal egalitarianism reject any appeal to moral considerations, and draw only on constitutional values such as liberty, equality, and **privacy**, the idea that political arguments must not appeal to individuals' moral values is not a view shared by all. Some liberals argue that taking up normative questions about the value of different forms of relationship is essential (Ball; Freeman). Communitarianism and New Natural Law theory both endorse the appropriateness of at least some appeals to morality in setting state policy. A political conception that is not rigidly neutral with respect to conceptions of the good also seems more compatible with actual political practice within liberal democracies. Some appeal to moral considerations would seem essential to explain why *marital* relationships are uniquely valuable, and thus the state's regulation of these relationships, including deciding who may enter them, is an especially vital issue.

Communitarianism. In the communitarian view, law and public policy should be framed with an eye to enabling individuals to sustain those relational bonds that make possible the individual's sense of self and moral value. Stable, long-term, committed marital relationships provide a particularly important source of individual self-definition, especially in highly mobile societies like the United States, where other relationships may be regularly disrupted by repeated job change and relocation (Eskridge, "Beyond"). Committed relationships also provide a particularly important context for individuals to acquire a sense of themselves as agents bound by moral requirements of fidelity, sexual self-restraint, and self-sacrifice (Macedo). Thus the state has a legitimate interest in protecting marital relationships.

In reasoning about whether marriage rights should be extended to same-sex couples, communitarian thinkers are deeply skeptical of liberal attempts to divorce the justification of public policy from moral or religious conceptions. On the communitarian view, citizens will find laws and public policies reasonable only if they are premised on values central to citizens' ways of life (Ball, 139–45). In liberal democracies, the values of privacy, liberty, and equality help define our national way of life and thus constitute an appropriate basis for law and public policy. But there will be other core values as well that contribute to our sense of sharing a single national community and having special duties of allegiance to fellow members of this national community. It is thus always relevant for the law to take into account "our" particular moral traditions and to be extremely cautious of legal innovations that might undermine the core values in terms of which individuals understand themselves as sharing the same community.

The values of equality and liberty will be relevant to communitarian thinking about same-sex marriage since these values are constitutive of our moral tradition. But it will also be relevant to take into account the 2,000-year-old understanding of marriage as the union of one man and one woman, a tradition that includes Greco-Roman, Judeo-Christian, western European, and American cultural histories (Witte). Given the extraordinary importance attached to heterosexual marriage within the cultural self-understandings of Western civilization and the absence of any comparable tradition of recognizing same-sex unions, some conclude that the state ought not to expand the current legal definition of marriage.

While agreeing on the importance of legally protecting stable, long-term, committed relationships that are a source of self-definition and a site for the development of important virtues, some argue that our marriage tradition does *not* in fact support restricting marriage to heterosexuals only (Boswell; Cott; Eskridge, *The Case*, 98–104). To begin, it is unclear that the Greco-Roman tradition is part of "our" tradition, particularly where framing current law is concerned. Even if taken as our tradition, the 2,000-year-old Judeo-Christian tradition includes more than heterosexual, monogamous marriage. **John Boswell** (1947–1994) documented union ceremonies for monks performed by the Roman Catholic Church in the Middle Ages; in the 1800s so-called Boston marriages between two women emerged as a recognized cultural phenomenon in the United States; and a variety of religious communities currently celebrate same-sex unions.

In addition, polygamy has a long history in the Judeo-Christian tradition. In the Old Testament, marital relationships included polygamy. Polygamy was not prohibited for European Jews until the eleventh century and then only to avoid Christian persecution. (Some non-European Jews continue to practice polygamy.) Martin Luther (1483–1546) observed in the 1500s that polygamy does not contradict Scripture and so cannot be prohibited, and at least one Christian sect, Mormonism, made polygamy a central practice until politically forced to abandon it in the 1800s. Under American slavery, African American marriages were often disrupted by the sale and forced separation of partners and, as a result, serial polygamy, where slaves remarried without divorcing the prior spouse, was common form. Finally, the United States and Canada are multinational states whose traditions include those of Amerindian nations—for whom monogamy was not the defining form of marriage and which sometimes recognized unions between same-sexed persons.

In short, tradition can justify a same-sex marriage bar if the appeal to tradition is selective and ignores both polygamous and same-sex marital practices. Further, tradition can justify a same-sex marriage bar if it ignores prominent features of traditional monogamous heterosexual marriage that are unacceptable to many people, including husbands' right to physically chastise their wives and force them to engage in intercourse.

One way of avoiding the appearance of selective attention to only some but not other features of "our" tradition is to take a shorter view of the tradition, focusing on the marriage tradition as it has emerged within, say, the last 100 years. But short-range views of the tradition do not clearly support a same-sex marriage bar. Expansionist communitarians have argued, for example, that the most recent marriage tradition within the United States is a tradition of companionate marriage, the principal function of which is to embody and express the emotional union of two persons rather than biological reproduction. It is also relevant to the communitarian argument from moral traditions that ours is a liberal tradition that values consent, privacy, self-fulfillment, equality, and (increasingly) tolerance of religious and cultural diversity. Taken together, one might argue that extending same-sex marriage rights is not only intelligible within our own culture but more consistent with our marriage tradition than continuing the bar. This would explain why some countries that share the Western tradition have already moved in this direction.

New Natural Law. One strength of the New Natural Law theory emerging from Catholic legal and political scholars is that it does not appeal uncritically to tradition but provides a substantive argument that attempts to show why marriage must be heterosexual and monogamous. New Natural Law scholars also try to show why sexual intimacy, commitment, reproduction, and child rearing are essential components of anything that qualifies as a marital relationship.

Natural Law theorists assert that the purpose of marriage is to unite two persons into one, spiritually, emotionally, *and* biologically. Because only reproductive sex biologically unites the male and female, heterosexual vaginal-penile sex is the only kind of sex that can unite two spouses into one flesh (Finnis; George; George and Bradley; Lee and George). "The distinctive unity of spouses is possible because human (like other mammalian) males and females, by mating, unite organically—they become a single reproductive principle. Although reproduction is a single act, in humans (and other mammals) the reproductive act is performed not by individual members of the species, but by a mated pair as an organic unit" (George, 121). Children produced through marital coupling (rather than, say, being adopted or created through donor insemination) actualize the couple's union. Long-term commitment to being unified as a mated pair, engagement in "marital acts" that unite them biologically, and the rearing of children who unite their biological material are thus all part of what it means to be united in marriage. Neither a same-sex couple nor a polygamous grouping can achieve this state of being two-in-one-flesh or produce children who express that union. On the New Natural Law view, then, same-sex unions and polygamous groupings could not possibly be marriages. Because marriage has an inherent nature and is not a creation of the law, no legal system has the authority to expand the definition of marriage.

The New Natural Law view faces the obvious difficulty that marriage licenses are currently issued to infertile couples, elderly couples, couples who choose not to have children and, in principle, couples who are disinterested in vaginal-penile sex (Macedo). New Natural Law theorists do not recommend expanding the marriage *bar* to exclude these couples from marriage licenses. In response to this objection, one might argue that legal verification of infertility, "deviant" sexual practice, and contraceptive use would be unreasonably invasive. The more standard Natural Law response is to argue that male-female couples who are unable to have children nevertheless can engage in sex that is procreative in *type* (vaginal-penile sex) and that this is sufficient to constitute them as a single reproductive unit. Same-sex couple's nonreproductive sex is of a different type; it involves sex acts that, for anyone, homosexual or heterosexual, are essentially nonreproductive.

While the Natural Law view has the merit of explaining why the definition of marriage cannot be expanded, Natural Law arguments are unlikely to make successful *legal* arguments. They are clearly sectarian, rooted in an explicitly Roman Catholic philosophical tradition. Even without agreeing with neutral liberalism that the law must not appeal to values other than constitutional ones, any argument that is compatible with a liberal democracy will refuse to found legal rights on a viewpoint that is so firmly tied to a single religious tradition. In addition, if we affirm the same-sex marriage bar on Natural Law grounds, consistency would require recriminalizing sodomy, **contraception**, and **abortion** and reinstituting both restrictive divorce laws and legal penalties for **adultery** and fornication.

We are likely to witness a wide variety of legal innovations: from same-sex marriage to civil unions that provide the rights and benefits of state (but not federal) marriage law to more limited legal packages offering same-sex couples some subset of the rights and benefits attached to marriage.

See also Adultery; Anscombe, G.E.M.; Casual Sex; Diseases, Sexually Transmitted; Feminism, Lesbian; Feminism, Liberal; Judaism, Twentieth- and Twenty-First-Century; Law, Sex and the; Liberalism; Love; Marriage; Natural Law (New); Privacy; Queer Theory; Wittgenstein, Ludwig

REFERENCES

Baehr v. Lewin. 74 Haw. 645, 852 P.2d 44 (1993); Ball, Carlos A. *The Morality of Gay Rights: An Exploration in Political Philosophy.* New York: Routledge, 2003; Boswell, John. *Same-Sex Unions in Premodern Europe.* New York: Villard Books, 1994; Calhoun, Cheshire. *Feminism, the Family, and the Politics of the Closet: Lesbian and Gay Displacement.* New York: Oxford University Press, 2000; Card, Claudia. "Against Marriage and Motherhood." *Hypatia* 11:3 (1996), 1–23; Coolidge, David Orgon. "The Question of Marriage." In Christopher Wolfe, ed., *Homosexuality and American Public Life.* Dallas, Tex.: Spence, 1999, 200–238; Cott, Nancy. *Public Vows: A History of Marriage and the Nation.* Cambridge, Mass.: Harvard University Press, 2000; Eskridge, William N., Jr. "Beyond Lesbian and Gay 'Families We Choose.'" In David M. Estlund and Martha C. Nussbaum, eds., *Sex, Preference, and Family: Essays on Law and Nature.* New York: Oxford University Press, 1996, 277–89; Eskridge, William N., Jr. *The Case for Same-Sex Marriage: From Sexual Liberty to Civilized*

Commitment. New York: Free Press, 1996; Ettelbrick, Paula L. "Since When Is Marriage a Path to Liberation?" In William B. Rubenstein, ed., *Lesbians, Gay Men, and the Law.* New York: New Press, 1993, 401–5; Finnis, John M. "The Good of Marriage and the Morality of Sexual Relations: Some Philosophical and Historical Observations." *American Journal of Jurisprudence* 42 (1997), 97–134; Freeman, M.D.A. "Not Such a Queer Idea: Is There a Case for Same Sex Marriages?" *Journal of Applied Philosophy* 16:1 (1999), 1–17; George, Robert P. "Neutrality, Equality, and 'Same-Sex Marriage.' " In Lynn D. Wardle, Mark Strasser, William C. Duncan, and David Orgon Coolidge, eds., *Marriage and Same-Sex Unions: A Debate.* Westport, Conn.: Praeger, 2003, 119–32; George, Robert P., and Gerard V. Bradley. "Marriage and the Liberal Imagination." *Georgetown Law Journal* 84 (1995): 301–20; Gerstmann, Evan. *Same-Sex Marriage and the Constitution.* Cambridge: Cambridge University Press, 2004; Hunter, Nan D. "Marriage, Law, and Gender: A Feminist Inquiry." In Lisa Duggan and Nan D. Hunter, *Sex Wars: Sexual Dissent and Political Culture.* New York: Routledge, 1995, 114–19; Kaplan, Morris B. "Intimacy and Equality: The Question of Lesbian and Gay Marriage." *Philosophical Forum* 25:4 (1994), 333–40; Koppelman, Andrew. "Why Discrimination against Lesbians and Gay Men Is Sex Discrimination." *New York University Law Review* 69:2 (1994), 197–287; Kymlicka, Will. "Rethinking the Family." *Philosophy and Public Affairs* 20:1 (1991), 77–97; Lee, Patrick, and Robert P. George. "What Sex Can Be: Self-Alienation, Illusion, or One-Flesh Union." *American Journal of Jurisprudence* 42 (1997), 135–57; *Loving v. Virginia.* 13 L.Ed 2d 1010; 388 U.S. 1; 87 S.Ct. 1817 (1967); Macedo, Stephen. "Homosexuality and the Conservative Mind." *Georgetown Law Journal* 84:2 (1995), 261–300; Mohr, Richard D. "The Case for Gay Marriage." *Notre Dame Journal of Law, Ethics, and Public Policy* 9:1 (1995), 215–39; Polikoff, Nancy D. "We Will Get What We Ask For: Why Legalizing Gay and Lesbian Marriage Will Not 'Dismantle the Legal Structure of Gender in Every Marriage.' " *Virginia Law Review* 79 (October 1993), 1535–50; Robson, Ruthann. "Resisting the Family: Repositioning Lesbians in Legal Theory." *Signs* 19 (Summer 1994), 975–96; *Romer v. Evans.* 517 U.S. 620 (1996); Strasser, Mark. *On Same-Sex Marriage, Civil Unions, and the Rule of Law: Constitutional Interpretation at the Crossroads.* Westport, Conn.: Praeger, 2002; Sunstein, Cass R. "Homosexuality and the Constitution." *Indiana Law Journal* 70 (Winter 1994), 5–28; Vanderheiden, Steve. "Why the State Should Stay Out of the Wedding Chapel." *Public Affairs Quarterly* 13:2 (1999), 175–90; Wedgwood, Ralph. "The Fundamental Argument for Same-Sex Marriage." *Journal of Political Philosophy* 7:3 (1999), 225–42; Witte, John Jr. "The Tradition of Traditional Marriage." In Lynn D. Wardle, Mark Strasser, William C. Duncan, and David Orgon Coolidge, eds., *Marriage and Same-Sex Unions: A Debate.* Westport, Conn.: Praeger, 2003, 47–49.

Cheshire Calhoun

ADDITIONAL READING

Alpert, Rebecca T. "Religious Liberty, Same-Sex Marriage, and the Case of Reconstructionist Judaism." In Kathleen M. Sands, ed., *God Forbid: Religion and Sex in American Public Life.* New York: Oxford University Press, 2000, 124–34; Appiah, K. Anthony. "The Marrying Kind." *New York Review of Books* (20 June 1996), 48–54; Benatar, David. "Same-Sex Marriage and Sex Discrimination." *American Philosophical Association Newsletters. Newsletter on Philosophy and Law* 97:1 (1997). <www.apa.udel.edu/apa/archive/newsletters/v97n1/law/samesex.asp> [accessed 17 June 2005]; Bolte, Angela. "Do Wedding Dresses Come in Lavender? The Prospects and Implications of Same-Sex Marriage." *Social Theory and Practice* 24:1 (1998), 111–31; Boonin, David. "Same-Sex Marriage and the Argument from Public Disagreement." *Journal of Social Philosophy* 30:3 (1999), 251–59; Bradley, Craig M. "The Right Not to Endorse Gay Rights: A Reply to Sunstein." *Indiana Law Journal* 70 (Winter 1994), 29–38; Bradley, Gerard V. "Same-Sex Marriage: Our Final Answer?" *Notre Dame Journal of Law, Ethics, and Public Policy* 14:2 (2000), 729–52; Butler, Judith. "Is Kinship Always Already Heterosexual?" *differences: A Journal of Feminist Cultural Studies* 15:1 (2002), 14–44; Calhoun, Cheshire. "Separating Lesbian Theory from Feminist Theory." *Ethics* 104:3 (1994),

558–81; Callahan, Sidney. "Why I Changed My Mind: Thinking about Gay Marriage." *Commonweal* (22 April 1994), 6–8; Canadian Conference of Bishops. "Pastoral Letter Regarding Same-Sex Marriage." *Origins* 32:27 (2002), 445–46; "Case Conference. Lesbian Couples: Should Help Extend to AID?" *Journal of Medical Ethics* 4:2 (1978), 91–95; Chambers, David L. "What If? The Legal Consequences of Marriage and the Legal Needs of Lesbian and Gay Male Couples." *Michigan Law Review* 95 (November 1996), 447–91; Cicovacki, Predrag. "Can Love Resolve the Problem of Marriage?" In Thomas Magnell, ed., *Explorations of Value*. Amsterdam, Holland: Rodopi, 1997, 221–33; Cicovacki, Predrag. "On Love and Fidelity in Marriage." *Journal of Social Philosophy* 24:3 (1993), 92–104; Collett, Teresa Stanton. "Should Marriage Be Privileged? The State's Interest in Childbearing Unions." In Lynn D. Wardle, Mark Strasser, William C. Duncan, and David Orgon Coolidge, eds., *Marriage and Same-Sex Unions: A Debate*. Westport, Conn.: Praeger, 2003, 152–61; Congregation for the Doctrine of the Faith. "Considerations Regarding Proposals to Give Legal Recognition to Unions between Homosexual Persons." *Origins* 33:14 (2003), 445–46; Cruz, David B. "Civil Marriage and the First Amendment." In Lynn D. Wardle, Mark Strasser, William C. Duncan, and David Orgon Coolidge, eds., *Marriage and Same-Sex Unions: A Debate*. Westport, Conn.: Praeger, 2003, 245–60; Dean, Craig R. "Fighting for Same Sex Marriage." In Anne Minas, ed., *Gender Basics: Feminist Perspectives on Women and Men*, 1st ed. Belmont, Calif.: Wadsworth, 1993, 275–77; Dean, Craig R. "Gay Marriage: A Civil Right." In Timothy F. Murphy, ed., *Gay Ethics: Controversies in Outing, Civil Rights, and Sexual Science*. Binghamton, N.Y.: Haworth, 1994, 111–15; Ellison, Marvin. *Same-Sex Marriage? A Christian Ethical Analysis*. Cleveland, Ohio: Pilgrim, 2004; Elliston, Frederick A. "Gay Marriage." In Robert B. Baker and Frederick A. Elliston, eds., *Philosophy and Sex*, 2nd ed. Buffalo, N.Y.: Prometheus, 1984, 146–66; Ertman, Martha M. "Marriage as a Trade: Bridging the Private/Private Distinction." *Harvard Civil Rights–Civil Liberties Law Review* 36:1 (2001), 79–132; Eskridge, William N., Jr. *Equality Practice: Civil Unions and the Future of Gay Rights*. New York: Routledge, 2002; Estlund, David M., and Martha C. Nussbaum, eds. *Sex, Preference, and Family: Essays on Law and Nature*. New York: Oxford University Press, 1996; Ettelbrick, Paula L. (1993) "Since When Is Marriage the Path to Liberation?" In Larry Gross and James D. Woods, eds., *The Columbia Reader on Lesbians and Gay Men in Media, Society, and Politics*. New York: Columbia University Press, 1999, 637–40; Finnis, John M. "Law, Morality, and 'Sexual Orientation.' " *Notre Dame Law Review* 69:5 (1994), 1049–76; Galeotti, Anna Elisabetta. "Same-Sex Marriage." In *Toleration as Recognition*. Cambridge: Cambridge University Press, 2002, 169–91; Haslett, Adam. "Love Supreme: Gay Nuptials and the Making of Modern Marriage." *The New Yorker* (31 May 2004), 76–80; Herman, Barbara. "Could It Be Worth Thinking about Kant on Sex and Marriage?" In Louise Antony and Charlotte Witt, eds., *A Mind of One's Own: Feminist Essays on Reason and Objectivity*. Boulder, Colo.: Westview, 1993, 49–67; Higgins, Kathleen Marie. "How Do I Love Thee? Let's Redefine a Term (A Response to Predrag Cicovacki)." *Journal of Social Philosophy* 24:3 (1993), 105–11; Jakobsen, Janet R. "Why Sexual Regulation? Family Values and Social Movements." In Kathleen M. Sands, ed., *God Forbid: Religion and Sex in American Public Life*. New York: Oxford University Press, 2000, 104–23; Jung, Patricia Beattie. Review of *Legally Wed: Same-Sex Marriage and the Constitution*, by Mark Strasser. *Theological Studies* 59:1 (1998), 187–88; Knight, Robert H. "How Domestic Partnerships and 'Gay Marriage' Threaten the Family." In John Corvino, ed., *Same Sex: Debating the Ethics, Science, and Culture of Homosexuality*. Lanham, Md.: Rowman and Littlefield, 1997, 289–303; Koppelman, Andrew. "Dumb and DOMA: Why the Defense of Marriage Act Is Unconstitutional." In *The Gay Rights Question in Contemporary American Law*. Chicago, Ill.: University of Chicago Press, 2002, 127–40; Koppelman, Andrew. "Is Marriage Inherently Heterosexual?" *American Journal of Jurisprudence* 42 (1997), 51–95; Kramer, Larry. "Same-Sex Marriage, Conflict of Laws, and the Unconstitutional Public Policy Exception." *Yale Law Journal* 106 (1997), 1965–2008; Kurtz, Stanley. "Beyond Gay Marriage: The Road to Polygamy." *The Weekly Standard* (4–11 August 2003), 26–33; Lodge, David. "Sick with Desire." *New York Review of Books* (5 July 2001), 28–32; Masters, R.E.L. "The Homosexual Revolution." In Henry Anatole Grunwald, ed., *Sex in America*. New York: Bantam, 1964, 256–82; Matter, E. Ann. "My Sister, My Spouse: Woman-Identified Women in Medieval Christianity." *Journal of Feminist Studies in*

Religion 2:2 (1986), 81–93; Mayo, David J., and Martin Gunderson. "Marriage: Same-Sex." In Timothy F. Murphy, ed., *Reader's Guide to Lesbian and Gay Studies*. Chicago, Ill.: Fitzroy Dearborn, 2000, 375–76; McCarthy, David Matzko. "The Relationship of Bodies: A Nuptial Hermeneutics of Same-Sex Unions." In Eugene F. Rogers, Jr., ed., *Theology and Sexuality: Classic and Contemporary Readings*. Oxford, U.K.: Blackwell, 2002, 200–216; Mohr, Richard D. "The Case for Gay Marriage." *Notre Dame Journal of Law, Ethics, and Public Policy* 9:1 (1995), 215–39. Reprinted in HS (231–55); P&S3 (190–211); Mohr, Richard D. *The Long Arc of Justice: Lesbian and Gay Marriage, Equality, and Rights*. New York: Columbia University Press, 2005; Mohr, Richard D. "Understanding Gay Marriage." In *A More Perfect Union: Why Straight America Must Stand Up for Gay Rights*. Boston, Mass.: Beacon Press, 1994, 31–53; Nussbaum, Martha C. "Lesbian and Gay Rights: Pro." In Michael Leahy and Dan Cohn-Sherbok, eds., *The Liberation Debate: Rights at Issue*. London: Routledge, 1996, 80–107; O'Donovan, Oliver. "Transsexualism and Christian Marriage." *Journal of Religious Ethics* 11:1 (1983), 135–62; Pakaluk, Michael. "Homosexuality and the Common Good." In Christopher Wolfe, ed., *Homosexuality and American Public Life*. Dallas, Tex.: Spence, 1999, 179–91; Palmer, David. "The Consolation of the Wedded." In Robert B. Baker and Frederick A. Elliston, eds., *Philosophy and Sex*, 1st ed. Buffalo, N.Y.: Prometheus, 1975, 178–89. Reprinted in P&S2 (119–29); Pascoe, Peggy. "Sex, Gender, and Same-Sex Marriage." In The Social Justice Group at The Center for Advanced Feminist Studies, University of Minnesota, ed., *Is Academic Feminism Dead? Theory in Practice*. New York: New York University Press, 2000, 86–136; Pierce, Christine. "Gay Marriage." *Journal of Social Philosophy* 26:2 (1995), 5–16; Polikoff, Nancy D. "This Child Does Have Two Mothers: Redefining Parenthood to Meet the Needs of Children in Lesbian-Mother and Other Nontraditional Families." *Georgetown Law Journal* 78 (February 1990), 459–575; Pontifical Council for the Family. "Family, Marriage, and 'De Facto' Unions." *Origins* 30:30 (2001), 473–88; Posner, Richard A. "Should There Be Homosexual Marriage? And If So, Who Should Decide?" *Michigan Law Review* 95:6 (1997), 1578–87; Ratzinger, Joseph (Cardinal). "Considerations Regarding Proposals to Give Legal Recognition to Unions between Homosexual Persons." *Origins* 33:11 (2003), 177, 179–82; Richards, David A. J. *Women, Gays, and the Constitution: The Grounds for Feminism and Gay Rights in Culture and Law*. Chicago, Ill.: University of Chicago Press, 1998; Robson, Ruthann. "Assimilation, Marriage, and Lesbian Liberation." *Temple Law Review* 75 (Winter 2002), 709–820; Rotello, Gabriel. "To Have and to Hold: The Case for Gay Marriage." *The Nation* (24 June 1996), 11–18; Schaff, Kory. "Kant, Political Liberalism, and the Ethics of Same-Sex Relations." *Journal of Social Philosophy* 32:3 (2001), 446–62; Shanley, Mary Lyndon. *Just Marriage*. Ed. Joshua Cohen and Deborah Chasman. New York: Oxford University Press, 2004; Shaw, Brent. "A Groom of One's Own? The Medieval Church and the Question of Gay Marriage." *The New Republic* (18–25 July 1994), 33–41; Singer, Irving. "Marriage: Same-Sex and Opposite-Sex." In *Sex: A Philosophical Primer*, expanded ed. Lanham, Md.: Rowman and Littlefield, 2004, ix–xxxii; Strasser, Mark. *Legally Wed: Same-Sex Marriage and the Constitution*. Ithaca, N.Y.: Cornell University Press, 1997; Sullivan, Andrew. *Love Undetectable: Reflections on Friendship, Sex, and Survival*. New York: Knopf, 1998; Sullivan, Andrew. *Virtually Normal: An Argument about Homosexuality*. New York: Knopf, 1995; Sullivan Andrew, ed. *Same-Sex Marriage, Pro and Con: A Reader*. New York: Vintage, 1997; Thomas, Laurence M., and Michael E. Levin. *Sexual Orientation and Human Rights*. Lanham, Md.: Rowman and Littlefield, 1999; Wardle, Lynn D. " 'Multiply and Replenish': Considering Same-Sex Marriage in Light of State Interests in Marital Procreation." *Harvard Journal of Law and Public Policy* 24 (June 2001), 771–814; Wardle, Lynn D., Mark Strasser, William C. Duncan, and David Orgon Coolidge, eds. *Marriage and Same-Sex Unions: A Debate*. Westport, Conn.: Praeger, 2003; Warner, Michael. *The Trouble with Normal: Sex, Politics, and the Ethics of Queer Life*. Cambridge, Mass.: Harvard University Press, 1999; Wedgwood, Ralph. "Same-Sex Marriage: A Philosophical Defense." In Robert B. Baker, Kathleen J. Wininger, and Frederick A. Elliston, eds., *Philosophy and Sex*, 3rd ed. Amherst, N.Y.: Prometheus, 1998, 212–30; Weston, Kath. *Families We Choose: Lesbians, Gays, Kinship*. New York: Columbia University Press, 1991; Yamin, Priscilla. "The Indie Interview: Nancy Cott." August 2001. <www.indiebride.com/interviews/cott/> [accessed 7 June 2005].

MARX, KARL. *See* Marxism

MARXISM. It is as difficult to exaggerate the influence of Karl Marx (1818–1883) on economics, sociology, and philosophy as it may be to connect him, at least in any convincing way, to the study of sexuality. This connection, however, is not only plausible but also vital to a comprehensive understanding of Marx's analysis of the relationship between human nature, labor, capital, and history.

Born into a "Christianized" Jewish family in Trier, Prussia, Karl Heinrich Marx began his education in an intellectually, politically, and economically stagnant Germany that had only fifteen years earlier been occupied by the French under Napoleon (Berlin, 17–18). Regarded even in childhood as intellectually gifted by his father, a lawyer, Marx completed his doctoral thesis at the University of Berlin in 1841. This achievement is particularly notable considering a cultural and political climate dominated by a government whose censorship, anti-Semitism, and reputation for encouraging exile had inspired a growing and deeply critical "underground" of radicals devoted to change. In this challenging atmosphere, Marx found his way to **G.W.F. Hegel** (1770–1831), **Johann Gottlieb Fichte** (1762–1814), Ludwig Feuerbach (1804–1872), and the "Young Hegelians."

Profoundly influenced by Hegel's historical dialectics, Marx began to articulate his view of the role of economy in human history in 1842 on the biting pages of a newspaper he edited, the *Rheinische Zeitung* (McLellan, 22–31). In an extremely productive period between 1842 and 1850, during which he broke away from the Young Hegelians, Marx wrote *Critique of Hegel's "Philosophy of Right"* (1843; *Early Writings*, 243–57; McLellan, 32–41; Tucker, 16–25, 53–65), *On the Jewish Question* (1843; *Early Writings*, 211–41; McLellan, 46–70; Tucker, 26–52), the *Economic and Philosophical Manuscripts* (1844; *Early Writings*, 279–400; McLellan, 83–121; Tucker, 66–125), *The Holy Family*, or "The Critique of Critical Critique" (with Engels, 1844; McLellan, 146–70; Tucker, 133–35), "Theses on Feuerbach" (1845; *Early Writings*, 421–23; McLellan, 171–74; Tucker, 143–45; the 11th Thesis is Marx's famous line, "The philosophers have only *interpreted* the world, in various ways; the point, however, is to *change* it"); *The German Ideology* (with Engels, 1845–1846; McLellan, 175–208; Tucker, 146–200), *The Poverty of Philosophy* (1846; McLellan, 212–33; Tucker, 136–42, 218–19), *The Communist Manifesto* (with Engels, 1848; McLellan, 245–72; Tucker, 469–500), "The Class Struggles in France" (1850; McLellan, 313–25; Tucker, 586–93), and other essays, articles, and speeches.

This body of philosophical writing is referred to as the work of the "humanist" or "young" Marx to distinguish it from the later, more economically analytical work of the *Grundrisse* (1857–1858; McLellan, 379–423; Tucker, 221–93), *Theories of Surplus Value* (1862–1863; McLellan, 429–51; Tucker, 443–65), and the first volume of *Capital* (1867; McLellan, 452–525; Tucker, 294–438). The significance of this distinction is that the weight of any argument whose aim is to connect Marx's critique of capitalism to his view of human sexuality will rest primarily on the dialectical materialism and the theory of alienation established by the "young" Marx—despite problems, a source of scholarly debate, of consistency between the earlier and later writings in Marx's huge corpus. It is no wonder that so many contemporary political theorists have a love/hate relationship with Marx.

Nevertheless, one does not have to go far beyond for Marx's idea that communism would eliminate the "community of women" (in which bourgeois men seduce each other's wives) or that the abolition of private property would release women from "prostitution, both public and private," that is, from both streetwalking and loveless marriages contracted out of economic necessity (*Communist Manifesto*, 72; McLellan, 259–60; Tucker, 488), to see how important sexuality and the status of women were to the utopian vision for which Marx agitated his entire life. Indeed, one might suspect that Marx was being more than merely metaphorical or whimsical when he wrote, "Prostitution is only a *particular* expression of the *universal* prostitution of the *worker*, and since prostitution is a relationship which includes not only the prostituted but also the prostitutor—whose infamy is even greater—the capitalist is also included in this category" (*Economic and Philosophic Manuscripts [EPM]*, 133, n.; *Early Writings*, 350, n.4). This is not an isolated use of this conspicuous sexual analogy by the "young" Marx. Consider these remarks on money: "*Money*, inasmuch as it possesses the *property* of being able to buy everything . . . is the *object* most worth possessing. . . . I *am* ugly, but I can buy the *most beautiful woman*. Which means to say that I am not *ugly*, for the effect of *ugliness*, its repelling power, is destroyed by money." And in this transaction by which the bourgeois male acquires his trophy wife, "Money is the *pimp* between need and object" (*Early Writings*, 375–77; *EPM*, 165).

This vision of the importance of sexuality and the relations between women and men was not principally broached or sustained by Marx but was singularly impressed on him by his friend and colleague Friedrich Engels (1820–1895), whose *Origin of the Family, Private Property, and the State* (1884) established links between the commodification of labor and the commodification of women's sexuality (where "commodification" means, at least, making something a fungible resource that can be bought and sold in the market). It seems reasonable to suggest that what limited sensitivity Marx does exhibit to the oppressive working conditions of women and to the commodification of women's reproductive capacities is due in large measure to Engels, who took pains to establish a relationship between private property and women's reproductive capacities. Women's ability to (re)produce laborers is the paradigm of an exploitable resource, and whoever controls this resource controls an essential element of production. Women's reproductive capacity constituted private property, for Engels, and the womb was the archetype of that which can be expropriated, owned, controlled, consumed, and used. And it is here that the patriarchal family originates. While the capacity to reproduce may "belong" to women, its products belong to men. But men can be guaranteed the paternity that is necessary to legitimate the inheritance of property only through the institutionalization of exclusive sexual access to the women who bear their children. Thus **marriage** is organized as a profit-seeking enterprise, functioning to fulfill a family's imperative to survive and control the disposition of its present and future acquisitions. What establishes the ties of the family's laborers to each other is not merely self-interest or mutual interest, and not even blood, but the inheritance required for the preservation of private property.

To what extent Marx agreed with Engels's analysis of women and the family can perhaps be decided by examining their jointly written *Communist Manifesto* (*CM*). What is clear is that later writers—for example, Russian political theorist and activist Alexandra Kollontai (1872–1952), historian Gerda Lerner, and contemporary feminist philosopher Alison Jaggar—are among the beneficiaries of both Marx and Engels. Kollontai prioritized class affiliation *over* sex and was opposed to a feminist movement that (on her view) aimed at the political enfranchisement of only bourgeois women, and she remarked that "only the evolution of those economic forms that once caused the enslavement of women, can effect a radical change in their social position" ("The Social Basis of the Women's Question" [1908], 19). By contrast, for Lerner the "appropriation by men of women's sexual and reproductive capacity occurred *prior* to the formation of private property and class society. Its commodification lies, in fact, at the foundation of private property" (8; emphasis added). Which came first, the commodification of women's sexuality (Engels) or private property (Marx)? Jaggar points out that no matter how we answer this question, what is crucial is Engels's insight that women's sexuality plays a decisive role in these dynamics (63–69). Indeed, without Engels the relevance of Marx to feminist political philosophy and activism might have waited until more recent times and at tremendous political, economic, and social cost to women.

Marx died thirty-four years before the 1917 October Revolution against the Romanov dynasty gave rise to the Soviet Union and many years before the civil rights, feminist, gay/lesbian, and environmental movements of the United States and western Europe pressed for expanded meanings of economic and social equality and justice. Nevertheless, Marx's influence can be seen throughout the twentieth century, particularly in the work of agitators such as Emma Goldman (1869–1940), Rosa Luxemburg (1871–1919) and, in his own way, Wilhelm Reich (1897–1957); historians such as Isaiah Berlin (1909–1997), Jacques Barzun (1907–   ), Edmund Wilson (1895–1972), and Jeffrey Weeks; critical theorists, including Hungarian Georg Lukács (1885–1971) and the Frankfurt School of Theodor Adorno (1903–1969), Max Horkheimer (1895–1973), and Herbert Marcuse (1898–1979); feminists such as Nancy Hartsock, Juliet Mitchell, and Ann Ferguson; and environmentalists John Foster, Gwyn Kirk, and Carolyn Merchant. This woefully incomplete list still hints at the breadth of Marx's influence.

Comprehending the role of sexuality within Marx's philosophy requires demonstrating its significance for Marx's central themes: species being (human nature), labor, praxis, reproduction of the proletariat, alienation, revolution, and utopia. This is a tall order. But it is made possible by revealing how the sexually determined differences that Marx assumes to characterize species being inform not only his conception of the human being but also the conceptual, economic, and political dynamics that follow from it. Important elements of Marx's critique of capitalism depend on his view of sexuality precisely because his concept of species being is so important to his understanding of labor. In two key respects, one tethered to species reproduction and the other to the division of labor, sexuality turns out to circumscribe not only what counts as labor but also who counts as a candidate for labor, alienation, membership in the proletariat, and membership in the postrevolution utopia.

For Marx, the unique species being of humanity (as distinguished from nonhuman animals) depends on human labor. While the natures of both humans and nonhuman animals *qua* animals demand the fulfillment of material needs, only human beings "objectify" themselves through the alteration of their environment in the course of meeting their needs. Nonhuman animals act on the world, but humans re-create the world by making objects (including themselves) in and from the material conditions that confront them. The point of labor, writes Marx, is

> *the objectification of man's species life*: for he duplicates himself not only, as in consciousness, intellectually, but also actively, in reality, and therefore he contemplates himself in a world that he has created. (*EPM*, 114)

Through the creation of this world, human beings develop a distinctly human consciousness that "takes the place of instinct" (Marx and Engels, *German Ideology* [*GI*], 51).

Well beyond exercising the capacity to meet material needs, humans create themselves as subjects capable of intention, reflection, and contemplation. Far from just inhabiting a world, human subjects create the world they inhabit. The development of consciousness, for Marx, is dialectical as well as materialist; species being overcomes or transcends itself by making its material conditions into its own image (Lee, 4). When humans interact with material nature, they negate nature in the sense that it is altered through human labor. But nature is also re-created, in that humans remake the natural world into the human one. Being able to conceive of both "self" and "nature," humans remake the natural world into the human one. Of course, the natural world supplies the material conditions for the emergence and expression of consciousness in humanity, without which no intentionality could exist. This human consciousness that remakes itself is the emergent product of a particular kind of material interaction: the labor of *Homo sapiens sapiens.*

Thus an essential component of Marx's philosophy is the idea of creative labor, or *praxis*, that labor through which the immediacy of material need is transcended by the continuity of the objects created by labor (including humans themselves and their remade consciousness). Praxis is labor by which humans individuate themselves as particular expressions of consciousness, that is, as *individuals*, and is possible only when subsistence needs have already been satisfied. On the basis of praxis, the artifacts out of which humans create a cultural world transform the bare, crude passage of time into the *historicity* of human species being. This is what it means to have *a world*, that is, to live in a past, a present, and a future represented by the enduring objects of the creative labor that is praxis (Lee, 4–5). It is not so much that humans simply have a history, or watch a history, a passage of time, as it flies by; they make their own history.

Praxis, as a result of being creative labor that issues in consciousness, is labor that allows human beings to represent themselves to themselves and to each other not only as members of a species, and not merely as animals, but as deliberating agents, that is, as *free* (*EPM*, 178–82). However, this happens not because praxis pertains to the mind and subsistence labor pertains to the body; Marx was neither a dualist nor a Hegelian idealist. Instead, it happens because praxis advances the development of human personality conceived, ontologically, as at once something embodied, experiential, and rational. Central to Marx's thought is the idea that freedom is not freedom *from* material constraint but rather freedom *to* pursue that **objectification** of the self represented in the creative praxis within which both the historicity of individuals and the histories of peoples originate (*EPM*, 179–82; Lee, 6).

Both subsistence labor and praxis are fully material activities of a specific kind of species being whose emergent consciousness and capacity for self-objectification are, unlike nonhuman animals, able to transform mere subsistence into both culture and history. In this respect, Marx had a distinctive and both admiring and uplifting vision of humanity. Further, human interactions are not mechanical, instinctive, or arbitrary, as they are among nonhuman animals. Rather, human interchanges are dialectical: One's recognition or consciousness of oneself as a free being is mediated through the acknowledgment of *that* in you by the other, whose own self-consciousness as a free being depends on and results from the same process (*EPM*, 112; Lee, 6; see Hegel, pars. 178–96).

But—and now we approach a problem in Marx's view of men and women—that which in Marx's philosophy distinguishes nonhuman animal life from human species life, the capacity for praxis, also figures into how Marx distinguishes male from female sexuality. According to Marx, life processes are phenomena "of the flesh" that include not only interchanges between humans and nonhuman nature but also interchanges, interactions, among human beings themselves. For Marx, the most fundamental human relationships are those mediated by what he calls "natural predisposition" (*GI*, 51), that is, the life processes involved in heterosexual intercourse. For first and foremost among human needs, on his view, is the propagation of human beings (*GI*, 49), a desire for which forms the foundation of the most basic of all human social relationships, "that of a man and a woman who, with their offspring, form the family" (*GI*, 49).

As the basis of the family, sexuality is nascent to the emergence of consciousness and thus to praxis itself. Even if we bracket our doubts about Marx's assumption that heterosexuality is natural, however, the nascence of sexuality does not imply that men and women are similarly situated with respect to the sexual act. On Marx's view, they are not. Indeed, not even acknowledging the other as self-conscious implies or requires that the other be situated similarly with respect to the human relationship between woman and man in sexuality. This point is perhaps best captured by Marx's analysis of what befalls the heterosexual relationship within capitalism. For although capitalism, according to Marx, distorts the sexual relationship between women and men, the way in which this occurs discloses his deeper assumptions about the structure of male/female sexual affiliation and the type of family that emerges from it.

Marx argues that within the constraints of capitalist labor the family is converted into a microcosmic unit of the production of laborers and the consumption and acquisition of goods, despite its original affiliative bonds or purposes. The family's condition under these oppressive conditions becomes one of estrangement both from itself *as a family* and the estrangement of its individual members from each other as not being connected by anything *other than* labor, competition, and subsistence. Capitalism so corrupts the family's affective bonds that its members come to identify its value solely in terms of the consumption accomplished under the father's name and title. Alienated from the original purpose of the family, but nonetheless responsible for its economic welfare, the family patriarch comes to see his actions within and outside the family structure as "not belonging to him" (*EPM*, 111). While he is the source of whatever status the family achieves, this status is measured in terms only of the production and consumption his own alienation can purchase. The greater his labor, the more extensive the family's consumption, and the more profound his alienation from himself, his wife, and his children.

Under these conditions, Marx argues, the worker comes to see his own "begetting as emasculating," as "an activity turned against him" (*EPM*, 111–12). What once was the natural expression of his species being is now a gelded and demoralized vestige of its former affirmation. Although the worker/husband/father retains unimpeded sexual access to his wife as a rite of patriarchal marriage, the sexual relationship is debased by his alienation from himself and from her. The products of their intercourse, for example, children *qua* future laborers and consumers, represent neither the worker himself, his future, nor his social/sexual relationship with his wife, for these products no more belong to him than his labor. Even the children belong to Moneybags. Under the authority of the capitalist, the most basic of human activities becomes little more than a fleeting respite from labor. Sex in capitalism, just like eating and sleeping, is reduced to an "animal function" denuded of its humanizing qualities. It becomes an activity that ultimately benefits the capitalist, either by restoring to the laborer a renewed capacity to labor (as eating and sleeping do) or by yielding future laborers. That sex should be experienced as *emasculating* is not surprising. Insofar as estrangement is emasculating, it would seem that the conditions under which any life activity is performed in capitalism could sire little else. Some recent Marxist thinkers have tried to expand the notion of alienation—or estrangement—to sexuality as a natural, animal function. Thus, one might claim that if people are not properly integrated with nature, including their own sexual nature, they are alienated from it. An example would be **sexual activity** done for its capitalistic functions and not as a life-affirming, naturally joyous experience. In such cases it would not be implausible to speak of "sexual alienation"

(Gendron, 114–33). Given this view of human-animal sexuality as life-affirming and joyous, it can be argued within such a Marxism that women, too, can be estranged, alienated, or emasculated with respect to their sexuality.

Underlying the analysis of marital sexuality in capitalism as serving economic functions (producing new laborers; providing relief from labor) is Marx's assumption that the emasculated laborer is a man who returns from work to his home where his wife awaits him. So whatever the position of women may be within the family, it is not that of wage worker, much less head of the household. Her sex determines a different course, for under any exploitative situation her role in the reproduction of offspring and in maintaining the conditions of daily life always remains the same. Regardless of the economic facts that characterize the world outside the home, the home and women's functions in it remain constant; their basic structure is dictated by natural propensity, maternal duty, and patriarchal interest. Even if the worker/husband/father is "at home" only in his "animal functions"—eating, sleeping, having sex—this alienated laborer still retains the privilege of the domestic service provided by the wife/mother that accrues to him in "his" dwelling (Lee, 31).

To understand why Marx conceives capitalist exploitation as sexually differentiated we need to confront his notion of the sexual division of labor. Originating in "nothing but the division of labor in the sexual act" itself (*GI*, 51)—already an astounding idea—Marx's sexual division of labor reiterates, within the materialist framework of species being, a long-standing Western tradition. It posits women as passive recipients of men's **sexual desire** and activity and men as the progenitors of *their* offspring. Although he does not go so far as to assert a dualist identification of women with the body and men with the mind, Marx's sexual division of labor establishes a difference so basic to species being that it permeates his analysis of capitalism. Indeed, the division between the sexes mirrors the distinction between subsistence labor and praxis labor, in that the heterosexual act of procreative intercourse reproduces the distinction between subsistence labor and creative labor. For while women's sexuality is presumed to be only the natural expression of their species being as passive recipients, men's sexuality contains the seeds of their future praxis activities precisely because it contains the seeds of the progeny who will carry *their* name. The similarity between Marx and a long line of male thinkers, beginning with **Aristotle** (384–322 BCE) and going through a stream of Catholic Fathers, is noteworthy.

On Marx's view, sexuality exhibits a division of labor that develops spontaneously or in virtue of a natural predisposition. But this is not, for Marx, a genuine division of labor, because it lacks the distinction between the mental and the material (*GI*, 51). For both women and men, sex is not an intellectual endeavor but only an "animal function" (*EPM*, 111). However, because sex contains the seeds of a commodifiable product, offspring who are to inherit and whose fate falls to the natural patriarchal authority of the family, sexual activity partakes of praxis *for the man*. The sexual division of labor is an ontologically necessary feature of labor because on its basis the most paradigmatic realization of praxis is made possible. Progeny are the archetypal *objectification of consciousness*. But sexuality is not praxis for women, regardless of the economic formation, be it capitalist or otherwise. For while sex is not a form of labor itself, it still decides the role of its participants in all future labor. Such participants are themselves presumed to be naturally divided into male and female and are attracted to each other only with respect to sexual disposition. The products of the sexual act further validate these roles and their culturally unmediated priority. Capitalism may distort these relationships, but it does not determine them. Indeed, for Marx what determines the division of labor is a heterosexuality presumed to be a feature of human nature. Capitalist production therefore simply exploits the naturalness of this division and in so doing both entrenches it as "natural" and profits from the distribution of labor the division provides.

In "The Social Basis of the Women's Question," Kollontai considers the question whether "working-class women should respond to the call of the feminists and participate actively and directly in the struggle for women's equality, or whether, faithful to the traditions of their class, they should go their own way and fight using other means to free not only women but all mankind from the oppression and enslavement of contemporary capitalist forms of social life" (18). Insisting that the latter course is the one most likely to achieve genuine emancipation, she argues, like Marx, that "the supporters of historical materialism fully recognize the naturally existing differences between the sexes and demand only one thing, namely that each individual, man or woman, be given the real possibility of achieving the freest and fullest self-determination, that the widest possible opportunities be provided for the development of all natural talents" (18). The primary issue, for Kollontai, is not whether a natural division of labor exists between the sexes; on her view, it does. Rather, it is whether emancipation from capitalist oppression can achieve for women the same degree of opportunity it can achieve for men, so that women can pursue their "natural talents" to whatever extent is possible given limitations imposed by sex.

Kollontai argues that the only viable answer to this question must be yes, because the feminist alternative to a Marxist movement of workers is "distinctly bourgeois in nature" and thus neither adequately outfitted for economic struggle nor aimed at the right goal, the freedom for all able humans to engage in praxis: "[B]y virtue of their class position, the feminists cannot struggle to achieve a fundamental restructuring of the present economic-social structure of society, and without this the emancipation of women cannot be complete" (32). Kollontai is, in fact, critical of feminists whose demands for political equality generates suspicion and hostility from those who might otherwise be allies in the struggle for economic justice:

> When arming ourselves against the indifference, or even hostility of men towards the question of female equality, feminists turn their attention only to the representatives of every shade of bourgeois liberalism, ignoring the existence of a large political party which, on the issue of women's equality, goes further than even the most fervent suffragettes. Since the appearance of the *Communist Manifesto* in 1848, Social-Democracy has always defended the interests of women. (30)

Because the feminist movement is intractably harnessed to the middle class and to middle-class aspirations, it cannot adequately represent the working class or attend to its issues, and thus it cannot represent either working-class men *or* working-class women. By Kollontai's lights, the feminist movement is not a true movement *for women*.

However sympathetic she is to the feminist plea for equality, Kollontai's choice of political movement is decisive—class comes before sex—so that men are not the woman's "enemy and oppressor but, on the contrary . . . a comrade in sharing a common, joyless lot, and a loyal comrade in arms in the struggle for a brighter future" (33). But while Kollontai may be right to recognize the importance of recruiting women into the working-class movement for economic justice, she may also seriously underestimate the obstacles women face with respect to achieving the benefits of this future revolution. According to her, women's economic and social status is unequal to men's because "certain specific characteristics of the present system weigh doubly upon the woman" (33). But, she continues, "the working class knows who is to blame for these unfortunate conditions," namely, the capitalist. As Engels observes, however, this doubled burden is not only capitalist but also patriarchal, so that overcoming class oppression does not necessarily imply freedom from patriarchal oppression. Whereas men are only commodified as wage laborers, women are commodified both in virtue of their reproductive capacities and as uncompensated domestic laborers.

A complication, then, for Marx's analysis of capitalist oppression and Kollontai's rendition is that being female means being subject to two independent yet mutually reinforcing systems of domination. Marxist-feminist Heidi Hartmann argues that "before capitalism a patriarchal system was established in which men controlled the labor of women and children in the family, and that in doing so men learned the techniques of hierarchical organization and control" ("Capitalism, Patriarchy," 147; see also her "Unhappy Marriage" and the essays in Sargent's *Women and Revolution*). Similarly, Lerner claims that "[m]en learned to institute dominance and hierarchy over other people by their earlier practice of dominance over the women of their own group" (9). If Hartmann and Lerner are right that capitalist domination derives from established patriarchal models of domination, then eradicating capitalist economic formations may have little or no effect on eradicating patriarchal oppression. Even if institutions like patriarchy, slavery, and primitive forms of capitalist exchange evolved more or less simultaneously, still the sexual commodification of women provides the archetype of a property that can be expropriated.

The question, then, is this: In virtue of the commodification of *what* are patriarchy and its consequent claim to private property in women established? The answer returns us to Marx's sexual dialectics: (1) What counts as creative labor or praxis largely discounts *as labor* women's procreative and domestic work and (2) however discounted, women's sexuality serves as the premier as well as original vehicle for all other forms of commodification (*CM*, 71–72; *EPM*, 110–12; Engels, *Origin*, 54–74). Women are the invisible but necessary ontological condition for the procreation and re-creation of labor *and* the maximally visible archetypal commodity whose exchange value resides precisely in the procreative and re-creative labor for which they receive no compensation (other than by reaping the "benefits" of "private," as opposed to suffering the destitution of "public," **prostitution**).

This is not to say that Marx does not recognize women as laborers but that, given his view of the role that sexuality plays in species being, his concept of labor not only does not but *cannot* accommodate traditionally uncompensated labor and cannot do so *because* it is performed by women. "Women's work" cannot be compensated as wage labor because doing so acknowledges that it is a source of self-creation or praxis from which women could *become alienated*. But this jeopardizes the very conditions that circumscribe the conditions of labor—the commodifiability of sexuality—in that it destabilizes the notion that sexual activity and the other activities presumed to accompany or follow from it are an aspect of our sexed animal natures, not of our creative natures. Hence Marx is saddled with the idea that women's animal nature is inalienable at least with respect to its two patriarchally established functions, re-creation (domestic labor) and procreation (future labor). If women's function in a patriarchal system of exchange is defined in terms of an inalienable capacity for reproductive service, we might posit ways in which capitalism appropriates the products of this service. But it is, according to Marx, the natural division of labor that defines it.

As many feminists, poststructuralists, and others have pointed out, the key to liberating Marx from this perhaps devastating critique of his sexual dialectics is to divorce his analysis of capitalism from his view of the sexual division of labor. But it might not be possible to do so. This division of labor makes the development of capitalist exchange dependent on the commodification of women's reproductive and domestic capacities, and so it commits Marx to sustaining a deeply traditional Western view of sexuality that confirms patriarchal prerogative even as it condemns capitalism (Lee, 13–17). Hence, such a divorce is not achievable without doing irrecoverable damage to his analysis. But, as Jaggar suggests, we could reassign what is traditionally seen as part of "nature" to "nurture" instead and argue that the sexual division of labor is an artifact of, and not a prerequisite for, the commodification of sexuality (369–77). Besides being plausible in light of historical research like Lerner's, this reading has received considerable support in the feminist literature because (among other reasons) it offers hope that patriarchal domination can be overcome.

Whatever the verdict is with respect to his sexual dialectics, Marx still has much to say to contemporary political theory. To feminist theory Marx offers a number of conceptual tools for analyzing oppression. Feminists have a similar love/hate relationship with **Sigmund Freud** (1856–1939), from whom they can still gather insights about the relations between the sexes. There remains much to learn from the ways in which sex and sexuality infuse Marx's thinking about exchange and commodification, even if there is much to be rejected or radically reinterpreted.

See also Existentialism; Feminism, Lesbian; Feminism, Liberal; Feminism, Men's; Fichte, Johann Gottlieb; Firestone, Shulamith; Foucault, Michel; Freudian Left, The; Hegel, G.W.F.; MacKinnon, Catharine; Poststructuralism; Prostitution; Social Constructionism; Utopianism; Westermarck, Edward

REFERENCES

Barzun, Jacques. (1941) *Darwin, Marx, Wagner: Critique of a Heritage*, 2nd ed. Garden City, N.Y.: Doubleday, 1958; Berlin, Isaiah. (1939) *Karl Marx: His Life and Environment*, 4th ed. Oxford, U.K.: Oxford University Press, 1978; Engels, Frederick. (1884) *The Origin of the Family, Private Property, and the State*. New York: International Publishers, 1942; Ferguson, Ann. *Sexual Democracy: Women, Oppression, and Revolution*. Boulder, Colo.: Westview, 1991; Foster, John Bellamy. *Marx's Ecology: Materialism and Nature*. New York: Monthly Review Press, 2000; Gendron, Bernard. *Technology and the Human Condition*. New York: St. Martin's Press, 1977; Goldman, Emma. (1910) *Anarchism and Other Essays*. New York: Dover, 1969; Hartmann, Heidi. (1976) "Capitalism, Patriarchy, and Job Segregation." In Karen V. Hanson and Ilene J. Philipson, eds., *Women, Class, and the Feminist Imagination: A Socialist Feminist Reader*. Philadelphia, Pa.: Temple University Press, 1990, 146–81; Hartmann, Heidi. "The Unhappy Marriage of Marxism and Feminism: Towards a More Progressive Union." In Lydia Sargent, ed., *Women and Revolution: A Discussion of the Unhappy Marriage of Marxism and Feminism*. Boston, Mass.: South End Press, 1981, 1–41; Hartsock, Nancy C. M. *Money, Sex, and Power: Toward a Feminist Historical Materialism*. New York: Longman, 1983; Hegel, G.W.F. (1807) *Phenomenology of Spirit*. Trans. Arnold V. Miller. Oxford, U.K.: Clarendon Press, 1977; Horkheimer, Max, and Theodor Adorno. (1944) *Dialectic of Enlightenment*. Trans. John Cumming. New York: Continuum, 1990; Jaggar, Alison M. *Feminist Politics and Human Nature*. Totowa, N.J.: Rowman and Allanheld, 1983; Kirk, Gwyn. "Standing on Solid Ground: A Materialist Ecological Feminism." In Rosemary Hennessy and Chrys Ingraham, eds., *Materialist Feminism: A Reader in Class, Difference, and Women's Lives*. New York: Routledge, 1997, 345–63; Kollontai, Alexandra. *Selected Articles and Speeches*. Trans. Cynthia Carlile. New York: International Publishers, 1984; Lee, Wendy Lynne. *On Marx*. Belmont, Calif.: Wadsworth, 2002; Lerner, Gerda. *The Creation of Patriarchy*. New York: Oxford University Press, 1986; Lukács, Georg. (1922) *History and Class Consciousness: Studies in Marxist Dialectics*. Trans. Rodney Livingstone. Cambridge, Mass.: MIT Press, 1971; Luxemburg, Rosa. [Various texts] In David McLellan, ed., *Marxism: Essential Writings*. Oxford, U.K.: Oxford University Press, 1988, 108–33; Marcuse, Herbert. (1955) *Eros and Civilization: A Philosophical Inquiry into Freud*. New York: Vintage, 1962;

Marx, Karl. *Early Writings*. Trans. Rodney Livingstone and Gregor Benton. New York: Vintage, 1975; Marx, Karl. *The Economic and Philosophic Manuscripts of 1844*. Trans. Martin Milligan. Ed. Dirk Struik. New York: International Publishers, 1964; Marx, Karl, and Friedrich Engels. *The Communist Manifesto*. Ed. Martin Malia. New York: Penguin Putnam, 1998; Marx, Karl, and Friedrich Engels. *The German Ideology*. Ed. C. J. Arthur. New York: International Publishers, 1981; McLellan, David, ed. (1977) *Karl Marx: Selected Writings*, 2nd ed. Oxford, U.K.: Oxford University Press, 2000; Merchant, Carolyn. *Radical Ecology: The Search for a Livable World*. New York: Routledge, 1992; Mitchell, Juliet. *Psychoanalysis and Feminism: Freud, Reich, Laing, and Women*. New York: Vintage, 1975; Reich, Wilhelm. *Sex-Pol: Essays 1929–1934*. Ed. Lee Baxandall. Trans. Anna Bostock, Tom DuBose, and Lee Baxandall. New York: Random House, 1972. New York: Columbia University Press, 1994; Sargent, Lydia, ed. *Women and Revolution: A Discussion of the Unhappy Marriage of Marxism and Feminism*. Boston, Mass.: South End Press, 1981; Tucker, Robert C., ed. (1972) *The Marx-Engels Reader*, 2nd ed. New York: Norton, 1978; Weeks, Jeffrey. *Sex, Politics and Society*. London: Longman, 1981; Weeks, Jeffrey. *Sexuality and Its Discontents: Meanings, Myths, and Modern Sexualities*. London: Routledge and Kegan Paul, 1985; Wilson, Edmund. (1940) *To the Finland Station: A Study in the Writing and Acting of History*. New York: Farrar, Straus and Giroux, 1972.

Wendy Lynne Lee

ADDITIONAL READING

Balbus, Isaac D. *Marxism and Domination: A Neo-Hegelian, Feminist, Psychoanalytic Theory of Sexual, Political, and Technological Liberation*. Princeton, N.J.: Princeton University Press, 1982; Bartky, Sandra Lee. "Narcissism, Femininity, and Alienation." *Social Theory and Practice* 8:2 (1982), 127–43; Bebel, August. *Woman and Socialism*. New York: Socialist Literature, 1910; Bebel, August. (1885) *Woman in the Past, Present, and Future*. New York: AMS Press, 1976; Belliotti, Raymond. "The Prostitution in Capitalist Marriage: Marxism." In *Good Sex: Perspectives on Sexual Ethics*. Lawrence: University Press of Kansas, 1993, 111–25; Bottomore, T. B., ed. and trans. *Karl Marx: Early Writings*. New York: McGraw-Hill, 1963. [Includes "Economic and Philosophical Manuscripts," 61–219]; Brod, Harry. "Pornography and the Alienation of Male Sexuality." *Social Theory and Practice* 14:3 (1988), 265–84. Reprinted in Michael S. Kimmel and Michael A. Messner, eds., *Men's Lives*, 3rd ed. Needham Heights, Mass.: Allyn and Bacon, 1995, 393–404; in Larry May, Robert Strikwerda, and Patrick D. Hopkins, eds., *Rethinking Masculinity: Philosophical Explorations in Light of Feminism*, 2nd ed. Lanham, Md.: Rowman and Littlefield, 1996, 237–53; POS2 (281–99); Cohen, G. A. *Karl Marx's Theory of History: A Defence*. Princeton, N.J.: Princeton University Press, 1978; Cohen, Marshall, Thomas Nagel, and Thomas Scanlon, eds. *Marx, Justice, and History*. Princeton, N.J.: Princeton University Press, 1980; Cornforth, Maurice. *The Open Philosophy and the Open Society: A Reply to Dr. Karl Popper's Refutation of Marxism*. New York: International Publishers, 1968; Dahmer, Helmut. "Sexual Economy Today." *Telos* 36 (Summer 1978), 111–26; Di Stephano, Christine. "Masculine Marx." In Mary Lyndon Shanley and Carole Pateman, eds., *Feminist Interpretation and Political Theory*. University Park: Pennsylvania State University Press, 1991, 146–63; Elshtain, Jean Bethke. "Marxist Feminism: Why Can't a Woman Be More Like a Proletarian?" In *Public Man, Private Woman: Women in Social and Political Thought*. Princeton, N.J.: Princeton University Press, 1981, 256–84; Elster, Jon. *Making Sense of Marx*. Cambridge: Cambridge University Press, 1985; Fisk, Milton. "Sex and Class." In *Ethics and Society: A Marxist Interpretation of Value*. Sussex, U.K.: Harvester, 1980, 51–53; Gendron, Bernard. "Sexual Alienation." In *Technology and the Human Condition*. New York: St. Martin's Press, 1977, 114–33. Reprinted in POS1 (281–98); Goldman, Emma. "The Traffic in Women." Anarchy Archives (Web site). <dwardmac.pitzer.edu/Anarchist_Archives/goldman/aando/traffic.html> [accessed 2 June 2005]; Goldstein, Leslie. "Mill, Marx, and Women's Liberation." *Journal of the History of Philosophy* 18 (1980), 319–34; Habermas, Jürgen. (1973) *Legitimation Crisis*. Trans. Thomas McCarthy. Boston, Mass.: Beacon Press, 1975; Hanson, Karen V., and Ilene J. Philipson, eds. *Women, Class, and the Feminist Imagination: A Socialist Feminist Reader*. Philadelphia, Pa.: Temple University Press,

1990; Hartsock, Nancy C. M. "Gender and Power: Masculinity, Violence, and Domination." In *Money, Sex, and Power: Toward a Feminist Historical Materialism*. New York: Longman, 1983, 155–85; Hegel, G.W.F. (1821) *Elements of the Philosophy of Right*. Ed. Allen W. Wood. Trans. Hugh B. Nisbet. Cambridge: Cambridge University Press, 1995; Heiss, Robert. *Hegel, Kierkegaard, Marx: Three Great Philosophers Whose Ideas Changed the Course of Civilization*. New York: Dell, 1975; Held, Virginia. "Marx, Sex, and the Transformation of Society." *Philosophical Forum* 5:1–2 (1973–1974), 168–84; Holmstrom, Nancy. "A Marxist Theory of Women's Nature." *Ethics* 94:3 (1984), 456–73; Hook, Sidney. (1936) *From Hegel to Marx: Studies in the Intellectual Development of Karl Marx*. Ann Arbor: University of Michigan Press, 1962; Horkheimer, Max, and Theodor Adorno. (1944) *Dialectic of Enlightenment*. Trans. John Cumming. New York: Continuum, 1990. Reprinted in W. McNeill and K. S. Feldman, eds., *Continental Philosophy: An Anthology*. Malden, Mass.: Blackwell, 1998, 253–59; Jaggar, Alison M. "Prostitution." In Alan Soble, ed., *The Philosophy of Sex: Contemporary Readings*, 1st ed. Totowa, N.J.: Rowman and Littlefield, 1980, 348–68. Reprinted in POS2 (259–80); Jaggar, Alison M., and Paula S. Rothenberg, eds. (1978) *Feminist Frameworks: Alternative Theoretical Accounts of the Relations between Women and Men*, 2nd ed. New York: McGraw-Hill, 1984; Kollontai, Alexandra. *Selections*. In Ellen K. Feder, Karmen Mac-Kendrick, and Sybol S. Cook, eds., *A Passion for Wisdom: Readings in Western Philosophy on Love and Desire*. Upper Saddle River, N.J.: Prentice Hall, 2004, 506–20; MacKinnon, Catharine A. "Desire and Power: A Feminist Perspective." In Cary Nelson and Lawrence Grossberg, eds., *Marxism and the Interpretation of Culture*. Urbana: University of Illinois Press, 1988, 105–21; MacKinnon, Catharine A. "Feminism and Marxism." In *Toward a Feminist Theory of the State*. Cambridge, Mass.: Harvard University Press, 1989, 1–80; Marx, Karl. (1867) *Capital: A Critique of Political Economy*, vol. 1: *The Process of Capitalist Production*. Trans. Samuel Moore and Edward Aveling. New York: International Publishers, 1967; McMurtry, John. "Monogamy: A Critique." In Robert B. Baker and Frederick A. Elliston, eds., *Philosophy and Sex*, 1st ed. Buffalo, N.Y.: Prometheus, 1975, 166–77. Reprinted in P&S2 (107–18). "Afterword," in Roger Libby and Robert Whitehurst, eds., *Marriage and Alternatives*. Glenview, Ill.: Scott, Foresman, 1977, 11–12; McMurtry, John. "Sex, Love, and Friendship." In Alan Soble, ed., *Sex, Love, and Friendship*. Amsterdam, Holland: Rodopi, 1997, 169–83; McMurtry, John. *The Structure of Marx's World-View*. Princeton, N.J.: Princeton University Press, 1978; Moon, S. Joan. "Feminism and Socialism: The Utopian Synthesis of Flora Tristan." In Marilyn A. Boxer and Jean H. Quataert, eds., *Socialist Women: European Socialist Feminism in the Nineteenth and Early Twentieth Centuries*. New York: Elsevier, 1978, 19–50; Ollman, Bertell. (1971) *Alienation: Marx's Conception of Man in Capitalistic Society*, 2nd ed. Cambridge: Cambridge University Press, 1976; Ollman, Bertell. *Social and Sexual Revolution: Essays on Marx and Reich*. Boston, Mass.: South End Press, 1979; Padgug, Robert. "Sexual Matters: On Conceptualizing Sexuality in History." *Radical History Review* 20 (Spring–Summer 1979), 3–23. Reprinted in Kathy Peiss and Christina Simmons, eds., *Passion and Power: Sexuality in History*. Philadelphia, Pa.: Temple University Press, 1989, 14–31; and Edward Stein, ed., *Forms of Desire: Sexual Orientation and the Social Constructionist Controversy*. New York: Routledge, 1992, 43–67; Popper, Karl R. (1945) *The Open Society and Its Enemies*, vol. 2: *The High Tide of Prophecy: Hegel, Marx, and the Aftermath*, 5th ed. Princeton, N.J.: Princeton University Press, 1966; Railton, Peter. "Alienation, Consequentialism, and the Demands of Morality." *Philosophy and Public Affairs* 13:2 (1984), 134–71; Reich, Wilhelm. (1930) *The Sexual Revolution: Toward a Self-Governing Character Structure* [*Die Sexualität im Kulturkampf*], 4th ed., rev. Trans. Theodore P. Wolfe. New York: Noonday, 1969; Ring, Jennifer. "Saving Objectivity for Feminism: MacKinnon, Marx, and Other Possibilities." *Review of Politics* 49 (Fall 1987), 467–89; Rowbotham, Sheila, and Jeffrey Weeks. *Socialism and the New Life: The Personal and Sexual Politics of Edward Carpenter and Havelock Ellis*. London: Pluto Press, 1977; Rubin, Gayle. "The Traffic in Women." In Ranya Reiter, ed., *Towards an Anthropology of Women*. New York: Monthly Review Press, 1975, 157–210; Schacht, Richard. *The Future of Alienation*. Urbana: University of Illinois Press, 1994; Shelby, Tommie. "Parasites, Pimps, and Capitalists: A Naturalistic Conception of Exploitation." *Social Theory and Practice* 28:3 (2002), 381–418; Singer, Peter. *Marx*. Oxford, U.K.: Oxford University Press, 1980; Soble, Alan. *Pornography: Marxism,*

Feminism, and the Future of Sexuality. New Haven, Conn.: Yale University Press, 1986; Turley, Donna. "The Feminist Debate on Pornography: An Unorthodox Interpretation." *Socialist Review* 16:3–4 (1986), 81–96; Wolff, Robert Paul. *Understanding Marx: A Reconstruction and Critique of Capital.* Princeton, N.J.: Princeton University Press, 1984.

MASOCHISM. *See* Sadomasochism

MASTURBATION. Masturbation, also called beating the beaver, brushing the beaver, buffing the bead, buffing the weasel, buttering the muffin, buttering the bagel, buzzing off (women), banging one out, bashing the Bishop, bashing the pear, basting the ham, beating off, beating the bologna, and beating the beagle (men), among many other even less probable expressions (see Green, 149–80; "Words"), is a perplexing phenomenon. Like sex that frequently occurs with an admired, compassionate, and intimate lover, masturbation is often sex with someone I care about and to whose satisfaction and welfare I am devoted. If I masturbate, the primping will be minimal and the date inexpensive. Further, I won't have to worry about finding a cab home. It is incestuous, since it happens with someone to whom I am blood-related, a person in my immediate family. If I am married, my masturbation (even if I have permission to do it) is adulterous, since it is sex with a person to whom I am not married, someone not my spouse. Masturbation is a same-sex, even homosexual, act: A man sexually pleases a man and/or is pleased by a man; a woman pleases a woman and/or is pleased by a woman. It is sex we can fall into inadvertently or nonconsciously. (Among the more intelligent men's bathroom graffiti is, "If you shake it more than twice, you're playing with it.") Hence some masturbation is sex that is not completely voluntary or consensual; it is not quite against my will yet not fully with it, either. And masturbating while entertaining a **fantasy** or virtual image of Britney Spears, J. Lo., Denzel Washington, or Adam Sandler involves using them, objectifying them. (This might be true even if, as a benefit, psychoanalyzing masturbatory fantasies provides a "royal road to the unconscious"; Francis, 96; see 107.)

The profound problem here—alternatively, the birdbrained pomo jokes—might reside in the concept "masturbation" *or* with the concepts "**incest**," "homosexual," "**adultery**," "**objectification**" (or with both). But many of these deconstructionist analogies have been taken seriously by someone or another, and each contains a grain of provocative truth. Betty Dodson avows that her "simple message"—and no hyperbole is intended—is that "self-sexuality is the ongoing love affair that each of us has with ourselves throughout our lifetime" (130). Robert Solomon points out that the "post-coital period" of masturbation, as opposed to paired sex, "is cleansed of . . . interpersonal hassles and arguments" ("Paradigms," 27). Robert of Sorbonne (1201–1274) long ago argued that "[b]ecause you are closer to yourself than to anyone else, having sex with yourself is the worst kind of incest—worse than copulating with your mother" (Jordan, 101). Psychological links between masturbation and **homosexuality** were sensed by **Sigmund Freud** (1856–1939; "On Narcissism," 87–88). The bathroom graffiti had been anticipated by the ancient Hebrews (or first scrawled by them): "As a precaution against masturbation, it was forbidden [in the *Zohar*] for a man to hold his penis even while urinating, except in the case of a married man whose wife was readily available for intercourse" (Glasner, 579). The idea that someone who engages in a fantasy during masturbation rapes (hence uses) his or her dream partner was dreamed up by **Jean-Jacques Rousseau** (1712–1778):

> This vice, which shame and timidity find so convenient, has a particular attraction for lively imaginations. It allows them to dispose, so to speak, of the whole female sex at their will, and to make any beauty who tempts them serve their pleasure without the need of first obtaining her consent. (*Confessions*, 109 [bk. 3]; see also *Emile*, 333–34)

And, finally, a connection between masturbation and adultery seems part of Jesus's message, at Matthew 5:27–30, which ends, "[I]f your right hand causes you to sin, cut it off and throw it away. It is better for you to lose one part of your body than for your whole body to go into hell." One reading is that if looking on a woman lustfully is already to commit adultery with her "in the heart," having masturbatory fantasies, also "in the heart," about her cannot be any better, and the offending hand should be dispatched straightaway. (What Matthew's Jesus does is to redefine looking lustfully "upward," making it more—adultery—than we usually think it is.) Hans Dieter Betz has written, "What the specific sin [of the hand] is we are not told directly, but the context of seduction and adultery suggests that the hand plays a role" (*Sermon on the Mount*, 238). Perhaps the correct reading of the passage, then, is more mundane: The hand that seduces a woman into adultery by manipulating her privates is the bad hand. But in a startling footnote (#335), Betz adds, "In semitic languages the hand can be a euphemism for the penis." Matthew's Jesus might have been advocating self-castration as the cure or punishment for looking at women lustfully. In **Plato**'s (427–347 BCE) *Symposium*, Diotima approvingly tells a young Socrates (469–399 BCE) that people will chop off their own hands and feet if they are diseased or evil (205e). Did Diotima also mean self-castration? How often could a foot be so sexually impertinent as to require amputation?

Perhaps such attitudes toward masturbation partly explain why we keep our masturbatory practices to ourselves (except anonymously, as in reports to Shere Hite). The sexual revolution, such as it was in the 1960s and 1970s, made living together and having sex outside matrimony socially acceptable; it encouraged the toleration, if not celebration, of lesbian and gay lifestyles; it breathed respectable life into the colorful practices of the sons and daughters of the **Marquis de Sade** (1740–1814). Adultery, homosexuality, **prostitution**, **pornography**, **sexual harassment**, **rape**, and premarital sex are standard fare as topics in television dramas and sitcoms, but except for one *Seinfeld* episode—who in this motley group can resist the temptation the longest? (the unlikely George won the bet)—masturbation is either MIA or POW. And to call a man a "jerk-off," or to insinuate that he jerks off, is still, in the civilized world in the twenty-first century, strongly derogatory. Bagel-buttering women avoid this condemnation, perhaps because (this kind of thinking has a long history) their masturbation is innocuous, not "wasting" any precious fluid, Neil Young's "silver seed" (see Epstein; Jordan, 101–2). Masturbation, at least the male variety, is one illustrious black sheep of the family of sex, though **bestiality** might be more literally the black sheep. Still, "dog fucker" and "turtle fucker" do not pack the punch of "mother fucker" and "jerk-off," and neither does "corpse fucker," which implies that incest and masturbation are more revolting to the vulgar mind than zoophilia and necrophilia, or that sexual play with animals or the bodies of dead persons never occurs to that foggy mind. Notice, though, that necrophiliac sexual acts are masturbatory, since only one animate being is involved. So for the vulgar mind "corpse fucker" *should* be intensely derogatory. That it is not suggests that this foggy mind actually *sees* two people having sex in necrophilia. In its vision necrophilia is little different from genuine coitus. Or genuine coitus is little different from necrophilia. (Ask the girlfriend of the vulgar, foggy-minded male.)

Defining It. What is masturbation? How should we define or analyze it? Once, when Bruno Bettelheim (1903–1990) was delivering a lecture, he said to a woman sitting in the first row of the auditorium, who was knitting while listening to the great man talk, something like, "You, madam, are engaged in sublimation for masturbation." The woman replied feistily (the comeback might be apocryphal): "No, sir, when I knit, I knit; when I masturbate, I masturbate" (Pollak, 213). What does this woman know to which philosophers ought to pay attention? Consider what is seemingly the paradigm case of masturbation: A person in a private place manually rubs the penis or clitoris and eventually reaches an orgasm. Most of the salient features of the paradigm case are, however, inessential. (1) One can brazenly masturbate in the waiting room of a bus terminal, erect penis or engorged vulva displayed for all to see. You are put away for such things. (2) The hands do not have to be used, as long as the sexually sensitive areas of the body can be pressed against a suitably shaped object of comfortable composition: the back of a horse or its saddle, the seat of a bicycle or motorcycle, a rug or pillows. (3) Orgasm need not be attained for a sexual act to be masturbatory, nor need it even be the goal. Prolonged sexual pleasure itself is often the point of masturbation, pleasure that is nipped in the bud by premature orgasm. (4) The clitoris or *glans penis* need not receive the most or even any attention. There are other sexually sensitive areas one can touch or probe for masturbatory pleasure: nipples, anus/rectum, thighs, lips, patellae. What remains in the paradigm case? (5) The person who, by touching or pressing the body's sexually sensitive areas, causally produces the sensations is the same person who experiences them. The rubber is the rubbed. The "solitary vice" of "self-abuse" or "self-pollution" is logically reflexive. ("Self-pollution," indeed: "When a man has a seminal discharge, he must wash his whole body with water and he shall be unclean until evening. Any clothing or leather touched by the seminal discharge must be washed and it will be unclean until evening" [Lev. 15:16–17]; good advice, ignored by William Jefferson Clinton.)

Can we masturbate others—is it conceptually possible? "To respect" and "to deceive" are both transitive and intransitive: We can respect or deceive others, and we can respect or deceive ourselves ("self-respect," "self-deception"). According to a **sexology** dictionary, one person can masturbate another. The entry defining "Masturbation" says:

> Self-stimulation of the genitalia (qv) by touch or pressure, usually with the hands or vibrator (qv), and with orgasm (qv) as a common but not inevitable or necessary outcome. In masturbating, many women may combine vaginal and breast stimulation with clitoral stimulation. . . . Mutual masturbation may be engaged in by a couple as an alternative to sexual intercourse (qv). (Francoeur et al., 381)

It is not a good idea to define "masturbation" using the word "vibrator." We should use more general terms that would also include in their extension stuffing oneself with an ivory dildo, for the ancients did not have batteries. Who knows what the technology of masturbation will be like in the middle of the twenty-first century?

But there is something more troubling about the definition: If "masturbation" is *defined* as "self-stimulation," there could not *be* any such phenomenon as "mutual" masturbation. What the dictionary authors might have in mind is that solitary masturbation often involves hand-genital contact, so when two people use their hands on each other's genitals that, too, is masturbation, albeit "mutual." Hence "to masturbate" can be transitive. The act can be done by one person on or to another; hence, two-party masturbation need not be *mutual*. Someone can use his or her hands on the other person, period. Reflexivity, then, is not a necessary condition for masturbation, even if it is sufficient. This way of understanding mutual masturbation, however, is inadequate, at least because the dictionary in effect grants, and must grant, that neither the hands nor the genitals are essential to masturbation. If so, mutual *masturbation* would include all sorts of acts between two people (for example, sucking on the other's nipples), most of which we do not *call* "mutual masturbation." The alternative is to reassert that reflexivity is both necessary and sufficient for a sexual act to be masturbatory and to jettison "mutual masturbation" as a misnomer.

The definition offered in another sexological reference book does not fare any better, although in part for a different reason. Psychologist Lester Dearborn, who begins his essay by reproducing **Havelock Ellis**'s (1859–1939) definition of "autoerotism"—"spontaneous sexual emotion . . . without any external stimulus" (Ellis, *Auto-Erotism*, 161; see Dixon and Dixon, 53)—proceeds to define a "subdivision" of this phenomenon, masturbation, "as any form of deliberate self-manipulation of, or application of pressure on, the sexual organs for pleasure and for the release of tension" (Dearborn, 204; Dearborn does not seem to notice the tension between the "spontaneous" of the larger class and the "deliberate" of the supposed subset). Among the various types of masturbation Dearborn lists (211–12) are: dual masturbation—X and Y masturbate themselves in the presence of the other (for a literary example, see Blackburn, 91); group masturbation—add a few more people to dual masturbation; nocturnal masturbation—*not* nocturnal emission but, instead, you wake up and find your hands busy in your crotch (not quite against your will but not fully with it); and psychic masturbation—orgasm from fantasy alone, *sans* manipulation of the genitals. (This type of masturbation seems to violate Dearborn's definition, unless a fantasy in some sense applies "pressure." But it also undercuts the "reflexivity" definition of masturbation provided above. For Ellis, this phenomenon counted, more precisely, as "auto-erotism.") The new difficulty is that Dearborn thinks that masturbation, by definition, is done "for pleasure and the release of tension." First, masturbation done for pleasure and masturbation done to release or relieve tension are already masturbations done for disparate reasons. Neither, however, needs to be the goal or the reason for masturbating. One might masturbate to produce a sperm sample, and one does not thereby try to release tension and might not even do so. Or in providing sperm for artificial insemination, one might masturbate into the collection dish quickly, not aiming for pleasure and even trying to minimize it. One might masturbate for lots of reasons, and even though pleasure may accompany these acts, that does not mean pleasure is the reason or purpose for masturbating. Why one masturbates, the motive behind the act, seems not to be part of the definition of the act. In discussing group masturbation, Dearborn himself says that it may be "a contest to see which [boy] ejaculates first."

About "mutual masturbation," which also seems to violate his definition, Dearborn writes: "This refers to two individuals, who practice manual masturbation of each other. Some laymen loosely use the term mutual masturbation to include any act other than penile-vaginal intercourse and would therefore consider fellation and cunnilinctus as masturbatory acts. But this is loose and inaccurate usage" (211). We can agree that this usage is suspicious, for we do not ordinarily take mutual oral sex as (mutual) masturbation, yet there may be some decent reasons for it. One has already been mentioned: Once we admit that the genitals and hands need not be involved in masturbation, then mutual masturbation cannot be restricted to the case in which the hands of X make contact with the genitals of Y. This allows oral sex to be transitive masturbation—*if* we want to continue to use "masturbation" to talk about two-person **sexual activity**.

Indeed, the contention that X's sucking the nipples of Y, as well as lots of other paired sexual activities, is masturbatory (mutually or two-party) might in some sense be right. Consider, to start, the exculpating redescription of adultery offered to his cheating father by the young, precocious, and helpful Alexander Portnoy: "What after all does it consist of? You put your dick some place and moved it back and forth and stuff came out the front. So, Jake, what's the big deal?" (Roth, 88). Adulterous coitus is redescribed, defined "downward," as if it were solitary masturbation: If you are a male, you put your penis someplace—in your clenched fingers—and move it, or your fingers, back and forth until ejaculation occurs. Every two-party sexual act is masturbatory because the rubbing of sensitive areas, the friction of skin against skin, that occurs during mutual masturbation is from this physicalistic perspective the same as any other mutual rubbing of skin against skin, including that which occurs during coitus. Further, there are no differences between solitary and mutual masturbation or between solitary sexual activity and any type of paired sexual activity, even coitus. All sex is the rubbing of surfaces; the only difference between some acts and others is the number of people—one, two, three, four—who possess these surfaces.

Note that as Alexander offers his father the gift of an exculpatory defense, he also achieves an exculpatory defense for himself, specifically for his own (prohibited and guilt-inducing) solitary masturbation. If adulterous coitus is *nothing but* masturbation, there cannot be much or anything wrong about masturbation: "What's the big deal?" Both the adulterous father and the masturbating son get off the hook. There is rich irony in Alex's saving the father by redescribing his suspicious activity as exactly that which the father has condemned. Alex's motive may be largely self-serving. Regardless, Alex's idea is not original, having been expressed many centuries earlier by Marcus Aurelius (121–180): "[S]exual intercourse [is] internal rubbing accompanied by a spasmodic ejection of mucus" (Grube, 6.13; 50); or "coitus . . . is but the attrition of an ordinary base entrail, and the excretion of a little vile snivel, with a certain kind of convulsion" (Casaubon, 6.11; 59; see Wills).

Here is another line of argument. Consider a person X who is engaging in coitus with a person Y but who deliberately conjures up private fantasies during the act, fantasies that add to X's sexual pleasure or even make it possible. In a not unreasonable sense, we could say that X is using Y's body to masturbate in or on. X's act in this case is significantly similar to the act X would be doing were X fantasizing yet masturbating reflexively. Similarly, we could say that the rapist who uses the body of his victim for his own pleasure, where she has no existence beyond supplying him with suitable body parts, is masturbating "in" or "on" her flesh (see Bogart, 264n.60). Much the same could be said about the inconsiderate husband who is thoroughly concerned with his own pleasure and is oblivious to what his partner is feeling or experiencing, as well as about the foggy-minded male who sees no difference between necrophilia and intercourse with his girlfriend. These men seem to be the authors of masturbatory sex acts. If so, what divides the nonmasturbatory from the masturbatory, at least in two-party cases, is not the physical nature of the act performed but whether the persons are sharing the activity or one person is employing it at the expense of the other. On such a view, any two-party act is masturbatory if it involves gross selfishness, and no two-party act that affords pleasure mutually or reciprocally is masturbatory. This might imply that solitary masturbation is essentially a selfish or at least a self-centered act. That may be true, but no moral judgment seems to follow from that fact alone, whereas in the two-party case it may be easier to derive moral judgments from the sex's being masturbatory.

Yet another way to argue that many two-party sexual acts are masturbatory emerges from the **New Natural Law** philosophy of John Finnis. On his view, the division between the sexually wholesome and the sexually worthless is that between potentially procreative "conjugal activity" and everything else sexual under the sexual sun. At the same time, Finnis advances a broad notion of masturbation that turns on a similar consideration: Even a married couple that performs oral sex, anal intercourse, *coitus interruptus*, or fellatio—nonprocreative sexual acts—are engaging in sex that is masturbatory (1068). Finnis is here offering a definition of masturbation that *does* depend on the nature of the act performed, for *even if* a sexual act between the spouses is thoroughly mutually pleasurable, it is still masturbatory if it is not a procreative kind of act. Indeed, were the spouses to pursue, deliberately, mutual sexual pleasure and wave good-bye to procreative potential (say, by using **contraception**), they would be joined together in a masturbatory (and worthless) sexual activity. It was **Augustine** (354–430) who said about this kind of conjugal sexual activity that the wife is the man's harlot and the man is the wife's adulterous lover (1.17). Reflexive masturbation, on such a view, would be equally condemned, to the extent (which is very often the case) that in this act pleasure is sought in a way incompatible with procreation.

What's Wrong with It. Alexander Portnoy, then, might not get off the hook (and his father would share his fate), were he to take seriously the long stream of antimasturbation condemnations issued throughout Western history of philosophy, theology, and medicine. In the middle of the thirteenth century, **Thomas Aquinas** (1224/25–1274) laid the foundation for Catholic **sexual ethics**. According to Thomas, intentional acts that are sexually unnatural are morally wrong, and a sexual act is unnatural if it is not procreative in form (*Summa theologiae*, 2a2ae, ques. 154, art. 1–12). It follows that nonprocreative sex—homosexual anal intercourse, heterosexual fellatio to orgasm ("completion"), masturbation—is unnatural and hence immoral. All such sexual activity was, for Aquinas, a mortal sin. (Consider an engaging rejoinder, in effect, from Ronald de Sousa: "Some things can be both valuable and useful, but only what is useless [say, nonprocreative, idle masturbation] can be purely valuable"; 219.) The secular philosopher **Immanuel Kant** (1724–1804) also asserted that masturbation and homosexuality were immoral because they are *crimina carnis contra naturam* (unnatural crimes of the flesh): "[O]nanism . . . is abuse of the sexual faculty without any object. . . . By it man sets aside his person and degrades himself below the level of animals. . . . [I]ntercourse between *sexus homogenii* . . . too is contrary to the ends of humanity; for the end of humanity in respect of sexuality is to preserve the species" (*Lectures*, 170). Kant culminates his denouncement of these sexual aberrations viciously: "He," the masturbator or the homosexual, "no longer deserves to be a person."

It has been suggested, with some truth, that Kant argued against masturbation in part by claiming that it "leads to sterility and early senility" (Ward, 109); masturbation, like gluttony and drunkenness, destroys the body and mind and hence undermines one's humanity. Kant's views about the debilitating effects of masturbation do not appear in the *Lectures on Ethics* (ca. 1780); his medical critique of masturbation is found, instead, in *Education* (117–18). It is arresting that Kant claims there (118) that if faced with the choice between masturbating and having unmarried sex with a girl, a young man would do much better opting for the girl (thereby violating the Second Formulation of the Categorical Imperative?), so severe are the effects of masturbation. **Arthur Schopenhauer** (1788–1860), in replying to Kant's moral condemnation of "self-abuse," wrote this obituary for the sexual ethics of masturbation:

> To combat [masturbation] is much more a matter of diet than ethics; for this reason works against it are written by medical men . . . and not by moralists. If morality now wishes to take a hand in this matter after dietetics and hygiene have done their part and crushed it with irrefutable arguments, she finds so much already done that there is little left for her to do. (60)

Schopenhauer must have been thinking about Kant's earlier moral condemnation of masturbation, not his later medical critique. But Schopenhauer was on to something: Medicine was quickly and firmly grabbing control over masturbation from religious institutions (see Szasz).

In an early foray into the medicine of masturbation, **Bernard Mandeville** (1670–1733) had already had outdone Kant. "[T]here are three Ways by which lewd young Men destroy their natural Vigour, and render themselves impotent: First, By Manufriction, *alias* Masturbation" (30). What happens to these boys?

> *Onanites* . . . so weaken their genitals, and accustom them to this violent Friction, that, tho' they have frequent Evacuations without an Erection, yet the common and ordinary Sensation which Females afford to those Parts, is not able of itself to promote this Evacuation: so that they are impotent to all Intents and Purposes of Generation. (31)

A few centuries later even Freud was to claim that "on the basis of my medical experience I cannot rule out a permanent reduction in potency as one among the results of masturbation" ("Contributions to a Discussion," 252; see also Whiteley and Whiteley, 87–88). Whereas Kant had relied on the frightful debilitating effects of masturbation to excuse (not bless) a young boy's engaging in sexual relations with an available girl, Mandeville used these effects to justify (and bless) houses of prostitution: "To put a stop therefore to these clandestine Practices, and prevent young Men from laying *violent Hands* upon themselves, we must have recourse to the *Publick Stews*" (31). The modern temper is quite different. It is frequently said that "there is not one shred of evidence that masturbation is harmful. . . . The only harm that can result from masturbation is if the individual [say, Alex] is plagued with feelings of guilt" (Haynes, 384). Or, if you prefer to hear it laced with sarcasm: "[M]ost students of sex think [masturbation] at least harmless, like chewing gum or backscratching" (Cameron, 19; but be mindful of "autoerotic asphyxiation" [Jenkins]). Indeed, masturbation is not only commonly judged innocuous; it is praised for its beneficial effect of "help[ing] teenagers abstain from intercourse" (Lewis Solomon, 54). Whereas from Kant and Mandeville we could extract the principle "*coitus ad remedium masturbationis*" (coitus is the remedy for masturbation), from the modern mind ironically emerges the Pauline "*masturbatio ad remedium concupiscentiae*" (masturbation cures lust). (**Saint Paul** [5–64?] thought that ***marriage*** would serve as the remedy against sinful sexuality: Engaging in satisfying sex with one person on demand—via the marriage debt—will prevent one from engaging in satisfying sex promiscuously; 1 Cor. 7:1–5.)

At the same time, however, the twentieth century has hardly been kind to masturbation. In Freud's picture, "The masturbator forsakes reality, hindering the development of strong character traits. Masturbatory fantasies, especially, preclude the formation of healthy sublimations. The masturbator lives in accordance with the principle of lust and so is caught in psychical infantilism" (Groenendijk, 87; Freud, "Contributions to a Discussion," 251–52). For their part, twentieth-century philosophers have frequently found esoteric faults with masturbation. (A notable exception is Russell Vannoy's humanist treatment of masturbation; see *Sex without Love*, 111–17.) For Alan Goldman, "Voyeurism or viewing a pornographic movie qualifies as a sexual activity, but only as an imaginative substitute for the real thing. . . . The same is true of masturbation as a sexual activity without a partner" (270). The "real thing" for Goldman, presumably, is penis-vagina intercourse or, more likely, any two-party sexual event. **Thomas Nagel**, another philosopher, thinks that solitary masturbation, unlike mutual masturbation, does not exhibit the **completeness** of psychologically natural sexuality: The masturbator is not aware of the embodiment of another person and is not sensed as embodied by another. (Mutual masturbators are so aware.) This is why Nagel claims that "narcissistic practices" are "truncated or incomplete" versions "of the complete [sexual] configuration" (16–17). Yet another philosopher, Robert Solomon, offers this ingenious account:

> If sexuality is essentially a language, it follows that masturbation, while not a perversion, is a deviation. . . . Masturbation is not "self-abuse" . . . but it is, in an important sense, self-denial. It represents an inability or a refusal to say what one wants to say. . . . Masturbation is . . . essential as an ultimate retreat, but empty and without content. Masturbation is the sexual equivalent of a Cartesian soliloquy. ("Perversion," 283)

Each of these views of masturbation has been criticized in a way that focuses on the particular details of each one (Soble, "Masturbation"; *Sexual Investigations*, chap. 2). There is, in addition, a global criticism, one that finds questionable something that each account shares with the others.

Depairing It. What they all assume is that two-party sex is the primary or paradigmatic case of sexual activity. Nagel, for instance, uses the word "intercourse," which is ordinarily reserved to talk about two-party coitus, in an odd way, when he says that "intercourse with . . . inanimate objects" (17), such as the masturbatory activity of the shoe fetishist (9), is psychologically incomplete. Nagel's philosophical or psychological commitment to the paradigmatic quality of paired sex is apparently so strong that he *sees* solitary masturbation with a shoe as in some way or another a paired sexual activity. (Recall the foggy-minded fellow who sees necrophilia as paired sexual activity.) Similarly, James Giles, who analyzes **sexual desire** as "the desire for mutual baring and caressing of bodies"—thereby explicitly building "pairedness" into his definition of sexual desire—interprets the fetish object as a "fantasized body" or a body "extension" (353). This move, which is motivated to save his theory from a counterexample, seems disingenuous or desperate: In masturbating with shoes, where is the "baring" of the fetish object? (In "Fetishism" [152–53], Freud proposed that a man's fetish object was a substitute for a woman's/his mother's penis; see Kaite for a grandiose elaboration of this theme in her analysis of the symbolism in pornography. Havelock Ellis *excluded* solitary sexual activities with fetish objects from "autoerotism"; *Auto-erotism*, 161.) **Irving Singer** engages in a maneuver similar to Giles's. In his view, masturbation is not "paradigmatic of human sexuality. For that is characteristically a way of using one's body to communicate—directly or indirectly—with some other person. . . . Even in autoeroticism, it is as if one has become a second person to oneself" (20). So *X*'s masturbating *X* is *really X*'s rubbing *Y*—unless it is, instead, *Y*'s rubbing *X*. An interesting implication: Solitary, reflexive masturbation is *mutual* masturbation. (Singer may be conflating "autoerot[ic]ism" in Freud's sense ["On Narcissism," 73] and Ellis's.) And how did Goldman arrive at the street proposition that masturbation is not "the real thing"? The notion is suggested by his definition of sexual desire that, like Giles's, incorporates pairedness: Sexual desire, writes Goldman, is the "desire for contact with another person's body and for the pleasure which such contact produces" (268).

The curious (not necessarily "nutty") implications of these accounts of sexuality can be avoided were it conceded that sexuality is not primarily or paradigmatically a two-party affair. Besides, there is some reason for taking that thesis seriously. Suppose we were to ask: Which is primary or paradigmatic, my respecting (deceiving) others or my respecting (deceiving) myself? One would be hard-pressed to answer the question in the absence of knowing what philosophical work "primary" and "paradigmatic" were doing. Do we mean "primary" in an ontological sense or an analytic sense? Or do we mean it psychologically-developmentally?

The latter type of primacy perhaps yields a clue. In terms of the development and growth of the human person, masturbation, solitary sexuality, precedes two-party sexuality. Further, probably more solitary, unpaired masturbation takes place in our lives than two-party sex. For both these reasons, we might want to understand paired sex in terms of masturbation instead of trying to understand masturbation in terms of two-party sex. William Masters (1915–2001) and Virginia Johnson, according to Paul Robinson, "made masturbation the ultimate criterion of correct sexual behavior," at least in their laboratory (13). It can be argued, not altogether in vain, that the success of modern sexological research, from Freud on, derived from the heuristic value of assuming that sexuality is, at root, a solitary matter. One upshot of this reversal, clearly, is that coitus can very well be conceived of as just another form of masturbation. Adam Phillips—to return to a question we were not fully able to answer, viz., why people are so critical of masturbation and masturbators—furnishes illumination by linking the question with the psychological primacy of solitary sexuality. "[W]e fear [that masturbation] may be the truth about sex: that sex is something we do on our own," even when we are in bed with a congenial partner, for "our lovers are just a prompt or a hint to remind us of our own erotic delirium" (*Monogamy*, aphorism 101). Admitting that fact is too dangerous, so we protect ourselves by condemning masturbation. But if that fact is true, we can understand the somewhat surprising conclusion reached by a psychologist, after he asked 421 undergraduate students about their fantasies during intercourse, that "fantasizing during coitus," which was reported by a *majority* of the subjects, "is a normal component of sexual behavior" (Sue, 299, 304)—neither perverted nor immoral. We fantasize during sex with our partners as if they were not there and as if we were, once again, beating off or buttering the bagel with our favorite images. And when both of the sexual partners X and Y do it at the same time, this would be *dual* masturbation, even with the physical contact.

See also Activity, Sexual; Bestiality; Bible, Sex and the; Buddhism; Communication Model; Completeness, Sexual; Desire, Sexual; Ellis, Albert; Ellis, Havelock; Existentialism; Fantasy; Freud, Sigmund; Kant, Immanuel; Lacan, Jacques; Language; Nagel, Thomas; Paraphilia; Perversion, Sexual; Pornography; Sex Education; Thomas Aquinas (Saint)

REFERENCES

Augustine. (418?–421) *On Marriage and Concupiscence*. Trans. Peter Holmes. In Marcus Dods, ed., *Works*, vol. 12. Edinburgh, Scot.: T. and T. Clark, 1874, 93–202; Aurelius (Antoninus), Marcus. (167 CE) *The Meditations*. Trans. G.M.A. Grube. Indianapolis, Ind.: Bobbs-Merrill, 1963; Aurelius (Antoninus), Marcus. *The Meditations of Marcus Aurelius*. Trans. Meric Casaubon (1906). London: J. M. Dent, 1935; Betz, Hans Dieter. *The Sermon on the Mount*. Minneapolis, Minn.: Augsburg Fortress, 1995; Blackburn, Simon. *Lust: The Seven Deadly Sins*. New York: Oxford University

Press/New York Public Library, 2004; Bogart, John. "Commodification and Phenomenology: Evading Consent in Theory Regarding Rape." *Legal Theory* 2:3 (1996), 253–64; Cameron, J. M. "Sex in the Head." *New York Review of Books* (13 May 1976), 19–28; de Sousa, Ronald. *The Rationality of Emotion.* Cambridge, Mass.: MIT Press, 1987; Dearborn, Lester W. "Autoerotism." In Albert Ellis and Albert Abarbanel, eds., *The Encyclopedia of Sexual Behavior.* New York: Jason Aronson, 1973, 204–15; Dixon, Dwight, and Joan K. Dixon. "Autoeroticism." In Vern L. Bullough and Bonnie Bullough, eds., *Human Sexuality: An Encyclopedia.* New York: Garland, 1994, 53–55; Dodson, Betty. "How I Became the Guru of Female Sexual Liberation." In Bonnie Bullough, Vern L. Bullough, Marilyn A. Fithian, William E. Hartman, and Randy Sue Klein, eds., *Personal Stories of "How I Got Into Sex": Leading Researchers, Sex Therapists, Educators, Prostitutes, Sex Toy Designers, Sex Surrogates, Transsexuals, Criminologists, Clergy, and More . . .* Amherst, N.Y.: Prometheus, 1997, 122–30; Ellis, Havelock. (1899, 1900, 1910) *The Evolution of Modesty/The Phenomena of Sexual Periodicity/Auto-erotism.* In *Studies in the Psychology of Sex (1897–1928).* New York: Random House, 1936; Epstein, Louis M. (1948) "Wasting Nature." In *Sex Laws and Customs in Judaism.* New York: Ktav, 1967, 144–47; Finnis, John. "Law, Morality, and 'Sexual Orientation.' " *Notre Dame Law Review* 69:5 (1994), 1049–76; Francis, John J. (reporter) "Masturbation." ["Panel Report"] *Journal of the American Psychoanalytic Association* 16:1 (1968), 95–112; Francoeur, Robert T., Timothy Perper, Norman A. Scherzer, George P. Sellmer, and Martha Cornog. *A Descriptive Dictionary and Atlas of Sexology.* New York: Greenwood Press, 1991; Freud, Sigmund. (1912) "Contributions to a Discussion on Masturbation." In *The Standard Edition of the Complete Psychological Works of Sigmund Freud,* vol. 12. Trans. James Strachey. London: Hogarth Press, 1953–1974, 243–54; Freud, Sigmund. (1927) "Fetishism." In *The Standard Edition of the Complete Psychological Works of Sigmund Freud,* vol. 21. Trans. James Strachey. London: Hogarth Press, 1953–1974, 152–57; Freud, Sigmund. (1914) "On Narcissism: An Introduction." In *The Standard Edition of the Complete Psychological Works of Sigmund Freud,* vol. 14. Trans. James Strachey. London: Hogarth Press, 1953–1974, 73–102; Giles, James. "A Theory of Love and Sexual Desire." *Journal for the Theory of Social Behaviour* 24:4 (1994), 339–57; Glasner, (Rabbi) Samuel. "Judaism and Sex." In Albert Ellis and Albert Abarbanel, eds., *The Encyclopedia of Sexual Behavior.* New York: Jason Aronson, 1973, 575–84; Goldman, Alan. "Plain Sex." *Philosophy and Public Affairs* 6:3 (1977), 267–87; Green, Jonathon. *The Big Book of Filth.* London: Cassell, 1999; Groenendijk, Leendert F. "Masturbation and Neurasthenia: Freud and Stekel in Debate on the Harmful Effects of Autoeroticism." *Journal of Psychology and Human Sexuality* 9:1 (1997), 71–94; Haynes, James. "Masturbation." In Vern L. Bullough and Bonnie Bullough, eds., *Human Sexuality: An Encyclopedia.* New York: Garland, 1994, 381–85; Hite, Shere. "Masturbation." In *The Hite Report on Male Sexuality.* New York: Knopf, 1981, 485–525; Jenkins, Andrew P. "When Self-Pleasuring Becomes Self-Destruction: Autoerotic Asphyxiation Paraphilia." *International Electronic Journal of Health Education* 3:3 (2000), 208–16. <www.aahperd.org/iejhe/archive/jenkins.pdf> [accessed 28 October 2004]; Jordan, Mark D. "Masturbation, or Identity in Solitude." In *The Ethics of Sex.* Oxford, U.K.: Blackwell, 2002, 95–104; Kaite, Berkeley. *Pornography and Difference.* Bloomington: Indiana University Press, 1995; Kant, Immanuel. (1803) *Education.* Trans. Annette Churton. Ann Arbor: University of Michigan Press, 1960; Kant, Immanuel. (ca. 1780) *Lectures on Ethics.* Trans. Louis Infield. Indianapolis, Ind.: Hackett, 1989; Mandeville, Bernard. (1724) *A Modest Defence of Publick Stews.* Ed. Richard I. Cook. Los Angeles, Calif.: Augustan Reprint Society, Publication No. 162, 1973; Nagel, Thomas. "Sexual Perversion." In Alan Soble, ed., *The Philosophy of Sex: Contemporary Readings,* 4th ed. Lanham, Md.: Rowman and Littlefield, 2002, 9–20; Phillips, Adam. *Monogamy.* New York: Pantheon, 1996; Plato. (ca. 380 BCE) *Symposium.* Trans. Alexander Nehamas and Paul Woodruff. Indianapolis, Ind.: Hackett, 1989; Pollak, Richard. *The Creation of Dr. B: A Biography of Bruno Bettelheim.* New York: Simon and Schuster, 1997; Robinson, Paul. *The Modernization of Sex: Havelock Ellis, Alfred Kinsey, William Masters and Virginia Johnson.* New York: Harper and Row, 1976; Roth, Philip. *Portnoy's Complaint.* New York: Random House, 1969; Rousseau, Jean-Jacques. (1782) *The Confessions of Jean-Jacques Rousseau.* Trans. J. M. Cohen. New York: Penguin, 1979; Rousseau, Jean-Jacques. (1761) *Emile, or On Education.* Trans. Allan Bloom. New York: Basic Books, 1979;

Schopenhauer, Arthur. (1841) *On the Basis of Morality*. Trans. E.F.J. Payne. Indianapolis, Ind.: Hackett, 1995; Singer, Irving. (1973) *The Goals of Human Sexuality*. New York: Schocken, 1974; Soble, Alan. "Masturbation: Conceptual and Ethical Matters." In Alan Soble, ed., *The Philosophy of Sex: Contemporary Readings*, 4th ed. Lanham, Md.: Rowman and Littlefield, 2002, 67–94; Soble, Alan. *Sexual Investigations*. New York: New York University Press, 1996; Solomon, Lewis D. *The Jewish Tradition, Sexuality, and Procreation*. Lanham, Md.: University Press of America, 2002; Solomon, Robert C. "Sex and Perversion." In Robert B. Baker and Frederick A. Elliston, eds., *Philosophy and Sex*, 1st ed. Buffalo, N.Y.: Prometheus, 1975, 268–87; Solomon, Robert C. "Sexual Paradigms." In Alan Soble, ed., *The Philosophy of Sex: Contemporary Readings*, 4th ed. Lanham, Md.: Rowman and Littlefield, 2002, 21–29; Sue, David. "Erotic Fantasies of College Students during Coitus." *Journal of Sex Research* 15:4 (1979), 299–305; Szasz, Thomas S. "The New Product— Masturbatory Insanity." In *The Manufacture of Madness: A Comparative Study of the Inquisition and the Mental Health Movement*. New York: Harper and Row, 1970, 180–206; Thomas Aquinas. (1265–1273) *Summa theologiae*, 60 vols. Trans. Blackfriars. Cambridge, U.K.: Blackfriars, 1964–1976; Vannoy, Russell. *Sex without Love: A Philosophical Exploration*. Buffalo, N.Y.: Prometheus, 1980; Ward, Keith. *The Development of Kant's View of Ethics*. Oxford, U.K.: Basil Blackwell, 1972; Whiteley, C. H., and Winifred N. Whiteley. *Sex and Morals*. New York: Basic Books, 1967; Wills, Garry. "Bill & the Emperor." *New York Review of Books* (8 October 1998), 53; "Words for Female Masturbation." <www.AdultToyReviews.com/words/fmstword.html> [accessed 15 February 2005]; "Words for Male Masturbation." <www.AdultToyReviews.com/words/mmstword.html> [accessed 15 February 2005].

Alan Soble

ADDITIONAL READING

Bennett, Paula, and Vernon A. Rosario, eds. *Solitary Pleasures: The Historical, Literary, and Artistic Discourses of Autoeroticism*. New York: Routledge, 1995; Budapest, Zsuzsanna E. "Self-Blessing Ritual." In Carol P. Christ and Judith Plaskow, eds., *Womanspirit Rising: A Feminist Reader in Religion*. San Francisco, Calif.: Harper and Row, 1979, 269–72; Burger, John R. *One-Handed Histories: The Eroto-Politics of Gay Male Video Pornography*. New York: Haworth Press, 1995; Butterworth, Dianne. (1993) "Wanking in Cyberspace: The Development of Computer Porn." In Stevi Jackson and Sue Scott, eds., *Feminism and Sexuality: A Reader*. New York: Columbia University Press, 1996, 314–20; Cornog, Martha. *The Big Book of Masturbation: From Angst to Zeal*. San Francisco, Calif.: Down There Press, 2003; Dodson, Betty. *Liberating Masturbation: A Meditation on Self Love*. New York: Betty Dodson, 1978; Dorff, Elliot N. "Masturbation." In *Matters of Life and Death: A Jewish Approach to Modern Medical Ethics*. Philadelphia, Pa.: Jewish Publication Society, 1998, 116–20; Elders, M. Joycelyn. "The Dreaded M Word[:] It's Not a Four-Letter Word." *Nerve* (26 June 1997). <www.nerve.com/dispatches/elders/mword/> [accessed 2 February 2005]; Ellis, Albert. "Masturbation." *Journal of Social Therapy* 1:3 (1955), 141–43. Reprinted, abridged, in Manfred F. DeMartino, ed., *Sexual Behavior and Personality Characteristics*. New York: Grove Press, 1963, 255–57; Ellis, Albert. (1958) "New Light on Masturbation." In *Sex without Guilt*. New York: Lyle Stuart, 1963, 15–25; Engelhardt, H. Tristram, Jr. "The Disease of Masturbation: Values and the Concept of Disease." *Bulletin of the History of Medicine* 48 (Summer 1974), 234–48. Reprinted in Tom Beauchamp and LeRoy Walters, eds., *Contemporary Issues in Bioethics*. Encino, Calif.: Dickenson, 1978, 109–13; Epstein, Louis M. *Sex Laws and Customs in Judaism*. New York: Bloch, 1948. Reprinted with new matter, New York: Ktav, 1967; Finnis, John M. "Law, Morality, and 'Sexual Orientation.'" *Notre Dame Law Review* 69:5 (1994), 1049–76. Reprinted, revised, in *Notre Dame Journal of Law, Ethics, and Public Policy* 9:1 (1995), 11–39; and John Corvino, ed., *Same Sex: Debating the Ethics, Science, and Culture of Homosexuality*. Lanham, Md.: Rowman and Littlefield, 1997, 31–43; Fortunata, Jacqueline. "Masturbation and Women's Sexuality." In Alan Soble, ed., *The Philosophy of Sex: Contemporary Readings*, 1st ed. Totowa, N.J.: Rowman and Littlefield, 1980, 389–408; Fracher, Jeffrey, and Michael S. Kimmel. "Hard Issues and Soft Spots: Counseling

Men about Sexuality." In Michael S. Kimmel and Michael A. Messner, eds., *Men's Lives*. New York: Macmillan, 1989, 471–82. 3rd ed., Needham Heights, Mass.: Allyn and Bacon, 1995, 365–74; Frijling-Schreuder, Elisabeth. "On Masturbation." In John Money and Herman Musaph, eds., *Handbook of Sexology*. Amsterdam, Holland: Excerpta Medica, 1977, 1139–44; Goldman, Alan. "Plain Sex." *Philosophy and Public Affairs* 6:3 (1977), 267–87. Reprinted in HS (103–23); POS1 (119–38); POS2 (73–92); POS3 (39–55); POS4 (39–55); Greenblatt, Stephen. "Me, Myself, and I." [Review of *Solitary Sex: A Cultural History of Masturbation*, by Thomas W. Laqueur] *New York Review of Books* (8 April 2004), 32–36; Kant, Immanuel. "Duties towards the Body in Respect of Sexual Impulse." In *Lectures on Ethics*. Trans. Louis Infield. New York: Methuen, 1930. Indianapolis, Ind.: Hackett, 1980, 162–71. Reprinted in POS4 (199–205); STW (140–45); Kielkopf, Charles. "Masturbation: A Kantian Condemnation." *Philosophia* 25:1–4 (1997), 223–46; Laqueur, Thomas W. *Solitary Sex: A Cultural History of Masturbation*. New York: Zone Books, 2003; Laumann, Edward O., John H. Gagnon, Robert T. Michael, and Stuart Michaels. "Masturbation." In *The Social Organization of Sexuality: Sexual Practices in the United States*. Chicago, Ill.: University of Chicago Press, 1994, 80–86; Macfadden, Bernarr. "Masturbation." In *Womanhood and Marriage*. New York: Physical Culture Corporation, 1918, 250–65; Maines, Rachel P. *The Technology of Orgasm: "Hysteria," the Vibrator, and Women's Sexual Satisfaction*. Baltimore, Md.: Johns Hopkins University Press, 1999; The Masturbation Home Page. "Frequently Asked Questions." <www.masturbationpage.com/asmfaq.html> [accessed 21 October 2004]; Nagel, Thomas. "Sexual Perversion." *Journal of Philosophy* 66:1 (1969), 5–17. Reprinted in P&S1 (247–60); P&S2 (268–79); POS1 (76–88). Reprinted, revised, in Thomas Nagel, *Mortal Questions*. Cambridge: Cambridge University Press, 1979, 39–52; Eugene F. Rogers, Jr., ed., *Theology and Sexuality: Classic and Contemporary Readings*. Oxford, U.K.: Blackwell, 2002, 125–36; and P&S3 (326–36); POS2 (39–51); POS3 (9–20); POS4 (9–20); STW (105–12); Nobus, Dany. "Over My Dead Body: On the Histories and Cultures of Necrophilia." In Robin Goodwin and Duncan Cramer, eds., *Inappropriate Relationships: The Unconventional, the Disapproved, and the Forbidden*. Mahwah, N.J.: Erlbaum, 2002, 171–89; Randall, Hilary E., and E. Sandra Byers. "What Is Sex? Students' Definitions of Having Sex, Sexual Partner, and Unfaithful Sexual Behaviour." *Canadian Journal of Human Sexuality* 12:2 (2003), 87–96; Roberta, Jean. Review of *The Big Book of Masturbation: From Angst to Zeal*, by Martha Cornog. *Cleansheets* (1 October 2003). <www.cleansheets.com/reviews/book_10.01.03.shtml> [accessed 16 February 2005]. Reprinted as "The Sound of One Hand Stroking." *Batteries Not Included* 11:2 (2004), 8–9; Roth, Philip. "Afterword to the Twenty-fifth-Anniversary Edition." In *Portnoy's Complaint*. New York: Vintage, 1994, 277–89; Russell, Bertrand. (1926) "Sex Education." In *On Education, Especially in Early Childhood*. London, U.K.: Unwin, 1973, 115–21; Sarnoff, Suzanne, and Irving Sarnoff. *Sexual Excitement/Sexual Peace: The Place of Masturbation in Adult Relationships*. New York: M. Evans, 1979; Satlow, Michael L. " 'Wasted Seed': The History of a Rabbinic Idea." *Hebrew Union College Annual* 65 (1994), 137–69; Soble, Alan. "Masturbation." *Pacific Philosophical Quarterly* 61:3 (1980), 233–44. Reprinted in HS (139–50). Revised as "Masturbation and Sexual Philosophy," POS2 (133–57). Revised again as "Masturbation," POS3 (67–85), and reprinted in David Benatar, ed., *Ethics for Everyday*. NY: McGraw-Hill, 2002, 180–96. Revised again as "Masturbation: Conceptual and Ethical Matters," POS4 (67–94); reprinted, abridged, as "Philosophies of Masturbation," in Martha Cornog, author and ed., *The Big Book of Masturbation: From Angst to Zeal*. San Francisco, Calif.: Down There Press, 2003, 149–66; Solomon, Robert C. "Sex, Contraception, and Conceptions of Sex." In S. F. Spicker, W. B. Bondeson, and H. T. Engelhardt, eds., *The Contraceptive Ethos*. Dordrecht, Holland: Reidel, 1987, 223–40. Reprinted in G. Lee Bowie, Meredith W. Michaels, and Kathleen Higgins, eds., *Thirteen Questions in Ethics*, 2nd ed. Fort Worth, Tex.: Harcourt Brace Jovanovich, 1992, 95–107; Solomon, Robert C. "Sexual Paradigms." *Journal of Philosophy* 71:11 (1974), 336–45. Reprinted in HS (81–90); POS1 (89–98); POS2 (53–62); POS3 (21–29); POS4 (21–29); Stengers, Jean, and Anne Van Neck. *Masturbation: The History of a Great Terror*. Trans. Kathryn A. Hoffman. New York: Palgrave, 2001; Tiefer, Leonore. Review of *Sexual Excitement/Sexual Peace: The Place of Masturbation in Adult Relationships*, by Suzanne Sarnoff and Irving Sarnoff. *Psychology of Women Quarterly* 8:1 (1983), 107–9.

MEAD, MARGARET (1901–1978). Margaret Mead, an American anthropologist and social commentator, was, at Columbia University, a student of Franz Boas (1858–1942), a founder of American anthropology. She was also a student (and eventual collaborator and lover) of anthropologist Ruth Benedict (1887–1948) (Banner, 3, 225–26). In the 1920s and 1930s, Mead did fieldwork in six societies in the Pacific Ocean, New Guinea, and Bali, Indonesia. Her work focused on hitherto neglected topics such as child rearing and women's role in society. Along with Gregory Bateson (1904–1980), her third husband, she pioneered the use of photography in ethnography (see Sullivan).

Mead's first book, *Coming of Age in Samoa* (1928), based on her field research, was a bestseller. Written to refute G. Stanley Hall's (1844–1924) account of adolescence as unavoidably troubled due to biological factors (see his *Adolescence*), *Coming of Age* pictured most Samoan youth as enjoying a period of relatively easy sexual and social exploration, despite a lack of cultural encouragement of "individuality" or personality differentiation.

In *Sex and Temperament in Three Primitive Societies* (1935), based on her field work in New Guinea and on the studies of Bateson and Reo Fortune (1903–1979), her second husband, Mead described cultures in which stereotypical American gender relations were not observed. Among the Arapesh, both men and women were socialized to act in "feminine" patterns; among the Mundugumor, they were to act according to broadly "masculine" gender roles; and among the Tchambuli, the patterns were generally the reverse of American gender roles. The argument that gender was largely the result of socialization and not biology was the theoretical importance of these studies.

Later, Mead developed a view of human sexuality in *Male and Female* (1949) that placed more emphasis on the role of biological sexual differences that are rooted in reproductive biology (see Sanday). Nonetheless, she advocated greater acceptance of social and cultural variation. For example, "The time has come . . . when we must recognize bisexuality as a normal form of human behavior" ("Bisexuality," 269). Mead wrote a column for the women's magazine *Redbook* for many years as well as a number of popular books on a variety of subjects. She eventually became a leading advocate of liberal and reformist social and political positions.

After her death, Australian anthropologist Derek Freeman (*Margaret Mead and Samoa*) attacked Mead's *Coming of Age* as based on substandard research. Considerable controversy ensued, both in academic anthropology and among the reading public. Freeman subsequently argued that Mead had taken too seriously the exaggerations and falsehoods related to her by her teenage research informants (*The Fateful Hoaxing*). Many outside anthropology, particularly among political conservatives and evolutionary psychologists, have accepted Freeman's studies as adequately debunking, as spurious and unwarranted, Mead's evidential support for the cultural determination of gender. Others, however, continue to cite Mead as an inspirational role model (for example, Newton). Sufficient evidence to resolve the controversy about Mead's studies may be unobtainable (see Orans).

See also Bisexuality; Feminism, Lesbian; Freud, Sigmund; Freudian Left, The; Herdt, Gilbert; Money, John; Orientation, Sexual; Social Constructionism

REFERENCES

Banner, Lois W. *Intertwined Lives: Margaret Mead, Ruth Benedict, and Their Circle*. New York: Knopf, 2003; Freeman, Derek. *The Fateful Hoaxing of Margaret Mead: A Historical Analysis of Her Samoan Research*. Boulder, Colo.: Westview, 1999; Freeman, Derek. *Margaret Mead and Samoa: The Making and Unmaking of an Anthropological Myth*. Cambridge, Mass.: Harvard University Press,

1983; Hall, G. Stanley. *Adolescence: Its Psychology and Its Relation to Physiology, Anthropology, Sociology, Sex, Crime, Religion, and Education.* New York: Appleton, 1904; Mead, Margaret. "Bisexuality: A New Awareness." In Margaret Mead and Rhoda Metraux, *Aspects of the Present.* New York: Morrow, 1980, 269–75. Reprinted from *Redbook* (January 1975); Mead, Margaret. (1928) *Coming of Age in Samoa: A Psychological Study of Primitive Youth for Western Civilization.* New York: Morrow, 1968; Mead, Margaret. *Male and Female: A Study of the Sexes in a Changing World.* New York: Morrow, 1949; Mead, Margaret. (1935) *Sex and Temperament in Three Primitive Societies.* New York: Morrow, 1963; Newton, Esther. *Margaret Mead Made Me Gay: Personal Essays, Public Ideas.* Durham, N.C.: Duke University Press, 2000; Orans, Martin. *Not Even Wrong: Margaret Mead, Derek Freeman, and the Samoans.* Novato, Calif.: Chandler and Sharp, 1996; Sanday, Peggy Reeves. "Margaret Mead's View of Sex Roles in Her Own and Other Societies." *American Anthropologist* 82:2 (1980), 340–48; Sullivan, Gerald. *Margaret Mead, Gregory Bateson, and Highland Bali: Fieldwork Photographs of Bayung Gedé, 1936–1939.* Chicago, Ill.: University of Chicago Press, 1999.

Robert A. Strikwerda

ADDITIONAL READING

Bateson, Mary Catherine. *With a Daughter's Eye: A Memoir of Margaret Mead and Gregory Bateson.* New York: Morrow, 1984; Davenport, William. "Sexual Patterns in a Southwest Pacific Society." In Ruth Brecher and Edward Brecher, eds., *An Analysis of* Human Sexual Response. New York: New American Library, 1966, 175–200; Library of Congress. "Margaret Mead: Human Nature and the Power of Culture." <www.loc.gov/exhibits/mead/> [accessed 1 July 2004]; Mead, Margaret. "On Freud's View of Female Psychology." In Jean Strouse, ed., *Women and Analysis: Dialogues on Psychoanalytic Views of Femininity.* New York: Grossman, 1974, 95–106; Mead, Margaret. (1962) "The Social Shotgun" ("Sex on the Campus"). In Henry Anatole Grunwald, ed., *Sex in America.* New York: Bantam, 1964, 108–11; Mead, Margaret. "What the Future Holds." In John Money and Herman Musaph, eds., *Handbook of Sexology.* Amsterdam, Holland: Excerpta Medica, 1977, 801–5; Mead, Margaret, and Rhoda Metraux. *Aspects of the Present.* New York: Morrow, 1980; Rapp, Linda. "Mead, Margaret (1901–1978)." *GLBTQ* Web site. <www.glbtq.com/social-sciences/mead_m,2.html> [accessed 15 February 2005].

MEN'S FEMINISM. *See* Feminism, Men's

MERLEAU-PONTY, MAURICE. *See* Phenomenology

MILITARY, SEX AND THE. There are three significant topics at the intersection of the philosophy of sex and the military: **homosexuality** (gays and lesbians as soldiers); **rape** (carried out by invading and victorious forces); and **sexual harassment** (made acute by the military's extensive hierarchy of authority).

Homosexuality. Randy Shilts (1951–1994) has suggested that "[f]or both men and women, the story of gays in the military is a story about manhood" (5). Throughout history, there have been shifts in conceptions of manhood (or masculinity) and thus varying attitudes about the suitability of homosexuals for military service. Around 378 BCE, for example, the elite unit of the army of Thebes, "the Sacred Band," was formed, composed exclusively of pairs of homosexual lovers (see **Plato** [427–347 BCE], *Symposium*, 178d–179b, and 10n.11). Following a pattern common in the Greek-speaking world, these pairs consisted of a boy in his teens (the *erōmenos*, the beloved) and an older man (the *erastēs*, the lover). The *erastēs* served as mentor, instructor, and guardian of the *erōmenos*; the *erastēs* also took sexual delight in the company of the *erōmenos*. In this dynamic, unbalanced relationship, "the desire of the erastes to excel in the eyes of his eromenos was a spur to his courage . . . [while] the eromenos wished to live up to example set by the erastes" (Dover, *Greek Homosexuality*, 191; "The Date of Plato's *Symposium*," 12–16). The homosexuality of these lovers did not impugn their manhood; nor did it make them unfit to be soldiers. Sparta was another Greek city-state in which the relationship between *erastēs* and *erōmenos* was put to military advantage, although whether this relationship had a sexual component is controversial. Official Spartan policy limited physical contact between *erastēs* and *erōmenos* to the clasping of right hands, and the Spartan legislator Lykourgos forbid sexual relations between *erastēs* and *erōmenos*, insisting that a beloved be chosen for his good character and not physical **beauty**. Nevertheless, "references to particular homosexual attachments of Spartans are conspicuous even by Greek standards" (Powell, 229; see Dover, *Greek*, chap. 4).

This same dynamic of man-boy **love** in a military context occurs in the Japanese samurai tradition. Ihara Saikaku devotes half of *The Great Mirror of Male Love* (1687) to stories about samurai and their teenage lovers. The roles played by the adult male samurai (*nenja*) and the teenage boy (*wakashu*) parallel those of the Greek *erastēs-erōmenos* relationship. The *nenja* "was supposed to provide social backing, emotional support, and a model of manliness" for the young *wakashu*, who in turn "was expected to be worthy of his lover by being a good student of samurai manhood" (Schalow, "Introduction," *Great Mirror*, 27). As with some of the Greeks, *nenja* and *wakashu* were also erotically involved.

At the end of the twentieth century, some Western countries loosened, to various degrees, restrictions on the presence of homosexuals in their armed forces. The facts that this loosening involved a reversal of long-standing policies against homosexuals serving in the military and that such changes were often fraught with acrimonious social controversy reveal how far removed modern thinking is from that of the ancients regarding homosexuality, masculinity, and military service. In most cases, the late-twentieth-century liberalization of participation by homosexuals in the military was part of a larger effort to ban discrimination against homosexuals in many other areas. It was buttressed by a wealth of evidence—from psychiatry, organizational and social psychology, and the experiences of homosexuals who have served in the military—showing that homosexuality does not preclude a person from serving effectively in the military (see the National Defense Research Institute's *Sexual Orientation and U.S. Military Personnel Policy*).

In 1993 the United States adopted what has come to be known as the "Don't Ask, Don't Tell" policy that suspended questioning a person about his or her **sexual orientation** as part of the process for determining an individual's suitability for military service. (The text of the law appears in the Appendix of Belkin and Bateman.) "Don't Ask, Don't Tell" constitutes a major departure from previous U.S. policy, which had viewed homosexuals serving in the military as threats to national security, good order, and discipline and as sexual predators (see Haggerty). Nevertheless, deep ambivalence about the suitability of homosexuals for military service remained into the twenty-first century: Open acknowledgment of one's homosexuality continued to be grounds for separation from the U.S. armed forces, and committing sodomy was grounds for court-martial.

Criticism of "Don't Ask, Don't Tell" came from conservatives who thought the policy too lenient. Criticism, however, was not limited to those who opposed admitting homosexuals into the military. Richard Mohr, a leading gay American philosopher, contends that the policy "is not one which can be morally acceptable to gays, or indeed to anyone who has respect for human beings" (112). For example, it perpetuates the debilitating closeting of gays and lesbians as much as did their outright prohibition from serving in the military (see Card, "Military Ban"). Further, by treating homosexuality as not worthy of being discussed openly or acknowledged, the "Don't Ask, Don't Tell" policy equates homosexuality with the "horrible, the disgusting, the loathsome, the unspeakably gross," since it is only "around these . . . abject matters that society sets up rituals of the form Don't Ask, Don't Tell (Mohr, 113). Some evidence for this thesis is provided by the fact that many heterosexual married couples implicitly adopt a domestic "Don't Ask, Don't Tell" policy about their extramarital sexual affairs—where, it might be assumed, they view **adultery** as one of those unspeakable, loathsome, horrible phenomena. (In reply, however, some have quipped that if "Don't Ask, Don't Tell" is good enough for heterosexual members of the institution of **marriage**, it is good enough for gay members of the institution of the military.)

Rape. During the World War II battle between U.S. and Japanese forces for the island of Okinawa, roughly 10,000 rapes occurred (see Mercier). According to conservative estimates, "110,000 women were raped in the Berlin area" in the first few months of Allied occupation of that city at the end of World War II (Seifert, 54). Within a nine-month period in 1971, up to 400,000 Bangladeshi women were raped by West Pakistani troops (Brownmiller, "War," 80). The mass rape of Bosnian and Croatian women, which occurred in camps set up for the purpose, appears to have been an integral part of the military tactics used by Serbian forces in the early 1990s (Allen, 41–86). During World War II, the Japanese established similar camps in which Korean and Southeast Asian "comfort women" were made available to soldiers (WordiQ; see Brownmiller, "War," 56–63). These and countless other cases testify to the fact that rape is endemic to warfare. A civilian population caught in a war zone is vulnerable to abuse: Law and order have broken down; most able-bodied men are preoccupied with fighting; and enemy troops, answerable only to commanding officers who might encourage the rapes, or do not care, or simply *look the other way*, have ample opportunity to terrorize unarmed, unprotected women. Women raped under such circumstances suffer physical and emotional trauma; some endure the further indignity of unwanted pregnancy. As a result, for example, the Serbian policy of mass rape drove many of its Muslim and Croatian victims to desperate measures: risky third-trimester abortions, infanticide, and suicide (Allen, 98–99; see Stiglmayer, "The Rapes," 131–37).

Feminist philosopher Claudia Card argues that a fundamental function of rape "is to display, communicate, and produce or maintain *dominance*" ("Rape," 7). In wartime, the rape of the women of one's enemies sends a message of domination not only to the female victims but also to male combatants. The rapes, and the message they carry, can be deeply demoralizing, causing great shame and humiliation. In this way rape becomes another weapon of war, one capable of psychologically weakening the enemy (see also Brownmiller, "Making Female Bodies the Battlefield"; Seifert, 59).

Robert Smith, arguing from a sociobiological perspective, offers a different explanation of the prevalence of rape during wartime. He analyzes it as one among many reproductive strategies available to men: It is a form of violent marital infidelity, an opportunity for the men to impregnate women and thereby reproduce, at little cost, outside their primary pair bond. Warfare facilitates rape because it affords access to vulnerable females and "the risks of punishment and detection are low" (634). In support of his theory, Smith cites evidence that rapes result in higher-than-average rates of pregnancy (see also Ridley, chap. 6; Shields and Shields; yet contrast Stanford). Opposing the notion that rape is an evolved male reproductive strategy is the fact that "one out of three has trouble performing sexually during the act" (Seifert, 56). Of course, the significance of rape (in or out of war) from the perspective of **evolution** has been a controversial area.

Beverly Allen argues that the conflict in Bosnia-Herzegovina in the 1990s is noteworthy for the role that rape played in Serbian "ethnic cleansing," a process whereby non-Serbs were removed, through force or intimidation, from land areas the Serbs wished to incorporate into "Greater Serbia." Allen describes the ways rape facilitated ethnic cleansing. Some women were killed after being raped. Others were raped in the presence of family and friends, who were then given the "opportunity" by Serbian soldiers to vacate the area to prevent further atrocities. And some women were raped until they became pregnant, held captive until the sixth or seventh month of gestation, and returned to their communities. In reasoning that defies both logic and science, the Serbian idea was that the children of these forced pregnancies would be purely Serb without a trace of the ethnic and cultural identities of their non-Serb mothers. The Serbian policy "whereby impregnation by rape equals genocide depends entirely on the rapists' capacity to deny any identity of their victims other than that as a sexual container" (97; see MacKinnon). By contrast, Susan Brownmiller denies that there is anything particularly unique about the Serbian policy of mass rape in Bosnia-Herzegovina. Women's bodies are customarily viewed as part of the spoils of war, booty to be plundered by conquering soldiers ("Making Female Bodies the Battlefield").

Sexual Harassment. In a survey of around 500 women veterans of the U.S. military (conducted from March 1992 to March 1993), 37 percent of those aged fifty or older and 90 percent of those under fifty reported having been sexually harassed (Murdoch and Nichol). In a U.S. Department of Defense (DoD) survey of 20,000 military personnel conducted in 1988, 64 percent of female respondents reported at least one incident of sexual harassment during the preceding year (Martindale, 11–15). In a similar survey conducted seven years later, 55 percent of female respondents reported having been sexually harassed in the preceding year (Bastian et al., iii–viii). The extent of sexual harassment in the U.S. military may be even greater than these numbers indicate (as in other venues where harassment occurs), since some women do not report the events to their superiors either because they are skeptical that anything will be done or they fear reprisal (Francke, chap. 6; Nelson, pt. 1). Over a third of the women who did report incidents of sexual harassment contended that either nothing was done or that their complaints were not taken seriously (Bastian et al.). Moreover, some female military personnel chose to endure sexual harassment and abuse without lodging a complaint because they feared being labeled a lesbian, a charge that could result in separation from the military (Francke, chap. 6; Shilts, 489–98).

All the service branches and the DoD have policies proscribing sexual harassment. The DoD issued its first policy directive in 1981 shortly after problems with sexual harassment in the military surfaced during congressional hearings. But these policies have been less than fully effective. Some critics have argued that this is not merely an accident. Sexual harassment is not a punishable offense under the Uniform Code of Military Justice. Further, the DoD policy locates primary responsibility for resolving complaints of sexual harassment within the chain of command, despite the abundance of documented incidents of female subordinates being sexually harassed by male superiors (Bastian et al.). Linda Francke blames the "masculine forces driving military culture" for the military's inability to deal effectively with sexual harassment. She also suggests that the "systematic denigration of feminine attributes in the making of a military man required the very harassment the directives were supposed to eradicate" (157). Francke's proposal for remedying the situation is for the military to rescind combat exclusion rules that prevent women from serving in assignments with a high likelihood of physical contact with the enemy; indeed, "the jobs and career fields closed to women are the very ones that lead to the highest levels of command and responsibility" (Whitman, 465). The net result is that women are condemned to a kind of second-class status within the military and fail to gain authority in the military hierarchy, on a par with men, that could effectively combat sexual harassment.

Unlike sexual harassment, fraternization (social and sexual mixing) does fall under the Uniform Code of Military Justice. Article 134 forbids fraternization between officers and enlisted personnel when such behavior threatens "good order and discipline" or threatens to bring discredit to the armed forces. The service branches have more stringent policies on fraternization than the DoD: They regulate "nonprofessional" relationships between any two persons of different grade or rank, and among the relationships they forbid are those that merely *appear* to undermine proper military authority (Whitman, 452). Respect for military authority is an essential feature of good order and discipline that, in turn, is indispensable to maintaining combat effectiveness. Stringent policies on fraternization may well be warranted "because senior personnel could influence if not virtually control a subordinate's assignments, promotions, even the degree of danger into which he or she could be sent." Hence "any perceived favoritism toward an individual [is] a cohesion and morale buster among other troops" (Franke, 263; see Whitman, 452). Although certain kinds of nonprofessional relationships must be strictly prohibited, such as that between an officer and an enlisted person under his or her direct command, human relationships are complex and variable. To determine the likelihood that a relationship might lessen respect for military authority, and to that extent undermine good order and discipline, "the full and particular circumstances need to be taken into account" (Whitman, 459). For this reason, policies on fraternization should be sufficiently "flexible" and "elastic" to allow commanders ample discretionary powers in enforcing them. Rigid, inflexible rules governing intimate relationships may place unrealistic and unjust demands on the private lives and loves of military personnel (Whitman, 458–59).

See also Adultery; Greek Sexuality and Philosophy, Ancient; Harassment, Sexual; Homosexuality, Ethics of; Marriage, Same-Sex; Plato; Privacy; Psychology, Evolutionary; Rape; Violence, Sexual

REFERENCES

Allen, Beverly. *Rape Warfare: The Hidden Genocide in Bosnia-Herzegovina and Croatia*. Minneapolis: University of Minnesota Press, 1996; Bastian, Linda, Anita Lancaster, and Heidi Reyst. *Department of Defense 1995 Sexual Harassment Survey* (Report No. 96–104). Arlington, Va.: Defense Manpower Center, 1996; Belkin, Aaron, and Geoffrey Bateman, eds. *Don't Ask, Don't Tell: Debating the Gay Ban in the Military*. Boulder, Colo.: Lynne Reinner, 2003; Brownmiller, Susan. "Making Female Bodies the Battlefield." *Newsweek* (4 January 1993), 37; Brownmiller, Susan. "War." In *Against Our Will: Men, Women, and Rape*. New York: Simon and Schuster, 1975, 31–113; Card, Claudia. "The Military Ban and the ROTC: A Study in Closeting." In Timothy F. Murphy, ed., *Gay Ethics: Controversies in Outing, Civil Rights, and Sexual Science*. Binghamton, N.Y.: Harrington Park Press, 1994, 117–46; Card, Claudia. "Rape as a Weapon of War." *Hypatia* 11:4 (1996), 5–18; Dover, Kenneth. "The Date of Plato's *Symposium*." *Phronesis* 10:1 (1965), 2–20; Dover, Kenneth. *Greek Homosexuality*. Cambridge, Mass.: Harvard University Press, 1978; Francke, Linda. *Ground Zero: The Gender Wars in the Military*. New York: Simon and Schuster, 1997; Haggerty, Timothy. "History Repeating Itself: A Historical Overview of Gay Men and Lesbians in the Military before 'Don't Ask, Don't Tell.'" In Aaron Belkin and Geoffrey Bateman, eds., *Don't Ask, Don't Tell: Debating the Gay Ban in the Military*. Boulder, Colo.: Lynne Reinner, 2003, 9–49; MacKinnon,

Catharine A. "Turning Rape into Pornography: Postmodern Genocide." *Ms.* (July–August 1993), 24–30; Martindale, Melanie. *Sexual Harassment in the Military: 1988.* Arlington, Va.: Defense Manpower Center, 1990; Mercier, Rick. "Way Off Base: The Shameful History of Military Rape in Okinawa." *On the Issues* 6:1 (1997), 29–31; Mohr, Richard. "Understanding Gays in the Military." In *A More Perfect Union: Why Straight America Must Stand Up for Gay Rights.* Boston, Mass.: Beacon Press, 1994, 112–19; Murdoch, Maureen, and Kristin Nichol. "Women Veterans' Experiences with Domestic Violence and Sexual Harassment While in the Military." *Archives of Family Medicine* 4 (May 1995), 411–18; National Defense Research Institute. *Sexual Orientation and U.S. Military Personnel Policy: Options and Assessment* (MR-323-OSD). Santa Monica, Calif.: Rand, 1993; Nelson, Terri Spahr. *For Love of Country: Confronting Rape and Sexual Harassment in the U.S. Military.* Binghamton, N.Y.: Haworth Maltreatment and Trauma Press, 2002; Plato. (ca. 380 BCE) *Symposium.* Trans. Alexander Nehamas and Paul Woodruff. Indianapolis, Ind.: Hackett, 1989; Powell, Anton. (1988) *Athens and Sparta: Constructing Greek Political and Social History from 478 B.C.*, 2nd ed. London: Routledge, 2001; Ridley, Matt. *The Red Queen: Sex and the Evolution of Human Nature.* New York: Macmillan, 1994; Saikaku, Ihara. (1687) *The Great Mirror of Male Love.* Trans. Paul Gordon Schalow. Stanford, Calif.: Stanford University Press, 1990; Seifert, Ruth. "War and Rape: A Preliminary Analysis." In Alexandra Stiglmayer, ed., *Mass Rape: The War against Women in Bosnia-Herzegovina.* Lincoln: University of Nebraska Press, 1994, 54–72; Shields, William, and Lea Shields. "Forcible Rape: An Evolutionary Perspective." *Ethology and Sociobiology* 4:3 (1983), 115–36; Shilts, Randy. *Conduct Unbecoming: Lesbians and Gays in the U.S. Military. Vietnam to the Persian Gulf.* New York: St. Martin's Press, 1993; Smith, Robert. "Human Sperm Competition." In Robert Smith, ed., *Sperm Competition and the Evolution of Animal Mating Systems.* Orlando, Fla.: Academic Press, 1984, 601–59; Stanford, Craig B. "Darwinians Look at Rape, Sex, and War." *American Scientist* 88:4 (2000), 360–68; Stiglmayer, Alexandra. "The Rapes in Bosnia-Herzegovina." In Alexandra Stiglmayer, ed., *Mass Rape: The War against Women in Bosnia-Herzegovina.* Lincoln: University of Nebraska Press, 1994, 82–173; Whitman, Jeffrey P. "Women, Sex, and the Military." *Public Affairs Quarterly* 12:4 (1998), 447–69; WordiQ. (Web site) "Comfort Women." <www.wordiq.com/definition/Comfort_women> [accessed 25 August 2004].

Jeffrey Hershfield

ADDITIONAL READING

Baird, Robert, and M. Katherine Baird, eds. *Homosexuality: Debating the Issues.* "Part Four: Homosexuality and the Military." Amherst, N.Y.: Prometheus, 1995, 151–99; Brownmiller, Susan. "Making Female Bodies the Battlefield." *Newsweek* (4 January 1993), 37. Reprinted in Alexandra Stiglmayer, ed., *Mass Rape: The War against Women in Bosnia-Herzegovina.* Lincoln: University of Nebraska Press, 1994, 180–82; Cammermeyer, Margarethe, and Chris Fisher. *Serving in Silence.* New York: Viking, 1994; Card, Claudia. "The Military Ban and the ROTC: A Study in Closeting." In Timothy F. Murphy, ed., *Gay Ethics: Controversies in Outing, Civil Rights, and Sexual Science.* Binghamton, N.Y.: Harrington Park Press, 1994, 117–46. [*Journal of Homosexuality* 27: 3–4 (1994), 117–46]; Chan, Connie S. "Don't Ask, Don't Tell, Don't Know: Sexual Identity and Expression among East Asian-American Lesbians." In B. Zimmerman and T.A.H. McNaron, eds., *The New Lesbian Studies: Into the Twenty-First Century.* New York: Feminist Press at CUNY, 1996, 91–97; Coyle, Bonnie, Diana Wolan, and Andrea Van Horn. "The Prevalence of Physical and Sexual Abuse in Women Veterans Seeking Care at a Veterans Affairs Medical Center." *Military Medicine* 161:10 (1996), 588–93; Davenport, Manuel M. "What We Do in Private." *Southwest Philosophy Review* 15:1 (1999), 177–83; Dover, Kenneth. *Greek Homosexuality.* Cambridge, Mass.: Harvard University Press, 1978. *Greek Homosexuality. Updated and with a New Postscript.* Cambridge, Mass.: Harvard University Press, 1989; Flinn, Kelly. *Proud to Be: My Life, the Airforce, the Controversy.* New York: Random House, 1997; Halley, Janet. *Don't: A Reader's Guide to the Military's Anti-Gay Policy.* Durham, N.C.: Duke University Press, 1999; Herek, Gregory, Jared Jobe, and Ralph Carney, eds. *Out in Force: Sexual Orientation and the Military.* Chicago, Ill.: University of Chicago Press, 1996;

Lehring, Gary. *Officially Gay: The Political Construction of Sexuality by the U.S. Military*. Philadelphia, Pa.: Temple University Press, 2003; MacKinnon, Catharine A. "Crimes of War, Crimes of Peace." In Stephen Shute and Susan Hurley, eds., *On Human Rights: The Oxford Amnesty Lectures 1993*. New York: Basic Books, 1993, 83–109; MacKinnon, Catharine A. "Rape, Genocide, and Women's Human Rights." *Harvard Women's Law Journal* 17 (Spring 1994), 5–16. Reprinted in Alexandra Stiglmayer, ed., *Mass Rape: The War against Women in Bosnia-Herzegovina*. Lincoln: University of Nebraska Press, 1994, 183–96; and Stanley French, Wanda Teays, and Laura Purdy, eds., *Violence against Women: Philosophical Perspectives*. Ithaca, N.Y.: Cornell University Press, 1998, 43–54; MacKinnon, Catharine A. "Turning Rape into Pornography: Postmodern Genocide." *Ms.* (July–August 1993), 24–30. Reprinted in Alexandra Stiglmayer, ed., *Mass Rape: The War against Women in Bosnia-Herzegovina*. Lincoln: University of Nebraska Press, 1994, 73–81; Murphy, Timothy F., ed. *Gay Ethics: Controversies in Outing, Civil Rights, and Sexual Science*. Binghamton, N.Y.: Harrington Park Press, 1994. Also published as *Journal of Homosexuality* 27:3–4 (1994); Philipose, Liz. "The Laws of War and Women's Human Rights." *Hypatia* 11:4 (1996), 46–62; Powell, Anton. *Athens and Sparta: Constructing Greek Political and Social History from 478 B.C.* London: Routledge, 1988. 2nd ed., 2001; Ray, Ronald. *Gays: In or Out? The U.S. Military and Homosexuals—A Sourcebook*. Washington, D.C.: Brassey's, 1993; Rivera, Rhonda R. "Sexual Orientation and the Law." In John C. Gonsoriek and James D. Weinrich, eds., *Homosexuality: Research Implications for Public Policy*. Newburk Park, Calif.: Sage, 1991, 81–100; Rodriguez, Richard. (1993) " 'Sissy' Warriors vs. 'Real' Men: A Perspective on Gays in the Military." In Michael S. Kimmel and Michael A. Messner, eds., *Men's Lives*, 3rd ed. Needham Heights, Mass.: Allyn and Bacon, 1995, 144–45; Russell, Bertrand. "Ostrich Code of Marriage." *Forum* 80 (1928), 7–10; Sadler, Anne, Brenda Booth, Deanna Nielson, and Bradley Doebbeling. "Health-Related Consequences of Physical and Sexual Violence: Women in the Military." *Obstetrics and Gynecology* 96:3 (2000), 473–80; Schalow, Paul Gordon. "Introduction" to Ihara Saikaku, *The Great Mirror of Male Love*. Stanford, Calif.: Stanford University Press, 1990, 1–46; Schalow, Paul Gordon. "Saikaku on 'Manly Love.' " *Stone Lion Review* 7 (Spring 1981), 3–7; Scott, Wilbur, and Sandra Carson Stanley, eds. *Gays and Lesbians in the Military: Issues, Concerns, and Contrasts*. New York: Aldine de Gruyter, 1994; Shilts, Randy. *And the Band Played On: Politics, People, and the AIDS Epidemic*. New York: St. Martin's Press, 1988; Siegel, Paul. "Dry-cleaning the Troops and Other Matters: A Critique of 'Don't Ask, Don't Tell.' " In John Corvino, ed., *Same Sex: Debating the Ethics, Science, and Culture of Homosexuality*. Lanham, Md.: Rowman and Littlefield, 1997, 274–80; Stiglmayer, Alexandra, ed. *Mass Rape: The War against Women in Bosnia-Herzegovina*. Lincoln: University of Nebraska Press, 1994; Sullivan, Andrew. *Love Undetectable: Reflections on Friendship, Sex, and Survival*. New York: Knopf, 1998; Sullivan, Andrew. *Virtually Normal: An Argument about Homosexuality*. New York: Knopf, 1995; West, Robin. "Unwelcome Sex: Toward a Harm-Based Analysis." In Catharine MacKinnon and Reva Siegel, eds., *Directions in Sexual Harassment Law*. New Haven, Conn.: Yale University Press, 2004, 138–52; Zeeland, Steven. *Barracks Buddies and Soldier Lovers: Dialogues with Gay Young Men in the U.S. Military*. New York: Harrington Park Press, 1993.

MILL, JOHN STUART. *See* Consequentialism; Liberalism

MOHAMMED. *See* Islam

MONEY, JOHN (1921–). John William Money, a controversial leader in the treatment of ambiguously sexed (intersexed or hermaphroditic) infants and transsexual adults, was born in Morrinsville, New Zealand. He received his bachelor's and master's degrees from Victoria University (Wellington) and his Ph.D. in psychology from Harvard (1952).

He spent most of his working life at Johns Hopkins University, where he was also appointed professor emeritus of medical psychology and pediatrics. Credited with introducing the term "gender" and its cognates into scientific writing about sexuality (*First Person*, 35–37; "Hermaphroditism," 254; "Linguistic Resources"; Bullough, 232), Money distinguished femininity and masculinity from biological (markers of) sex and developed a **sexology** that combined biological and social components. Drawing on new techniques for identifying and counting chromosomes, and experiments in which female animals were made to behave in stereotypically male ways by *in utero* injections of androgens, Money concluded that persons with intersexed or hermaphroditic conditions constituted "experiments of nature" whose study could help explain normal human sexuality (*Adam Principle*, 11; *Gay, Straight*, 28).

Biologists in the mid-twentieth century hypothesized an organizational theory to explain the prenatal developmental sequence through which the presence or absence of sexual hormones governed animals' acquisition of coherent, dimorphic, and complementary male or female genital morphologies, neural processes, and reproductive behaviors. The sequence begins at fertilization with the laying down of a male or female chromosomal profile, thereby precipitating gonadal differentiation, hormonal secretions, the growth of sex distinctive genitals, and the acquisition of dimorphic sexual behaviors. This organizational hypothesis included one or more critical periods in the sequence during which hormones were maximally effective and after which developmental reversals were difficult or impossible to induce (Goy and McEwen, 1–12).

Money applied this organizing theory to individuals with ambiguously sexed conditions. These included persons with abnormal numbers of sex chromosomes: Instead of the usual two, XX for females and XY for males, some persons have either one chromosome (always X) or three (either XXY or XYY). Other individuals have hormonal abnormalities, such as virilizing congenital adrenal hyperplasia, which afflicts both males and females but which in females can result in masculinization of the external genitals, and androgen insensitivity syndrome, in which XY males can be born with feminized genitals.

The birth of an intersexed infant, often marked by visibly ambiguous genitalia, is considered a "psychosocial emergency" (Grumbach and Conte, 1400). Money rejects relying on any single criterion, such as chromosomal or gonadal sex, to assign an intersexed infant to a particular sex. He believes that the most important factor in assigning sex is the functional capacity of the external genitals, either as they exist at birth or as they can be reconstructed surgically. On his view, any individual can live as either man or woman, regardless of the person's chromosomal or gonadal sex and independently of the prenatal influence of hormones. Thus an XY boy born with testes but with agenesis or microgenesis of the penis (micropenis) should probably be morphologically reconstructed as a female and raised as a girl (*Adam*, 167, 176). Similarly, a virilized chromosomal female born with an anatomically normal penis instead of a clitoris, even though lacking testes, can be raised as a boy and can function effectively as an infertile male.

Money distinguishes between an individual's sense of self as masculine, feminine, or androgynous, which he calls gender identity, and gender role, which he sees as the public performance or disclosure of gender-coded behaviors (*Sin*, 123–24). One way in which individuals are disadvantaged is if genital morphology does not match gender identity. A boy who has a micropenis or lacks a penis (his genital morphology) suffers because he cannot, in accordance with his masculine identity, urinate standing up or perform penetrative sex.

Money believes that psychological health demands concordance among all three—genital morphology, gender identity, and gender role. These factors can be manipulated independently of chromosomal, gonadal, or hormonal sex. He acknowledges hormonal influences on feminine and masculine brain differentiation but believes that these influences are weaker than those of early gender socialization (mediated by the brain), provided children receive, from the earliest possible age, clear and consistent messages about whether they are boys or girls (*Gay*, 31–32). Money postulates a critical postnatal period (up to an age of eighteen to twenty-four months) during which a child's gender identity and role are socially malleable. He thereby extends the organizational hypothesis of biologists to include social influences on development. Gender acquisition parallels **language** learning. Every child is genetically programmed to learn a language, but the language the child actually speaks is socially determined. Similarly, while every child is programmed to learn gender, which gender is acquired depends on rearing. Human development is organized biologically to allow this sort of social construction of gender (*Sex Errors*, 64).

Even though the child's acquisition of a particular gender is socially driven, gender itself is a natural necessity. The malleability of gender, coupled with the surgical correctability of genitals deemed defective, gives hope to intersexed infants, who otherwise would be doomed to identity problems, **sexual dysfunction**, and impaired role performance.

While intersexed cases proved to Money that a person could live contentedly in a gender identity and role discordant with chromosomal and gonadal sex, transsexuals present a converse problem. These are individuals whose gender identities and role preferences are contrary to their consistent chromosomal, gonadal, and morphological constitutions; they think they are men in women's bodies, or vice versa. Money believes transsexualism is caused by many factors, including personal experience. He recognizes the suffering of transsexuals and has worked to develop therapeutic counseling and planning for surgical reconstruction of their bodies. He believes that in many cases—especially when a transsexual can "pass"—it is easier to change morphology than gender identity (*First Person*, 38–39; Money and Walker, "Counseling").

Money also devised the theory of "lovemaps" to explain human sexual attractions and behaviors. A lovemap is "a developmental schema or template in the mind and brain [about] the idealized lover and the projected sexuoerotic activity with that lover" (*Sin*, 25). All sexually reproducing species have lovemaps, though in subprimate species lovemaps are restricted to biologically determined courtship rituals and copulatory acts. Human lovemaps are grounded in prenatal brain hormonalization, but the details of individual maps develop postnatally through interaction between environmental influences and species-wide biological forces. Under "optimal conditions," human lovemaps develop heterosexually and include genital copulation (*Lovemaps*, xvi).

Money rejects the notion that individuals choose their **sexual orientation** or erotic interests. Lovemaps govern all sexual attractions and activities, including **paraphilia**s (what some call "**sexual perversion**s"), which Money defined as syndromes "in which a person is reiteratively responsive to and dependent on atypical or forbidden stimulus imagery, in fantasy or in practice, for initiation and maintenance of erotosexual arousal and achievement or facilitation of orgasm" ("Paraphilias," 75; see *Gay*, 133). Paraphilias arise from associations that individuals make, based on specific experiences, between erotic lust and nonerotic evolutionary traits, such as tendencies to attack when threatened or to seek dominance over others (hence sadism). Money postulates another critical period, around age eight, during which heterosexual lovemaps can be displaced from their optimal development (*First Person*, 85–88). Homosexual and bisexual maps are unusual displacements but not objectionable; some paraphilic lovemaps, such as **rape**, are criminal when enacted.

Money's critics fall into two groups. One holds that he underestimates the prenatal effects on the brain and nervous system of sex chromosomes and hormones (Blizzard, 616–21; Diamond and Sigmundson, "Management," 1047). These critics focus on Money's much publicized clinical case in which a male child had his penis destroyed during circumcision. Money recommended that the boy's testes be removed, an artificial vagina constructed postpubertally, and that the boy be reared as a girl (*First Person*, 72–73; Colapinto, 64; Money and Ehrhardt, 118–23). The child lived as a girl with mixed results until, as a teenager, "she" rejected her female identity and had "her" breasts (gained through estrogens) removed and a penis constructed by plastic surgery. With a masculine gender identity and role orientation, **marriage** to a woman (and three children) ensued. Critics claim this case refutes Money's assertion that gender identity and role depend primarily on what sex the child is reared to be (Diamond and Sigmundson, "Sex Reassignment"), because socialization as a girl did not overcome what they presume was intense prenatal brain masculinization. However, the case does not provide conclusive evidence; it is not known whether the child received consistent messages supporting feminine gender development at home or in the community. (For a view of the case that calls it a "sham" on Money's part, see Feder, 308–9.)

Another group of critics fault Money for restricting the impact of society to individual gender and not extending it to the production of gender itself (Fausto-Sterling, 63; Kessler, 7, 13, 120–21). He acknowledges that, except for genetically determined, dimorphic functions (gamete production, fertilization, child bearing, lactation), conventional gender roles are socially arbitrary. But the existence of dimorphic gender roles and the possession of one gender identity/role by every individual are, for Money, a natural necessity for species survival.

It seems to follow from Money's theories that every infant could be raised in either gender (although it must be raised in *some* gender). Which gender an infant should acquire is not in doubt in normal births, and only psychotic caregivers would contravene normal genital morphology (*Sex Errors*, 65). Because the possession of a gender is important, an ambiguously sexed birth sometimes justifies surgical and hormonal interventions for the sake of the infant. Acquiring a gender presupposes visible sexual anatomy that triggers differential social responses to the child. (**Sigmund Freud** [1856–1939], for example, pointed out how mothers and fathers respond differently to their children, depending on the child's sex; *Introductory Lecture* 21, 333.) Genital surgery on intersexed infants creates the morphologies that launch the social construction of the gender of these infants and promotes their psychological health.

Some feminists deny that gender is naturally necessary and reject medical interventions in **intersexuality** and transsexuality as needlessly shaping individuals to fit contingent and oppressive dimorphic patterns. They hold that unless their condition is life-threatening, intersexed neonates should not be treated as suffering from errors of bodily development but as exhibiting morphological variations that society should accept. If society fails to accept these variations, we should work to change social attitudes about them, rather than cutting bodies, like Procrustes, to match social demands (Heyes, 1102; Raymond, xvi).

Money believes these critics condemn intersexed children to ridicule and misery. In other contexts, he does oppose social attitudes and practices that he judges developmentally detrimental. He emphasizes, for example, the value of childhood sex rehearsal play and the damage done by suppressing children's sexual explorations ("Need"). At the same time, however, he stresses the socially driven need for children to have conventional genitals to display to their peers. Possession of unambiguously male or female genitals is "the sign, above all others, which gives a growing child assuredness of his or her gender" (Money et al., 159). Ambiguous genitals are "unsightly and wrong" (Money and Ehrhardt, 97), and their exhibition leads to taunts from others, especially among children, and doubts about personal identity.

Money's dispute with advocates for the intersexed reflects his belief that while gender is socially constructed in the individual, it is naturally determined in the species. Abandoning gender because it has served oppressive purposes would be, for him, like rejecting language because the speakers of some languages historically have dominated those of others.

See also Bisexuality; Bullough, Vern L.; Dysfunction, Sexual; Ellis, Albert; Ellis, Havelock; Freud, Sigmund; Genital Mutilation; Homosexuality and Science; Intersexuality; Orientation, Sexual; Paraphilia; Perversion, Sexual; Psychology, Twentieth- and Twenty-First-Century; Reproductive Technology; Sexology; Social Constructionism; Wittgenstein, Ludwig

REFERENCES

Blizzard, Robert M. "Intersex Issues: A Series of Continuing Conundrums." *Pediatrics* 110:3 (2002), 616–21; Bullough, Vern L. "The Contributions of John Money: A Personal View." *Journal of Sex Research* 40:3 (2003), 230–36; Colapinto, John. "The True Story of John Joan." *Rolling Stone* (11 December 1997), 54–97; Diamond, Milton, and Keith Sigmundson. "Management of Intersexuality." *Archives of Pediatric and Adolescent Medicine* 151:10 (1997), 1046–50; Diamond, Milton, and Keith Sigmundson. "Sex Reassignment at Birth." *Archives of Pediatric and Adolescent Medicine* 151:3 (1997), 298–304; Fausto-Sterling, Anne. *Sexing the Body: Gender Politics and the Construction of Sexuality.* New York: Basic Books, 2000; Feder, Ellen K. " 'Doctors' Orders': Parents and Intersexed Children." In Eva Feder Kittay and Ellen K. Feder, eds., *The Subject of Care: Feminist Perspectives on Dependency.* Lanham, Md.: Rowman and Littlefield, 2002, 294–320; Freud, Sigmund. (1916–1917) *Introductory Lectures on Psycho-Analysis.* In *The Standard Edition of the Complete Psychological Works of Sigmund Freud*, vol. 16. Trans. James Strachey. London: Hogarth Press, 1953–1974; Goy, Robert W., and Bruce S. McEwen. *Sexual Differentiation of the Brain.* Cambridge, Mass.: MIT Press, 1980; Grumbach, Melvin M., and Felix A. Conte. "Disorders of Sex Differentiation." In Jean D. Wilson, Daniel W. Foster, Henry M. Kronenberg, and P. Reed Larson, eds., *Williams Textbook of Endocrinology*, 9th ed. Philadelphia, Pa.: W. B. Saunders, 1998, 1303–1425; Heyes, Cressida J. "Feminist Solidarity after Queer Theory: The Case of Transgender." *Signs* 28:4 (2003), 1093–1120; Kessler, Suzanne J. *Lessons from the Intersexed.* New Brunswick, N.J.: Rutgers University Press, 1998; Money, John. *The Adam Principle. Genes, Genitals, Hormones, & Gender: Selected Readings in Sexology.* Buffalo, N.Y.: Prometheus, 1993; Money, John. *A First Person History of Pediatric Psychoendocrinology.* New York: Kluwer, 2002; Money, John. *Gay, Straight, and In-Between: The Sexology of Erotic Orientation.* New York: Oxford University Press, 1988; Money, John. "Hermaphroditism, Gender, and Precocity in Hyperadrenocorticism: Psychologic Findings." *Bulletin of the Johns Hopkins Hospital* 96 (1955), 253–64; Money, John. "Linguistic Resources and Psychodynamic Theory." *British Journal of Medical Psychology* 28:4 (1955), 264–66; Money, John. *Lovemaps: Clinical Concepts of Sexual/Erotic Health and Pathology, Paraphilia, and Gender Transposition in Childhood, Adolescence, and Maturity.* New York: Irvington, 1986; Money, John. "The Need for Sexual Rehearsal Play." *Sexology* 49:9 (1980), 21–24; Money, John. "Paraphilias: Phyletic Origins of Erotosexual Dysfunction." *International Journal of Mental Health* 10:2–3 (1981), 75–109; Money, John. *Sex Errors of the Body and Related Syndromes.* Baltimore, Md.: Paul H. Brookes, 1994; Money, John. *Sin, Science, and the Sex Police.* Buffalo, N.Y.: Prometheus, 1998; Money, John, and Anke Ehrhardt. *Man and Woman, Boy and Girl: The Differentiation and Dimorphism of Gender Identity from Conception to Maturity.* Baltimore, Md.: Johns Hopkins University Press, 1972; Money, John, J. G. Hampson, and J. L. Hampson. "An Examination of Some Basic Sexual Concepts: The Evidence of Human Hermaphroditism." In John Money, *Venuses Penuses: Sexology, Sexosophy, and Exigency Theory.* Buffalo, N.Y.: Prometheus, 1986, 152–71; Money, John, and Paul A. Walker. "Counseling the Transexual." In John Money and Herman Musaph, eds., *Handbook of Sexology.* Amsterdam, Holland: Excerpta Medica, 1977, 1289–1301; Raymond, Janice G. *The Transsexual Empire: The Making of the She-male.* Boston, Mass.: Beacon Press, 1979.

Joseph A. Diorio

ADDITIONAL READING

American Academy of Pediatrics, Committee on Genetics/Section on Endocrinology/Section on Urology. "Evaluation of the Newborn with Developmental Anomalies of the External Genitalia." *Pediatrics* 106:1 (2000), 138–42; Baker, Susan W. "Biological Influences on Human Sex and Gender." *Signs* 6:1 (1980), 80–96; Benjamin, Harry. *The Transsexual Phenomenon.* New York: Julian Press, 1966; Bergner, Raymond M. "Money's 'Lovemap' Account of the Paraphilias: A Critique and Reformulation." *American Journal of Psychotherapy* 42:2 (1988), 254–59; Bradley, Susan J., Gillian D. Oliver, Avinoam B. Chernick, and Kenneth J. Zucker. "Experiment of Nurture: Ablatio Penis at 2 Months, Sex Reassignment at 7 Months, and a Psychosexual Follow-up in Young Adulthood." *Pediatrics* 102:1 (July 1998). <pediatrics.aappublications.org/cgi/content/full/102/1/e9> [accessed 18 June 2005]; Brecher, Edward M. "Males, Females, and Others." In *The Sex Researchers.* Boston, Mass.: Little, Brown, 1969, 198–229; Bullough, Vern L. "Transgenderism and the Concept of Gender." *International Journal of Transgenderism* 4:3 (2000). <www.symposion.com/ijt/gilbert/bullough.htm> [accessed 16 February 2005]; Catlin, Anita J. "Ethical Commentary on Gender Reassignment: A Complex and Provocative Modern Issue." *Pediatric Nursing* 24:1 (1998), 63–65, 99; Colapinto, John. *As Nature Made Him: The Boy Who Was Raised as a Girl.* New York: HarperCollins, 2000; Coleman, Eli, ed. *John Money: A Tribute.* New York: Haworth Press, 1991; Coleman, Eli, Louis Gooren, and Michael Ross. "Theories of Gender Transpositions: A Critique and Suggestions for Further Research." *Journal of Sex Research* 26:4 (1989), 525–38; Creighton, Sarah. "Surgery for Intersex." *Journal of the Royal Society of Medicine* 94:5 (2001), 218–20; Creighton, Sarah, and Catharine Minto. "Managing Intersex." *British Medical Journal* 323:7324 (2001), 1264–65; Diamond, Milton, Teresa Binstock, and James V. Kohl. "From Fertilization to Adult Sexual Behavior." *Hormones and Behavior* 30:4 (1996), 333–53; Diamond, Milton, and Keith Sigmundson. "Management of Intersexuality." *Archives of Pediatric and Adolescent Medicine* 151:10 (1997), 1046–50; Diamond, Milton, and Keith Sigmundson. "Sex Reassignment at Birth." *Archives of Pediatric and Adolescent Medicine* 151:3 (1997), 298–304; Dreger, Alice Domurat. *Hermaphrodites and the Medical Invention of Sex.* Cambridge, Mass.: Harvard University Press, 1998; Dreger, Alice Domurat, ed. *Intersex in the Age of Ethics.* Hagerstown, Md.: University Publishing Group, 1999; Fausto-Sterling, Anne. "The Five Sexes." *The Sciences* 33 (March–April 1993), 20–24; Fausto-Sterling, Anne. *Myths of Gender: Biological Theories about Women and Men.* New York: Basic Books, 1985; Feder, Ellen K. "Disciplining the Family: The Case of Gender Identity Disorder." *Philosophical Studies* 85:2–3 (1997), 195–211; Feder, Ellen K. " 'Doctors' Orders': Parents and Intersexed Children." In Eva Feder Kittay and Ellen K. Feder, eds., *The Subject of Care: Feminist Perspectives on Dependency.* Lanham, Md.: Rowman and Littlefield, 2002, 294–320. <www.bodieslikeours.org/research-and-studies/feder-docsorders-2.html> and <www.bodieslikeours.org/respdf/Feder2002.pdf> [accessed 16 February 2005]; Goy, Robert W., and Bruce S. McEwen. *Sexual Differentiation of the Brain.* Cambridge, Mass.: MIT Press, 1980; Green, Robert, and John Money, eds. *Transsexualism and Sex Reassignment.* Baltimore, Md.: Johns Hopkins University Press, 1969; Grumbach, Melvin M., and Felix A. Conte. "Disorders of Sex Differentiation." In Jean D. Wilson, Daniel W. Foster, Henry M. Kronenberg, and P. Reed Larson, eds., *Williams Textbook of Endocrinology,* 9th ed. Philadelphia, Pa.: W. B. Saunders, 1998, 1303–1425; Hausman, Bernice. *Changing Sex: Transsexualism, Technology, and the Idea of Gender.* Durham, N.C.: Duke University Press, 1995; Heinämaa, Sara. "Woman—Nature, Product, Style? Rethinking the Foundations of Feminist Philosophy of Science." In Lynn Hankinson Nelson and Jack Nelson, eds., *Feminism, Science, and the Philosophy of Science.* Dordrecht, Holland: Kluwer, 1997, 289–308; Hendricks, Melissa. "Into the Hands of Babes." *Johns Hopkins Magazine* (September 2000). <www.jhu.edu/~jhumag/0900web/babes.html> [accessed 15 February 2004]; Herdt, Gilbert, ed. *Third Sex. Third Gender: Beyond Sexual Dimorphism in Culture and History.* New York: Zone

Books, 1994; Holden, Constance. "Doctor of Sexology." *Psychology Today* (May 1998), 45–48; Hubbard, Ruth. "Gender and Genitals." *Social Text* 14:1–2 (1996), 157–65; Kaplan, Alexandra G. "Human Sex-Hormone Abnormalities Viewed from an Androgynous Perspective: A Reconsideration of the Work of John Money." In Jacquelynne Parsons, ed., *The Psychobiology of Sex Differences and Sex Roles*. Washington, D.C.: Hemisphere, 1980, 81–91; Kessler, Suzanne J. "Evaluating Genital Surgery." In *Lessons from the Intersexed*. New Brunswick, N.J.: Rutgers University Press, 1998, 52–76; Kessler, Suzanne J. "The Medical Construction of Gender: Case Management of Intersexed Infants." *Signs* 16:1 (1990), 3–26. Reprinted in Barbara Laslett, Sally Gregory Kohlstedt, Helen Longino, and Evelynn Hammonds, eds., *Gender and Scientific Authority*. Chicago, Ill.: University of Chicago Press, 1996, 340–63; King, Michael. "The Duke of Dysfunction." *New Zealand Listener* (4 April 1998), 18–21; Kirby, Dahlian. "Transsexualism." In Ruth Chadwick, ed., *Encyclopedia of Applied Ethics*, vol. 4. San Diego, Calif.: Academic Press, 1998, 409–12; Locker, Sari. "Money, John William." In Vern L. Bullough and Bonnie Bullough, eds., *Human Sexuality: An Encyclopedia*. New York: Garland, 1994, 397–98; Meyer-Bahlburg, Heino F. L. "Biographies of Gender and Hermaphroditism in Paired Comparisons: Clinical Supplement of the *Handbook of Sexology*." *Archives of Sexual Behavior* 26:1 (1997), 97–102; Migeon, Claude J., Amy B. Wisniewski, Terry R. Brown, John A. Rock, Heino F. L. Meyer-Bahlburg, John Money, and Gary D. Berkovitz. "46,XY Intersex Individuals: Phenotypic and Etiologic Classification, Knowledge of Condition, and Satisfaction with Knowledge in Adulthood." *Pediatrics* 110:3 (September 2002). <pediatrics.aappublications.org/cgi/content/full/110/3/e32> [accessed 18 June 2005]; Migeon, Claude J., Amy B. Wisniewski, John P. Gearhart, Heino F. L. Meyer-Bahlburg, John A. Rock, Terry R. Brown, Samuel J. Casella, Alexander Maret, Ka Ming Ngai, John Money, and Gary D. Berkowitz. "Ambiguous Genitalia with Perineoscrotal Hypospadias in 46,XY Individuals: Long-Term Medical, Surgical, and Psychosexual Outcome." *Pediatrics* 110:3 (September 2002). <pediatrics.aappublications.org/cgi/content/full/110/3/e31> [accessed 18 June 2005]; Money, John. *Clinical Concepts of Sexual/Erotic Health and Pathology, Paraphilia, and Gender Transposition in Childhood, Adolescence, and Maturity*. New York: Irvington, 1986; Money, John. "Components of Eroticism in Man: The Hormones in Relation to Sexual Morphology and Sexual Desire." *Journal of Nervous and Mental Disease* 132:3 (1961), 239–48; Money, John. "Determinants of Human Gender Identity/Role." In John Money and Herman Musaph, eds., *Handbook of Sexology*. Amsterdam, Holland: Excerpta Medica, 1977, 57–79; Money, John. *Gendermaps: Social Constructionism, Feminism, and Sexosophical History*. New York: Continuum, 1995; Money, John. "History, Causality, and Sexology." *Journal of Sex Research* 40:3 (2003), 237–39; Money, John. "Homosexuality: Bipotentiality, Terminology, and History." In Erwin Haeberle and Rolf Gindorf, eds., *Bisexualities: The Ideology and Practice of Sexual Contact with Both Men and Women*. New York: Continuum, 1998; Money, John. *Love and Love Sickness: The Science of Sex, Gender Difference, and Pairbonding*. Baltimore, Md.: Johns Hopkins University Press, 1980; Money, John. *The Lovemap Guidebook: A Definitive Statement*. New York: Continuum, 1999; Money, John. "Lovemaps." In Vern L. Bullough and Bonnie Bullough, eds., *Human Sexuality: An Encyclopedia*. New York: Garland, 1994, 373–76; Money, John. *Lovemaps: Clinical Concepts of Sexual/Erotic Health and Pathology, Paraphilia, and Gender Transposition in Childhood, Adolescence, and Maturity*. New York: Irvington, 1986. Paperback reprint, Buffalo, N.Y.: Prometheus, 1988; Money, John. "Paraphilias." In John Money and Herman Musaph, eds., *Handbook of Sexology*. Amsterdam, Holland: Excerpta Medica, 1977, 917–28; Money, John. *Principles of Developmental Sexology*. New York: Continuum, 1999; Money, John. *Reinterpreting the Unspeakable: Human Sexuality 2000. The Complete Interviewer and Clinical Biographer, Exigency Theory, and Sexology for the Third Millennium*. New York: Continuum, 1994; Money, John. *Sex Errors of the Body: Dilemmas, Education, Counselling*. Baltimore, Md.: Johns Hopkins University Press, 1968. *Sex Errors of the Body and Related Syndromes*. Baltimore, Md.: Paul H. Brookes, 1994; Money, John. *Venuses Penuses: Sexology, Sexosophy, and Exigency Theory*. Buffalo, N.Y.: Prometheus, 1986; Money, John, and Anke Ehrhardt. "Prenatal Hormonal Exposure: Possible Effects on Behavior in Man." In Richard P. Michael, ed., *Endocrinology and Human Behavior*. London: Oxford University Press, 1968, 32–48; Money, John, J. G. Hampson, and J. L. Hampson. "An Examination of Some Basic Sexual Concepts: The Evidence of Human Hermaphroditism." *Bulletin of the Johns Hopkins Hospital* 97 (1995), 301–19. Reprinted in John Money, *Venuses Penuses: Sexology, Sexosophy, and Exigency Theory.* Buffalo, N.Y.: Prometheus, 1986, 152–71; Money, John, J. G. Hampson, and J. L. Hampson. "Hermaphroditism: Recommendations Concerning Assignment of Sex, Change of Sex, and Psychologic Management." *Bulletin of the Johns Hopkins Hospital* 97 (1955), 284–300; Money, John, and Herman Musaph, eds. *Handbook of Sexology.* Amsterdam, Holland: Excerpta Medica, 1977; Money John, and Patricia Tucker. *Sexual Signatures: On Being a Man or a Woman.* Boston, Mass.: Little, Brown, 1975; Morland, Ian. "Is Intersexuality Real?" *Textual Practice* 15:3 (2001), 527–47; Phoenix, C. H., R. W. Goy, A. A. Gerall, and W. C. Young. "Organizational Action of Prenatally Administered Testosterone Propionate on the Tissues Mediating Behavior in the Female Guinea Pig." *Endocrinology* 65 (1959), 369–82; Preves, Sharon. "Negotiating the Constraints of Gender Binarism: Intersexuals' Challenge to Gender Categorization." *Current Sociology* 48:3 (2000), 27–50; Sax, Leonard. "How Common Is Intersex? A Response to Anne Fausto-Sterling." *Journal of Sex Research* 39:3 (2002), 174–78; Simon, William. *Postmodern Sexualities.* New York: Routledge, 1996; Young, W. C., R. W. Goy, and C. H. Phoenix. "Hormones and Sexual Behavior." *Science* 143 (17 January 1964), 212–18; Yudkin, Marcia. "Transsexualism and Women: A Critical Perspective." *Feminist Studies* 4:3 (1978), 97–106; Zucker, Kenneth. "Intersexuality and Gender Identity Differentiation." *Annual Review of Sex Research* 10 (1999), 1–69.

MORALITY, SEXUAL. *See* Ethics, Sexual

MORALITY AND THE LAW. *See* Law, Sex and the; Liberalism

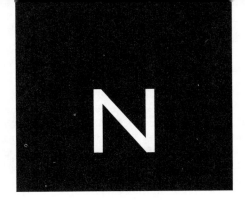

NAGEL, THOMAS (1937–). Born in Belgrade, Yugoslavia, Thomas Nagel studied at Cornell (B.A., 1958), at Oxford (B.Phil., 1960), and at Harvard (Ph.D., 1963). He has taught at the University of California at Berkeley (1963–1966), Princeton University (1966–1980), and New York University, where he has been Fiorello La Guardia Professor of Law, University Professor, and Professor of Philosophy. The author of several highly regarded books and articles (e.g., *The Possibility of Altruism*, *The View from Nowhere*, "What Is It Like to Be a Bat?"), Nagel's interests embrace metaethics, ethics, and philosophy of mind. A pervasive theme in his research concerns the character of and relationship between subjective and objective orientations toward the world.

Nagel's essay "Sexual Perversion" was published in 1969 in *Journal of Philosophy*, one of the most prestigious philosophy journals in the English-speaking world. This publication was a watershed event in the development of the philosophy of sex in the late twentieth century (see, for example, Trevas et al., 1), due to the visibility of the article's venue, its author's reputation, and the intriguing character of its argument. Discussions of Nagel's essay appeared in subsequent numbers of the same journal by Robert Solomon, Janice Moulton, and Robert Gray, which further solidified the intellectual credentials of the field. An importantly emended version of Nagel's essay appeared ten years later in his *Mortal Questions*. In the revision, Nagel's account of **sexual perversion** includes the role played by causal influences in distorting normal sexual development (cf. 13–16 in the original, 48–51 in the revision).

In "Sexual Perversion," Nagel defends the concept of sexual perversion against the claim that it is empty, confused, or incoherent, and he accepts the traditional connection between the (un)natural and the sexually perverted. The natural, however, is to be understood in psychological rather than anatomical or physiological terms. Nagel's account of sexual perversion rests on a theory of desire and human interaction, not on what facilitates or stymies reproduction or on which organs are placed in proximity to other organs (as in, for example, **Thomas Aquinas** [1224/25–1274], *Summa theologiae* 2a2ae, ques. 154, art. 1–12). Thus Nagel's approach to understanding natural sexuality and sexual perversion places him in the camp of either the Enlightenment or the Freudian "psychological turn" and separates him from ancient Greek and medieval thought. It coheres as well with the emphasis on the significance of consciousness that is characteristic of his work in the philosophy of mind.

Nagel's conception of natural sexuality is developed through a phenomenological description of a somewhat unusually structured but otherwise paradigmatic instance of sexual arousal, a human experience typically characterized by a "complex system of superimposed mutual perceptions" (1969, 10; 1979, 44). He identifies the features of the episode that are essential to natural **sexual desire** and arousal and then considers whether forms of sexuality commonly considered perverted possess or lack these features. His driving example is provided by his protagonists "Romeo" and "Juliet," who are sipping martinis in a cocktail lounge while observing each other in the room's strategically placed mirrors. Romeo becomes aroused by looking at Juliet, and Juliet by looking at Romeo. Romeo notices ("senses") her arousal, which itself adds to his desire for her. Eventually Romeo realizes that the arousal he notices in Juliet is caused by her looking at him, which adds another dimension to his sexual experience: His sense of his own embodiment now stems not only from his visceral reactions of desiring Juliet but also from noticing the sexual reactions of another person to him.

Juliet, going through the same process, picks up on her role in Romeo's excitement, which further arouses her. Romeo is now aroused by her response of arousal to his being aroused by her. And so on. Nagel mentions that this process could (logically, if not practically) escalate indefinitely. Its "natural extension" is physical contact between them, which can encompass all the psychological complexity of the awareness of self and other present in the visual interaction, but with "a far greater range of subtlety and acuteness" (1969, 11; 1979, 46).

Romeo and Juliet's mutual sensing of each other's desire and arousal serves for Nagel as the paradigm of psychologically natural or "complete" sexuality. He finds in Jean-Paul Sartre's (1905–1980) writings on sexuality inspiration for the central features of his account (*Being and Nothingness*, 391). Nagel is particularly impressed by the French philosopher's stress on the role of reciprocal awareness in achieving distinctively sexual perceptions of one's own body. Nagel also detects in the complex structure of sexual interaction an echo of H. P. Grice's theory of meaning, which involves a person's intention to instill beliefs in others, or cause certain effects, by way of bringing about their recognizing the person's intention to instill that belief or cause that effect. By analogy, natural sexuality involves the desire that one's partner be aroused by the recognition that one desires that she or he be aroused.

The elements essential to natural sexuality, for Nagel, include (1) sexual attraction is an attraction to an individual person, not to the properties she happens to instantiate; (2) sexual desire is importunate (an "assault"); and (3) sexuality involves a reciprocal pattern of awareness that impresses on those related by it a sense of their own and their partner's embodiment. Normal sexuality involves a distinctive perceptual experience of one's own body that requires for its achievement an awareness of the other's awareness of oneself under a sexual aspect. This complex perception gives rise to (or constitutes) a desire for "unity and possession." Nagel says that "physical possession must eventuate in the creation of the sexual object in the image of one's desire, and not merely in the object's recognition of that desire, or in his or her own private arousal" (1969, 13; 1979, 48). (In the original essay, Nagel confesses here that this feature of his account "may reveal a male bias," perhaps because he understands possession in terms of regarding the object of one's sexual attention through, or under the aspect of, one's own conception of that object rather than by being more receptive to the object's features that are not mere projections. Nagel's language here is unusually obscure. In any event, whatever scruples he had about "male bias" were apparently overcome by the time of the reprinting. See Pierce, 500.)

Nagel admits that it would be implausible to regard every sexual encounter that does not correspond to his model as perverted. Unadorned heterosexual intercourse during which the parties fantasize about other people may be defective, but judging it perverted is counterintuitive. Thus sex cannot be divided in any comprehensive and straightforward way into the normal and the perverted. Nagel largely regards people whose sexual activities fail to achieve the multilayered form of awareness described here, due to causally distorting influences, as manifesting perverted sexuality. His idea might be that constitutional, as opposed to what might be called "elective," sadism, masochism, and **pedophilia** are perversions. About **homosexuality**, Nagel is diffident; his considered opinion is that nothing seems to rule out that the reciprocal pattern of arousal and awareness of embodiment characteristic of natural sexuality is experienced by same-sex partners.

Nagel concludes his essay by noting that while to label a sexual phenomenon "perverted" is an evaluative judgment, it is not a moral evaluation. Indeed, on his view nothing prevents given instances of perverted sex from being better (for example, more satisfying) than unperverted sex. And he suggests that even when perverted sex is bad, it is, like bad food or bad music, generally better than none at all. Nagel says that this idea should not be controversial (1969, 17; 1979, 52), which suggests that he thinks it would be widely accepted even by those who reject his account of perversion. But this seems overconfident. If, for example, a person's conception of good sex requires a particularly rich kind of interpersonal acknowledgment, she might not regard anonymous sexual experiences as worth having. (See also Ketchum.) In "Personal Rights and Public Space" (99–102), Nagel discusses sexuality and social policy and observes:

> Sex is the source of the most intense pleasure of which humans are capable, and one of the few sources of human ecstasy. It is also the realm of adult life in which the defining and inhibiting structures of civilization are permitted to dissolve, and our deepest presocial, animal, and infantile natures can be fully released and expressed, offering a form of physical and emotional completion that is not available elsewhere.

He claims, on this basis, "The case for toleration and an area of protected privacy . . . is especially strong" regarding sexuality (100; see "Concealment and Exposure," 19).

It is not clear that Nagel's effort to vindicate and analyze the concept of sexual perversion has any practical implications. He allows that there is no good reason to think that perverted sex is *eo ipso* of lower quality than natural sex, either morally or nonmorally. Nor is it clear that the analysis is convincing. Michael Slote argues that any effort to rescue or rehabilitate the concept of "unnatural" must misfire. Sara Ruddick argues that Nagel's notion of **completeness** does not analyze *perversion* but illuminates a different dimension of sexuality and that perversion cannot be understood apart from physiological and procreative considerations (although she agrees that perversion alone yields no moral judgments). Solomon wonders why Romeo and Juliet go through Nagel's psychological process and (drawing on Sartre himself) proposes that it cannot be just for the eventual pleasure of physical contact. Janice Moulton claims that Nagel conflates **flirting** and **seduction** with sexual behavior as such. And Alan Goldman thinks that Nagel overintellectualizes sex (277–78). Nevertheless, Nagel's essay had a germinal influence on the development of philosophical discussions of sex, and his essay remains of philosophical, and not merely historical, interest.

See also Anscombe, G.E.M.; Arts, Sex and the; Communication Model; Completeness, Sexual; Cybersex; Ethics, Sexual; Existentialism; Leibniz, Gottfried; Masturbation; Perversion, Sexual; Privacy; Scruton, Roger; Thomas Aquinas (Saint)

REFERENCES

Goldman, Alan. "Plain Sex." *Philosophy and Public Affairs* 6:3 (1977), 267–87; Gray, Robert. "Sex and Sexual Perversion." *Journal of Philosophy* 75:4 (1978), 189–99; Grice, H. P. "Meaning." *Philosophical Review* 66:3 (1957), 377–88; Ketchum, Sara Ann. "The Good, the Bad, and the Perverted:

Sexual Paradigms Revisited." In Alan Soble, ed., *The Philosophy of Sex: Contemporary Readings*, 1st ed. Totowa, N.J.: Rowman and Littlefield, 1980, 139–57; Moulton, Janice. "Sexual Behavior: Another Position." *Journal of Philosophy* 73:16 (1976), 537–46; Nagel, Thomas. "Concealment and Exposure." *Philosophy and Public Affairs* 27:1 (1998), 3–30; Nagel, Thomas. *Mortal Questions*. Cambridge: Cambridge University Press, 1979; Nagel, Thomas. "Personal Rights and Public Space." *Philosophy and Public Affairs* 24:2 (1995), 83–107; Nagel, Thomas. *The Possibility of Altruism*. Oxford, U.K.: Oxford University Press, 1970; Nagel, Thomas. "Sexual Perversion." *Journal of Philosophy* 66:1 (1969), 5–17; Nagel, Thomas. *The View from Nowhere*. Oxford, U.K.: Oxford University Press, 1986; Nagel, Thomas. "What Is It Like to Be a Bat?" *Philosophical Review* 83:4 (1974), 435–50; Pierce, Christine. "Review Essay: Philosophy." *Signs* 1:2 (1975), 487–503; Ruddick, Sara. "Better Sex." In Robert B. Baker and Frederick A. Elliston, eds., *Philosophy and Sex*, 1st ed. Buffalo, N.Y.: Prometheus, 1975, 83–104; Sartre, Jean-Paul. (1943) *Being and Nothingness: An Essay on Phenomenological Ontology*. Trans. Hazel E. Barnes. New York: Philosophical Library, 1956; Slote, Michael. "Inapplicable Concepts and Sexual Perversion." In Robert B. Baker and Frederick A. Elliston, eds., *Philosophy and Sex*, 1st ed. Buffalo, N.Y.: Prometheus, 1975, 261–67; Solomon, Robert C. "Sexual Paradigms." *Journal of Philosophy* 71:11 (1974), 336–45; Thomas Aquinas. (1265–1273) *Summa theologiae*, 60 vols. Cambridge, U.K.: Blackfriars, 1964–1976; Trevas, Robert, Arthur Zucker, and Donald Borchert, eds. *Philosophy of Sex and Love: A Reader*. Upper Saddle River, N.J.: Prentice-Hall, 1997.

James Lindemann Nelson

ADDITIONAL READING

Blackburn, Simon. "Hobbesian Unity." In *Lust: The Seven Deadly Sins*. New York: New York Public Library/Oxford University Press, 2004, 87–92; Cornell, Drucilla. "Dropped Drawers: A Viewpoint." In Leonard V. Kaplan and Beverly I. Moran, eds., *Aftermath: The Clinton Impeachment and the Presidency in the Age of Political Spectacle*. New York: New York University Press, 2001, 312–20; Davidson, Arnold I. "Styles of Reasoning, Conceptual History, and the Emergence of Psychiatry." In Peter Galison and David J. Strump, eds., *The Disunity of Science: Boundaries, Contexts, and Power*. Stanford, Calif.: Stanford University Press, 1996, 75–100. Reprinted, edited and abridged, as "Conceptual History and Conceptions of Perversions," in P&S2 (476–86); Goldman, Alan. "Plain Sex." *Philosophy and Public Affairs* 6:3 (1977), 267–87. Reprinted in HS (103–23); POS1 (119–38); POS2 (73–92); POS3 (39–55); POS4 (39–55); Gray, Robert. "Sex and Sexual Perversion." *Journal of Philosophy* 75:4 (1978), 189–99. Reprinted in POS1 (158–68); POS3 (57–66); POS4 (57–66); Moulton, Janice. "Sexual Behavior: Another Position." *Journal of Philosophy* 73:16 (1976), 537–46. Reprinted in HS (91–100); POS1 (110–18); POS2 (63–71); POS3 (31–38); POS4 (31–38); Nagel, Thomas. "Concealment and Exposure." *Philosophy and Public Affairs* 27:1 (1998), 3–30. Reprinted in *Concealment and Exposure and Other Essays*. Oxford, U.K.: Oxford University Press, 2002, 3–26; Nagel, Thomas. *Concealment and Exposure and Other Essays*. Oxford, U.K.: Oxford University Press, 2002; Nagel, Thomas. "Personal Rights and Public Space." *Philosophy and Public Affairs* 24:2 (1995), 83–107. Reprinted in *Concealment and Exposure and Other Essays*. Oxford, U.K.: Oxford University Press, 2002, 31–52; Nagel, Thomas. *The Possibility of Altruism*. Oxford, U.K.: Oxford University Press, 1970. Reprinted, Princeton, N.J.: Princeton University Press, 1978; Nagel, Thomas. "Sexual Perversion." *Journal of Philosophy* 66:1 (1969), 5–17. Reprinted in P&S1 (247–60); P&S2 (268–79); POS1 (76–88). Reprinted, revised, in Thomas Nagel, *Mortal Questions*. Cambridge: Cambridge University Press, 1979, 39–52; in Eugene F. Rogers, Jr., ed., *Theology and Sexuality: Classic and Contemporary Readings*. Oxford, U.K.: Blackwell, 2002, 125–36; and P&S3 (326–36); POS2 (39–51); POS3 (9–20); POS4 (9–20); STW (105–12); Ruddick, Sara. "On Sexual Morality." In James Rachels, ed., *Moral Problems: A Collection of Philosophical Essays*, 2nd ed. New York: Harper and Row, 1971, 16–34. Reprinted, revised, as "Better Sex," in Robert B. Baker and Frederick A. Elliston, eds., *Philosophy and Sex*, 1st ed. Buffalo, N.Y.: Prometheus, 1975, 83–104; P&S2 (280–99); Scruton, Roger. "Sartre's Paradox." In *Sexual Desire: A Moral Philosophy of the Erotic*. New York: Free Press, 1986, 120–25; Solomon, Robert C. "Sexual Paradigms." *Journal of Philosophy* 71:11 (1974), 336–45. Reprinted in HS (81–90); POS1 (89–98); POS2 (53–62); POS3 (21–29); POS4 (21–29). Solomon, Robert C., and Kathleen Higgins, eds., *The Philosophy of (Erotic) Love.* Lawrence: University Press of Kansas, 1991.

NATURAL LAW (NEW). One traditional view about sexual morality has its roots in classical philosophy and Judeo-Christian religion. It holds that sexual behaviors are morally wrong if they are contrary to nature. The view is perhaps most intelligible if understood theologically. The apparent purposiveness of natural entities, including organic bodies and their organs, indicates the design of the artificer who created them: The natural order of things reflects God's will. Further, God commands that humans act in accordance with the patterns he established in nature, and so departures from the natural order are sinful. If we add to this theological background the claim, commonly made in this tradition (for example, **Thomas Aquinas** [1224/25–1274], *Summa contra gentiles*, chap. 122), that sexuality and the genitals were designed by God solely for reproduction, it follows that employing them in a deliberately nonreproductive way constitutes sin. This judgment appears to apply directly to contracepted heterosexual coitus, **masturbation**, homosexual relations, and other sexual behaviors.

Inferring divine intentions from the apparent purposes of natural entities is intellectually problematic. We can infer almost any intention about God or His plan from observations of natural entities. One contemporary Christian theologian, for example, concludes that God designed the sexual organs to produce pleasure (Gudorf, 65). Observations of nature alone, furthermore, cannot prove a central claim of traditional Natural Law philosophy, that deviating from the natural order is necessarily objectionable. The notions that human behavior can (conceptually) deviate from nature to begin with and that acts inconsistent with nature are questionable depend heavily on religious faith or (as in **Aristotle** [384–322 BCE]) a speculative teleological metaphysics (see Baltzly; Koppelman, 74–75; Priest).

The most influential attempt to rehabilitate this tradition is called "New Natural Law" (NNL) philosophy. The arguments developed by theologian Germain Grisez and legal scholar and philosopher John Finnis, as well as contributions made by Robert George, Gerard Bradley, and Patrick Lee, comprise a body of literature that seriously bolsters the Natural Law tradition. Consistent with the religious (usually Catholic) tradition from which it emerges, NNL condemns ubiquitous sexual behaviors that are widely regarded in the West as morally innocuous, such as contracepted heterosexual coitus and masturbation. But NNL theorists also defend many popular moral intuitions, including the condemnation of homosexual activity and perversions. One of NNL's central claims is that **marriage** is necessarily a relation between one male person and one female person. NNL argues that whatever (nonsexual) goods a same-sex couple is capable of achieving, marriage is impossible for them, because of the kind of thing that marriage is. Many Americans agree. Even people who are friendly to gays and their claims for social recognition and legal protection often draw the line at **same-sex marriage**. So NNL's views are not idiosyncratic. On the contrary, NNL is the most fully worked out statement of a position that is widely held and politically powerful.

A foundational theme of NNL is that particular identifiable goods are intrinsically and not merely instrumentally worthy of being pursued. These "basic goods" are intelligible ends, valuable in themselves, and capable of motivating us to act. Such goods are worth pursuing even at the price of discomfort or pain. In the early work of Grisez and Finnis, the reasons "for acting which need no further reason" include life, health, knowledge, aesthetic experience, excellence in work and play, **friendship**, inner peace, peace of conscience, and peace with God (Grisez et al., 103, 107–8; Finnis, *Natural Law*, chap. 4, sec. 2; for variations of this list in Finnis, see Alkire, 76). Each good, as an end, can provide a sufficient explanation of human action: Being told that an action is done for the sake of these goods is answer enough (George, 45–48). Note that bodily pleasure for its own sake is not a basic good (Finnis, *Natural Law*, 95–96; see Black, 11–12). Declining to acknowledge the intrinsic value of pleasure makes it easier for NNL to reject nonprocreative sexuality like masturbation and homosexual relations.

The basic goods are "incommensurable": None is reducible to any other or to a common factor, such as utility, that they essentially share. Further, as incommensurable "[n]o basic good considered precisely as such can be meaningfully said to be better than another" (Grisez et al., 110). Hence they cannot be arranged hierarchically (Finnis, *Natural Law*, 92). It follows from this that it can never be morally justified to act in a way directly contrary to one of the basic goods. For Finnis, a

> proposed destroying, damaging, or blocking of some basic aspect of some person's reality provides, of itself, a reason not to choose that option. . . . [T]hat reason could be set aside . . . only if one could . . . identify some rationally preferable reason for choosing that option: that is, some greater good . . . promised by that option than is . . . promised by the options which do not include that choice to destroy, damage, or block a basic human good. But . . . such a commensurating of goods is rationally impossible. (*Moral Absolutes*, 54–55)

Basic goods may never be sacrificed for less valuable advantages or states of affairs, and this is how NNL grounds the wrongness of, for example, **contraception**, "acts whose exclusive intention is to impede the coming-to-be of a human life" (Finnis, *Moral Absolutes*, 87). Life is a basic good, and sexual acts employing contraception impede this good: "[T]he choice to exclude the possibility of procreation while engaging in intercourse is always, and in an obvious and unambiguous way (which it requires no Christian weighting of the value of procreation to see), a choice directly and immediately against a basic value" ("Natural Law," 384). Similarly, for NNL, **casual sex**, masturbation, and homosexual acts are wrong, because they, too, damage or block basic goods.

The integrity of the self, "harmony among all the parts of a person which can be engaged in freely chosen action" (Grisez, *The Way*, vol. 1, 124), is a basic good; it is better to be a single, coherent self rather than a heap of conflicting desires and impulses. Integrity is violated when one acts for the sake of bodily pleasure in, for example, masturbating or using psychoactive drugs. In these cases, "one separates in one's choice oneself as bodily from oneself as an intentional agent. The content of such a choice includes the disintegration attendant upon a reduction of one's bodily self to the level of an extrinsic instrument" (Lee and George, 139). Similarly, Finnis claims that "in masturbating, as in being . . . sodomized," the body is a mere tool of satisfaction. As a result, a person undergoes disintegration. In these activities "one's choosing self [becomes] the quasi-slave of the experiencing self which is demanding gratification" ("Homosexual Conduct"). The danger of disintegration is especially prominent in sexuality, since sexual conduct aims at bodily pleasure.

For NNL, the only morally permissible sexual acts are those of married couples (even here there are many restrictions). In their more recent work, Grisez and Finnis add another basic good to those enumerated above, claiming that marriage is among them (Finnis, "Law, Morality," 1064–65; Grisez, *The Way*, vol. 2, 556). Marriage is a basic good because it constitutes "a full communion of persons: a communion of will by mutual covenantal commitment, and of organism by the generative act they share in" (Grisez, *The Way*, vol. 2, 580). Communion of will consists of a mutual commitment to an exclusive and indissoluble partnership, while organic communion consists in the fact that when husband and wife engage in procreative marital intercourse, they become a single organism.

For NNL "each animal is incomplete, for a male or a female . . . is only a potential part of the mated pair, which is the complete organism . . . capable of reproducing sexually. This is true also of men and women: as mates who engage in sexual intercourse suited to initiate new life, they complete each other and become an organic unit. In doing so, it is literally true that 'they become one flesh' (Gn 2.24)" (*The Way*, vol. 2, 570). For the married couple, sexual union is not extrinsic to their mutual friendship. It is not merely a means to their experience of bodily pleasure, and so does not violate their integrity the way other sexual acts would. On the contrary, according to Lee and George (144), sexual union preserves their integrity:

> In sexual intercourse they unite (become one) precisely in that respect in which their community is distinct and naturally fulfilled. So this bodily unity is not extrinsic to their emotional and spiritual unity. The bodily, emotional, and spiritual are the different levels of a unitary, multi-leveled personal communion. Therefore, in such a community sexual intercourse actualizes the multi-leveled personal communion.

Nonmarital sexual acts, whether homosexual or heterosexual, cannot achieve this bodily unity. At best, they achieve the *illusory experience* of unity (on this, see Perry; Weithman, "A Propos"). "For a truly common good, there must be more than experience; the experiences must be subordinated to a truly common act that is genuinely fulfilling." When gay couples (or heterosexual couples, for that matter) achieve sexual satisfaction by means other than marital intercourse, the act "is really an instance of mutual masturbation, and is as self-alienating as any other instance of masturbation" (Lee and George, 146). Thus Finnis writes ("Law, Morality," 1066–67) about sex between unmarried people that

> their reproductive organs cannot make them a biological (and therefore personal) unit. . . . Because their activation of . . . their reproductive organs cannot be an actualizing and experiencing of the *marital* good . . . it can do no more than provide each partner with an individual gratification. For want of a *common good* that could be actualized . . . *by and in this bodily union*, that conduct involves the partners in treating their bodies as instruments to be used in the service of their consciously experiencing selves; their choice to engage in such conduct thus dis-integrates each of them precisely as acting persons.

Homosexual acts are wrong not only because they violate integrity but also because they "violate the good of marriage" (Grisez, *The Way*, vol. 2, 633). Choosing nonmarital sex "damages the body's capacity for the marital act as an act of self-giving which constitutes a communion of bodily persons" (650). This damage is "a damage to the person as an integrated, acting being; it consists principally in that disposition of the will which is initiated by the choice to engage in" such **sexual activity** (Finnis, "Good of Marriage," 119). Consider a married man who has never committed **adultery** but who might be willing to do so if, say, his wife were unavailable when he felt strong **sexual desire**. The exclusivity of the man's sex with his wife is not an expression of commitment, because conditional willingness to commit adultery precludes commitment. He is thus motivated even in marital intercourse by something other than the good of marriage. This is why Finnis claims that the "complete exclusion of nonmarital sex acts from the range of acceptable and valuable human options is existentially, if not logically, a precondition for the truly marital character of one's intercourse as and with a spouse" ("Good of Marriage," 123). When one damages that precondition, one damages marriage, since "to damage an intrinsic and necessary condition for attaining a good is to damage that good itself" (Grisez, *The Way*, vol. 2, 650–51).

Thus, the NNL case against sexual acts that are not of the procreative kind (including masturbation, homosexual sex, and any marital sex involving male ejaculation outside the vagina) can be summarized as follows:

1. It is always wrong to act directly contrary to a basic good.
2. Performing sex acts not of the procreative kind is always directly contrary to the basic good of integrity.
3. Performing sex acts not of the procreative kind is always directly contrary to the basic good of marriage.
4. Therefore, it is always wrong to perform sex acts not of the procreative kind.

For the argument to succeed, the premises (1 and 2, or 1 and 3) must be true. There is, however, reason to think that none of them is.

First, from NNL's claim that the basic goods are incommensurable, it does not follow that acting directly contrary to a basic good is always wrong. Even if there is no airtight argument that can justify any particular trade-off of incommensurable goods, it might still be possible to compare these goods intuitively and to feel reasonably confident of one's conclusions. NNL concedes that even after honoring the rule against "doing evil that good might come of it" there are still choices to be made between goods, for example, between pursuing graduate programs in psychology or in medicine (George, 117–18). The choice against a basic good might rest on just this kind of intuitive weighing. NNL, which constrains choice regardless of the consequences, might in some circumstances require one to endure very bad consequences. For example, one might be required to surrender to a totalitarian state if the only defense against that state is the use of nuclear weapons, which is prohibited because doing so directly targets the innocent, contrary to the basic good of life. Charles Larmore has argued that deontology's indifference to consequences is acceptable only if we have theological guarantees, so that we are assured that the damage we tolerate or suffer will be corrected, ultimately, by divine providence (134–39). NNL theorists are divided over whether their moral theory makes sense without this theology. Finnis places great weight on faith in providence (*Moral Absolutes*, 9–20; see Finnis on Aquinas, *Aquinas*, 315–19), while Grisez suggests that the theory holds together without such faith, that "a generous and reasonable love of human goods will lead one to act in a way compatible with this ideal" (*The Way*, vol. 1, 186).

The second premise is also weak. Now, even if nonmarital sex acts cannot realize the good of marriage, it does not follow that such acts "can do no more than provide each partner with an individual gratification" (Finnis, "Law, Morality," 1066). Weithman, for one, thinks that homosexual activity "provides the occasion of, and thus serves the function of, promoting emotional intimacy" ("A Propos," 87; "Natural Law, Morality," 239–40). In this way, loving homosexual activity could fail to damage and even support integrity. If so, loving homosexual activity is a counterexample to the second premise. There are other reasons the premise fails.

NNL claims that it is always wrong to manipulate one's body, or another's, for the sole purpose of pleasure, in part because doing so involves disintegration. Hence NNL concludes, in effect, that most sexual activity engaged in by human beings is wrong. Were bodily pleasure a basic good, this conclusion could be avoided. Of course, we often do act solely for the sake of pleasure, and it is extraordinarily difficult to comprehend how this is morally problematic. Many would agree that "bodily pleasure is itself an important human good" and that "absolutely nothing [is] wrong with using one's body for the purpose of getting pleasure" (Nussbaum and Dover, 1649; see Biggar, 286–87). Finnis admits that pleasure is a good, but he qualifies that concession: "when it is the experienced aspect of one's participation in some intelligible good" ("Homosexual Conduct"). This piggybacking of pleasure onto other goods underestimates the value of pleasure.

Further, and perhaps more to the point, it is not obvious that pursuing pleasure for its own sake always disrupts integrity. The pursuit of pleasure is often a response to a bodily need. In scratching an itch, I am not abusing my body or regarding it as "a lower form of life with its own dynamism" (Grisez, *The Way*, vol. 1, 139). I am tending to its needs, which are *my* needs, the needs of an integrated person, not the needs of a body detached from or distinct from me. And when A gives B sexual pleasure, A is tending to the needs of at least B's body (if not also B's mind), which are B's needs, the needs of a similarly integrated person. Such considerations seem not to move NNL. Even a married couple, according to NNL, might fail to achieve unity if their sexual pleasure is divorced from marital acts. "If Susan, for example, masturbates John to orgasm or applies oral stimulation to him to bring him to orgasm, no real unity has been effected" (Lee and George, 146). But a case can be made that their joint sexual activity, even if neither coital nor procreative, can still deepen their union and preserve their integrity. One might even suggest that solitary masturbation, too, involves no disintegration: "An experience of masturbation . . . is not an experience of a conscious self but of a whole person. . . . There is no existential alienation from the body" (Moore, 232; see Koppelman, 85–86).

Seeking pleasure for its own sake in sexuality also runs counter, for NNL, to the basic good of marriage (premise three). What about a young married couple that has intercourse when and only when it gives them pleasure to do so—is their intercourse morally licit? On Finnis's sympathetic account of Aquinas's sexual ethics, "there is nothing wrong at all with our welcoming assent to such pleasure in the marital act, nor in our being motivated towards such an act by the prospect of giving and sharing in that delight *as token of* our marital commitment" (*Aquinas*, 147, italics added; see "Good of Marriage," 102). Moreover, it is appropriate for spouses to refrain from intercourse when, for example, "either of them is disinclined or unwell" ("Good of Marriage," 109n.47; *Aquinas*, 151n.86; see **Saint Paul** [5–64?], 1 Cor. 7:3). But it is morally illicit for spouses to desire coitus solely for its pleasure, even if they are wholly unwilling to have sex with anyone else (*Aquinas*, 148–49). What is wrong is one's having an attitude in which "one is not interested in or concerned with anything about one's spouse other than what one would be concerned with in a prostitute" ("Good of Marriage," 103). Some pretty fine line-drawing seems at work here. How could one tell whether the young married couple is engaging in sex for the sake of the good of marriage, or as a token of their commitment (in which case the pleasure of the act is innocent), or just for the sake of their mutual pleasure? Probably not even the couple will know. Another implication is that an elderly married couple that no longer experiences pleasure in intercourse still has reason, for NNL, to engage in it—to actualize their unity (George and Bradley, 310). It is a curious view that blesses "unitive" intercourse without pleasure but condemns pleasure for its own sake even within marriage.

Many object to NNL's prohibition of contraception not only because the purported harm done to the basic goods seems strained but also because the emphasis placed on the value of procreative coitus would seem to rule out, in addition to contraception, not just masturbation and homosexual activity but any coitus engaged in by infertile heterosexual couples (whether due to advanced age or a medical condition). NNL's answer focuses on the capacity of the heterosexual couple to engage in acts of the reproductive *kind*. Even when a heterosexual couple cannot reproduce, the "union of the reproductive organs of husband and wife really unites them biologically (and their biological reality is part of, not merely an instrument of, their *personal* reality)" (Finnis, "Law, Morality," 1066). The gay couple is different: "[T]heir reproductive organs cannot make them a biological (and therefore personal) unit." Finnis also writes ("Law, Morality," 1068) that the infertile married couple

> who unite their reproductive organs in an act of sexual intercourse which, so far as they can make it, is of a kind suitable for generation, do function as a biological (and thus personal) unit and thus can be actualizing . . . the two-in-one-flesh common good and reality of marriage, even when some biological condition happens to prevent that unity resulting in generation of a child. Their conduct thus differs radically from the acts of a husband and wife whose intercourse is . . . sodomitic or by fellatio or coitus interruptus.

The *radical* difference here is difficult to discern. That sterile heterosexual coitus could have been procreative in some other possible world does not distinguish it from homosexual sex.

The NNL distinction turns on the *form* of the act, about which Lee and George write:

> People who are not temporarily or permanently infertile could procreate by performing exactly the same type of act which the infertile married couple perform and by which they consummate or actualize their marital communion. The difference between sterile and fertile married couples is not a difference in what they do. Rather it is a difference in a distinct condition which affects what may result from what they do. (150)

What sense, however, does it make to say that heterosexual intercourse is an act of a reproductive type or kind even if reproduction cannot be intended and is known to be impossible? It would seem to be equally plausible to say that all acts of seminal ejaculation are reproductive in kind (even masturbatory acts) or even that no ejaculatory acts are reproductive in kind (since no mere ejaculation, by itself, results in procreation). Reproduction would then be merely an accidental effect that occurs only under certain conditions. Nothing in nature dictates that the lines should be drawn one way or another.

The distinctive good of marriage that NNL advocates appears to be incoherent. Gareth Moore has argued that the idea of a "two-in-one-flesh" cannot do the necessary work in NNL's argument unless it is understood literally (since even gay and lesbian couples might unite metaphorically). But it cannot be so understood, because a heterosexual couple does not in fact unite biologically: "We might at a pinch speak of male and female reproductive organs as incomplete, if by that is meant that one cannot achieve reproduction without the other, but the male and female animals are in no sense incomplete. So neither is a mating pair a single complete organism: it is simply two organisms cooperating in a joint activity of mating" (Moore, 225–26).

NNL's argument might be salvaged by presupposing an Aristotelian metaphysics in which infertile heterosexual married couples participate imperfectly in the *idea* of one-flesh unity, but same-sex couples do not participate at all. The infertile heterosexual couple does become one organism, albeit a handicapped organism that cannot do what a normally functioning organism can do. The heterosexual couple is only accidentally infertile, while the same-sex couple is essentially so. In what sense, however, is an infertile couple one flesh, since in them procreative unity is not realized? Their unity, if it exists outside the symbolic community in which they participate, and in which the same-sex couple could also participate, consists in their membership in a class, a natural kind composed of those who ideally *could* procreate. But why think that this natural kind is a real thing, rather than a construct? An unloaded but otherwise functional gun remains a gun, a device designed for and capable of shooting. In contrast, the genital organs of a sterile man cannot be called reproductive organs at all. They are not fit for reproduction. They are more like a gun with a busted firing pin that is, as a result, unfit for shooting.

Finnis recognizes that not every ejaculation of normal male genitalia will successfully lead to conception, and perhaps this is meant to minimize the difference between the organs of normal and infertile males. "Biological union between humans is the inseminatory union of male genital organ with female genital organ; in most circumstances it does not result in generation, but it is the behavior that unites biologically because it is the behavior which, as behavior, is suitable for generation" ("Law, Morality," 1066n.46). But whether such behavior "is suitable for generation" depends on whether the organs are in fact suitable for generation. A sterile person's genitals are no more suitable for generation than a gun with a broken firing pin is suitable for shooting. The gun's pin might be repairable, perhaps not; perhaps medicine can in some cases cure infertility. It is, however, a conceptual stretch to insist that the sexual acts of the incurably infertile are of the same kind as the sexual acts of fertile organs that occasionally fail to deliver the goods.

NNL might, finally, appeal to the essentialism implied by the ordinary meaning of words. A dead man's heart, which will never beat again, is still a heart, and his stomach is still a digestive organ. (So to speak! Don't put lasagna in it.) So the penis of a sterile man is still a reproductive organ. But the only aspect of reproductiveness relevant to NNL's argument—the reproductive power of the organ—does not inhere in this particular organ. It is not reproductive in the sense of power or potential, even if it is a reproductive organ in the taxonomic sense. It is mysterious why its being taxonomically a reproductive organ should have any moral significance (see Koppelman, 86–93).

The claims of NNL theorists may sometimes be obscure, but they are significant. Only NNL theorists, among defenders of traditional views about the morality of **homosexuality**, justify those views without invoking false factual claims about gay people. Intellectually candid, they recognize that the task is to identify something of value in the sexuality of married, infertile heterosexual couples that is absent from homosexual relations. A fair assessment of NNL is important, because it may be the last respectable stronghold of the beliefs that homosexual conduct is intrinsically wrong and marriage is necessarily heterosexual.

See also Anscombe, G.E.M.; Aristotle; Augustine (Saint); Catholicism, History of; Catholicism, Twentieth- and Twenty-First-Century; Contraception; Ethics, Sexual; Homosexuality, Ethics of; Marriage; Marriage, Same-Sex; Masturbation; Perversion, Sexual; Plato; Scruton, Roger; Thomas Aquinas (Saint); Wojtyła, Karol (Pope John Paul II)

REFERENCES

Alkire, Sabina. "The Basic Dimensions of Human Flourishing: A Comparison of Accounts." In Nigel Biggar and Rufus Black, eds., *The Revival of Natural Law* (q.v.), 73–110; Baltzly, Dirk. "Peripatetic Perversions: A Neo-Aristotelian Account of the Nature of Sexual Perversion." *The Monist* 85:1 (2003), 3–29; Biggar, Nigel. "Conclusion." In Nigel Biggar and Rufus Black, eds., *The Revival of Natural Law* (q.v.), 283–94; Biggar, Nigel, and Rufus Black, eds. *The Revival of Natural Law: Philosophical, Theological, and Ethical Responses to the Finnis-Grisez School.* Aldershot, U.K.: Ashgate, 2000; Black, Rufus. "Introduction: The New Natural Law Theory." In Nigel Biggar and Rufus Black, eds., *The Revival of Natural Law* (q.v.), 1–25; Finnis, John M. *Aquinas: Moral, Political, and Legal Theory.* Oxford, U.K.: Oxford University Press, 1998; Finnis, John M. "The Good of Marriage and the Morality of Sexual Relations: Some Philosophical and Historical Observations." *American Journal of Jurisprudence* 42 (1997), 97–134; Finnis, John M. "Law, Morality, and 'Sexual Orientation.'" *Notre Dame Law Review* 69:5 (1994), 1049–76; Finnis, John M. *Moral Absolutes: Tradition, Revision, and Truth.* Washington, D.C.: Catholic University of America, 1991; Finnis, John M. *Natural Law and Natural Rights.* Oxford, U.K.: Clarendon Press, 1980; Finnis, John M. "Natural Law and Unnatural Acts." *The Heythrop Journal* 11 (1970), 365–87; Finnis, John M., with Martha C. Nussbaum. "Is Homosexual Conduct Wrong? A Philosophical Exchange." *The New Republic* (15 November 1993), 12–13; George, Robert P. *In Defense of Natural Law.* Oxford, U.K.: Oxford University Press, 1999; George, Robert P., and Gerard V. Bradley. "Marriage and the Liberal Imagination." *Georgetown Law Journal* 84:2 (1995): 301–20; Grisez, Germain. *The Way of the Lord Jesus,* vol. 1: *Christian Moral Principles.* Chicago, Ill.: Franciscan Herald Press, 1983; Grisez, Germain. *The Way of the Lord Jesus,* vol. 2: *Living a Christian Life.* Quincy, Ill.: Franciscan Press, 1993; Grisez, Germain, Joseph Boyle, and John Finnis. "Practical Principles, Moral Truth, and Ultimate Ends." *American Journal of Jurisprudence* 32 (1987), 99–151; Gudorf, Christine E. *Body, Sex, and Pleasure: Reconstructing Christian Sexual Ethics.* Cleveland, Ohio: Pilgrim Press, 1994; Koppelman, Andrew. "Why Discriminate?" In *The Gay Rights Question in Contemporary American Law.* Chicago, Ill.: University of Chicago Press, 2002, 72–93; Larmore, Charles. *Patterns of Moral Complexity.* Cambridge: Cambridge University Press, 1987; Lee, Patrick, and Robert P. George. "What Sex Can Be: Self-Alienation, Illusion, or One-Flesh Union." *American Journal of Jurisprudence* 42 (1997), 135–57; Moore, Gareth. "Natural Sex: Germain Grisez, Sex, and Natural Law." In Nigel Biggar and Rufus Black, eds., *The Revival of Natural Law* (q.v.), 223–41; Nussbaum, Martha C., and Kenneth J. Dover. "Appendix 4" (1641–51). In Martha C. Nussbaum, "Platonic Love and Colorado Law: The Relevance of Ancient Greek Norms to Modern Sexual Controversies." *Virginia Law Review* 80:7 (1994), 1515–1651; Perry, Michael J. "The Morality of Homosexual Conduct: A Response to John Finnis." *Notre Dame Journal of Law, Ethics, and Public Policy* 9:1 (1995), 41–74; Priest, Graham. "Sexual Perversion." *Australasian Journal of Philosophy* 75:3 (1997), 360–72; Thomas Aquinas. (1258–1264) *On the Truth of the Catholic Faith. Summa contra gentiles. Book Three: Providence. Part II.* Trans. Vernon J. Bourke. Garden City, N.Y.: Image Books, 1956; Weithman, Paul J. "A Propos of Professor Perry: A Plea for Philosophy in Sexual Ethics." *Notre Dame Journal of Law, Ethics, and Public Policy* 9:1 (1995), 75–92; Weithman, Paul J. "Natural Law, Morality, and Sexual Complementarity." In David M. Estlund and Martha C. Nussbaum, eds., *Sex, Preference, and Family: Essays on Law and Nature.* New York: Oxford University Press, 1997, 227–46.

Andrew Koppelman

ADDITIONAL READING

Anscombe, G.E.M. [Elizabeth]. "Contraception and Chastity." *The Human World,* no. 7 (1972), 9–30. Reprinted in Michael D. Bayles, ed., *Ethics and Population.* Cambridge, Mass.: Schenkman, 1976, 134–53; HS (29–50); Cahill, Lisa Sowle. "Grisez on Sex and Gender: A Feminist Theological Perspective." In Nigel Biggar and Rufus Black, eds., *The Revival of Natural Law: Philosophical, Theological, and Ethical Responses to the Finnis-Grisez School.* Aldershot, U.K.: Ashgate, 2000, 242–61; Chang, Ruth, ed. *Incommensurability, Incomparability, and Practical Reason.* Cambridge,

Mass.: Harvard University Press, 1997; Cohen, Carl. "Sex, Birth Control, and Human Life." *Ethics* 79:4 (1969), 251–63. Reprinted in P&S1 (150–65); P&S2 (185–99); Cooper, John M. "Aristotle on Natural Teleology." In Malcolm Schofield and Martha Nussbaum, eds., *Language and Logos: Studies in Ancient Greek Philosophy Presented to G.E.L. Owen.* Cambridge: Cambridge University Press, 1982, 197–222; Estlund, David M., and Martha C. Nussbaum, eds. *Sex, Preference, and Family: Essays on Law and Nature.* New York: Oxford University Press, 1997; Feldman, Fred. "On the Intrinsic Value of Pleasures." *Ethics* 107:3 (1997), 448–66; Finnis, John M. "Law, Morality, and 'Sexual Orientation.' " *Notre Dame Law Review* 69:5 (1994), 1049–76. Reprinted, revised, in *Notre Dame Journal of Law, Ethics, and Public Policy* 9:1 (1995), 11–39; and John Corvino, ed., *Same Sex: Debating the Ethics, Science, and Culture of Homosexuality.* Lanham, Md.: Rowman and Littlefield, 1997, 31–43; Finnis, John M. "Natural Law and Unnatural Acts." *The Heythrop Journal* 11 (1970), 365–87. Reprinted in HS (5–27); Finnis, John M. "The Rights and Wrongs of Abortion: A Reply to Judith Thomson." *Philosophy and Public Affairs* 2:2 (1973), 117–45; Finnis, John M., with Martha C. Nussbaum. "Is Homosexual Conduct Wrong? A Philosophical Exchange." *The New Republic* (15 November 1993), 12–13. Reprinted in POS3 (89–94); POS4 (97–100); Fuchs, Josef. "Natural Law." In Judith Dwyer, ed., *The New Dictionary of Catholic Social Thought.* Collegeville, Minn.: Liturgical Press, 1994, 669–75; George, Robert P. "Neutrality, Equality, and 'Same-Sex Marriage.' " In Lynn D. Wardle, Mark Strasser, William C. Duncan, and David Orgon Coolidge, eds., *Marriage and Same-Sex Unions: A Debate.* Westport, Conn.: Praeger, 2003, 119–32; George, Robert P., ed. *Natural Law and Moral Inquiry: Ethics, Metaphysics, and Politics in the Work of Germain Grisez.* Washington, D.C.: Georgetown University Press, 1998; George, Robert P., ed. *Natural Law Theory.* Oxford, U.K.: Clarendon Press, 1992; Grisez, Germain. *Abortion: The Myths, the Realities, the Arguments.* New York: Corpus Books, 1970; Grisez, Germain. *Contraception and the Natural Law.* Milwaukee, Wis.: Bruce, 1964; Grisez, Germain. *The Way of the Lord Jesus*, vol. 3: *Difficult Moral Questions.* Quincy, Ill.: Franciscan Press, 1997; Grisez, Germain, Joseph Boyle, John Finnis, William E. May, and John C. Ford. *The Teaching of "Humanae Vitae": A Defense.* San Francisco, Calif.: Ignatius Press, 1988; Haakonssen, Knud. "Natural Law." In Lawrence C. Becker and Charlotte B. Becker, eds., *Encyclopedia of Ethics*, 2nd ed., vol. 2. New York: Routledge, 2001, 1205–12; Hittinger, Russell. *A Critique of the New Natural Law Theory.* Notre Dame, Ind.: University of Notre Dame Press, 1987; Koppelman, Andrew. *Antidiscrimination Law and Social Equality.* New Haven, Conn.: Yale University Press, 1996; Koppelman, Andrew. "Homosexual Conduct: A Reply to the New Natural Lawyers." In John Corvino, ed., *Same Sex: Debating the Ethics, Science, and Culture of Homosexuality.* Lanham, Md.: Rowman and Littlefield, 1997, 44–57; Koppelman, Andrew. "Is Marriage Inherently Heterosexual?" *American Journal of Jurisprudence* 42 (1997), 51–95; Koppelman, Andrew. "Sexual and Religious Pluralism." In Saul M. Olyan and Martha C. Nussbaum, eds., *Sexual Orientation and Human Rights in American Religious Discourse.* New York: Oxford University Press, 1998, 215–33; Koppelman, Andrew. "Why Discrimination against Lesbians and Gay Men Is Sex Discrimination." *New York University Law Review* 69:2 (1994), 197–287; Kosnick, Anthony, William Carroll, Agnes Cunningham, Ronald Modras, and James Schulte. *Human Sexuality: New Directions in American Catholic Thought.* New York: Paulist Press, 1977; Kuhn, Thomas S. "Objectivity, Value Judgment, and Theory Choice." In *The Essential Tension: Selected Studies in Scientific Tradition and Change.* Chicago, Ill.: University of Chicago Press, 1977, 320–39; Levy, Donald. "Perversion and the Unnatural as Moral Categories." *Ethics* 90:2 (1980), 191–202. Reprinted, revised, in POS1 (169–89); Macedo, Stephen. "Homosexuality and the Conservative Mind." *Georgetown Law Journal* 84:2 (1995), 261–300; McCarthy, David Matzko. "The Relationship of Bodies: A Nuptial Hermeneutics of Same-Sex Unions." In Eugene F. Rogers, Jr., ed., *Theology and Sexuality: Classic and Contemporary Readings.* Oxford, U.K.: Blackwell, 2002, 200–216; Pope, Stephen J. "Primate Sociality and Natural Law Theory." In Robert W. Sussman and Audrey R. Chapman, eds., *The Origins and Nature of Sociality.* New York: Aldine de Gruyter, 2004, 313–31; Richardson, Henry S. "Commensurability." In Lawrence C. Becker and Charlotte B. Becker, eds., *Encyclopedia of Ethics*, 2nd ed., vol. 1. New York: Routledge, 2001, 258–62; Sullivan, Andrew. "Unnatural Law: We're All Sodomists Now." *The New Republic* (24 March 2003), 18–23; Vacek, Edward

C. "Contraception Again—A Conclusion in Search of Convincing Arguments: One Proportionalist's [Mis?]understanding of a Text." In Robert P. George, ed., *Natural Law and Moral Inquiry: Ethics, Metaphysics, and Politics in the Work of Germain Grisez*. Washington, D.C.: Georgetown University Press, 1998, 50–81; Vacek, Edward C. Proportionalism: One View of the Debate." *Theological Studies* 46:2 (1985), 287–314. Reprinted in Christopher Kaczor, ed., *Proportionalism: For and Against*. Milwaukee, Wis.: Marquette University Press, 2000, 406–35; Watt, E. D. "Professor Cohen's Encyclical." *Ethics* 80:3 (1970), 218–21; Westerman, Pauline C. *The Disintegration of Natural Law Theory: Aquinas to Finnis*. Leiden, Holland: Brill, 1998.

NEW NATURAL LAW. *See* Natural Law (New)

NIETZSCHE, FRIEDRICH (1844–1900). Friedrich Wilhelm Nietzsche was born at Röcken in Prussian Saxony. He was educated at Schula Pforta (1858–1864), the University of Bonn (1864–1865), and Leipzig University (1865–1869), where he studied classical philology (and discovered the writings of **Arthur Schopenhauer** [1788–1860]). In 1869 he was appointed to a professorship at the University of Basel. Nietzsche was originally sent to school to follow in the ecclesiastical tradition of his family. His father, Karl Ludwig, was a Lutheran pastor, his grandfather a superintendent, and his great-grandfather an archdeacon of the Lutheran church. His mother, Franziska, was the daughter of a Lutheran pastor. Nietzsche's own rebellion from his family destiny came fairly early. By 1865 he had abandoned theology as his course of study.

Nietzsche's resistance to family pressure allowed him to feel the weight of the cultural strictures he would be so fond of exposing in his adult work. His reputation is built on his role as "cultural physician": He considered European culture sick and set for himself an enormous task of moral and cultural reform. His notion of the "re-evaluation of all values" was aimed at the specific problems of the culture of his age. To gage the health of contemporary European culture, Nietzsche engaged in comparisons with ancient and contemporary cultures. Philosophy was for him a process of reclamation and invention. We reclaim the healthy philosophies of the past, and we invent a new culture for the future. A culture's view of sexuality becomes a barometer for its health; the illness of culture rests on its suppression of instinct. A healthy culture requires the reintegration of drives and impulses.

Nietzsche's views about sex can be gleaned from several strands in his thought: his remarks on passion and the philosophers who are its enemies; his powerful and prevalent sexual metaphors, including his masculine and feminine imagery; and his remarks on reproduction. What he wrote about gender ranges from the merely conventional to the enigmatic, and in these writings can be found much of what he thought about sexuality. Despite a veritable cottage industry on Nietzsche's views of women (see, for example, Pearsall and Oliver), not many scholarly studies of his sexual views exist. Like his allusions to art, his allusions to sexuality and passion are scattered throughout his works.

Nietzsche's most philosophically profound remarks about sexuality occur in his opposition to various fleshless philosophies of the past, especially those that suppress the passions. The objects of these critiques range from Euripides (ca. 485–406 BCE) and Socrates (469–399 BCE), who are accused of removing passion from art and thought (see *The Birth of Tragedy*, passim; and " 'Reason' in Philosophy" and "The Problem of Socrates," in *Twilight of the Idols*), to his positivist and utilitarian contemporaries, who exhibited the same tendency (see *The Gay Science* and *Genealogy of Morals*, passim). The bloodless tenor of these works, their admitted escape from the transitoriness of feeling, and the very smallness of their goals are what damn them in Nietzsche's eyes. These features signaled a philosophy motivated not only by fear of the unknown but also by fear of passions and impulses natural to and important for the full experience of life. In this sense, Nietzsche's entire philosophy, from start to finish, is an indictment of those who fear the erotic.

The resurrection of the erotic motivates Nietzsche's interest in the underside of ancient Greek cultures. *The Birth of Tragedy* (1872) moves the high point of antiquity back prior to the golden age, and it does this precisely to capture the Dionysian elements of ecstatic and orgiastic cults. The book counters the trend to whitewash Greek culture to make it palatable to an age of Christianity and positivism. Nietzsche turns back to the Greeks for a legacy that includes the sensual and sexual: "It is here I set the Dionysus of the Greeks: the religious affirmation of life, life whole and not denied or in part; (typical—that the sexual act arouses profundity, mystery, reverence)" (*Will to Power*, §1052). In stark contrast to Dionysian culture, there is the philosophy of Socrates and **Plato** (427–347 BCE), who substitute for Dionysian affirmation of life a metaphysics that bases its projects on obtaining truths with mathematical precision and certainty. This is, for Nietzsche, *anti*erotic. The flight to reason claims to be motivated by truth, yet it is ultimately motivated by fear, a fear of the unknown, a discomfort with change, and (as an expectable result) a distrust of the (disorderly) physical and emotional passions.

Nietzsche sees Christianity as the natural heir to the Socratic/Platonic project. The Other World, created by Christianity, is based on rejecting the realities of this life.

> The Christian priest is from the first a mortal enemy of sensuality: no greater antithesis can be imagined than the innocently awed and solemn attitude by, e.g., the most honorable women's cults of Athens in presence of the symbols of sex. The act of procreation is the mystery as such in all non-ascetic religions: a sort of symbol of perfection and of the mysterious design of the future: rebirth, immortality. (*Will*, §184)

In the earlier Greek view the presence of the phallus, to which Nietzsche alludes, is a natural part of spiritual life. "It was Christianity, on the basis of its *ressentiment against* life, that first made something unclean out of sexuality" (*Twilight of the Idols*, 90). In most of his writing on antiquity he concentrates on a masculine, phallic, view of sexuality: "The church fights passion by cutting it out, in every sense; its practice, its therapy, is *castration*" (*Twilight*, 25). Notice how Nietzsche's passionate and forceful writing uses strong sensual and sexual imagery; its goal is serious criticism of the sterility of many philosophies. To extend his criticism: Positivism too, retains the puritanism of Christianity on matters sexual.

As the early Greek thinkers said, and Nietzsche reiterated, much of life is frightening and ugly. Rather than veil it, as Schopenhauer did, Nietzsche transfigures it. Sexual physiology will then require transfiguration. " 'The human being under the skin' is for all lovers a horror and unthinkable, a blasphemy against God and love" (*Gay Science*, §59). What the masculine artist does is transform what he finds (like philosophy is cultural creation). Nietzsche imagines this transformation in **love**, too. Like Schopenhauer, for whom the actual physical reality of the female form and function inspires revulsion, Nietzsche laments the very reality of women's embodied nature: "When we love a woman, we easily conceive a hatred for nature on account of all the repulsive natural functions to which every woman is subject. We prefer not to think of all this. . . . Then we refuse to pay any heed to physiology and decree secretly: 'I want to hear nothing about the fact that a human being is something more than soul and form' " (*Gay*, §59). Here women are addressed as the object of attraction, but their actual functioning at all stages of life is viewed with condescension and contempt.

Nietzsche's physiological explanations of women's purposes echo essentialism. Women are breeders, helpmates to men, "the recreation of the warrior." "Everything about woman is a riddle, and everything in woman has one solution: that is pregnancy" (*Thus Spoke Zarathustra*, 178). Once they are mothers, "females find in their children satisfaction for their desire to dominate, a possession, an occupation, something that is wholly intelligible to them and can be chattered with. . . . Pregnancy has made women kinder, more patient, more timid, more pleased to submit" (*Gay*, §72). Women are condemned to submit (physiology is destiny), yet pregnancy and birth become the noblest of virtues that are, however, enlisted as the most potent metaphors for masculine creativity. Nietzsche's conventionalism in expropriating women's reproductive powers in the service of men's creativity is what Plato did in the *Symposium* (but not only Plato). As with other thinkers of this ilk, the old (or older) woman presents a problem. She appears as a panderer or as one who advises that man bring a whip when he comes to women. ("You are going to women? Do not forget the whip!" *Thus Spoke*, 179.) As one critic puts it, Nietzsche "is decidedly critical of older women and feminists (who devalue their childbearing abilities and want to be seen as equal to men)" (Scott, 69).

As much as Nietzsche finds the image of Dionysus sexually freeing, he still takes his models of sexual unions and heterosexuality from what are basically Pre-Socratic ideas. His book *Philosophy in the Tragic Age of the Greeks* refers to a view of the world that is divided in sexual terms into the passive and active. "For lovers in the complete and strong sense of the word sexual gratification is not essential and is really no more than a symbol: for one party . . . a symbol of unconditional submission, for the other a symbol of assent to this, a sign of taking a possession" (*Will*, §732). Females receive; males give. "It is the same here as with the difference between the sexes: One ought not to demand of the artist, who gives, that he should become a woman—that he should receive" (*Will*, §811). This theme is continued into the discussion of male **homosexuality**: The male who receives is the lower of the two men; he is subject to the other. So to come across Nietzsche using the language of submission in considering mature women is not shocking. Nietzsche, who smashed so many philosophical and conceptual dichotomies, seemingly accepted these essentializing notions. He promises a Dionysian sexuality, a new coupling that should (in following the method of his other works) not only give us something new but also deny the reality of the preexisting dichotomies. The true and apparent worlds disappear together, as do objectivity and subjectivity; and "good" and "evil" are exposed as equally limited in their ability to shed light on the world in which we live. With these dichotomies dismantled, Nietzsche usually engages in a tripartite analysis. He shows how these dichotomies were only constructs; he shows next what they were able to do when they functioned helpfully; finally, he shows how they are retrogressive to contemporary philosophical thought. Yet in his writings about sex, we seem to be teased by his metaphorical promises; it is unclear that he delivers on the suggestions for a new sexuality. Further, thinking of a new heterosexual sexuality is difficult without rethinking gender, and that he did not do. His views of sexuality are hypermasculinized: "[S]exual love, too, belongs here: it desires to overpower, to take possession, and it appears as self-surrender. Fundamentally it is only love of one's 'instrument,' of one's 'steed'—the conviction that this or that belongs to one because one is in a position to use it" (*Will*, §776). Such metaphors abound in his work.

Since Nietzsche's perspective is so profoundly masculine, what he fears—emasculation and castration—is predictable. Nietzsche's criticism of Christianity can be extended in an important way, by injecting fear into all contemporary morality:

> Affect, great desire, the passion for power, love, revenge, possessions: moralists want to extinguish and uproot them, to "purify" the soul of them. . . . [T]he founder of Christianity, recommended this practice to his disciples, the case of sexual excitation, the consequence is, unfortunately, not only the loss of an organ but the *emasculation* of a man's character.—And the same applies to the moralist's madness that demands, instead of restraining of the passions, their extirpation. Its conclusion is always: only the castrated man is a good man. (*Will*, §383)

Nietzsche's point is powerful. But in his writings the woman is left "castrated," her passion extirpated.

In a sense Nietzsche is dealing with a great conundrum, that of the European man's heterosexuality. Indeed he at times alludes to the social superiority of the homosexual and the homosocial cultures of ancient Greece. Part of the riddle of Socrates can be explained by his erotic nature. "All great achievements on the part of the man of antiquity were supported by the fact that man stood beside man, and that a woman was not allowed to claim to be the nearest or highest, let alone sole object of his love" (*Daybreak*, 204–5). "All great achievements," says Nietzsche, have an erotic component. This has the profound consequence that "the degree and kind of a man's sexuality reach up into the ultimate pinnacle of his spirit" (*Beyond Good and Evil*, §75). In contrast to these virile images from antiquity, Christian culture is weak, effeminate; its sexual impulse is merely the tamed and moralized sexual impulse of **marriage** (*Will*, §62). This Christian suppression of masculine passion harms not only men but also culture. Their "great achievements" get weighed down by domesticity.

But breeding, in the sense of producing a new generation of humans, is no trivial matter for Nietzsche (nor was it trivial for Schopenhauer). "In marriage in the aristocratic, old aristocratic sense of the word it was a question of the breeding of a race. . . . [M]an and woman were sacrificed to this point of view. It is obvious that love was not the first consideration here; on the contrary!" (*Will*, §732). Marriage within such cultures is a proposition about procreation and property. It is not a place of sensuality or sexuality. "The tremendous importance the individual accords to the sexual instinct is not a result of its importance for the species, but arises because procreation is the real achievement of the individual" (*Will*, §680). Because he so often presents women conventionally, what Nietzsche might have had in mind about the type of women with whom Dionysian men would breed remains a serious question.

For one thing, the physiological woman has to be transfigured; she must be improved, made more perfect:

> That making perfect, seeing as perfect, . . . characterizes the cerebral system bursting with sexual energy. . . . [E]very perfection, all the beauty of things, revives through contiguity this aphrodisiac bliss. . . . Physiologically: the creative instinct of the artist and the distribution of semen in his blood. . . . The demand for art and beauty is an indirect demand for the ecstasies of sexuality communicated to the brain. The world become perfect, through "love." (*Will*, §805)

Although Nietzsche describes these phenomena physiologically, the artist and the philosopher of culture must transform these physical realities. As one critic puts it, "*Where things are not beautiful, attractive, desirable . . . The Gay Science* turns to art . . . for the erotic transfiguration that is love" (Babich, 163).

Nietzsche's early remarks on women are conventional and full of stereotypes: "[I]n the Orient women regard chastisements and the secret seclusion of their person from the world as a sign of their husband's love, and complain if this sign is lacking" (*Daybreak*, 9). Women want to be passive. Further, women's sexual passions must nevertheless be held in check, lest "ignorant young wives . . . become accustomed to the frequent enjoyment of sex and miss it greatly later if their husbands become ill or prematurely feeble; it is precisely this innocent and credulous idea that frequent intercourse is thoroughly right and proper that it produces in them a need which later expose them to violent temptations or worse" (*Daybreak*, 159). But on a few occasions he does try to figure out what love and sex could be for women, and he states one conundrum with some perspicacity:

> There is something quite amazing and monstrous about the education of upper-class women. . . . All the world is agreed that they are to be brought up as ignorant as possible of erotic matters, and that one has to imbue their souls with a profound sense of shame in such matters . . . [and] then to be hurled, as by a gruesome lightning bolt, into reality and knowledge, by marriage— precisely by the man they love and esteem most! . . . Thus a psychic knot has been tied that may have no equal. Even the compassionate curiosity of the wisest student of humanity is inadequate for guessing how this or that woman manages to accommodate herself to this solution of the riddle, and to the riddle of a solution, and what dreadful, far-reaching suspicions must stir in her poor, unhinged soul. (*Gay*, §71)

In spite of his conventionalism, Nietzsche shows some sensitivity to the plight of women in a culture that cannot quite come to grips even with the existence of female sexuality, let alone its various manifestations. Sounding already a bit like the **Sigmund Freud** (1856–1939) who often complained about the repression and suppression of female **sexual desire** in Victorian culture, Nietzsche wrote, "The enormous expectation in sexual love and the sense of shame in this expectation spoils all perspective for women from the start" (*Beyond*, §114). This does not take us very far, however, in imagining or creating a woman equal to the man whose sexuality reaches up "into the ultimate pinnacle of his spirit."

See also Existentialism; Greek Sexuality and Philosophy, Ancient; Hobbes, Thomas; Kierkegaard, Søren; Lacan, Jacques; Language; Paglia, Camille; Poststructuralism; Sade, Marquis de; Schopenhauer, Arthur

REFERENCES

Babich, Babette E. "Nietzsche and Eros between the Devil and God's Deep Blue Sea: The Problem of the Artist as Actor—Jew—Woman." *Continental Philosophy Review* 33 (April 2000), 159–88; Nietzsche, Friedrich. (1886) *Beyond Good and Evil*. Trans. Walter Kaufmann. New York: Random House, 1966; Nietzsche, Friedrich. (1872, 1888) *The Birth of Tragedy* and *The Case of Wagner*. Trans. Walter Kaufmann. New York: Random House, 1967; Nietzsche, Friedrich. (1881) *Daybreak: Thoughts on the Prejudices of Morality*. Trans. R. J. Hollingdale. Cambridge: Cambridge University Press, 1982; Nietzsche, Friedrich. (1882, 1887) *The Gay Science, with a Prelude of Rhymes and an Appendix of Songs*. Trans. Walter Kaufmann. New York: Random House, 1974; Nietzsche, Friedrich. (1887, 1908) *On the Genealogy of Morals* and *Ecce Homo*. Trans. Walter Kaufmann and R. J. Hollingdale. New York: Random House, 1967; Nietzsche, Friedrich. *Philosophy in the Tragic Age of the Greeks.* Trans. Marianne Cowan. Chicago, Ill.: Henry Regnery Company, 1962; Nietzsche, Friedrich. (1883/1892) *Thus Spoke Zarathustra.* Trans. Walter Kaufmann. In *The Portable Nietzsche.* New York: Viking, 1954, 121–439; Nietzsche, Friedrich. (1889) *Twilight of the Idols, or, How to Philosophize with a Hammer.* Trans. Richard Polt. Indianapolis, Ind.: Hackett, 1997; Nietzsche, Friedrich. (1901) *The Will to Power.* Trans. Walter Kaufmann. New York: Random House, 1967; Pearsall, Marilyn, and Kelly Oliver, eds. *Feminist Interpretations of Friedrich Nietzsche.* University Park: Pennsylvania State University Press, 1998; Plato. (ca. 380 BCE) *Symposium.* Trans. Alexander Nehamas and Paul Woodruff. Indianapolis, Ind.: Hackett, 1989; Schopenhauer, Arthur. (1818, 1844, 1859) *The World as Will and Representation,* 2 vols. Trans. E.F.J. Payne. New York: Dover, 1966; Scott, Jacqueline R. "Nietzsche and the Problem of Women's Bodies." *International Studies in Philosophy* 31:3 (1999), 65–75; Sedgwick, Peter R., ed. *Nietzsche: A Critical Reader.* Oxford, U.K.: Blackwell, 1995; Solomon, Robert C., and Kathleen M. Higgins, eds. *Reading Nietzsche.* New York: Oxford University Press, 1988.

Kathleen J. Wininger

ADDITIONAL READING

Abbey, Ruth. "Odd Bedfellows: Nietzsche and Mill on Marriage." *History of European Ideas* 23:2–4 (1997), 81–104; Acampora, Christa Davis, and Ralph R. Acampora, eds. *A Nietzschean Bestiary: Becoming Animal Beyond Docile and Brutal.* Lanham, Md.: Rowman and Littlefield, 2004; Allison, David B., ed. *The New Nietzsche: Contemporary Styles of Interpretation.* Cambridge, Mass.: MIT Press, 1985; Ansell-Pearson, Keith. "Who Is the Übermensch? Time, Truth, and Woman in Nietzsche." *Journal of the History of Ideas* 53 (April–June 1992), 326–48; Aschheim, Steven E. *The Nietzsche Legacy in Germany, 1890–1990.* Berkeley: University of California Press, 1992; Babich, Babette E. "Nietzsche and Eros between the Devil and God's Deep Blue Sea: The Problem of the Artist as Actor—Jew—Woman." *Continental Philosophy Review* 33 (April 2000), 159–88. <www.fordham.edu/philosophy/lc/babich/Babich.Erotic-Valence-of-Art.kluwer.htm> [accessed 15 February 2005]; Bataille, Georges. (1945) *On Nietzsche.* Trans. Bruce Boone. London: Athlone, 1992; Bloom, Harold, ed. *Modern Critical Views: Friedrich Nietzsche.* New York: Chelsea House, 1987; Clark, Maudemarie. *Nietzsche on Truth and Philosophy.* Cambridge: Cambridge University Press, 1990; Conant, James. "Nietzsche, Kierkegaard, and Anscombe on Moral Unintelligibility." In D. Z. Phillips, ed., *Religion and Morality.* New York: St. Martin's Press, 1996, 250–98; Danto, Arthur C. *Nietzsche as Philosopher: An Original Study.* New York: Columbia University Press, 1965; Deleuze, Gilles. (1962) *Nietzsche and Philosophy.* Trans. Hugh Tomlinson. New York: Columbia University Press, 1983; Derrida, Jacques. (1978) *Spurs: Nietzsche's Styles.* Trans. Barbara Harlow. Chicago, Ill.: University of Chicago Press, 1979; Foucault, Michel. (1971) "Nietzsche, Genealogy, History." Trans. Donald Bouchard and Sherry Simon. In Donald Bouchard, ed., *Michel Foucault: Language, Counter-Memory, Practice. Selected Essays and Interviews.* Ithaca, N.Y.: Cornell University Press, 1977, 139–64; Gallop, Jane. " 'Women' in *Spurs* and Nineties Feminism." *Diacritics* 25:2 (1995), 126–34; Gilman, Sander L., ed. *Conversations with Nietzsche: A Life in the Words of His Contemporaries.* Trans. David J. Parent. New York: Oxford University Press, 1987; Hayman, Ronald. *Nietzsche: A Critical Life.* New York: Oxford University Press, 1980; Heidegger, Martin. (1961) *Nietzsche,* vol. 1: *The Will to Power as Art.* Trans. David F. Krell. New York: Harper and Row, 1979; Heidegger, Martin. (1961) *Nietzsche,* vol. 2: *The Eternal Recurrence of the Same.* Trans. David F. Krell. San Francisco, Calif.: Harper and Row, 1984; Heidegger, Martin. (1961) *Nietzsche,* vol. 3: *Will to Power as Knowledge and as Metaphysics.* Trans. Joan Stambaugh and Frank Capuzzi. San Francisco, Calif.: Harper and Row, 1986; Heidegger, Martin. (1961) *Nietzsche,* vol. 4: *Nihilism.* Trans. David F. Krell. New York: Harper and Row, 1982. San Francisco, Calif.: Harper and Row, 1986; Higgins, Kathleen Marie. *Nietzsche's "Zarathustra."* Philadelphia, Pa.: Temple University Press, 1987; Higgins, Kathleen Marie. "Schopenhauer and Nietzsche: Temperament and Temporality." In Christopher Janaway, ed., *Willing and Nothingness: Schopenhauer as Nietzsche's Educator.* Oxford, U.K.: Clarendon Press, 1998, 151–77; Hollingdale, R. J. *Nietzsche.* London: Routledge and

Kegan Paul, 1973; Hubben, William. *Dostoevsky, Kierkegaard, Nietzsche, and Kafka: Four Prophets of Our Destiny*. New York: Collier, 1962; Hunt, Lester H. *Nietzsche and the Origin of Virtue*. London: Routledge, 1991; Irigaray, Luce. (1980) *Marine Lover of Friedrich Nietzsche*. Trans. Gillian C. Gill. New York: Columbia University Press, 1991; Janz, Curt Paul. *Friedrich Nietzsche Biographie*, 3 vols. Munich, Ger.: Deutscher Taschenbuch Verlag, 1981; Kaufmann, Walter. *Nietzsche: Philosopher, Psychologist, Antichrist*. Princeton, N.J.: Princeton University Press, 1950; Kennedy, Ellen, and Susan Mendus, eds. *Women in Western Political Philosophy: Kant to Nietzsche*. New York: St. Martin's Press, 1987; Klossowski, Pierre. (1969) *Nietzsche and the Vicious Circle*. Trans. Daniel W. Smith. London: Athlone, 1993; Koelb, Clayton, ed. *Nietzsche as Postmodernist: Essays Pro and Contra*. Albany: State University of New York Press, 1990; Kofman, Sarah. "Baubô: Theological Perversion and Fetishism." Trans. Tracy B. Strong. In Michael Allen Gillespie and Tracy B. Strong, eds., *Nietzsche's New Seas: Explorations in Philosophy, Aesthetics, and Politics*. Chicago, Ill.: University of Chicago Press, 1988, 175–202; Kofman, Sarah. "Explosion I: Of Nietzsche's *Ecce Homo*." Trans. Duncan Large. *Diacritics* 24:4 (1994), 51–70; Kofman, Sarah. (1972) *Nietzsche and Metaphor*. Trans. Duncan Large. London: Athlone Press, 1993. Stanford, Calif.: Stanford University Press, 1993; Krell, David Farrell. *Postponements: Women, Sensuality, and Death in Nietzsche*. Bloomington: Indiana University Press, 1986; Krell, David Farrell, and Donald L. Bates. *The Good European: Nietzsche's Work Sites in Word and Image*. Chicago, Ill.: University of Chicago Press, 1997; Lambert, Laurence. *Nietzsche's Teaching: An Interpretation of "Thus Spoke Zarathustra."* New Haven, Conn.: Yale University Press, 1987; Löwith, Karl. (1956) *Nietzsche's Philosophy of the Eternal Recurrence of the Same*. Trans. J. Harvey Lomax. Berkeley: University of California Press, 1997; Macintyre, Ben. *Forgotten Fatherland: The Search for Elisabeth Nietzsche*. London: Macmillan, 1992; Magnus, Bernd. (1978) *Nietzsche's Existential Imperative*. Bloomington: Indiana University Press, 1993; Magnus, Bernd, and Kathleen M. Higgins, eds. *The Cambridge Companion to Nietzsche*. Cambridge: Cambridge University Press, 1996; Magnus, Bernd, Stanley Stewart, and Jean-Pierre Mileur. *Nietzsche's Case: Philosophy as/and Literature*. New York: Routledge, 1992; Mandel, Siegfried. *Nietzsche and the Jews*. Amherst, N.Y.: Prometheus, 1998; Nehamas, Alexander. *Nietzsche: Life as Literature*. Cambridge, Mass.: Harvard University Press, 1985; Nietzsche, Friedrich (1895) *The Antichrist*. Trans. Walter Kaufmann. In *The Portable Nietzsche*. New York: Viking Press, 1954, 568–656; Nietzsche, Friedrich. (1878) *Human, All Too Human: A Book for Free Spirits*. Trans. R. J. Hollingdale. Cambridge: Cambridge University Press, 1986; Nietzsche, Friedrich. *Kritische Gesamtausgabe Briefwechsel*, 24 vols. Ed. Georgio Colli and Mazzino Montinari. Berlin, Ger.: Walter de Gruyter, 1975; Nietzsche, Friedrich. *My Sister and I*. New York: Amok, 1990; Nietzsche, Friedrich. *Philosophy and Truth: Selections from Nietzsche's Notebooks of the Early 1870's*. Trans. and ed. Daniel Breazeale. Atlantic Highlands, N.J.: Humanities Press, 1979; Nietzsche, Friedrich. *Sämtliche Werke: Kritische Studienausgabe*. Ed. Georgio Colli and Mazzino Montinari. Berlin, Ger.: Walter de Gruyter, 1967– ; Nietzsche, Friedrich. (1873, 1874, 1876) *Untimely Meditations*. Trans. R. J. Hollingdale. Cambridge: Cambridge University Press, 1983; Oliver, Kelly. "Woman as Truth in Nietzsche's Writings." *Social Theory and Practice* 10:2 (1984), 185–99; Oliver, Kelly. *Womanizing Nietzsche: Philosophy's Relation to the "Feminine."* New York: Routledge, 1995; Parkes, Graham. *Composing the Soul: Reaches of Nietzsche's Psychology*. Chicago, Ill.: University of Chicago Press, 1994; Parkes, Graham. *Nietzsche and Asian Thought*. Chicago, Ill.: University of Chicago Press, 1991; Patton, Paul, ed. *Nietzsche, Feminism and Political Theory*. Sydney, Australia: Allen and Unwin, 1993; Picart, Caroline Joan. *Resentment and the "Feminine" in Nietzsche's Politico-Aesthetics*. University Park: Pennsylvania State University Press, 1999; Pletch, Carl. *Young Nietzsche: Becoming a Genius*. New York: Free Press, 1991; Prose, Francine. "Lou Andreas-Salomé." In *The Lives of the Muses: Nine Women and the Artists They Inspired*. New York: HarperCollins, 2002, 139–85; Rosen, Stanley. *The Mask of Enlightenment: Nietzsche's Zarathustra*. Cambridge: Cambridge University Press, 1995; [Andreas-]Salomé, Lou. (1894) *Nietzsche*. Trans. Siegfried Mandel. Redding Ridge, Conn.: Black Swan Books, 1988, Urbana: University of Illinois Press, 2001; Schacht, Richard. (1983) *Nietzsche*. London: Routledge, 1999; Schacht, Richard, ed. *Nietzsche, Genealogy, Morality: Essays on Nietzsche's Genealogy of Morals*. Berkeley: University of California Press,

1994; Schrift, Alan D. *Nietzsche and the Question of Interpretation: Between Hermeneutics and Deconstruction.* New York: Routledge, 1990; Shapiro, Gary. *Nietzschean Narratives.* Bloomington: Indiana University Press, 1989; Simmel, Georg. (1907) *Schopenhauer and Nietzsche.* Trans. Helmut Loiskandle, Deena Weinstein, and Michael Weinstein. Urbana: University of Illinois Press, 1991; Singer, Irving. "Anti-Romantic Romantics: Kierkegaard, Tolstoy, Nietzsche." In *The Nature of Love,* vol. 3: *The Modern World.* Chicago, Ill.: University of Chicago Press, 1987, 38–94; Solomon, Robert C. *Living with Nietzsche: What the Great "Immoralist" Has to Teach Us.* New York: Oxford University Press, 2004; Solomon, Robert C., ed. *Nietzsche: A Collection of Critical Essays.* Garden City, N.Y.: Anchor Books, 1973; Stambaugh, Joan. (1959) *The Problem of Time in Nietzsche.* Trans. John F. Humphrey. Philadelphia, Pa.: Bucknell University Press, 1987; Steinbuch, Thomas. *A Commentary on Nietzsche's Ecce Homo.* Lanham, Md.: University Press of America, 1994; Taylor, Charles Senn. "Nietzsche's Schopenhauerianism." *Nietzsche-Studien* 17 (1988), 45–73; White, Alan. *Within Nietzsche's Labyrinth.* New York: Routledge, 1990; Wilcox, John T. *Truth and Value in Nietzsche.* Ann Arbor: University of Michigan Press, 1990; Wininger, Kathleen J. *Nietzsche and the Reclamation of Philosophy.* Amsterdam, Holland: Rodopi, 1997; Young, Julian. *Nietzsche's Philosophy of Art.* Cambridge: Cambridge University Press, 1992; Yovel, Yirmiyahu, ed. *Nietzsche as Affirmative Thinker.* Dordrecht, Holland: Martinus Nijhoff, 1986.

NUDISM. Nudism (or naturism) is the practice of nonsexualized social nudity. Organized nudism has been part of North American culture since the late 1920s (Cinder, 505–627). Nudists believe that nudity engaged in with family, friends, or others is physically, psychologically, and socially beneficial. They often argue for greater social tolerance of their practices, seeking greater freedom for themselves and others to be naked in private and in appropriate public settings.

Many lawmakers accept some version of John Stuart Mill's (1806–1873) harm principle (from *On Liberty*) as justification for laws prohibiting behavior. But legislators have difficulty showing that public nudity harms anyone. Further, legislators are unable to show that mere nudity in public is immoral (see Storey). Nudists have endlessly combated the fiction that mere social nudity leads to sexual promiscuity. As **Camille Paglia** has said, "There is nothing less erotic than a nudist colony" (36; see Posner, 359; Shalit, 173–74, 176). So lawmakers often advance a third argument, which appeals to *offense*: Nudity seriously offends many people and hence may be legally prohibited. Of course, some offensive behaviors are morally permissible. Jesus offended those around him in ways that left his followers incredulous (Matt. 15:12); Mary Wollstonecraft (1759–1797) offended Britons as she fought for women's rights; Martin Luther King, Jr. (1929–1968) offended many when, in 1963, he led marches in Birmingham; many find **homosexuality** offensive, but that might not be legally decisive (Thomas and Levin, 142–45, 162–64). Legislators must determine what offending behaviors warrant legal sanction. Recall that in 1967 the Supreme Court struck down antimiscegenation laws (*Loving v. Virginia*) even though many Americans found interracial **marriage** (as well as dating) offensive.

A flippant nudist might say, "We have the right to be naked when and where we wish. Because people can be offended by *anything*, being offensive should not be legally relevant." This view fails to acknowledge the complexities of offense, ignoring sensible principles that judges and lawmakers can rewardingly bring to the discussion. Joel Feinberg (1926–2004), who often uses nudity as an example of nonharmful offensive behavior (*Moral Limits,* 12, 14, 17–20, 40, 41, 58), articulates principles for weighing the seriousness of offensive behavior against its reasonableness. He thereby provides a useful context for investigating the social and legal aspects of nudism.

That which we need to function fully and fruitfully as humans is that in which we have an interest. We have an interest in being alive, remaining healthy, retaining our possessions, moving about freely, learning, and associating with friends. According to Feinberg, harmful acts are those that set back these interests (*Moral Limits*, x). By contrast, offensive acts cause uncomfortable psychological states: sensory affronts (by ugly sights, noxious odors, grating noises), disgust, revulsion, shame, embarrassment, anxiety, annoyance, resentment, and humiliation (10–13). We prefer not to experience these states. But acts that cause them cannot be prohibited as harmful, as they do not frustrate our interests. The difference between nonharmful offensiveness and harmful acts (on which, see Shoemaker, 545n.2, 547–51) mirrors the Model Penal Code's distinction between mere nude sunbathing, which it would not prohibit, and sexual aggression (Posner and Silbaugh, 83).

Various factors are relevant in determining whether offensive behavior is serious enough to warrant legal sanction. One is *intensity*. The offense of a neighbor practicing drums indoors is not as intense as the offense of practicing outdoors beneath your bedroom window. Witnessing public nudity seems not to have this intensity for most observers. The offense of nudity is not like that of acts that produce powerful reactions, such as public defecation (Feinberg, "Reply," 134).

The seriousness of offense also depends on *duration*. When we pass a smelly man on the street, the odor may be offensive, but not for long. Once out of olfactory range, we might recall the sensation but no longer suffer it. By contrast, if a woman walks past men who shout offensive remarks at her, her suffering might last for days. The duration of experiencing discomfort from seeing naked sunbathers or swimmers, however, is likely to be short.

Another factor is *extent*. The larger the number of people offended by an act, the greater the justification for discouraging it. Most people find loud, piercing noises to be irritating; few find elevator music more than mildly annoying. According to the Naturist Education Foundation's 2000 Roper-Starch poll, most Americans (80 percent) think people should be permitted to sunbathe nude in designated locations, and 25 percent have engaged in mixed-sex skinny-dipping (Storey and Baxandall). The poll did not address people's being offended by public nudity, but it does suggest that its extent is low.

In terms of its seriousness, public nudity seems unworthy of legal sanction. Nevertheless, without being overdramatic ("Surely there have been a few automobile accidents and a few drinks spilled because of reactions to public nudity" [VanDeVeer, 176n.3]), it can be admitted that some people are offended by seeing others naked and experience genuine shock, embarrassment, annoyance, and anxiety (Feinberg, "Harmless Immoralities," 101; see Bayles, 118–19). To be weighed against the factors making an offense serious and perhaps warranting legal sanction are factors showing the offensive conduct to be acceptable or reasonable.

The *standard of reasonable avoidability* states one counterbalancing factor. If people can avoid offensive behavior without undue inconvenience, the state should not intervene (Feinberg, *Moral Limits*, 32). When people are not compelled to experience offensive, nonharmful behavior, others should be free to behave that way. Communities often allow erotic magazines to be sold in general stores even if they are offensive, partly on the ground of the importance of free speech. But, further, people who wish to avoid being offended can ignore these magazines. Some communities require that magazine stands include arrangements to shield people from nudity on magazine covers, for even if perusing a magazine's pages is easily avoidable, it is hard to avoid seeing displayed covers. Defenders of nudism appeal to "reasonable avoidability": Signs at the entrance of clothing-optional beaches and private parks allow people to avoid offense. The *volenti maxim* ("*volenti non fit injuria*") also applies here. This legal principle holds that those who freely and knowingly **consent** to experiencing a behavior cannot be wronged by it. If signs are posted informing people that an area is used for nude sunbathing, anyone who continues past the sign cannot complain.

Another factor is the *personal importance* of the offensive conduct. An act that offends others might provide economic support, maintain health, or be critical for relationships with loved ones (recall Feinberg's interests). These benefits provide grounds for not prohibiting the behavior. Because playing CDs at ear-piercing levels in public does not serve an interest, communities are justified in discouraging it. By contrast, even though bagpipes might sound to some like the wail of dying animals, a professional bagpipe player must have opportunity to master her craft while doing so as unobtrusively as possible. The importance of public nudity to the interest some people have in health, pleasure, and association with like-minded friends counts in favor of allowing it (Feinberg, *Moral Limits*, 40). It is now clear that *locality* is also relevant in judging offensive behavior. A secluded woodland area is a more appropriate place for playing bagpipes than the lawn outside a hospital. Similarly, a secluded beach, out of view of roads and homes and signed effectively to alert people to its use, is an appropriate place for social nudity.

The *social value* of offensive conduct is also relevant. Nudists point to problems people have with self-concept and body image, to bulimia and anorexia caused by poor body acceptance, and to the spurious connection the entertainment industry makes between nudity and sex. They argue that more widespread social nudity at beaches, hot springs, and private nudist camps can help alleviate these social and psychological ills. "Nudists contend that the removal of clothing brings about greater honesty between people . . . and creates greater equality between the sexes and weakens sexual segregation and discrimination. Research . . . tends to support such claims" (Hartman and Fithian, 421).

One other social value that tends to protect offensive behavior is *free expression*. Without the freedom to debate political, religious, or sexual issues in ways that some find offensive, people will not be sufficiently informed to play their role in democracy (Mill, chap. 2). When offensive conduct expresses ideas, the state should therefore be reluctant to prohibit it (VanDeVeer, 189–90; *Cohen v. California*). Courts have rarely recognized a link between nudity and free speech (*Naturist Society, Inc. v. Fillyaw*), however, and have ruled more often that nudity is not speech but activity (*Barnes v. Glen Theatre, Inc.*; *City of Erie v. Pap's A.M.*).

Another factor in favor of allowing offensive behavior is the actor's lacking *alternative opportunities*. Because some laws prohibit nudity even in one's own backyard, nudists have little opportunity to be naked socially outdoors. Limiting nudity to the inside of homes eliminates the fresh air, water, and communion with nature that are inherent to nudism. Many people live too far from private nudist parks to make them an option for daylong or weekend visits. Nudist parks were once inexpensive, so even low-income families could enjoy them. But many clubs have raised the price of admission and membership fees (Woodall). Younger families and retired people on fixed incomes thus do not have private nudist parks as an alternative opportunity for social nudity. Further, private clubs are unrewarding for nudists who prefer undeveloped areas such as beaches, hot springs, rivers, and lakes. Nudists argue that select public sites, not the entire coastline, should be open for clothing-optional recreation.

A weighing of these various factors might imply that public nudity is defensible, yet it is often discouraged. According to Montana Code 45-5-504, on a third conviction of indecent exposure, skinny-dippers "shall be punished by life imprisonment or by imprisonment in a state prison for a term of not less than 5 years or more than 100 years and may be fined not more than $10,000" (Naturist Action Committee). But the prohibition of nudity by the criminal law should be a last resort. As Feinberg argues, the law should not treat mild offenses as if they were harmful (*Moral Limits*, 3, 5). More appropriate discouragement is achievable by nuisance laws with, say, penalties no greater than parking tickets (Feinberg, "Reply," 130; Bayles, 124).

See also Bestiality; Consequentialism; Law, Sex and the; Liberalism; Pornography; Privacy; Prostitution

REFERENCES

Barnes v. Glen Theatre, Inc. 115 L.Ed. 2d 504; 501 U.S. 560; 111 S.Ct. 2456 (1991); Bayles, Michael D. "Comments [on Feinberg]: Offensive Conduct and the Law." In Norman S. Care and Thomas K. Trelogan, eds., *Issues in Law and Morality*. Cleveland, Ohio: Press of Case Western Reserve University, 1973, 111–26; Cinder, Cec. *The Nudist Idea*. Riverside, Calif.: Ultraviolet Press, 1998; *City of Erie v. Pap's A.M.* 529 U.S. 277; 120 S.Ct. 1382 (2000); *Cohen v. California*. 29 L.Ed. 2d 284; 403 U.S. 15; 91 S.Ct. 1780 (1971); Feinberg, Joel. " 'Harmless Immoralities' and Offensive Nuisances." In Norman S. Care and Thomas K. Trelogan, eds., *Issues in Law and Morality*. Cleveland, Ohio: Press of Case Western Reserve University, 1973, 83–109; Feinberg, Joel. *The Moral Limits of the Criminal Law*, vol. 2: *Offense to Others*. New York: Oxford University Press, 1985; Feinberg, Joel. "Reply [to Bayles]." In Norman S. Care and Thomas K. Trelogan, eds., *Issues in Law and Morality*. Cleveland, Ohio: Press of Case Western Reserve University, 1973, 127–40; Hartman, William E., and Marilyn A. Fithian. "Nudism." In Vern L. Bullough and Bonnie Bullough, eds., *Human Sexuality: An Encyclopedia*. New York: Garland, 1994, 419–21; *Loving v. Virginia*. 13 L.Ed 2d 1010; 388 U.S. 1; 87 S.Ct. 1817 (1967); Mill, John Stuart. (1859) *On Liberty*. Ed. Elizabeth Rapaport. Indianapolis, Ind.: Hackett, 1978; Naturist Action Committee. (Web site) <www.nac.oshkosh.net> [accessed 15 February 2005]; *Naturist Society, Inc. v. Fillyaw*. 958 F.2d 1515 (11th Cir. 1992); Paglia, Camille. *Sexual Personae: Art and Decadence from Nefertiti to Emily Dickinson*. New Haven, Conn.: Yale University Press, 1990; Posner, Richard A. *Sex and Reason*. Cambridge, Mass.: Harvard University Press, 1992; Posner, Richard A., and Katharine B. Silbaugh. "Public Nudity and Indecency." In *A Guide to America's Sex Laws*. Chicago, Ill.: University of Chicago Press, 1996, 83–97; Shalit, Wendy. "Modesty and the Erotic." In *A Return to Modesty: Discovering the Lost Virtue*. New York: Free Press, 1999, 171–93; Shoemaker, David W. " 'Dirty Words' and the Offense Principle." *Law and Philosophy* 19 (December 2000), 545–84; Storey, Mark. "Cultural Relativism and the Morality of Naturism." *Naturist LIFE International*, no. 14 (Summer 1995), 28–29; Storey, Mark, and Lee Baxandall. "A Growing Nude Attitude in America." *Nude & Natural* 20:2 (2000), 4–5; Thomas, Laurence M., and Michael E. Levin. *Sexual Orientation and Human Rights*. Lanham, Md.: Rowman and Littlefield, 1999; VanDeVeer, Donald. "Coercive Restraint of Offensive Actions." *Philosophy and Public Affairs* 8:2 (1979), 175–93; Woodall, Ellen E. "The American Nudist Movement: From Cooperative to Capital, the Song Remains the Same." *Journal of Popular Culture* 36:2 (2002), 264–84.

Mark Storey

ADDITIONAL READING

Bacher, K. "205 Arguments and Observations in Support of Naturism." *Nude & Natural* 16:1 (1996), 61–95. <www.naturistsociety.com/resources/PDF/205ARGUE.pdf> [accessed 16 February 2005]; Barcan, Ruth. "The Moral Bath of Bodily Unconsciousness: Female Nudism, Bodily Exposure, and the Gaze." *Continuum: Journal of Media and Cultural Studies* 15:3 (2001), 303–17; Bell, Alan P. "Attitudes towards Nudity by Social Class." *Medical Aspects of Human Sexuality* 3:9 (1969), 101, 105–8; Bork, Robert H. "Of Moralism, Moral Relativism, and the Constitution." In *The Tempting of America: The Political Seduction of the Law*. New York: Free Press, 1990, 241–50; Casler,

Lawrence. "Some Sociopsychological Observations in a Nudist Camp: A Preliminary Study." *Journal of Social Psychology* 64 (December 1964), 307–23; Clark, Kenneth. (1953) *The Nude: A Study in Ideal Form*. New York: Pantheon, 1956; *Cohen v. California*. 29 L.Ed. 2d 284; 403 U.S. 15; 91 S.Ct. 1780 (1971). <www.bc.edu/bc_org/avp/cas/comm/free_speech/cohen.html> [accessed 4 February 2004]; Cunningham, Jim C. "A Dialog of Conscience." *Naturist LIFE International*, no. 8 (Summer 1993), 22–24; DeMartino, Manfred F. *The New Female Sexuality: The Sexual Practices and Experiences of Social Nudists, "Potential" Nudists, and Lesbians*. New York: Julian Press, 1969; Eliade, Mircea. "Eschatological Nudism." In *Mephistopheles and the Androgyne: Studies in Religious Myth and Symbol*. Trans. J. M. Cohen. New York: Sheed and Ward, 1965, 125–28; Ellis, Anthony. "Offense and the Liberal Conception of the Law." *Philosophy and Public Affairs* 13:1 (1984), 3–23; Feinberg, Joel. "Harm and Offense." In Lawrence C. Becker and Charlotte B. Becker, eds., *Encyclopedia of Ethics*, 2nd ed., vol. 2. New York: Routledge, 2001, 652–55; Feinberg, Joel. " 'Harmless Immoralities' and Offensive Nuisances." In Norman S. Care and Thomas K. Trelogan, eds., *Issues in Law and Morality*. Cleveland, Ohio: Press of Case Western Reserve University, 1973, 83–109. Reprinted in Joel Feinberg, *Rights, Justice, and the Bounds of Liberty: Essays in Social Philosophy*. Princeton, N.J.: Princeton University Press, 1980, 69–109; Feinberg, Joel. *The Moral Limits of the Criminal Law*, 4 vols. New York: Oxford University Press, 1984–1988; Gill, Gordon, ed. *Recreational Nudity and the Law: Abstracts of Cases*. Macomb, Ill.: Dr. Leisure, 1987; Hartman, William E., and Marilyn A. Fithian. "Enhancing Sexuality Through Nudism." In Herbert A. Otto, ed., *The New Sexuality*. Palo Alto, Calif.: Science and Behavior Books, 1971, 122–39; Hartman, William E., Marilyn A. Fithian, and Donald Johnson. (1970) *Nudist Society: The Controversial Study of the Clothes-Free Naturist Movement in America*. Revised by I. Bancroft. Los Angeles, Calif.: Elysium Growth Press, 1991; Heinze, Eric. "Victimless Crimes." In Ruth Chadwick, ed., *Encyclopedia of Applied Ethics*, vol. 4. San Diego, Calif.: Academic Press, 1998, 463–75; Hyde, Alan. *Bodies of Law*. Princeton, N.J.: Princeton University Press, 1997; Ilfeld, Fred, Jr., and Roger Lauer. *Social Nudism in America*. New Haven, Conn.: College and University Press, 1964; Johnson, Donald. *The Nudists*. New York: Duell, Sloan, and Pearce, 1959; Kozlowski, James C. "Does the Constitution Protect Nude Bathing at a Public Beach?" *Parks and Recreation* 25:5 (1990), 16; Lewis, Robin J., and Louis H. Janda. "The Relationship between Adult Sexual Adjustment and Childhood Experiences Regarding Exposure to Nudity, Sleeping in the Parental Bed, and Parental Attitudes toward Sexuality." *Archives of Sexual Behavior* 17:4 (1988), 349–62; Naturist Education Foundation. (Web site) <www.nef.oshkosh.net> [accessed 15 February 2005]; *People v. Cohen*. 1 C.A. 3d 94; 81 Cal. Rptr. 503 (1969). Reprinted in Richard A. Wasserstrom, ed., *Morality and the Law*. Belmont, Calif.: Wadsworth, 1971, 132–39; Storey, Mark. *Cinema Au Naturel: A History of Nudist Film*. Oshkosh, Wis.: Naturist Education Foundation, 2003; Storey, Mark. "The Offense of Public Nudity." *Nude & Natural* 22:2 (2002), 82–88; Story, Marilyn D. "Comparisons of Body Self-Concept between Social Nudists and Nonnudists." *Journal of Psychology* 118:1 (1984), 99–112; Weinberg, Martin S. "Becoming a Nudist." *Psychiatry: Journal for the Study of Interpersonal Processes* 29:1 (1966), 15–24; Weinberg, Martin S. "The Nudist Camp: Way of Life and Social Structure." *Human Organization* 26:3 (1967), 91–99; Weinberg, Martin S. "The Nudist Management of Respectability." In Martin S. Weinberg, ed., *Sex Research: Studies from the Kinsey Institute*. New York: Oxford University Press, 1976, 217–32; Weinberg, Martin S. "Sexual Modesty, Social Meaning, and the Nudist Camp." *Social Problems* 12:3 (1965), 311–18; Williams, Carl Easton. *The Psychology of Nudism: A Study of Mental Health and the Techniques of Happiness*. Mays Landing, N.J.: Sunshine, 1941; Woycke, James. *Au Naturel: The History of Nudism in Canada*. Etobicoke, Ont.: Federation of Canadian Naturists and Anecdote Productions, 2003; Wyner, ToniAnne. "MacArthur, Man, and Beach." *Nude & Natural* 10:4 (1991), 61–64; Wyner, ToniAnne. "Wyner's Winning Strategy." *Nude & Natural* 13:4 (1994), 71–73.

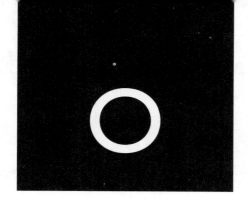

OBJECTIFICATION, SEXUAL. People are objectified when they are treated like objects rather than subjects. Someone is *sexually* objectified when she is reduced to the level of an object in a sexual manner or for sexual purposes. On Sandra Bartky's view, a woman is objectified sexually if "her sexual parts or sexual functions are separated out from the rest of her personality and reduced to the status of mere instruments or else regarded as if they were capable of representing her" (26). On this account, the prostitute, the *Playboy* centerfold, the **beauty** queen, and the **rape** victim may all be illustrations (to different degrees) of sexually objectified women. Linda LeMoncheck points out that treating someone as a sex object can involve either *conceiving* of her as a sex object or *acting* toward her as a sex object, or both (*Dehumanizing*, 5). Defined in such blunt terms, sexual objectification seems morally unsavory; indeed, sexual objectification can be harmful and demeaning. However, some people do not condemn all sexual objectification and may enjoy at least some types of it.

There is a central, even if stereotypical, example of sexual objectification: A woman, walking on the street along a construction site, is whistled at by the men and taunted with their sexually suggestive comments. Bartky claims that in this encounter the woman is "made to know" through the men's behavior that she is merely or primarily "a nice piece of ass" (27). In noticing and recognizing their intention to cause her distress and demean her by taunting her, the woman unwillingly sees herself as the workers see her: She may feel shamed, embarrassed, as well as angry at being put down. She may not know how to react—as if she were paralyzed, like a deer caught in a car's headlights—and so be afraid and feel vulnerable. (Catcalling is similar, in some ways, to hostile environment **sexual harassment**.) Some women claim to enjoy this sort of catcalling or whistling attention from men. But their enjoying it does not make the men's behavior any less a case of sexual objectification, although their enjoying it might (or might not) influence our overall moral judgment of it.

LeMoncheck describes other cases of sexual objectification. A store manager is attracted to his younger assistant manager, but he doubts that she is interested in him. He connives to get her to sleep with him in exchange for a promotion. The assistant agrees because she desires the promotion, good jobs are hard to come by, and she does not want to resign. Here the assistant manager is both being conceived of as a sex object and acted toward as a sex object, so she is being sexually objectified (*Dehumanizing*, 9). It may well be true that the woman is being sexually objectified if the manager's attitude and behavior toward her are such that her sexual capacities are for him detached from and take precedence over her personality (as in Bartky's account).

It is arguable, however, that more is going on in this case than sexual objectification and that the objectification might not be the worst of it. To start, the woman appears to be entangled in *quid pro quo* sexual harassment, especially if she is in danger of losing her job if she refuses her manager's offer. Further, she may be sexually exploited. On Raymond

Belliotti's view, to exploit someone sexually is to capitalize on the person's vulnerabilities or inferior bargaining power to bring about **sexual activity** with that person (202–3; see also Mappes). Sexual objectification and sexual exploitation are related but not the same. Sexual exploitation apparently requires sexual objectification; one cannot sexually exploit another without first objectifying her, without seeing her as someone to be manipulated as a object. But not all sexual objectification is sexual exploitation. One can sexually objectify someone but not exploit her, as in the construction worker example. Or suppose a powerful woman wants to have her way sexually with one of her male employees. She might conceive of him as a mere piece of meat and go out of her way to connive him into sexual activity. But even though she treats him as a sexual object, she does not necessary exploit him, despite his lower position. The fact that he might well be very eager to engage in sex with his female boss—for psychological reasons having to do with his sense of masculinity, for social reasons relating to his status among his colleagues, as well as for the pure sensual pleasure of it—makes it more difficult for us, and for him, to think of this as exploitation. (This does not mean that powerful or aggressive women could never sexually exploit men or treat them as sex objects.)

Why is sexual objectification morally wrong? Martha Nussbaum's Kantian view is that in objectification we are "treating *as an object* what is really not an object, what is, in fact, a human being" (257). According to the Second Formulation of **Immanuel Kant**'s (1724–1804) Categorical Imperative, one must act so "that one treats humanity, whether in one's own person or in that of another, always at the same time as an end and never simply as a means" (*Grounding*, 36; see Ak 4:428, 4:429). This principle is often glossed as a principle of respect, which asserts that we must never treat ourselves and others merely as objects (i.e., as a means) but always as persons (i.e., as ends), with the respect that rational, autonomous beings deserve. One can easily see, with Nussbaum, how sexual objectification, treating another not as a full person but only as a sexual being, might run afoul of the Second Formulation. On Kant's own, idiosyncratic metaphysics of human sexuality, **sexual desire** itself *always* breeds treating the other as a thing, merely as a means for attaining sexual satisfaction. Sexual desire, for Kant, necessarily focuses on the body and body parts, not the person, and hence is always objectifying (*Lectures*, 162–63). Thus sexuality is, for Kant, always morally problematic. (For discussion, see Soble, "Sexual Use"; and for a different, non-Kantian account of sexual desire, see Scruton, 78–82, 84.)

Many feminists have written about sexual objectification, especially but not only as it occurs in or relates to heterosexual relationships, **pornography**, sexual advertising, and both media and real violence against women. **Catharine MacKinnon**, for one, has written about objectification in all these areas and dramatically condemns it: "Sexual objectification is the primary process of the subjection of women. It unites act with word, construction with expression, perception with enforcement, myth with reality. Man fucks woman; subject verb object" (124). Although it is not difficult to interpret much of MacKinnon's analysis of sexuality in a Kantian way (see Nussbaum and Herman, who explore links between Kant's sexual metaphysics and MacKinnon's **feminism**), MacKinnon, unlike Kant, does not claim that sexual desire and activity are, by their very nature, objectifying. Instead, sexual objectification is constitutive of sexuality as it exists and functions in a male-dominated society. Our sexuality has been socialized in terms of hierarchy and domination: Men have been socialized to be "active-fucker-conqueror," women to be "passive-fucked-victim" (Zweig, 100; see Baker). In such a cultural context, much sexuality will be, or have the appearance of being, objectifying.

In *Dehumanizing Women* (66 ff.), LeMoncheck examines this culture of objectification and tries to uncover why some women participate in their own objectification, why some women complain about being treated as sex objects, and why others do not, perhaps even finding it agreeable. On her view, many women uncritically accept objectification because they have been indoctrinated, in subtle and deceptive ways, to be sex objects; some women may even believe that women are the natural sexual subordinates of men. Through marketing techniques and with the encouragement of other women (mothers, kin, friends), women are persuaded to buy and wear clothing and cosmetics that contribute to or reinforce their status as sex objects. Many women dress in sexy ways for men, deliberately drawing attention to their bodies, because it is through men that they are assigned their value. (Or because, in some cases, it is through men that women attain what they may want in life, including wealth and power.) Women's preoccupation with their appearance is often unreflectively accepted as normal and even natural, and women compete against each other for men's attention, dressing according to male-defined standards of beauty and sexiness (*Dehumanizing*, 62). But the cultural system does not have a stranglehold, nor does it *need* one: "[M]en can have voyeur-fetishist reactions to *any* female self-presentation, without regard to the sign system, or in perverse reversal of its conventional meanings. Straight male sexuality, as we have constructed it, locks women into the role of performer no matter what they do to avoid it" (Kennedy, 166–67).

Even though some ordinary people and scholars see women's preoccupation with their appearance as a normal or natural state of affairs (perhaps the result of **evolution**, in particular sexual selection; see Etcoff), others, feminists in particular, believe it is the result of restrictive social indoctrination that manipulates women (or coerces them; see Burgess-Jackson) into leading subordinate lives, thereby denying them fully self-determined lives.

> To become the object, [a woman] takes herself and transforms herself into a thing: all freedoms are diminished and she is caged. . . . In becoming an object so [a man] can objectify her so that he can fuck her, [a woman] begins a political collaboration with his dominance; and then when he enters her, he confirms for himself and for her what she is: that she is *something*, not someone; certainly not someone equal. (**Andrea Dworkin** [1946–2005], 56; emphasis added)

Women who **consent** to or collaborate in their own sexual objectification are not only harming themselves but other women as well, by perpetuating this restrictive social indoctrination.

Some women understand that they consent to their own objectification and might not be especially happy about it but nevertheless continue to participate. Some women thrive on men's sexual attention and work hard to get it, because this enhances their self-image and self-esteem. Others say that the fine dining, theater tickets, cocktail parties, and jewelry are worth being treated as sex objects. Pornography models or prostitutes might tolerate sexual objectification because the money is good. Women with more traditional jobs might dress up for work, thereby contributing to their objectification, either because they do not want to lose their jobs or because they want to move up the corporate ladder. A woman might strip on stage in a tavern (or model for photographs or prostitute herself) simply because she needs the money for necessities of all kinds (food for her children; medical care for her mother) and has no other source of income. Some strippers, however, or others who engage in **sex work**, claim that they *are* leading lives of self-determination in which they freely choose to use their bodies in sexual ways, and this neither demeans them nor diminishes their self-respect (LeMoncheck, *Dehumanizing*, 67–69; *Loose Women*, 110 ff.).

The possibility of engaging in sex work or other job-related self-objectification that might not be morally abominable suggests that our judgments about objectification can be context-sensitive and that objectification comes in degrees or has different types (for a catalog of the various senses or types of "objectification," see Nussbaum, 257 ff.). This is why Avedon Carol and Nettie Pollard argue that the use of the term "objectification" in the late twentieth century went overboard, beyond its original feminist political meaning. Whereas the term originally referred to evaluating women in virtue merely of their sexual functions or sexuality and to projecting male fantasies or idealized versions of women onto real women, the term was eventually robbed of its politics and began to mean (with a derogatory connotation) finding women physically or sexually attractive and admiring them for their physical or sexual attributes. Under this redefinition, finding a feature of a woman or man physically or sexually compelling is to devalue that person. (See also LeMoncheck on the moral distinction between treating a person as a sex object and considering a person only as an object of sexual attraction; "What's Wrong," 138–39.) Carol and Pollard argue that one defect of the redefinition is that it facilitates inappropriate attitudes of "paternalistic protectiveness toward women and children" (47). Some objectification is unquestionably bad. But other behavior that is objectifying might not be bad, and it might not even be objectifying in any interesting sense. It could be, instead, a healthy appreciation of the other person.

Indeed, Martha Nussbaum argues that in the context of a mutually respectful relationship, sexual objectification is morally permissible and in some ways wonderful. In part, Nussbaum grounds this view in her reading of D. H. Lawrence's (1885–1930) *Lady Chatterley's Lover* (1928), in which both Oliver Mellors and Constance Chatterley become identified with and see each other in terms of their sexual organs. Because this objectification is reciprocal and occurs in a context of mutual respect, it is not disgraceful. The lovers only *sometimes* objectify each other, but otherwise their relationship is replete with equal respect and regard, which implies that Oliver and Constance have avoided Kantian moral objections. Further, the immersion of the pair in their bodies adds tremendously to their enjoying each other sexually, so that objectification is not merely permissible but "wonderful" (275, 277). By contrast, *Playboy* exemplifies unacceptable objectification, for Nussbaum, since it "encourages the idea that an easy satisfaction can be had in [an] uncomplicated way, without the difficulties attendant on recognizing women's subjectivity and autonomy in a more full-blooded way" (284). It seems to follow from Nussbaum's account that **casual sex**, or sexual activity that occurs between two people before they have established a relationship replete with equal respect and regard, would be morally wrong, since the specific "narrative" context that makes objectification permissible is absent (see Soble). Of course, many would agree here with Nussbaum, and many would reject her view as too restrictive.

See also Beauty; Casual Sex; Coercion (by Sexually Aggressive Women); Consent; Desire, Sexual; Existentialism; Feminism, French; Feminism, History of; Feminism, Lesbian; Feminism, Liberal; Feminism, Men's; Harassment, Sexual; Kant, Immanuel; Language; MacKinnon, Catharine; Personification, Sexual; Pornography; Prostitution; Rape; Rape, Acquaintance and Date; Sadomasochism; Scruton, Roger; Sex Work; Violence, Sexual

REFERENCES

Baker, Robert B. " 'Pricks' and 'Chicks': A Plea for 'Persons.' " In Robert B. Baker and Frederick A. Elliston, eds., *Philosophy and Sex*, 1st ed. Buffalo, N.Y.: Prometheus, 1975, 45–64; Bartky, Sandra

Lee. "On Psychological Oppression." In *Femininity and Domination: Studies in the Phenomenology of Oppression*. New York: Routledge, 1990, 22–32; Belliotti, Raymond. *Good Sex: Perspectives on Sexual Ethics*. Lawrence: University Press of Kansas, 1993; Burgess-Jackson, Keith. "On the Coerciveness of Sexist Socialization." *Public Affairs Quarterly* 9:1 (1995), 15–27; Carol, Avedon, and Nettie Pollard. "Changing Perceptions in the Feminist Debate." In Alison Assister and Avedon Carol, eds., *Bad Girls and Dirty Pictures: The Challenge to Reclaim Feminism*. London: Pluto Press, 1993, 45–56; Dworkin, Andrea. *Intercourse*. New York: Free Press, 1987; Etcoff, Nancy. *Survival of the Prettiest: The Science of Beauty*. New York: Doubleday, 1999; Herman, Barbara. "Could It Be Worth Thinking about Kant on Sex and Marriage?" In Louise M. Antony and Charlotte Witt, eds., *A Mind of One's Own: Feminist Essays on Reason and Objectivity*. Boulder, Colo.: Westview, 1993, 49–67; Kant, Immanuel. (1785) *Grounding for the Metaphysics of Morals*. Trans. Arnulf Zweig. New York: Oxford University Press, 2002; Kant, Immanuel. (ca. 1780) *Lecture on Ethics*. Trans. Louis Infield. New York: Harper and Row, 1963; Kennedy, Duncan. "Sexual Abuse, Sexy Dressing, and the Eroticization of Domination." In *Sexy Dressing Etc.: Essays on the Power and Politics of Cultural Identity*. Cambridge, Mass.: Harvard University Press, 1993, 126–213; LeMoncheck, Linda. *Dehumanizing Women: Treating Persons as Sex Objects*. Totowa, N.J.: Rowman and Allanheld, 1984; LeMoncheck, Linda. *Loose Women, Lecherous Men: A Feminist Philosophy of Sex*. New York: Oxford University Press, 1997; LeMoncheck, Linda. "What's Wrong with Treating Women as Sex Objects?" In Alan Soble, ed., *Sex, Love, and Friendship*. Amsterdam, Holland: Rodopi, 1997, 137–45; MacKinnon, Catharine A. *Toward a Feminist Theory of the State*. Cambridge, Mass.: Harvard University Press, 1989; Mappes, Thomas A. (1985) "Sexual Morality and the Concept of Using Another Person." In Thomas A. Mappes and Jane S. Zembaty, eds., *Social Ethics: Morality and Social Policy*, 3rd ed. New York: McGraw-Hill, 1987, 248–62; Nussbaum, Martha C. "Objectification." *Philosophy and Public Affairs* 24:4 (1995), 249–91; Scruton, Roger. *Sexual Desire: A Moral Philosophy of the Erotic*. New York: Free Press, 1986; Soble, Alan. "Sexual Use and What to Do about It: Internalist and Externalist Sexual Ethics." *Essays in Philosophy* 2:2 (2001). <www.humboldt.edu/~essays/soble.html> [accessed 4 February 2005]; Zweig, Bella. "The Mute Nude Female Characters in Aristophanes' Plays." In Amy Richlin, ed., *Pornography and Representation in Greece and Rome*. New York: Oxford University Press, 1992, 73–111.

Carol V. Quinn

ADDITIONAL READING

Anderson, Clelia Smyth, and Yolanda Estes. "The Myth of the Happy Hooker: Kantian Moral Reflections on a Phenomenology of Prostitution." In Stanley G. French, Wanda Teays, and Laura M. Purdy, eds., *Violence against Women: Philosophical Perspectives*. Ithaca, N.Y.: Cornell University Press, 1998, 152–58; Baker, Robert B. " 'Pricks' and 'Chicks': A Plea for 'Persons.' " In Robert B. Baker and Frederick A. Elliston, eds., *Philosophy and Sex*, 1st ed. Buffalo, N.Y.: Prometheus, 1975, 45–64. Reprinted in P&S2 (249–67); P&S3 (281–97), with " 'Pricks' and 'Chicks': A Postscript after Twenty-Five Years" (297–305); Bartky, Sandra Lee. "Narcissism, Femininity, and Alienation." *Social Theory and Practice* 8:2 (1982), 127–43; Benson, Paul. "Autonomy and Oppressive Socialization." *Social Theory and Practice* 17:3 (1991), 385–408; Dworkin, Andrea. *Woman Hating*. New York: Dutton, 1974; Eames, Elizabeth R. "Sexism and Woman as Sex Object." *Journal of Thought* 11:2 (1976), 140–43; Earle, W. J. "Depersonalized Sex and Moral Perfection." *International Journal of Moral and Social Studies* 2:3 (1987), 203–10. Reprinted in HS (67–74); Freud, Sigmund. (1912) "On the Universal Tendency to Debasement in the Sphere of Love." In *The Standard Edition of the Complete Psychological Works of Sigmund Freud*, vol. 11. Trans. James Strachey. London: Hogarth Press, 1953–1974, 179–90; Garry, Ann. "Pornography and Respect for Women." *Social Theory and Practice* 4:4 (1978), 395–421. Reprinted in Sharon Bishop and Marjorie Weinzweig, eds., *Philosophy and Women*. Belmont, Calif.: Wadsworth, 1979, 128–39; Garry, Ann. "Sex (and Other) Objects." In Alan Soble, ed., *Sex, Love, and Friendship*. Amsterdam, Holland: Rodopi, 1997, 163–67; Garry, Ann. "Sex, Lies, and Pornography." In Hugh LaFollette, ed., *Ethics in Practice: An*

Anthology, 2nd ed. Malden, Mass.: Blackwell, 2002, 344–55; Gramich, Katie. "Stripping Off the 'Civilized Body': Lawrence's *nostalgie de la boue* in *Lady Chatterley's Lover*." In Paul Poplawski, ed., *Writing the Body in D. H. Lawrence: Essays on Language, Representation, and Sexuality*. Westport, Conn.: Greenwood Press, 2001, 149–61; Haslanger, Sally. "On Being Objective and Being Objectified." In Louise Antony and Charlotte Witt, eds., *A Mind of One's Own: Feminist Essays on Reason and Objectivity*. Boulder, Colo.: Westview, 1993, 85–125; Hill, Judith M. "Pornography and Degradation." *Hypatia* 2:2 (1987), 39–54; Jarvie, Ian C. "Pornography and/as Degradation." *International Journal of Law and Psychiatry* 14 (1991), 13–27; Landry, Donna. "Treating Him Like an Object: William Beatty Warner's 'Di(va)lution.'" In Linda Kauffman, ed., *Feminism and Institutions: Dialogues on Feminist Theory*. Cambridge, Mass.: Blackwell, 1989, 126–38; Lawrence, D. H. (1929) "A Propos of *Lady Chatterley's Lover*." In *Sex, Literature, and Censorship*. Ed. Harry T. Moore. New York: Twayne, 1953, 89–122; Lawrence, D. H. (1928) *Lady Chatterley's Lover*. New York: New American Library, 1962; LeMoncheck, Linda. "Feminist Politics and Feminist Ethics: Treating Women as Sex Objects." In Robert M. Stewart, ed., *Philosophical Perspectives on Sex and Love*. New York: Oxford University Press, 1995, 29–38; LeMoncheck, Linda. "I Only Do It for the Money: Pornography, Prostitution, and the Business of Sex." In *Loose Women, Lecherous Men: A Feminist Philosophy of Sex*. New York: Oxford University Press, 1997, 110–54; MacKinnon, Catharine A. *Feminism Unmodified: Discourses on Life and Law*. Cambridge, Mass.: Harvard University Press, 1987; Mappes, Thomas A. (1985) "Sexual Morality and the Concept of Using Another Person." In Thomas A. Mappes and Jane S. Zembaty, eds., *Social Ethics: Morality and Social Policy*, 3rd ed. New York: McGraw-Hill, 1987, 248–62. 4th ed., 1992, 203–16. 5th ed., 1997, 163–76. 6th ed., 2002, 170–83. Reprinted in POS4 (207–23); Moscovici, Claudia. *From Sex Objects to Sexual Subjects*. New York: Routledge, 1996; Nagel, Thomas. (1999) "Nussbaum on Sexual Injustice." In *Concealment and Exposure and Other Essays*. New York: Oxford University Press, 2002, 56–62; Nussbaum, Martha C. "Objectification." *Philosophy and Public Affairs* 24:4 (1995), 249–91. Reprinted in POS3 (283–321); POS4 (381–419). Reprinted, revised, in *Sex and Social Justice*. New York: Oxford University Press, 1999, 213–39; Richards, Richard C. "Objections to Sex Objectification." In Alan Soble, ed., *Sex, Love, and Friendship*. Amsterdam, Holland: Rodopi, 1997, 147–55; Richlin, Amy, ed. *Pornography and Representation in Greece and Rome*. New York: Oxford University Press, 1992; Soble, Alan. "Sexual Use and What to Do about It: Internalist and Externalist Sexual Ethics." *Essays in Philosophy* 2:2 (2001). <www.humboldt.edu/~essays/soble.html> [accessed 4 February 2005]. Reprinted, revised, in POS4 (225–58); Stoltenberg, John. *Refusing to Be a Man: Essays on Sex and Justice*. Portland, Ore.: Breitenbush Books, 1989; Sullivan, John. "Women as Sex Objects." In Alan Soble, ed., *Sex, Love, and Friendship*. Amsterdam, Holland: Rodopi, 1997, 157–60; Tewksbury, Richard. "Male Strippers: Men Objectifying Men." In Christine L. Williams, ed., *Doing "Women's Work": Men in Nontraditional Occupations*. Newbury Park, Calif.: Sage, 1993, 168–81; Warner, William Beatty. "Treating Me Like an Object: Reading Catharine MacKinnon's Feminism." In Linda Kauffman, ed., *Feminism and Institutions: Dialogues on Feminist Theory*. Cambridge, Mass.: Blackwell, 1989, 90–125; Wertheimer, Alan. *Exploitation*. Princeton, N.J.: Princeton University Press, 1996.

ORIENTATION, SEXUAL. A person has a sexual orientation by virtue of the sex of his or her actual or preferred sexual partners. Roughly, persons with a *heterosexual* orientation are predominantly attracted to or sexually active with persons of the other sex, persons with a *homosexual* orientation are predominantly attracted to or sexually active with persons of the same sex, and persons with a *bisexual* orientation are attracted to or sexually active with persons of both sexes (see De Cecco).

While the foregoing suffices as a preliminary definition, numerous questions can be raised. Does sexual orientation fall into discrete categories (the three mentioned above), or does it exist on a continuum? What is the relative importance, in defining a particular sexual orientation, of dispositions as opposed to behaviors? Might sexual orientation encompass features beyond sex, such as age, specific body characteristics, or personality types? Might it even include factors such as preferred sexual position or arousal patterns? How should we classify sexual acts done by or with ambiguously sexed persons? The philosophical literature on sexual orientation has attempted to resolve these and other conceptual questions. It has also addressed other issues, such as the metaphysical status of sexual orientation and the ethics of sexual orientation research.

Sexual orientation is defined sometimes in terms of sex, sometimes in terms of gender, and sometimes in terms of both ("sex/gender"). Part of the problem is that the distinction between sex and gender has been drawn in various and often incompatible ways (see, for example, Shively and De Cecco). Let us say that "sex" refers not only to chromosomes and other underlying biological features but also to anatomical features typically associated with a person's being a man or a woman (body hair, genitalia, breasts, and so on). Some of these features may be classified as gender characteristics, and insofar as such classification is preferable, sexual orientation may be defined in terms of gender as well as sex. There are also "gray areas." If Jack, a biological male, is attracted to Jill, a transgendered person who appears female but whose biological sex (male) Jack knows, is Jack's attraction heterosexual or homosexual? Difficult cases like these raise interesting conceptual questions.

Sexual orientation is sometimes called "sexual preference." Some gay rights advocates have objected to the term "preference" on the grounds that it implies something arbitrary, rather than a deep and relatively fixed feature of human personality. But the objection is at least partially misplaced, for many "preferences" appear to lie beyond voluntary control: Someone who prefers jazz to opera, for example, cannot simply will herself to change her preferences. On the other hand, we often do have preferences in which we are not deeply invested: I might be perfectly satisfied eating vanilla ice cream even though I prefer chocolate. Such casual preferences explain why the term "preference" is sometimes thought to diminish the importance of sexual orientation as a feature of human identity, especially given its connection with life-defining relationships.

A central question about sexual orientation is whether it is best defined by behavior or by mental states (feelings, dispositions, or fantasies). Those who adopt a *behavioral* view (see Stein, *Mismeasure*, 41–44) claim that people are heterosexual if and only if they engage in sex with people of the other sex; homosexual if and only if they engage in sex with people of the same sex; and bisexual if and only if they engage in sex with both. (Replacing "if and only if" with "to the extent that" suggests continuous instead of discrete categories; see LeVay, 46–52.) The behavioral view yields counterintuitive results. People who are confined to single-sex environments (prisons, boarding schools) sometimes engage in homosexual conduct even though they strongly prefer heterosexual conduct. Although we might refer to such persons as "situational" or "opportunistic" homosexuals, it is not clear that, merely given their behavior, they should be classified homosexual (or bisexual) at all. Consider, too, fully "closeted" homosexuals. On the behavioral view, if they conform to social pressure and thus engage only in heterosexual sex, then they *are* heterosexual, despite their sexual fantasies or feelings.

Most theorists therefore favor a *dispositional* approach to sexual orientation (see Stein, *Mismeasure*, 45–49), which classifies people according to their desires and preferences instead of actual behavior. (Behavior is still relevant on the dispositional view, since it not only manifests but also clarifies and reinforces dispositions.) On this view, people are heterosexual if and only if (or to the extent that) they are attracted to, and thus disposed toward **sexual activity** with, members of the other sex—and so on. Some versions of the dispositional view classify people according to their dispositions under *ideal conditions*. We are to ask, counterfactually, what a person would choose to do if various social constraints and pressure were absent, if personal inhibitions were removed, and suitable partners of different types were abundantly available. These questions are often entertaining ("what would you do if?"), but as in other areas of philosophy, counterfactual claims about sexuality are beset with epistemological difficulties (Stein, *Mismeasure*, 46).

Are orientations discrete, or do they comprise a continuum? Alfred Kinsey (1894–1956) is credited with advancing a continuum view in *Sexual Behavior in the Human Male* (1948) and *Sexual Behavior in the Human Female* (1953). Kinsey located subjects on a scale, ranging from 0 (exclusively heterosexual) to 6 (exclusively homosexual), in terms of their sexual experiences and psychosexual reactions. He also had a category, X, for people with no sexual experiences or reactions, though he found that few adults fell into this category. Kinsey and his colleagues created controversy by claiming that nearly half (46 percent) of the population was neither exclusively heterosexual (Kinsey 0s) nor exclusively homosexual (Kinsey 6s) but fell somewhere between these extremes (Kinsey, *Human Female*, 656). Some subset of these people—centering on Kinsey 3s, and perhaps including 2s and 4s—may properly be termed "bisexual." While Kinsey's studies have occasionally been criticized, his importance in sexual orientation research seems undeniable.

Location on Kinsey's scale depends on heterosexual and homosexual attractions and behaviors but not their intensity. Some have objected to Kinsey on this point, noting that someone *intensely* attracted to both same-sex and other-sex partners would fall on the same point on Kinsey's scale as someone only *mildly* attracted to both, provided they had the same proportion of heterosexual and homosexual attraction (Stein, *Mismeasure*, 53–61). In tracking only proportions and not intensity of hetero- and homosexual attraction, Kinsey's scale is one-dimensional. Michael Storms has proposed an alternative two-dimensional scale in which one vector tracks heterosexual attraction and another homosexual attraction. Kinsey 3s, whose heterosexual and homosexual attractions are roughly equal, would fall on the same diagonal 45-degree line on Storms's scale but at different points along that line, depending on the intensity of their attractions.

Storms's scale, like Kinsey's, is organized around heterosexual and homosexual attraction, rather than attraction to men and attraction to women. On the first approach, lesbians and gay men (both of whom are attracted to the same sex) are grouped together, in contrast to male and female heterosexuals (both of whom are attracted to the other sex). On the second approach, lesbians and heterosexual men (both of whom are attracted to women) are grouped together, in contrast to gay men and heterosexual women (both of whom are attracted to men). The difference between the two approaches might seem to reflect mere organizational convenience, yet it makes us ask whether heterosexual males are more like heterosexual females (since both are attracted to the other sex) or more like homosexual females (both are attracted to females). Such questions are at once conceptual and empirical.

The attempt to categorize people according to their sexual interests appears to have ancient roots, although considerable debate exists over the uniformity, extent, and significance of such categorizing throughout history. In the *Symposium*, **Plato** (427–347 BCE) portrays the comic poet Aristophanes as relating a myth of three primordial "gender" types, each consisting of a double body: male-male, female-female, and male-female (the androgyne or hermaphrodite). After being split in two by Zeus (as punishment for not sufficiently respecting the gods), the resulting halves desperately sought to cling to their former counterparts. Plato's Aristophanes claims that the differences in sexual interest among his "postlapsarian" contemporaries can be explained by their having descended from different original types (*Symposium*, 189e–93d). The account is widely read as an early etiology of the modern categories of male **homosexuality**, lesbianism, and heterosexuality. Notice, however, that **bisexuality** is excluded and that male homosexuality and lesbianism are treated as separate categories, while male and female heterosexuality share one category. There is controversy over whether Aristophanes's myth and similar texts support or undermine the metaphysical view that our modern categories of sexual orientation are objective and "real" rather than socially constructed. (See Neu, 177n.1, on the similarities between Plato's Aristophanes and **Sigmund Freud** [1856–1939] on the etiology of sexual orientation.)

This debate over the metaphysical status of sexual orientation categories is known as the essentialist-constructionist debate (see Stein, *Forms of Desire*). Essentialists hold that sexual orientation is an objective, intrinsic, culturally independent property of persons, while **social constructionism** denies this. Following **John Boswell** (1947–1994), one might say that essentialists are realists about sexual orientation and social constructionists are nominalists.

The concept of sexual orientation might well be expanded beyond the standard categories of heterosexual, homosexual, and bisexual. If it makes any sense at all to classify people into types of sexual beings, then why not count "females attracted to much older men" and "men arousable only in the presence of high heels" as distinct sexual orientations? Perhaps what we can learn from this potential proliferation is not only that human sexuality is extraordinarily variable but also that (regardless of whether essentialism or constructionism is right) it might not be very illuminating or worthwhile to classify people according to their sexual interests.

See also Bible, Sex and the; Bisexuality; Boswell, John; Cybersex; Greek Sexuality and Philosophy, Ancient; Herdt, Gilbert; Homosexuality and Science; Intersexuality; Money, John; Paraphilia; Plato; Psychology, Twentieth- and Twenty-First-Century; Queer Theory; Sexology; Social Constructionism

REFERENCES

Boswell, John. "Revolutions, Universals, and Sexual Categories." *Salmagundi*, nos. 58–59 (Fall 1982–Winter 1983), 89–113; De Cecco, John P. "Definition and Meaning of Sexual Orientation." *Journal of Homosexuality* 6:4 (1981), 51–67; Kinsey, Alfred, Wardell Pomeroy, and Clyde Martin. *Sexual Behavior in the Human Male*. Philadelphia, Pa.: W. B. Saunders, 1948; Kinsey, Alfred, Wardell Pomeroy, Clyde Martin, and Paul Gebhard. *Sexual Behavior in the Human Female*. Philadelphia, Pa.: W. B. Saunders, 1953; LeVay, Simon. "The Nature and Prevalence of Homosexuality." In *Queer Science: The Use and Abuse of Research on Homosexuality*. Cambridge, Mass.: MIT Press, 1996, 41–65; Neu, Jerome. "Freud and Perversion." In Earl E. Shelp, ed., *Sexuality and Medicine*, vol. 1: *Conceptual Roots*. Dordrecht, Holland: Reidel, 1987, 153–84; Plato. (ca. 380 BCE) *Symposium*. Trans. Alexander Nehamas and Paul Woodruff. Indianapolis, Ind.: Hackett, 1989; Shively, Michael G., and John P. De Cecco. "Components of Sexual Identity." *Journal of Homosexuality* 3:1 (1977), 41–48; Stein, Edward. *The Mismeasure of Desire: The Science, Theory, and Ethics of Sexual Orientation*. New York: Oxford University Press, 1999; Stein, Edward, ed. (1990) *Forms of Desire: Sexual Orientation and the Social Constructionist Controversy*. New York: Routledge, 1992; Storms, Michael D. "Theories of Sexual Orientation." *Journal of Personality and Social Psychology* 38:4 (1980), 783–92.

John Corvino

ADDITIONAL READING

Abelove, Henry, Michèle Aina Barale, and David M. Halperin, eds. *The Lesbian and Gay Studies Reader*. New York: Routledge, 1993; Bell, Alan, and Martin Weinberg. *Homosexualities: A Study of*

Diversity among Men and Women. New York: Simon and Schuster, 1978; Bell, Alan, Martin Weinberg, and Susan Hammersmith. *Sexual Preference: Its Development in Men and Women*. Bloomington: Indiana University Press, 1981; Bem, Daryl. "Exotic Becomes Erotic: A Developmental Theory of Sexual Orientation." *Psychological Review* 103:2 (1996), 320–35; Berky, Branden Robert, T. Perelman-Hall, and L. A. Kurdek. "The Multidimensional Scale of Sexuality." *Journal of Homosexuality* 19:4 (1990), 67–97; Bohan, Janice. *Psychology and Sexual Orientation: Coming to Terms*. New York: Routledge, 1996; Boswell, John. "Revolutions, Universals, and Sexual Categories." *Salmagundi*, nos. 58–59 (Fall 1982–Winter 1983), 89–113. Reprinted, with "Postscript" (1988), in Martin Duberman, Martha Vicinus, and George Chauncey, Jr., eds., *Hidden from History: Reclaiming the Gay and Lesbian Past*. New York: New American Library, 1989, 17–36; and John Corvino, ed., *Same Sex: Debating the Ethics, Science, and Culture of Homosexuality*. Lanham, Md.: Rowman and Littlefield, 1997, 185–202; Bruckman, Amy S. "Gender Swapping on the Internet." In Peter Ludlow, ed., *High Noon on the Electronic Frontier: Conceptual Issues in Cyberspace*. Cambridge, Mass.: MIT Press, 1996, 317–25; Byne, William, and Mitchell Lasco. "The Origins of Sexual Orientation: Possible Biological Contributions." In John Corvino, ed., *Same Sex: Debating the Ethics, Science, and Culture of Homosexuality*. Lanham, Md.: Rowman and Littlefield, 1997, 107–20; Byne, William, and Edward Stein. "The Ethical Implications of Medical and Biological Research on the Causes of Sexual Orientation." *Health Care Analysis* 5 (1997), 136–48; Califia, Pat [Patrick Califia-Rice]. "Sex Changes: The Politics of Transgenderism." *sexuality.org: society for human sexuality*. <www.sexuality.org/l/trangen/scpc.html> [accessed 3 September 2004]; Carr, Brian. "Sexual Orientation: Gender Identity Disorders." In Timothy F. Murphy, ed., *Reader's Guide to Lesbian and Gay Studies*. Chicago, Ill.: Fitzroy Dearborn, 2000, 538–39; Coleman, Eli. "Bisexuality: Challenging Our Understanding of Human Sexuality and Sexual Orientation." In Earl E. Shelp, ed., *Sexuality and Medicine*, vol. 1: *Conceptual Roots*. Dordrecht, Holland: Reidel, 1987, 225–42; Corvino, John. "How Not to Argue for Gay Rights." In Juha Räikkä, ed., *Do We Need Minority Rights? Conceptual Issues*. The Hague, Holland: Martinus Nijhoff, 1996, 215–35; Corvino, John. "Justice for Glenn and Stacy: On Gender, Morality, and Gay Rights." In James P. Sterba, ed., *Social and Political Philosophy: Contemporary Perspectives*. New York: Routledge, 2001, 300–318; Corvino, John, ed. *Same Sex: Debating the Ethics, Science, and Culture of Homosexuality*. Lanham, Md.: Rowman and Littlefield, 1997; De Cecco, John P. "Definition and Meaning of Sexual Orientation." *Journal of Homosexuality* 6:4 (1981), 51–67. Reprinted in Noretta Koertge, ed., *Philosophy and Homosexuality*. New York: Harrington Park Press, 1985, 51–67; De Cecco, John P., and Michael Shively, eds. *Origins of Sexuality and Homosexuality*. New York: Harrington Park Press, 1985; Duberman, Martin, Martha Vicinus, and George Chauncey, eds. *Hidden from History: Reclaiming the Gay and Lesbian Past*. New York: New American Library, 1989. New York: Penguin, 1990; Epstein, Julia, and Kristin Straub, eds. *Body Guards: The Cultural Politics of Gender Ambiguity*. New York: Routledge, 1991; Fausto-Sterling, Anne. "The Five Sexes: Why Male and Female Are Not Enough." *The Sciences* (March–April 1993), 20–24; Fausto-Sterling, Anne. (1985) *Myths of Gender: Biological Theories about Men and Women*, rev. ed. New York: Basic Books, 1992; Golden, Carla. "Diversity and Variability in Women's Sexual Identities." In Boston Women's Psychologies Collective, ed., *Lesbian Psychologies: Explorations and Challenges*. Urbana: University of Illinois Press, 1987, 18–34. Reprinted in John Corvino, ed., *Same Sex: Debating the Ethics, Science, and Culture of Homosexuality*. Lanham, Md.: Rowman and Littlefield, 1997, 149–66; Gonsiorek, John C., and James D. Weinrich. "The Definition and Scope of Sexual Orientation." In John C. Gonsiorek and James D. Weinrich, eds., *Homosexuality: Research Implications for Public Policy*. Newbury Park, Calif.: Sage, 1991, 1–12; Halberstam, Judith. *Female Masculinity*. Durham, N.C.: Duke University Press, 1998; Hale, C. Jacob. "Leatherdyke Boys and Their Daddies: How to Have Sex without Women or Men." *Social Text* 15:3–4 (1997), 222–36. Reprinted in Robert J. Corber and Stephen Valocchi, eds., *Queer Studies: An Interdisciplinary Reader*. Malden, Mass.: Blackwell, 2003, 61–70; Halley, Janet E. "The Sexual Economist and Legal Regulation of the Sexual Orientations." In David M. Estlund and Martha C. Nussbaum, eds., *Sex, Preference, and Family: Essays on Law and Nature*. New York: Oxford University Press, 1997, 173–91; Halperin, David. *One Hundred Years of Homosexuality: And*

Other Essays on Greek Love. New York: Routledge, 1990; Halperin, David. "Sex before Sexuality." In Martin Duberman, Martha Vicinus, and George Chauncey, eds., *Hidden from History: Reclaiming the Gay and Lesbian Past.* New York: Penguin, 1990, 37–53. Reprinted in John Corvino, ed., *Same Sex: Debating the Ethics, Science, and Culture of Homosexuality.* Lanham, Md.: Rowman and Littlefield, 1997, 203–19; Halwani, Raja. "Essentialism, Social Constructionism, and the History of Homosexuality." *Journal of Homosexuality* 35:1 (1998), 25–51; Halwani, Raja. "Prolegomena to Any Future Metaphysics of Sexual Identity: Recasting the Essentialism and Social Constructionism Debate." In Linda Alcoff, Michael Hames-Garcia, Satya Mohanty, and Paula Moya, eds., *Redefining Identity Politics.* New York: Palgrave, 2005; Hamer, Dean, and Peter Copeland. "Who's Gay?" In *The Science of Desire: The Search for the Gay Gene and the Biology of Behavior.* New York: Simon and Schuster, 1994, 52–73; Hotvedt, Mary. "Gender Identity and Sexual Orientation: The Anthropological Perspective." In Mark Schwartz, Albert Moraczewski, and James Monteleone, eds., *Sex and Gender: A Theological and Scientific Inquiry.* St. Louis, Mo.: Pope John Center, 1983, 144–76; Klein, Fritz. "The Need to View Sexual Orientation as a Multivariable Dynamic Process: A Theoretical Perspective." In David P. McWhirter, Stephanie A. Sanders, and June M. Reinisch, eds., *Homosexuality/Heterosexuality: Concepts of Sexual Orientation.* New York: Oxford University Press, 1990, 277–82; Klein, Fritz, Barry Sepekoff, and Timothy Wolf. "Sexual Orientation: A Multi-Variable Dynamic Process." *Journal of Homosexuality* 11:1–2 (1985), 35–50; Koertge, Noretta. "Constructing Concepts of Sexuality: A Philosophical Commentary." In David P. McWhirter, Stephanie A. Sanders, and June M. Reinisch, eds., *Homosexuality/Heterosexuality: Concepts of Sexual Orientation.* New York: Oxford University Press, 1990, 387–97; Koertge, Noretta, ed. *Philosophy and Homosexuality.* New York: Harrington Park Press, 1985; Mass, Lawrence. "*Homosexual* as Acts or Persons: A Conversation with John De Cecco." In *Homosexuality as Behavior and Identity: Dialogues of the Sexual Revolution*, vol. 2. New York: Haworth, 1990, 132–69; McWhirter, David, Stephanie Sanders, and June Reinisch, eds. *Homosexuality/Heterosexuality: Concepts of Sexual Orientation.* New York: Oxford University Press, 1990; Mohr, Richard D. "The Thing of It Is: Some Problems with Models for the Social Construction of Homosexuality." In *Gay Ideas: Outing and Other Controversies.* Boston, Mass.: Beacon Press, 1992, 221–42; Mondschein, Ken. "Surpassing the Love of Women: Male Homosexuality in the Pre-Modern World." *Renaissance* 9:6, no. 40 (2004), 43–50; Money, John. *Gay, Straight, and In-Between: The Sexology of Erotic Orientation.* New York: Oxford University Press, 1988; Murphy, Timothy F. "Sexual Orientation: Therapy." In Timothy F. Murphy, ed., *Reader's Guide to Lesbian and Gay Studies.* Chicago, Ill.: Fitzroy Dearborn, 2000, 544–46; Neu, Jerome. "Freud and Perversion." In Jerome Neu, ed., *The Cambridge Companion to Freud.* Cambridge: Cambridge University Press, 1991, 175–208. Reprinted in *A Tear Is an Intellectual Thing: The Meanings of Emotion.* New York: Oxford University Press, 2000, 144–65; and Robert Stewart, ed., *Philosophical Perspectives on Sex and Love.* New York: Oxford University Press, 1995, 87–104. Original publication in Earl E. Shelp, ed., *Sexuality and Medicine*, vol. 1: *Conceptual Roots.* Dordrecht, Holland: Reidel, 1987, 153–84; Okin, Susan Moller. (1996) "Sexual Orientation and Gender: Dichotomizing Differences." In David M. Estlund and Martha C. Nussbaum, eds., *Sex, Preference, and Family: Essays on Law and Nature.* New York: Oxford University Press, 1997, 44–59; Ortner, Sherry, and Harriet Whitehead, eds. *Sexual Meanings: The Cultural Construction of Gender and Sexuality.* Cambridge: Cambridge University Press, 1981; Pattatucci, Angela M. L., and Dean H. Hamer. "The Genetics of Sexual Orientation: From Fruit Flies to Humans." In Paul R. Abramson and Steven D. Pinkerton, eds., *Sexual Nature Sexual Culture.* Chicago, Ill.: University of Chicago Press, 1995, 154–74; Peplau, Letitia, Linda Garnets, Leah Spalding, Terri Conley, and Rosemary Veniegas. "A Critique of Bem's 'Exotic Becomes Erotic' Theory of Sexual Orientation." *Psychological Review* 105:2 (1998), 387–94; Rich, Adrienne. "Compulsory Heterosexuality and Lesbian Existence." *Signs* 5:4 (1980), 631–60. Reprinted in *Blood, Bread, and Poetry: Selected Prose 1979–1985.* New York: Norton, 1986, 23–75; and Henry Abelove, Michèle Aina Barale, and David M. Halperin, eds., *The Lesbian and Gay Studies Reader.* New York: Routledge, 1993, 227–54; Ruse, Michael. *Homosexuality: A Philosophical Inquiry.* New York: Blackwell, 1988; Sánchez, María C., and Linda Schlossberg. *Passing: Identity and Interpretation in Sexuality, Race, and Religion.* New York: New

York University Press, 2001; Shively, Michael G., Christopher Jones, and John P. De Cecco. "Research on Sexual Orientation: Definitions and Methods." In John P. De Cecco and Michael Shively, eds., *Origins of Sexuality and Homosexuality*. New York: Harrington Park Press, 1985, 127–36; Silverstein, Charles. "The Ethical and Moral Implications of Sexual Classification: A Commentary." *Journal of Homosexuality* 9:4 (1984), 29–38; Simon, William. "The Oppressions of Object Choice." In *Postmodern Sexualities*. New York: Routledge, 1996, 34–36; Stein, Edward. "Essentialism and Constructionism in Sexual Orientation." In Robert B. Baker, Kathleen J. Wininger, and Frederick A. Elliston, eds., *Philosophy and Sex*, 3rd ed. Amherst, N.Y.: Prometheus, 1998, 393–96; Stein, Edward. "The Relevance of Scientific Research about Sexual Orientation to Lesbian and Gay Rights." *Journal of Homosexuality* 27:3–4 (1994), 269–308. Reprinted in HS (191–230); Stein, Edward, ed. *Forms of Desire: Sexual Orientation and the Social Constructionist Controversy*, 1st pnt. New York: Garland, 1990. 2nd pnt., New York: Routledge, 1992; Stein, Edward, Jacinta Kevin, and Udo Schüklenk. "Sexual Orientation." In Ruth Chadwick, ed., *Encyclopedia of Applied Ethics*, vol. 4. San Diego, Calif.: Academic Press, 1998, 101–8; Stoller, Robert J. "Problems with the Term 'Homosexuality.'" In *Observing the Erotic Imagination*. New Haven, Conn.: Yale University Press, 1985, 93–103; Stone, Sandy [Allucquère Rosanne Stone]. "The Empire Strikes Back: A Posttranssexual Manifesto." In Julia Epstein and Kristin Straub, eds., *Body Guards: The Cultural Politics of Gender Ambiguity*. New York: Routledge, 1991, 280–304. Revised version, *Camera Obscura* 29 (May 1992), 151–76; Suppe, Frederick. "Curing Homosexuality." In Robert B. Baker and Frederick A. Elliston, eds., *Philosophy and Sex*, 2nd ed. Buffalo, N.Y.: Prometheus, 1984, 391–420; Suppe, Frederick. "Explaining Homosexuality: Philosophical Issues, and Who Cares Anyhow?" *Journal of Homosexuality* 27: 3–4 (1984), 223–68. Also in Timothy F. Murphy, ed., *Gay Ethics: Controversies in Outing, Civil Rights, and Sexual Science*. New York: Haworth Press, 1994, 223–68. Reprinted, abridged, and retitled "Explaining Homosexuality: Who Cares Anyhow?" in John Corvino, ed., *Same Sex: Debating the Ethics, Science, and Culture of Homosexuality*. Lanham, Md.: Rowman and Littlefield, 1997, 167–75; Weeks, Jeffrey. "Necessary Fictions: Sexual Identities and the Politics of Diversity." In *Invented Moralities: Sexual Values in an Age of Uncertainty*. New York: Columbia University Press, 1995, 82–123.

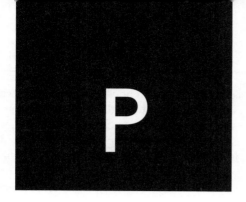

PAGLIA, CAMILLE (1947–). A leading culture critic and feminist dissident, Camille Paglia grew up in an Italian American working-class section of Endicott, New York, and later lived in Syracuse, where her father was a professor of Romance languages at Le Moyne College. Reacting to 1950s conformism, Paglia embraced the sexual **liberalism** and emerging feminist movement of the following decade, in part because she was bisexual. She studied literature and art history, eventually taking her Ph.D. at Yale. Paglia first taught at Bennington College and moved on to Wesleyan University, Yale University, and Philadelphia's University of the Arts (in 1984), where she became University Professor of Humanities and Media Studies and a major figure in her field, a provocative and widely discussed scholar.

Paglia's first book, *Sexual Personae* (*SP*), was published in 1990. Based on her doctoral dissertation, it argues that there is unity and continuity in Western culture, through examination of art and literature from antiquity to the late nineteenth century (ranging from Egyptian sculpture through Edmund Spenser's [1552–1599] *The Faerie Queene* to Emily Dickinson's [1830–1886] poetry). A second volume (written by 1981) of this massive work has not yet been published. It covers twentieth-century popular culture, a major preoccupation of the author, who believes it to be "the great heir of the Western past" as a result of the "neurotic nihilism" of recent high culture (*SP*, 31). In the 1990s, Paglia published two collections of essays, book reviews, film transcripts, and a monograph on Alfred Hitchcock's (1899–1980) film *The Birds*.

In "Sex and Violence, or Nature and Art," chapter 1 of *Sexual Personae*, and in the book's previously unpublished preface (included in *Sex, Art, and American Culture* (*SAAC*), 101–24), Paglia airs a view of sexuality and sex differences that is consistent with **evolutionary psychology** and biology (she refers to Charles Darwin [1809–1882]), yet one that is primarily influenced by the **Marquis de Sade** (1740–1814), Charles Baudelaire (1821–1867), **Friedrich Nietzsche** (1844–1900), and **Sigmund Freud** (1856–1939). Existing at the intersection of nature and culture, eroticism is dark, irrational, with an underlying current of **sadomasochism**. "Sadomasochism is a sacred cult, a pagan religion that reveals the dark secrets of nature. The bondage of sadomasochism expresses our own bondage by the body, our subservience to its brute laws, concealed by our myths of romantic love" (*SAAC*, 44–45). Sexuality is neither nurturing nor loving but both predatory (as in Darwinian struggles) and violent (as in the Freudian link between *eros* and *thanatos*). Its meaning should be comprehended psychologically as the playing out of the turbulent and risky Freudian "family romance." Sexuality has its own mysterious agenda. We usually have little understanding of how it determines our choices and shapes our identity (a theme reminiscent of **Arthur Schopenhauer**'s [1788–1860] conception of the ultimate processes of nature to which we are individually blind).

Male sexuality is Apollonian, Paglia maintains, in its striving for separation from nature, its seeking purity of form. It is opposed to the Dionysian or chthonian (of the earth) character of the feminine, as ancient sky-cults are opposed to earth-cults and mother-worship. Concentration and projection are the salient features of masculine sexual energy, just as they are of the male genitals. Maleness, with its quest for objectivity (however deluded) and preference for logic over emotion, is history's muscular creative force, from which flows most science, art, and philosophy (*SP*, 9, 12–13, 17–21, 30–32). Men must become men, while women simply need to be. In the struggle to distinguish themselves from their mothers and women in general through deeds, men define themselves as men. Women are more self-contained, their sexuality hidden and internal, their sensitivity more diffuse. Thus, Paglia suggests, we can understand the appeal and meaning of striptease, which always leaves something shrouded in mystery. ("There is nothing less erotic than a nudist colony"; *SP*, 36.) Most women are receptive and intuitive rather than aggressively penetrating, subjective and accepting of ambiguity: Witness their less-defined sexual organs. They entrap men, often infantilizing them if allowed to do so. Women's **beauty** and the **love** men have for them are devices for reconciling men to what they must do to satisfy their heterosexual impulses (see Schopenhauer, 538–40). The grossness of the female body, its liquidity and odors, subliminally reminds us of the primeval swamp. Chthonian nature, with its dark horrors from which our remote ancestors emerged, must be disguised. Drag queens do not mock but glorify female allure in its disguised, civilized form.

Our identities as men and women are heavily defined by biology; neither sex nor gender is a mere social construct. "[N]ature, not society, . . . is our greatest oppressor" (*SAAC*, 45), and nature is remarkably hierarchical (as are most societies, whatever their egalitarian professions). We are in bondage to inegalitarian nature, and this is especially true of women, whose bodies are "chthonian machines" formed to conceive and bear children. Monthly cycles and premenstrual tension do not permit women to forget it, and "no role may be more important than bearing and raising children" (*Vamps and Tramps* [*V&T*], 29). But for those who do not choose motherhood, there should be the full range of opportunities for education and the careers open to men. What we should not expect is equal outcomes in the social and economic positions filled by the sexes. Too many innate differences of aptitude will prevent this even without invidious sex discrimination. Attempts to bring about equal outcomes through preferential treatment for women are unfair to men, harmful to institutions, and paternalistic and condescending to women, who are thereby infantilized and disabled (*V&T*, x–xii, 53–56).

The denigration of traditional female roles by feminists is also wrong, in Paglia's view. Equal political rights and economic opportunities should be the aim of **feminism**, which is what feminism was originally about in the 1960s and earlier. Contemporary gender feminism, with its pollution from language-driven French philosophy (Paglia cites, among others, **Jacques Lacan** [1901–1981], **Michel Foucault** [1926–1984], Hélène Cixous, and Luce Irigaray), downplays biology and hence misconceives the nature of sexuality, masculinity, and femininity. ("As a flunky of Saussure, Foucault has to keep nature invisible at all times"; *SAAC*, 229.) For Paglia, what is most valid in feminist thought stems from nineteenth-century liberal, utilitarian philosophy, largely the work of men (for example, John Stuart Mill's [1806–1873] *The Subjection of Women*).

Paglia's feminism is a philosophy of self-reliance and independent action. She considers the labels "liberal" and "conservative" obsolete: She is a registered Democrat and supporter of Ralph Nader and other liberal candidates, yet also has much affinity with the libertarian Right and shares some beliefs of traditional conservativism. The personal overlaps the political, in her view, but the first should not be reduced to the second. Despite her paganism/atheism, Paglia has considerable respect for the Judeo-Christian tradition (indeed for all religions as symbol-systems) and the institutions of modern capitalism that Protestantism helped to shape. Private property and the free market have made possible freedom for women and equality with men. Intellectuals in particular should acknowledge their debt to capitalism; they would otherwise lack the freedom and leisure to live and work as they do (*SP*, 36–38).

Paglia's libertarian feminism is outlined in her two collections. Of special importance are her pieces on **rape** and **date rape** (in *SAAC*) and "No Law in the Arena: A Pagan Theory of Sexuality" (in *V&T*). Paglia's unorthodox opinions have caused backlash against her from both mainstream and radical feminist quarters: She has been attacked as antifeminist, antiwoman, and homophobic (see Bright, 76–79; Pollitt, 21–23). Her position is that when physical violence is not in question, sexual conduct should be free of regulation by church and state. Women and homosexuals must take personal responsibility for their actions within this sphere of protected liberty. (In part for this reason, Linda LeMoncheck characterizes Paglia as a "sex radical feminist" instead of a "cultural feminist"; 193–96.) Because "she that gives life [the mother] also blocks the way to [men's] freedom," Paglia agrees "with Sade that we have the right to thwart nature's procreative compulsions, through sodomy or abortion" (*SP*, 14).

One of Paglia's most controversial positions, from the standpoint of orthodox feminism, is on rape and how to deal with it. Her assertion that "[r]ape is the sexual expression of the will-to-power" (*SP*, 23) is meant to expose the naivete of the feminist cliché that rape is a crime of power, not sex. Sexuality itself is power, both in men and women. (**Catharine MacKinnon** agrees, but for reasons distinct from Paglia's, and she evaluates the phenomenon quite differently; 172–79.) Seeking sexual gratification is a warlike competition with serious risks and physical danger. These aspects of sex often heighten its appeal, just as restraint, whether moral or legal, real or imagined, can increase erotic intensity, as in bondage and discipline. "Sex is not the pleasure principle but the Dionysian bondage of pleasure-pain" (*SP*, 27). Sexuality is therefore not a route to freedom; sexual liberation is always succeeded by sadomasochism (*SP*, 39).

The aggression of the rapist is uncivilized, "piggish." He is desperate, conflicted, ashamed of his vulnerable need and dependence on women. His crime might even be interpreted as "a confession of envy and exclusion," having more to do with "unbridled lust" than the politics of dominating women (*V&T*, 32, 41; see **Richard Posner**, 385). Real rape is by an acquaintance or a stranger who injects sexuality into a situation where it does not belong. **Consent** to sex need not, she claims, be verbal, and seductive persuasion is not coercion. The feminist notion that rape includes "date rape" is, for her, a serious mistake, one that absolves women of personal responsibility, the other side of the freedom they now have, and reduces them to victim status. (See especially Paglia's 1991 *Newsday* article, reprinted in *SAAC*, 49–54.) A woman's "no" does not always mean no, and sometimes placing oneself in a certain situation does constitute an invitation to intercourse. We have the right to deny sex, just as we have the right not to be robbed, but women must take it on themselves to avoid circumstances where such violations are likely. This is why Paglia writes, sounding like many a mother, "A girl who lets herself get dead drunk at a fraternity party is a fool. A girl who goes upstairs with a brother at a fraternity party is an idiot. Feminists call this 'blaming the victim.' I call it common sense" (*SAAC*, 51; see LeMoncheck, 201).

The misconceptions of orthodox feminism about rape underlie its attitude toward **sexual harassment**, the extreme forms of which are stalking and unwanted touching. Moderate sexual harassment policies are appropriate in educational institutions and the workplace, but they should include harsh penalties for false accusations and be suitably framed for the kind of place they are intended to regulate. (Paglia condemns what she sees as a restoration on college campuses of the *in loco parentis* mentality against which her generation fought; see *SAAC*, 52.) Attempts to guarantee a "non-hostile workplace" will fail, because most places of employment are hostile by their very nature: Power and competition are part of the territory. Further, attempts to separate sex and power cannot succeed, for they assume simplistic notions of sexuality and human behavior. Treating women as childlike, needing protection from words and pictures that some find offensive, not only infringes coworkers' free speech but is paternalistic and patronizing: It underestimates women's ability to handle common situations and defend themselves with words and actions. Given the frequency of contact between the sexes, office romances, and women's erotic clothing, "a sex-free workplace is neither possible nor desirable" (*V&T*, 51). Paglia's prescription for women entering the professional world where they compete with men and women is to study football. They must acquire strategic abilities and rough-and-tumble virtues to attain leadership positions.

Paglia's independent and iconoclastic politics ("Leaving sex to the feminists is like letting your dog vacation at the taxidermist's"; *SAAC*, 50) are apparent in her views about other controversial sexual subjects. **Prostitution** and **pornography** are often condemned by white, middle-class feminists who think women in these industries are exploited. For Paglia, successful prostitutes are invisible, not the pathetic cases seen on the streets or television programs hosted by would-be therapists. The expert prostitute is a "shrewd entrepreneur," "a performance artist of hyper-developed sexual imagination." Women who sell sexual services are "pagan goddesses" like the temple prostitutes of ancient societies (see Fabian). They provide a needed social service under very difficult conditions, which makes them "among the strongest and most formidable women on the planet" (*V&T*, 57–59; see Califia). Prostitution, like recreational drug use, should be decriminalized with reasonable regulation.

Pornography should remain legal, Paglia maintains, rejecting the antipornography measures of both religious conservatives and feminists such as MacKinnon and **Andrea Dworkin** (1946–2005). Pornography is an art form that "forces a radical reassessment of sexual value" and "shows the deepest truth about sexuality, stripped of romantic veneer" (*V&T*, 66–67). The "artifice and animality," the "dynamic interplay of nature and culture" in human sexuality, is evident in pornography (*V&T*, 19). **Sexual objectification**, which orthodox feminists condemn, is "intertwined" with the artistic impulse and so cannot or must not be eliminated (*SP*, 30). Youth, beauty, and strength are revered in pornography, but even ugly or perverse images can be revelatory. Men are drawn to pornography not only because their arousal is more visual but also because their conceptual and objectifying mentality makes them more susceptible to **perversion**, especially fetishism with its rich symbolic associations (*SP*, 20–25; cf. Posner, 98–99).

Paglia's libertarian feminism, her encyclopedic knowledge of art, literature, history, philosophy, politics, and popular culture, her thorough and original scholarship, and her courageous willingness to confront the feminist establishment—together with her unique and colorful personality—make her a figure of exceptional distinction. In the writings of Katie Roiphe, Wendy McElroy, Rene Denfeld, and Tammy Bruce one can see her influence among a younger generation of feminists who question the dogmatic attitudes of orthodox feminism.

See also Beauty; Coercion (by Sexually Aggressive Women); Dworkin, Andrea; Feminism, French; Feminism, Liberal; Harassment, Sexual; MacKinnon, Catharine; Nietzsche, Friedrich; Objectification,

Sexual; Pornography; Posner, Richard; Prostitution; Psychology, Evolutionary; Rape; Rape, Acquaintance and Date; Sadomasochism; Schopenhauer, Arthur; Violence, Sexual

REFERENCES

Bright, Susie. *Susie Bright's Sexwise*. San Francisco, Calif.: Cleis Press, 1995; Bruce, Tammy. *The New Thought Police: Inside the Left's Assault on Free Speech and Free Minds*. Roseville, Calif.: Prima, 2003; Califia, Pat. "Whoring in Utopia." In *Public Sex: The Culture of Radical Sex*. Pittsburgh, Pa.: Cleis Press, 1994, 242–48; Denfeld, Rene. *The New Victorians: A Young Woman's Challenge to the Old Feminist Order*. New York: Warner, 1995; Fabian, Cosi. "The Holy Whore: A Woman's Gateway to Power." In Jill Nagle, ed., *Whores and Other Feminists*. New York: Routledge, 1997, 44–54; LeMoncheck, Linda. *Loose Women, Lecherous Men: A Feminist Philosophy of Sex*. New York: Oxford University Press, 1997; MacKinnon, Catharine A. *Toward a Feminist Theory of the State*. Cambridge, Mass.: Harvard University Press, 1989; McElroy, Wendy. *Sexual Correctness: The Gender-Feminist Attack on Women*. Jefferson, N.C.: McFarland, 1996; Mill, John Stuart. (1869) *The Subjection of Women*. In Alice Rossi, ed., *Essays on Sex Equality: John Stuart Mill and Harriet Taylor Mill*. Chicago, Ill.: University of Chicago Press, 1970, 123–242; Paglia, Camille. *The Birds*. London: British Film Institute, 1998; Paglia, Camille. *Sex, Art, and American Culture: Essays*. New York: Vintage, 1992; Paglia, Camille. *Sexual Personae: Art and Decadence from Nefertiti to Emily Dickinson*. New Haven, Conn.: Yale University Press, 1990; Paglia, Camille. *Vamps and Tramps: New Essays*. New York: Vintage, 1994; Pollitt, Katha. *Subject to Debate: Sense and Dissents on Women, Politics and Culture*. New York: Random House, 2001; Posner, Richard A. *Sex and Reason*. Cambridge, Mass.: Harvard University Press, 1992; Roiphe, Katie. *The Morning After: Sex, Fear, and Feminism on Campus*. New York: Little, Brown, 1993; Schopenhauer, Arthur. (1818, 1844, 1859) *The World as Will and Representation*, vol 2. Trans. E.F.J. Payne. Indian Hills, Colo.: Falcon's Wing Press, 1958.

Robert M. Stewart

ADDITIONAL READING

Arner, Michael. "Opinions after the Cancelled Preface to *Sexual Personae*." *The Autodidact's Journal*, no. 1. <www.monad.com/sdg/Journal/sexual.html> [accessed 31 August 2004]; Califia, Pat. "Radical Assessment." [Review of *Sex, Art, and American Culture: Essays*, by Camille Paglia] *Philadelphia Inquirer* (4 October 1992); Califia, Pat. "Whoring in Utopia." In *Public Sex: The Culture of Radical Sex*. Pittsburgh, Pa.: Cleis Press, 1994, 242–48. Reprinted in POS4 (475–81); Craghead, S. Elaine. "Camille Paglia and the Problematics of Sexuality and Subversion." In Karla Jay, ed., *Lesbians Erotics*. New York: New York University Press, 1995, 85–100; Friend, Tad. "Yes." *Esquire* (February 1994), 48–56; Hersey, George L. *The Evolution of Allure: Sexual Selection from the Medici Venus to the Incredible Hulk*. Cambridge, Mass.: MIT Press, 1996; Maglin, Nan Bauer, and Donna Perry, eds. *"Bad Girls"/"Good Girls": Women, Sex, and Power in the Nineties*. New Brunswick, N.J.: Rutgers University Press, 1996; McElroy, Wendy. *XXX: A Woman's Right to Pornography*. New York: St. Martin's Press, 1995; Nietzsche, Friedrich. (1872) *The Birth of Tragedy or Hellenism and Pessimism*. Trans. Walter Kaufmann. In Walter Kaufmann, ed., *Basic Writings of Nietzsche*. New York: Modern Library, 1968, 1–144; Paglia, Camille. "Cults and Cosmic Consciousness: Religious Vision in the American 1960s." *Arion* 10:3 (2003), 58–111. <www.bu.edu/arion/paglia_cults1.htm> [accessed 6 July 2004]; Paglia, Camille. "The Magic of Images: Word and Picture in a Media Age." *Arion* 11:3 (2004), 1–22; Paglia, Camille. Review of *Same-Sex Unions in Premodern Europe*, by John Boswell. *Washington Post* (17 July 1994). <www.fordham.edu/halsall/pwh/bosrev-paglia.html> [accessed 16 February 2005]; Paglia, Camille, and Neil Postman. "Dinner Conversation: She Wants Her TV! He Wants His Book!" *Harper's Magazine* (March 1991), 44–55; Patai, Daphne. *Heterophobia: Sexual Harassment and the Future of Feminism*. Lanham, Md.: Rowman and Littlefield, 1998; Patai, Daphne. "Women on Top." [Review essay] *Academic Questions* 16:2 (2003), 70–82; Patai, Daphne, and Noretta Koertge. *Professing Feminism: Cautionary Tales from the Strange World of Women's Studies.* New York: Basic Books, 1994. *Professing Feminism: Education and Indoctrination in Women's Studies,* new and expanded ed. Lanham, Md.: Lexington, 2003; Sommers, Christina Hoff. "A Genie Strikes Back: Correctness, Subversion, and the Risks of Freedom." *The Times Literary Supplement* (8 January 1993), 3–4; Sommers, Christina Hoff. *Who Stole Feminism? How Women Have Betrayed Women.* New York: Simon and Schuster, 1994. Expanded paperback ed., 1995; Stein, Harry. "*Penthouse* Interview, Christina Hoff Sommers." *Penthouse* (January 1965), 66–74, 181; Synnevåg, Marit. "Camille Paglia: Resources on the WWW." <privat.ub.uib.no/BUBSY/nomore.htm> [accessed 16 February 2005]; Wattenberg, Ben. "Has Feminism Gone Too Far?" [Interview with Camille Paglia and Christina Sommers] *PBS Think Tank* (4 November 1994). <www.pbs.org/thinktank/show_132.html> [accessed 4 January 2005]; Wells, Melanie. "Woman as Goddess: Camille Paglia Tours Strip Clubs." *Penthouse* (October 1994), 56–61, 132; West, Robin. "Unwelcome Sex: Toward a Harm-Based Analysis." In Catharine A. MacKinnon and Reva B. Siegel, eds., *Directions in Sexual Harassment Law.* New Haven, Conn.: Yale University Press, 2004, 138–52.

PARAPHILIA. There exists in the field of psychiatry a set of sexual conditions, once called "perversions" but more recently labeled "paraphilias" by the American Psychiatric Association (APA), whose malady status and defining criteria have often changed since at least the 1960s. Diagnostic uncertainty is not unknown in psychiatry—witness, for example, the discussion about whether premenstrual dysphoria should be counted as a psychiatric disorder—but probably with respect to no other condition(s) has it been more pronounced.

Are the paraphilias listed by the APA in the various editions of its *Diagnostic and Statistical Manual of Mental Disorders* actually mental disorders? At first blush there seems a straightforward way to answer this question: The DSM supplies a general definition of mental disorder, so the questions are whether (or to what extent) this definition is adequate and how well the paraphilias listed in DSM satisfy the definition.

We begin with the definition of "mental disorder" from DSM-IV-TR (xxxi):

> In DSM-IV, each of the mental disorders is conceptualized as a clinically significant behavioral or psychological syndrome or pattern that occurs in an individual and that is associated with present distress (e.g., a painful symptom) or disability (i.e., impairment in one or more important areas of functioning) or with a significantly increased risk of suffering death, pain, disability, or an important loss of freedom. In addition, this syndrome or pattern must not be merely an expectable and culturally sanctioned response to a particular event, for example, the loss of a loved one. Whatever its original cause, it must currently be considered a manifestation of a behavioral, psychological, or biological dysfunction in the individual. Neither deviant behavior (e.g., political, religious, or sexual) nor conflicts that are primarily between the individual and society are mental disorders unless the deviance or conflict is a symptom of a dysfunction in the individual, as described above.

The first sentence in the definition provides the essential features of mental disorders and distinguishes them from physical disorders. The definition makes clear that mental disorders involve behavioral or psychological features rather than the physical features of the person. Normally, what makes a disorder a mental disorder is its symptoms, not its cause or etiology.

For both mental and physical disorders, the symptoms must be associated with present distress or disability (or functional impairment) or with an increased risk of distress, disability, death, and so forth. For example, arthritis is a physical disorder that involves both present distress and disability. High blood pressure is a physical disorder that may not involve present distress or disability but does involve an increased risk of death or disability in the future. Phobias are mental disorders that are associated with both present distress and disability. It is extremely important that no condition is a disorder, either mental or physical, unless it is associated with present distress or disability (or a significantly increased risk), for it helps to establish the objectivity of the concept of a disorder: The presence or absence of these symptoms can in general be objectively verified. Mental disorders, properly understood, like physical disorders, are not merely labels for conditions that some culture or society has arbitrarily picked out for special calumny or treatment.

Mental disorders, since they involve distress, disability, or significant risks, are conditions that no one wants for himself or herself (or for a beloved person), at least not without an adequate reason. Sometimes one might choose or want to suffer a minor disorder to gain an advantage; for example, mild asthma may result in a deferment from a wartime draft. But, as the example shows, although social circumstances may make it advantageous to have a disorder, having a disorder nevertheless involves at least an increased risk of suffering some harm or evil that one (*ceteris paribus*) would prefer to do without.

According to this notion of a disorder, suffering, distress, disability (and so forth), though necessary features of a mental or physical disorder, are not sufficient: More things cause suffering than mental or physical disorders. We often suffer because something has gone wrong—not with us but with the world outside us. A loved one dies; someone threatens us with serious physical harm; poverty prevents us from providing adequate food or clothing for our children. All these circumstances cause one to experience distress, but this distress is not a symptom of mental disorder if it is "merely an expectable and culturally sanctioned response to a particular event."

However, these conditions, especially if prolonged, can bring about changes in a person. The point is that even were the original cause of the symptoms to cease, the individual may still feel distress. The distress brought about by the strains or tensions of real world events can cause a dysfunction in the individual that persists even after these strains or tensions have been removed. One example is posttraumatic stress disorder. The parallel here with physical disorders is exact. For example, prolonged exposure to extreme heat or cold may not only make a person experience distress but may cause a change in the person so that he or she now has a dysfunction that involves being afflicted with symptoms even after the external temperature has returned to normal (see Culver and Gert, 72–74).

Sometimes external conditions may not cause present distress or disability but may affect the individual in such a way that he or she suffers significantly increased risk of death, pain, and so forth. Continuing strain and tension may cause high blood pressure. Continuing to smoke, to drink alcohol, or to take various drugs recreationally may result in a person acquiring a substance abuse disorder that significantly increases his or her risk of distress or disability. Substance abuse, like the physical disorder of high blood pressure, undoubtedly is sometimes made more likely by a person's genetic predisposition. This fact reinforces the view that what distinguishes mental from physical disorders is their symptoms, not their etiology.

The DSM definition of mental disorder concludes by asserting that merely "deviant behavior" (political, religious, even sexual) and "conflicts" between an individual and his or her society are not mental disorders—"unless the deviance or conflict is a symptom of a dysfunction in the person." Simply holding, even promulgating, unpopular or strange political or religious ideas is not a mental disorder. But most important, and not made sufficiently explicit by the definition, nothing is a *dysfunction* unless it is associated with present distress or disability or increased risk. It is not as if some dysfunctions are associated with these harms and risks, but others are benign dysfunctions that have no harms or risks at all. A mild dysfunction is associated with mild symptoms or lower risks, but there can be no dysfunction that has no symptoms or no increased risks. Rigorous adherence to this definition of mental disorder frees psychiatry from any temptation to enforce social conformity and contributes to psychiatry's simply being one more medical speciality. But rigorous adherence requires that deviant behavior (in the absence of a painful symptom or impairment in functioning) is no more a mental disorder than asymptomatic *situs inversus* or being able to wiggle one's ears are physical disorders. However, when discussing the paraphilias the various editions of DSM over the years have not always abided by their own definition of mental disorder.

The definition of mental disorder has remained essentially the same from DSM-III-R (1987) to DSM-IV-TR (2000), but the discussion of the various paraphilias and the defining characteristics necessary to diagnose them have significantly changed. In particular, the diagnostic roles of *behavioral deviance* and of *the suffering of harms* have varied. Sometimes, especially in DSM-III (1980) and DSM-III-R, the existence of behavioral deviancy alone is sufficient to diagnose a paraphilia (and thus a mental disorder). By contrast, in DSM-IV (1994) distress plays a major and necessary role in defining all the paraphilias. DSM-IV-TR offers a more complex picture: It continues to stipulate (in the fashion of DSM-IV) that the suffering of harms is necessary—but only for *some* paraphilias; thus DSM-IV-TR asserts that the suffering of harms is *not* necessary for others (in the fashion of DSM-III-R).

Examine, for example, the defining criteria of the paraphilia "Transvestic Fetishism" ("Transvestism" in DSM-III), the DSM term for men who experience sexual excitement by dressing in women's clothing. Compare three sets of defining criteria:

DSM-III (1980; 270):

    A. Recurrent and persistent cross-dressing by a heterosexual male.

    B. Use of cross-dressing for the purpose of sexual excitement, at least initially in the course of the disorder.

    C. Intense frustration when cross-dressing is interfered with.

    D. Does not meet criteria for Transsexualism.

DSM-III-R (1987; 288–89):

    A. Over a period of at least six months, in a heterosexual male, recurrent intense sexual urges and sexually arousing fantasies involving cross-dressing.

    B. The person has acted on these urges, or is markedly distressed by them.

    C. Does not meet the criteria for Gender Identity Disorder of Adolescence or Adulthood, Nontranssexual Type, or Transsexualism.

DSM-IV (1994; 530–31), DMS-IV-TR (2000; 574–75):

    A. Over a period of at least six months, in a heterosexual male, recurrent, intense sexually arousing fantasies, sexual urges, or behaviors involving cross-dressing.

B. The fantasies, sexual urges, or behaviors cause clinically significant distress or impairment in social, occupational, or other important areas of functioning.

Now consider Mr. X, a forty-year-old man who for years has found it sexually arousing to put on women's underwear. Once or twice a month, in the privacy of his bedroom, he dresses in lingerie, becomes sexually excited, and masturbates to orgasm. He considers himself heterosexual and has had reasonably satisfying sexual relations during his two marriages and more recently with several women he has dated. He finds cross-dressing exciting and has no desire to change. He has never engaged in any **homosexuality** and has never desired to be in public fully dressed as a woman. His social demeanor is (to use DSM-IV-TR's term) "unremarkably masculine." No acquaintance, male or female, knows about his cross-dressing, except one girlfriend. He once vaguely described his activities to her, but she seemed mostly amused, and the subject never came up again. Mr. X is usually able to cross-dress when he has the urge. There was once, however, a two-month family summer vacation during which he became highly frustrated; he never had a chance to cross-dress.

How would Mr. X be diagnosed? According to DSM-III, Mr. X has a mental disorder: He has cross-dressed persistently over the years (criterion A) to become sexually excited (criterion B) and, on rare occasions when he has not been able to cross-dress, he has been intensely frustrated (criterion C). Mr. X would also have a disorder according to DSM-III-R, although its criteria are different. In fact, essentially all cross-dressers would have a disorder because they would satisfy not only criterion A but also the first part of B: It would be highly unusual to find a man with "recurrent intense sexual urges and sexually arousing fantasies involving cross-dressing" who never acted on them. Thus criterion B would be satisfied even if its second half—being markedly distressed—were not satisfied. Deviance without distress, as in DSM-III, could constitute a mental disorder. However, according to DSM-IV and DSM-IV-TR, Mr. X does not have a mental disorder. He satisfies criterion A: He has become sexually aroused through cross-dressing for a period of at least six months. He does not, however, satisfy criterion B: His cross-dressing fantasies, urges, and behaviors have not over the years caused him "clinically significant" distress or functional impairment. Indeed, they have caused him little, if any, distress or impairment of any kind, and he would not want to eliminate his urge to cross-dress, even if doing so were possible.

An important difference between the two sets of DSM criteria (between DSM-III and DSM-III-R, on the one hand, and DSM-IV and DSM-IV-TR, on the other) is that behavioral deviance or abnormality alone is sufficient to warrant a diagnosis of mental disorder in the first set. This is true despite the fact that the DSM-III-R definition of mental disorder clearly states that deviance alone is *not* sufficient for mental disorder. The authors of the DSM-III-R criteria of transvestism seemingly ignored DSM-III-R's own definition of mental disorder (see Gert on this problem). In DSM-IV and DSM-IV-TR, by contrast, deviance is not sufficient for the diagnosis; the behavior must be accompanied by significant distress or dysfunction. Even so, it would have been useful for the authors of DSM-IV and DSM-IV-TR to have been more precise. Suppose Mr. X feels comfortable with his transvestite experiences, but his cross-dressing is accidentally discovered by a friend who tells other people about it, and Mr. X suffers significant social rejection as a result. On one interpretation of criterion B, it could be said that Mr. X's behavior *has* led to (i.e., caused) his experiencing significant social distress. This interpretation is almost certainly not what the DSM-IV and DSM-IV-TR authors would endorse—otherwise a gay person who was distressed by encountering hostile homophobic behaviors would have to be said to have a mental disorder. DSM-IV and DSM-IV-TR should have stated that the transvestite behavior, urges, or fantasies *directly* cause the distress and that the person feels significant distress that exists independently of whether anyone else knows about his or her sexual behavior, urges, or fantasies. "Cause" in the criterion is ambiguous and needs to be carefully defined. The notion (or the many examples) of nonparaphiliac cross-dressing men nicely captures the important distinctions that need to be made. The situation seems entirely analogous to that of ego-syntonic homosexuality, which the APA removed from the list of DSM mental disorders in the 1970s (see Conrad and Schneider; Gonsiorek). Why this was done for distress-free homosexuality, but not for any other conditions involving statistically unusual sexual behaviors, is a mystery that DSM never addresses (see Soble; Suppe).

Although the defining criteria for transvestism in DSM-IV and DSM-IV-TR come closer to the DSM definition of mental disorder, the same cannot be said for all the paraphilias. Although DSM-IV stipulated that distress was a necessary component of all the paraphilias, DSM-IV-TR has regressed. In DSM-IV-TR, the diagnosis of five of the eight paraphilias does not require distress: exhibitionism, frotteurism, **pedophilia**, sadism, and voyeurism. For each of these five paraphilias, criterion B states, "The person has acted on these sexual urges, or the sexual urges or fantasies cause marked distress or interpersonal difficulty." The first "or" makes it clear that just acting, without distress or difficulty, constitutes a disorder.

Why did DSM-IV-TR go back to the DSM-III-R form of criterion B for five paraphilias? DSM-IV-TR does not say. Consider a voyeur who is not distressed by his voyeurism. In 1987 he had a disorder (he "acted on his urges"; DSM-III-R); in 1994 he did not have a disorder (he did not suffer "clinically significant distress"; DSM-IV); but in 2000 he once again has a disorder (he "acts on his urges"; DSM-IV-TR). If the psychiatric profession's authoritative diagnostic manual changes a condition's disorder status every time a revised edition is issued, one would think that significant theoretical or empirical reasons for doing so existed and they would be fully discussed. Not so. Appendix D in DSM-IV-TR ("Highlights of Changes in DSM-IV Text Revision," at 840) notes this change in diagnosing some of the paraphilias, but no attempt is made to explain or justify it.

This regression to the DSM-III-R criterion for these five paraphilias may well be a mistake because it confuses criminal or immoral behavior with having a mental disorder. For a person to have a mental disorder, the individual suffering harm must be the person with the disorder, not someone else (the "victim" in the criminal or moral sense). This is abundantly clear from DSM's definition of mental disorder. Once again it appears that the crafters of DSM have ignored their own definition of mental disorder.

An examination of the description and discussion of the paraphilias found in psychiatric textbooks illustrates a lack of agreement within the profession about the correct definition of these conditions. One text is trenchant and to the point:

> Paraphilias include sexual disorders related to culturally unusual sexual activity. A key criterion for the diagnosis of a paraphilia (as in all psychiatric disorders) is that the disorder must cause an individual to experience significant distress or impairment in social or occupational functioning. In other words, an individual with unusual sexual practices who does not suffer significant distress or impairment would not be diagnosed with a psychiatric illness. (Murphy et al., 51)

However, another text states, "These patients [paraphiliacs] may not be troubled by their desires (ego syntonic) and thus are difficult to treat, although depression, anxiety, and guilt do occur" (Tomb, 180–81). Yet another states, "Individuals with paraphilias may not report feeling distress and may justify their sexual interests as variant sexualities" (Goldman, 372). These last two authors fail to see that persons who are not distressed by having or acting on their unusual **sexual desire**s do not satisfy the DSM definition of mental disorder.

The American Psychiatric Association, in its DSM volumes, has supplied over the years a valid and useful definition of mental disorder. However, the specific criteria listed for the various paraphilias have not always conformed with that definition. The DSM-IV criteria came reasonably close, but the DSM-IV-TR criteria regressed significantly. The lack of conformity between definition and criteria centers on the issue of whether deviant (statistically unusual) sexual behavior in and of itself constitutes a disorder or whether the unusual sexual behavior must be intrinsically distressing to the individual. The DSM definition of mental disorder makes it clear that deviance, although necessary for the diagnosis, is not sufficient, while the various DSM criteria of the paraphilias fall short, to differing degrees, of this principle. Descriptions and discussions of the paraphilias in psychiatric textbooks reflect this persistent ambiguity in the profession.

See also Addiction, Sexual; Bestiality; Bullough, Vern L.; Orientation, Sexual; Perversion, Sexual; Sadomasochism; Sexology

REFERENCES

American Psychiatric Association. *Diagnostic and Statistical Manual of Mental Disorders*, 3rd ed. [DSM-III] Washington, D.C.: Author, 1980; American Psychiatric Association. *Diagnostic and Statistical Manual of Mental Disorders*, 3rd ed., revised. [DSM-III-R] Washington, D.C.: Author, 1987; American Psychiatric Association. *Diagnostic and Statistical Manual of Mental Disorders*, 4th ed. [DSM-IV] Washington, D.C.: Author, 1994; American Psychiatric Association. *Diagnostic and Statistical Manual of Mental Disorders*, 4th ed., text revision. [DSM-IV-TR] Washington, D.C.: Author, 2000; Conrad, Peter, and Joseph W. Schneider. "Homosexuality: From Sin to Sickness to Life-Style." In *Deviance and Medicalization: From Badness to Sickness*. St. Louis, Mo.: C. V. Mosby, 1980, 172–214; Culver, Charles M., and Bernard Gert. *Philosophy in Medicine: Conceptual and Ethical Issues in Medicine and Psychiatry*. New York: Oxford University Press, 1982; Gert, Bernard. "A Sex Caused Inconsistency in DSM-III-R: The Definition of Mental Disorder and the Definition of Paraphilias." *Journal of Medicine and Philosophy* 17:2 (1992), 155–71; Gert, Bernard, and Charles M. Culver. "Defining Mental Disorder." In Jennifer Radden, ed., *The Philosophy of Psychiatry: A Companion*. New York: Oxford University Press, 2004, 415–25; Goldman, Howard H. *Review of General Psychiatry*, 5th ed. New York: Lange, 2000; Gonsiorek, John C. "The Empirical Basis for the Demise of the Illness Model of Homosexuality." In John C. Gonsiorek and James D. Weinrich, eds., *Homosexuality: Research Implications for Public Policy*. Newbury Park, Calif.: Sage, 1991, 115–36; Murphy, Michael J., Ronald L. Cowan, and Lloyd I. Sederer. *Blueprints in Psychiatry*, 2nd ed. Malden, Mass.: Blackwell, 2001; Soble, Alan. "Desire: Paraphilia and Distress in *DSM-IV*." In Jennifer Radden, ed., *The Philosophy of Psychiatry: A Companion*. New York: Oxford University Press, 2004, 54–63; Suppe, Frederick. "The Diagnostic and Statistical Manual of the American Psychiatric Association: Classifying Sexual Disorders." In Earl E. Shelp, ed., *Sexuality and Medicine*, vol. 2: *Ethical Viewpoints in Transition*. Dordrecht, Holland: Reidel, 1987, 111–35; Tomb, David A. *Psychiatry*, 6th ed. Philadelphia, Pa.: Lippincott Williams and Wilkins, 1999.

Charles M. Culver and Bernard Gert

ADDITIONAL READING

Allen, Clifford. (1940, 1949) *The Sexual Perversions and Abnormalities: A Study in the Psychology of Paraphilia*. Westport, Conn.: Greenwood Press, 1979; American Psychiatric Association. *Diagnostic and Statistical Manual of Mental Disorders*, 1st ed. Washington, D.C.: Author, 1952;

American Psychiatric Association. *Diagnostic and Statistical Manual of Mental Disorders*, 2nd ed. Washington, D.C.: Author, 1968; American Psychiatric Association. "Sexual and Gender Identity Disorders." In *Diagnostic and Statistical Manual of Mental Disorders*, 4th ed. [DSM-IV] Washington, D.C.: Author, 1994, 493–538; Bancroft, John. (1983) *Human Sexuality and Its Problems*, 2nd ed. Edinburgh, Scot.: Churchill Livingstone, 1989; Bergner, Raymond M. "Money's 'Lovemap' Account of the Paraphilias: A Critique and Reformulation." *American Journal of Psychotherapy* 42:2 (1988), 254–59; Bullough, Vern L., and Bonnie Bullough. *Cross Dressing, Sex, and Gender*. Philadelphia: University of Pennsylvania Press, 1993; Carnes, Patrick. *Out of the Shadows: Understanding Sexual Addiction*, 3rd ed. Center City, Minn.: Hazelden, 2001; Carr, Brian. "Sexual Orientation: Gender Identity Disorders." In Timothy F. Murphy, ed., *Reader's Guide to Lesbian and Gay Studies*. Chicago, Ill.: Fitzroy Dearborn, 2000, 538–39; Chauncey, George, Jr. (1983) "From Sexual Inversion to Homosexuality: The Changing Medical Conceptualization of Female Deviance." In Kathy Peiss and Christina Simmons, eds., *Passion and Power: Sexuality in History*. Philadelphia, Pa.: Temple University Press, 1989, 87–117; Coleman, Eli. "Treatment of Compulsive Sexual Behavior." In Raymond C. Rosen and Sandra R. Leiblum, eds., *Case Studies in Sex Therapy*. New York: Guilford, 1995, 333–39; Conrad, Peter, and Joseph W. Schneider. *Deviance and Medicalization: From Badness to Sickness*. St. Louis, Mo.: C. V. Mosby, 1980. Expanded edition, Philadelphia, Pa.: Temple University Press, 1992; Cooper, Arnold M. "The Unconscious Core of Perversion." In Gerald I. Fogel and Wayne A. Myers, eds., *Perversions and Near-Perversions in Clinical Practice: New Psychoanalytic Perspectives*. New Haven, Conn.: Yale University Press, 1991, 17–35; Davis, Dona, and Gilbert Herdt. "Cultural Issues and Sexual Disorders." In Thomas A. Widiger, Allen J. Francis, Harold Alan Pincus, Ruth Ross, Michael B. First, and Wendy Davis, eds., *DSM-IV Sourcebook*, vol. 3. Washington, D.C.: American Psychiatric Association, 1997, 951–57; Davis, L. J. "The Encyclopedia of Insanity." *Harper's Magazine* (February 1997), 61–66. See "Letters." *Harper's Magazine* (May 1997), 4–7; DeVito, Scott. "On the Value-Neutrality of the Concepts of Health and Disease: Unto the Breach Again." *Journal of Medicine and Philosophy* 25:5 (2000), 539–67; Feder, Ellen K. "Disciplining the Family: The Case of Gender Identity Disorder." *Philosophical Studies* 85:2–3 (1997), 195–211; Galbreath, Nathan W., Fred S. Berlin, and Denise Sawyer. "Paraphilias and the Internet." In Al Cooper, ed., *Sex and the Internet: A Guide Book for Clinicians*. New York: Brunner-Routledge, 2002, 187–205; Gates, Katharine. *Deviant Desires: Incredibly Strange Sex*. New York: Juno Books, 2000. Web site, <www.deviantdesires.com> [accessed 28 October 2004]; Groneman, Carol. *Nymphomania: A History*. New York: Norton, 2000; House of Sissify. "DSM-IV Labeling of a Community." <www.sissify.com/juice/dsm4.html> [accessed 28 October 2004]; Irons, Richard, and Jennifer P. Schneider. "Differential Diagnosis of Addictive Sexual Disorders Using the DSM-IV." *Sexual Addiction and Compulsivity* 3 (1996): 7–21. <www.jenniferschneider.com/articles/diagnos.html> [accessed 28 October 2004]; Irvine, Janice M. "Reinventing Perversion: Sex Addiction and Cultural Anxieties." *Journal of the History of Sexuality* 5:3 (1995), 429–50; Jenkins, Andrew P. "When Self-Pleasuring Becomes Self-Destruction: Autoerotic Asphyxiation Paraphilia." *International Electronic Journal of Health Education* 3:3 (2000), 208–16. <www.aahperd.org/iejhe/archive/jenkins.pdf> [accessed 28 October 2004]; Kaplan, Louise J. "Women Masquerading as Women." In Gerald I. Fogel and Wayne A. Myers, eds., *Perversions and Near-Perversions in Clinical Practice: New Psychoanalytic Perspectives*. New Haven, Conn.: Yale University Press, 1991, 127–52; Leiblum, Sandra R., and Raymond C. Rosen, eds. *Sexual Desire Disorders*. New York: Guilford Press, 1988; Margolis, Joseph. "The Question of Homosexuality." In Robert B. Baker and Frederick A. Elliston, eds., *Philosophy and Sex*, 1st ed. Buffalo, N.Y.: Prometheus, 1975, 288–302; Mead, Rebecca. "Sex and Sensibility: The Histories of Nymphomania and Celibacy." *The New Yorker* (18 September 2000), 146–48; Meisenkothen, Christopher. "Chemical Castration: Breaking the Cycle of Paraphiliac Recidivism." *Social Justice* 26:1 (1999), 139–55; Money, John. *Lovemaps: Clinical Concepts of Sexual/Erotic Health and Pathology, Paraphilia, and Gender Transposition in Childhood, Adolescence, and Maturity*. New York: Irvington, 1986. Paperback reprint, Buffalo, N.Y.: Prometheus, 1988; Money, John. "Paraphilias." In John Money and Herman Musaph, eds., *Handbook of Sexology*.

Amsterdam, Holland: Excerpta Medica, 1977, 917–28; Money, John. "Paraphilias: Phyletic Origins of Erotosexual Dysfunction." *International Journal of Mental Health* 10:2–3 (1981), 75–109; Money, John. "Prologue." In James J. Krivacska and John Money, eds., *The Handbook of Forensic Sexology: Biomedical and Criminological Perspectives*. Amherst, N.Y.: Prometheus, 1994, 21–28; Money, John. "Transcultural Sexology: Formicophilia, a Newly Named Paraphilia in a Young Buddhist Male." In *The Adam Principle. Genes, Genitals, Hormones, & Gender: Selected Readings in Sexology*. Buffalo, N.Y.: Prometheus, 1993, 334–40; Moser, Charles. "Paraphilia: Another Confused Sexological Concept." In Peggy J. Kleinplatz, ed., *New Directions in Sex Therapy: Innovations and Alternatives*. Philadelphia, Pa.: Brunner-Routledge, 2001, 91–108; Moser, Charles, and Peggy J. Kleinplatz. (2003) "DSM-IV-TR and the Paraphilias: An Argument for Removal." <www.home.netcom .com/~docx2/mk.html> [accessed 10 February 2005]; National Organization for Women. "Testimony from Physicians and Psychiatrists for the S/M Policy Reform Statement" (22 March 1997). <members.aol.com/NOWSM/Psychiatrists.html> [accessed 28 October 2004]; Neu, Jerome. "Boring from Within: Endogenous versus Reactive Boredom." In W. F. Flack, Jr., and J. D. Laird, eds., *Emotions in Psychopathology: Theory and Research*. Oxford, U.K.: Oxford University Press, 1998. Reprinted in *A Tear Is an Intellectual Thing: The Meanings of Emotion*. New York: Oxford University Press, 2000, 95–107; Neu, Jerome. "Freud and Perversion." In Earl E. Shelp, ed., *Sexuality and Medicine*, vol. 1: *Conceptual Roots*. Dordrecht, Holland: Reidel, 1987, 153–84. Reprinted in Jerome Neu, ed., *The Cambridge Companion to Freud*. Cambridge: Cambridge University Press, 1991, 175–208; STW (87–104); "Psychiatric Diagnosis: Manufacturing Madness." In *Psychiatry: Destroying Religion*. Los Angeles, Calif.: Citizens Commission on Human Rights, 1997, 44–47; Reiersol, Odd. "SM: Causes and Diagnoses." <www.revisef65.org/reiersol1.html> [accessed 28 October 2004]; Roth, Philip. *Portnoy's Complaint*. New York: Random House, 1969; Russell, Denise. "Female Bodies and Food: A Case of Ethics and Psychiatry." In Paul A. Komesaroff, ed., *Troubled Bodies: Critical Perspectives on Postmodernism, Medical Ethics, and the Body*. Durham, N.C.: Duke University Press, 1995, 222–34; Russell, J. Michael. "Perversion, Eating Disorders, and Sex Roles." *International Forum for Psychoanalysis* 1 (1992), 98–103. <members.aol.com/jmrussell/perversi.htm> [accessed 28 October 2004]; Schmidt, Chester W., Jr., Raul C. Schiavi, Leslie R. Schover, R. Taylor Segraves, and Thomas N. Wise. "DSM-IV Sexual Disorders: Final Overview." In Thomas Widiger, Allen Frances, Harold Pincus, Ruth Ross, Michael First, Wendy Davis, and Myriam Kline, eds., *DSM-IV Sourcebook*, vol. 4. Washington, D.C.: American Psychiatric Association, 1998, 1087–95; Schmidt, Chester W., Jr., Raul C. Schiavi, Leslie R. Schover, R. Taylor Segraves, and Thomas N. Wise. "Introduction to Section VI: Sexual Disorders." In Thomas Widiger, Allen Frances, Harold Pincus, Ruth Ross, Michael First, and Wendy Davis, eds., *DSM-IV Sourcebook*, vol. 2. Washington, D.C.: American Psychiatric Association, 1996, 1081–89; Silverstein, Charles. "The Ethical and Moral Implications of Sexual Classification: A Commentary." *Journal of Homosexuality* 9:4 (1984), 29–38; Soble, Alan. "Health." In *Sexual Investigations*. New York: New York University Press, 1996, 143–74; Stoller, Robert, Judd Marmor, Irving Bieber, Ronald Gold, Charles W. Socarides, Richard Green, and Robert L. Spitzer. "A Symposium: Should Homosexuality Be in the APA Nomenclature?" *American Journal of Psychiatry* 130:11 (1973), 1207–16; Suppe, Frederick. "Classifying Sexual Disorders: The *Diagnostic and Statistical Manual* of the American Psychiatric Association." *Journal of Homosexuality* 9:4 (1984), 9–28; Suppe, Frederick. "Explaining Homosexuality: Philosophical Issues, and Who Cares Anyhow?" In Timothy F. Murphy, ed., *Gay Ethics: Controversies in Outing, Civil Rights, and Sexual Science*. New York: Haworth Press, 1994, 223–68; Suppe, Frederick. "Medical and Psychiatric Perspectives on Human Sexual Behavior." In Earl E. Shelp, ed., *Sexuality and Medicine*, vol. 1: *Conceptual Roots*. Dordrecht, Holland: Reidel, 1987, 17–37; Szasz, Thomas S. *The Manufacture of Madness: A Comparative Study of the Inquisition and the Mental Health Movement*. New York: Harper and Row, 1970; Wise, Thomas N., and Chester W. Schmidt, Jr. "Paraphilias." In Thomas Widiger, Allen Frances, Harold Pincus, Ruth Ross, Michael First, and Wendy Davis, eds., *DSM-IV Sourcebook*, vol. 2. Washington, D.C.: American Psychiatric Association, 1996, 1133–47.

PAUL (SAINT) (5–64?). The epistles of Paul, the earliest Christian writer, have had an incalculable influence on Christian theology and ethics, including **sexual ethics**. Born in Tarsus, in southern Asia Minor, Paul was raised in an Orthodox Jewish family. It is probable, although debated, that he was a Roman citizen. His relations with Jews in Jerusalem, and his possible education there, were already debated in his lifetime. He also received a Hellenic education. Whereas Jesus, who died around 30 CE, taught Jewish peasants in rural Galilee in Aramaic, Paul traveled extensively and founded believing worshiping communities among Greek-speaking pagans in urban settings between Syria and Rome. Paul thereby internationalized Jewish Christianity. He was martyred under the Roman emperor Nero in the 60s.

Greco-Roman medical handbooks, frescoes on Pompeii walls, and literature contemporary to Paul help us place the debates about sex in Paul's first letter to the Corinthians in their cultural context (Clarke; Deming, 50–107; Osiek and Balch, 103–18). Medical handbooks by doctors and laymen "helped men take possession of the female body" (Rouselle, 21–22). "Sexual intercourse, [Epicurean philosophers] say, has never done a man good, and he is lucky if it has not harmed him" (Diogenes Laertius [10.118], in a handbook composed of earlier handbooks, from around 200 CE). Celsus (born ca. 25 BCE) advised, during the reign of Tiberius (14–37 CE), that "sexual intercourse neither should be avidly desired, nor should it be feared very much. Rarely performed, it revives the body, performed frequently, it weakens. . . . The weak, however, among whom are a large portion of townspeople, and almost all those fond of letters, need greater precaution" (1.1.4; 2.1). The physician Soranus (under Trajan and Hadrian, 98–138 CE) reports a late-first-century debate between two medical schools over sexual **abstinence**, but both parties agreed with Epicurus's (341–270 BCE) opinion that abstinence is ideal. Soranus, too, argued that "permanent virginity is healthful, because intercourse is harmful in itself " (1.7.32). Few medical sources illuminate why physicians thought sexual intercourse was harmful, but the physician Galen (129–199/216? CE) explained that because sperm is identical with spirit, the person becomes spiritually and physically weaker when it is ejected (Rouselle, 14–15). Given these medical opinions, Corinthian Christian ascetics might have rejected sex from their desire for spiritual gifts (1 Cor. 6–7, 12, 14).

The sexually ascetic Jewish Therapeutae described by the Alexandrian Jewish philosopher Philo (ca. 20 BCE–50 CE) are similar to the Pauline Christian ascetics. Philo writes of aged virgins who, because they yearned for wisdom, freely remained chaste. Males, too, possessed like bacchanals and desiring the vision of God, soar above the senses: They abandon property, leave their families, and retire to Jewish monasteries (*Contemplative Life*, 23–39, 89). Philo perhaps wrote in response to the Stoic philosopher and Egyptian priest Chaeremon (a teacher of Nero, mid-first century CE), who similarly praised Egyptian priests for renouncing their income and devoting themselves to contemplating the divine. These priests practiced self-control, did not drink wine, abstained from animal food, vegetables, and above all, sexual intercourse with women or men (Van der Horst, 16–17, 22–23). Philo and Chaeremon wrote near the date of 1 Corinthians (ca. 55), expecting their readers to admire sexual ascetics seeking a vision of the divine. Jesus himself may have been sexually ascetic (Matt 19:12). After Christianity became (321) a state-sponsored cult under the emperor Constantine (272 [or 288]–337), many radical disciples went to the desert to become ascetics, a lifestyle supported by Jerome (347–419/20).

These first-century literary, philosophical, and theological values match those of medical handbooks and provide a context for understanding Corinthian Christian sexual ascetics.

They had written to Paul their opinion that "it is well for a man not to touch a woman" (1 Cor. 7:1b). Paul also had an oral report that "a [Christian] man is living with his father's wife" (5:1). Paul demands that they "hand this man over to Satan for the destruction [*olethron*] of the flesh, so that his spirit may be saved in the day of the Lord" (5:5). Adela Collins cites 1 Thessalonians 5:2–3, where Paul refers to the "sudden [eschatological] destruction that will come upon them" (259). But Paul is not judging the eternal fate of the incestuous son. He is insisting, in view of the coming eschatological crisis, that those who are sanctified should act that way. This is a typical indicative/imperative in Paul.

Paul also condemns Christians going to court before the "unjust," concluding that the "unjust," pagan or Christian, will not inherit the kingdom of God (1 Cor. 6:1, 7a, 8, 9a). Linking the topics with the term "unjust," Paul repeats the six vices of 5:11 (sexual immorality, greed, idolatry, slander, drunkenness, swindling) and adds four more in 6:9–10, including *malakoi* and *arsenokoitai*, terms of uncertain meaning. The first can be understood in terms of ancient biology, which contrasted male and female nature. In *History of Animals* (IX.1, 608a32–b18), **Aristotle** (384–322 BCE) had written:

> All females are less spirited than the males, except the bear and leopard: in these the female is held to be braver. But in the other kinds the females are softer [*malakotera*], more vicious, less simple, more impetuous, more attentive to the feeding of the young, while the males on the contrary are more spirited, wilder, simpler, less cunning. . . . [M]an's nature [*physin*] is the most complete, so that these dispositions too are more evident in humans. Hence a wife is more compassionate than a husband and more given to tears, but also more jealous and complaining and more apt to scold and fight. . . . The male, on the other hand, as we have said, is a readier ally and is braver than the female.

Women are by nature softer, men stronger. Paul does not argue this but assumes it and its ethical corollary, that males should not act in a feminine way. This assumption is in tension both with the baptismal confession employed in his churches ("there is no longer . . . male and female"; Gal. 3:28) and with modern biology.

Paul then quotes Corinthian Christian slogans, "all things are lawful for me" (1 Cor. 6:12a) and "food is meant for the stomach and the stomach for food" (6:13a), which he wants to nuance. Although Greeks typically drew parallels between the passions for food and sex, Paul rejects it. Food is irrelevant to one's relationship to God. However, "the body is meant not for fornication [*porneia*], but for the Lord, and the Lord for the body" (6:13b). The phrase "the Lord for the *body*" is astounding in Middle Platonic culture. True, Paul agrees, neither a kosher Jewish diet (Lev. 11) nor Hellenistic vegetarianism (Plutarch [ca. 45–125 CE], *Eating of Flesh*) will present a person to God. Paul exhorts Corinthian Christian males to cling to the Lord and His body, the church, not to prostitutes (6:15–18). For men in the Greek world, it was unremarkable to be sexually active with more than one woman. Plutarch advises Pollianus, soon to be Eurydice's husband, to send her away after dinner if he is going to impose himself sexually on a slave woman, to which Eurydice should not object (*Advice to Bride and Groom*, 140B). To explain male Christians' continuing to use prostitutes, we can refer to their slogan "all things are lawful" (1 Cor. 6:12), which might have been their interpretation of Paul's earlier preaching that the Gospel saves apart from the law (1 Cor. 7:19; 15:56), as well as, perhaps, to their Plutarchian defensiveness about sexual partners. Paul, however, rejects husbands' sex with prostitutes or slaves as entertainment after meals.

In considering the Corinthian Christians' ascetic thought that "it is well not to touch a woman" (1 Cor. 7:1), Paul argues the opposite, doing so in gender-neutral language: "but because of cases of sexual immorality, each man should have his own wife and each woman her own husband" (7:2). He famously concludes, "It is better to marry than to burn" (7:9). Barré (195) observes that although "to burn" might mean to be aflame with passion, it is not used absolutely with this meaning (only so in association with a noun that specifies the emotion, which is absent). Paul is referring, rather, to the "fiery" eschatological judgment of Yahweh. Thus 7:9 is not proposing **marriage** as a cure for being passionately "inflamed" but is warning converts with ascetic ideals about the eschatological consequences.

According to Paul, the husband and wife mutually have each other's body (1 Cor. 7:3–4), a Stoic idea opposed to the widespread assumption that the man unilaterally owns the woman. Compare the Stoic Musonius Rufus (ca. 25–95 CE): "The husband and wife . . . should come together for the purpose of making a life in common and of procreating children, and furthermore, of regarding all things in common between them, and nothing peculiar or private to one or the other, not even their own bodies" (frag. 13A). There was a contemporary debate about the relationship between **friendship** and sex. In Plutarch's *Amatorius*, Protogenes praises pederasty because it includes friendship (750D) but denounces the house-bound **love** of women as devoid of it (*aphiloi*; 751B). Daphnaeus and Plutarch himself argue the opposite, against older views of friendship with boys (as found, perhaps, in **Plato**'s [427–347 BCE] *Symposium*), that a wife is a suitable, more graceful, and constant friend (769A–D, 751C). Paul's exhortations correspond to the domestication of friendship.

One conclusive sign that the relationship of women to men was changing in the first century is architectural. In Republican times (ca. 500–31 BCE), men and women were segregated in public baths; during the Empire (beginning 31 BCE) the baths were remodeled so that men and woman bathed nude together; but in the fourth century men and women were again separated (Ward, 131–34). The cultural development of greater friendship between men and women and the acts that symbolized it (bathing together; women's charismatic speech in Corinthian Christian worship) generated conflict, which occurred in the early Pauline Corinthian house churches. Paul was ambivalent. He accepted Christian women's charismatic speech (1 Cor. 11:5) and their leadership of house churches (Rom. 16:1, 3–5, 6, 12; Phil. 4:2) but rejected women's removing their veils in worship (1 Cor. 11:5–16). The claim that women were leaders in early Pauline house churches assumes that 1 Corinthians 14:33b–36 is an interpolation by a deutero-Pauline editor (Osiek and Balch, 117; contrast Wire, 237–69).

The preference for celibacy might have motivated some Corinthian Christians to separate from their spouses (1 Cor. 7:10–16), as among Philo's Therapeutae. In response, Paul cites the Lord's prohibition (Mark 10:2–12), interpreting this as a prohibition not of divorce but of separation. He is, however, not focused on legal rules: "but if she does separate, let her remain unmarried or else be reconciled to her husband" (1 Cor. 7:11). Although Paul repeatedly uses gender-neutral language in 1 Corinthians 7, this specific exhortation concerns a particular woman, who might have been seeking social and religious freedom. Paul reverses the usual understanding of purity and argues that her sanctity would make her spouse holy, as it has her children (7:14). But if the unbelieving spouse separates, the brother or sister is not "enslaved" (7:15).

Later in Corinthians Paul insists that the husband and wife are not to be enmeshed (1 Cor. 7:29), that the relationship is to reduce anxiety, that each is to make efforts to please the other, that marriage is for the benefit of both, and that it should not distract (*aperispastos*) from the affairs of the Lord (7:32–35; see Balch). Contemporary Stoic philosophers debated whether marriage is a "distraction." Epictetus (ca. 55–135 CE) discussed whether in a city of wise persons the Cynic might marry one like himself (3.22.63) and have children:

> But in such an order of things as the present, which is like that of a battle-field, it is a question, perhaps if the Cynic ought not to be free from distraction (*aperispaston*), wholly devoted to the service of god, . . . not tied down by the private duties of men; . . . if he observes them, he will destroy the messenger, the scout, the herald of the gods. . . . [H]e must get a kettle to heat water for the baby, for washing it in a bathtub; wood for his wife when she has a child, . . . not to speak of . . . his distraction (*perispasmon*). Where, I beseech you, is left now our king, the man who has leisure for the public interest? (3.22.69–72)

But the same value could be employed among Stoics to argue otherwise. Antipater of Tarsus (second century BCE), head of the Stoic school, reasons:

> But for a male who loves the good and wishes to lead a life of leisure devoted to reason or to political deeds or both, the matter is just the same. The more he is turned away from household management, the more he must take a wife to do the housekeeping for him and make himself free from distraction [*eauton aperispaston*] about daily necessities. (Von Arnim, vol. 3, 256 [line 33]–257 [l. 3])

According to the popular philosophical handbook by Stobaeus (ca. 400 CE), the Stoic discussion of marriage could conclude that "marriage is best," "marriage is not good," or that "the paired style of life makes marriage helpful for some but not advantageous for others" (*Anthologium*, vol. 4: 494 [line 2]; 513 [l. 2]; 524 [ll. 2–3]). Antipater, Epictetus, and Paul agree that one should be "undistracted" from one's primary duty. Antipater argues that for this marriage is best, while Epictetus and Paul argue that it is sometimes helpful, sometimes not.

Further, Paul observes that "anxiety" is negative, so he writes, "I want you to be free from anxieties" (1 Cor. 7:32):

> The unmarried man is *anxious* about the affairs of the Lord, how to please the Lord; the married man is *anxious* about the affairs of the world, how to please his wife, and his interests are divided. And the unmarried woman and the virgin are *anxious* about the affairs of the Lord, so that they may be holy in body and spirit; but the married woman is *anxious* about the affairs of the world, how to please her husband. (1 Cor. 7:32b–34, New Revised Standard Version; emphasis added)

Paul observes that celibacy makes some men and women anxious and distracted; marriage makes others anxious and distracted. Paul avoids the Stoic conclusions that marriage is best or that marriage is not good. Depending on the particular person involved, the one who marries does well, and the one who refrains from marriage does better (1 Cor. 7:38).

Paul's approach, encouraging each believer to decide whether marriage or celibacy makes him or her anxious, and to act accordingly (compare 1 Cor. 7:7b; 10:15; 11:13, 28; 2 Cor. 8:8, 10; 9:7; 13:5; Rom. 14:2–6, 10, 12, 23), contrasts with the Roman emperors' concern (beginning with Augustus [63 BCE–14 CE]) that all citizens marry and have children and with the Corinthian Christian ascetics' concern that sex is a sin (1 Cor. 7:36). For Paul there is more than one manner in which to live a sanctified life: both celibacy and married, mutually active sex are holy (7:34; 7:3–4). Paul prefers celibacy (7:7, 38) because, as he says about the impending (apocalyptic) crisis (7:26), "the time has grown short" (7:29), and because, we may surmise, Paul has this ascetic "gift" from God (7:7), which makes him less "anxious" (7:32).

Another key text for understanding Paul is Romans 1. Focusing on ways of conceiving sexual matters in Paul's Greco-Roman philosophic and literary environment, we may conclude, "in Rom. 1:24–27 Paul points to the problem of passion without introducing the modern dichotomy of homo-heterosexuality" (Fredrickson, 199). Like his contemporaries, Paul writes about the "natural use" (*physiken chresin*) and "unnatural use" (*chresin . . . ten para physin*) of **sexual desire** (Rom. 1:26, 27), which was thought analogous to the "natural use" of hunger. Plutarch, in *Eating of Flesh*, argues much as Paul does in Romans, but in relation to compulsive eating of food. He asks what passion (*pathos*) the first man had who ate animal meat (993AB), the question Paul asks in relation to sex (see Fredrickson, 204–15). The first humans "made use of" (*chraomai*) animal flesh, contrary to nature, because their hunger gave them no respite (993E, 996F). Humans act impiously (*asebeite*; Rom. 1:18) against Demeter and bring shame (*aischunete*; Rom. 1:26, 27) on Dionysus, as if humans did not receive enough from them (994A, 996F). Nature (*physis*) produced tame creatures for **beauty** and grace, not for food (994B). Humans are not naturally carnivorous; they have no hooked beaks, sharp nails, or jagged teeth (994F). When the body is burdened with improper food, the soul errs (*planasthai*; 995F, 997B; compare Rom. 1:27). Human souls are imprisoned in mortal bodies as punishment (*dike*) for eating animal flesh (996B; compare Rom. 1:21–28). Plutarch writes (*Eating*, 997B):

> Then, just as with women [cf. Rom. 1:26] who are insatiable in seeking pleasure, their lust tries everything, goes astray [*planomenos*; errs] and explores the gamut of profligacy until at last it ends in unspeakable practices, so intemperance in eating passes beyond the necessary ends of nature [*to physikon*] and resorts to cruelty and lawlessness [*paranomia*] to give variety to appetite [*orexin*; cf. Rom. 1:27]. . . . [O]rgans of sense are infected and won over and become licentious when they do not keep to natural standards.

The pleasure of sex should be limited by satisfaction, just as a wise person with a full stomach stops eating.

This use of "natural" does not raise the question of the gender of the subject or object of sexual desire. Plutarch (*Advice to Bride and Groom*, 144B) also refers to the wife's "use" of the husband in heterosexual marriage, to which Paul probably refers in Romans 1:26 ("Their females exchanged natural use for that which is against nature"), which was not then a reference to lesbian sexuality (Fredrickson, 201). Greco-Roman discussions of household management are one source of this terminology, which advised the householder about the "use" of possessions, including the "use" of a wife (not a modern value). "Use" focuses on "the psychological significance of the act for the subject," not the object, "of sexual desire" (Fredrickson, 205). By "against nature" (*para physin*), Paul means not "disoriented desire" but "inordinate desire" (Martin, *Corinthian Body*, 6–37, 198–228; "Heterosexism," 342). When desire is insatiable, addictive, it is "against nature." Paul uses a string of terms that point toward the problem of *eros*: "desire" (*epithumia*, Rom. 1:24), "passion" (*pathos*; 1:26), "inflame," "appetite," and "error" (*ekkaio, orexis, plane*; 1:27). Each terms plays a role in the contemporary discussion of erotic love (Fredrickson, 208–15). The Greek emphasis on the insatiability of passion gives the word a qualitatively different nuance than the modern English word, which does not denote disease. When humans refuse to give God glory and gratitude, God is wronged and dishonored, which provokes God's anger, according to Paul. God delivers into dishonor those who dishonor the creator. Insatiable (therefore diseased) passion brings lovers into dishonor, which itself is punishment (1:27; Fredrickson 216). **Saint Augustine** (354–430) eventually elaborated this theme significantly (14.15).

See also Abstinence; Bible, Sex and the; Boswell, John; Catholicism, History of; Friendship; Greek Sexuality and Philosophy, Ancient; Judaism, History of; Kierkegaard, Søren; Marriage; Roman Sexuality and Philosophy, Ancient; Thomas Aquinas (Saint)

REFERENCES

Aristotle. (ca. 345–342 BCE) *Aristotle*, vol. 11: *History of Animals: Books VII–X*. Trans. David M. Balme. Loeb Classical Library. Cambridge, Mass.: Harvard University Press, 1991; Augustine. (413–427) *The City of God*. Trans. Marcus Dods. New York: Modern Library, 1950; Balch, David L. "1 Cor. 7:32–35 and Stoic Debates about Marriage, Anxiety, and Distraction." *Journal of Biblical Literature* 102:3 (1983), 429–39; Barré, Michael L. "To Marry or to Burn: *Purousthai* in 1 Cor. 7:9." *Catholic Biblical Quarterly* 36:2 (1974), 193–202; Celsus. (14–37 CE) *De medicina*, 3 vols. Trans. Walter G. Spencer. Loeb Classical Library. Cambridge, Mass.: Harvard University Press, 1935–1938, 1960–1963; Clarke, John R. *Looking at Lovemaking: Constructions of Sexuality in Roman Art 100 B.C.–A.D. 250*. Berkeley: University of California Press, 1998; Collins, Adela Y. "The Function of 'Excommunication' in Paul." *Harvard Theological Review* 73:1–2 (1980), 251–63; Deming, Will. (1995) *Paul on Marriage and Celibacy: The Hellenistic Background of 1 Corinthians 7*, 2nd ed. Grand Rapids, Mich.: Eerdmans, 2004; Diogenes Laertius. *Lives of Eminent Philosophers*, 2 vols. Trans. Robert D. Hicks. Loeb Classical Library. Cambridge, Mass.: Harvard University Press, 1966, 1970; Epictetus. *Epictetus*, vol. 2: *Discourses: Books 3–4*. Trans. William A. Oldfather. Loeb Classical Library. Cambridge, Mass.: Harvard University Press, 1969; Fredrickson, David E. "Natural and Unnatural Use in Romans 1:24–27." In David L. Balch, ed., *Homosexuality, Science, and the "Plain Sense" of Scripture*. Grand Rapids, Mich.: Eerdmans, 2000, 197–222; Martin, Dale. *The Corinthian Body*. New Haven, Conn.: Yale University Press, 1995; Martin, Dale. "Heterosexism and the Interpretation of Romans 1:18–32." *Biblical Interpretation* 3:3 (1995), 332–55; Musonius Rufus. "The Roman Socrates." Ed. and trans. Cora E. Lutz. *Yale Classical Studies* 10. New Haven, Conn.: Yale University Press, 1947, 3–147; Osiek, Carolyn, and David L. Balch. *Families in the New Testament World: Households and House Churches*. Louisville, Ky.: Westminster/John Knox, 1997; Philo. *Philo*, vol. 9: *The Contemplative Life*. Trans. Francis H. Colson. Loeb Classical Library. Cambridge, Mass.: Harvard University Press, 1969; Plato. (ca. 380 BCE) *The Symposium*. Trans. Christopher Gill. London: Penguin, 1999; Plutarch. *Plutarch Moralia*, vol. 2: *Advice to Bride and Groom* (*Moralia* 138B–146A). Trans. Frank C. Babbitt. Loeb Classical Library. Cambridge, Mass.: Harvard University Press, 1928, 1969; Plutarch. *Plutarch Moralia*, vol. 9: *Dialogue on Love* [*Amatorius*] (*Moralia* 748E–771E). Trans. P. A. Clement and H. B. Hoffleit. Loeb Classical Library. Cambridge, Mass.: Harvard University Press, 1969; Plutarch. *Plutarch Moralia*, vol. 12: *The Eating of Flesh* (*Moralia* 993A–999B). Trans. Harold Cherniss and William C. Helmbold. Loeb Classical Library. Cambridge, Mass.: Harvard University Press, 1969; Rouselle, Aline. *Porneia: On Desire and the Body in Antiquity*. Oxford, U.K.: Blackwell, 1988; Soranus. *Soranus' Gynecology*. Trans. Owsei Tempkin. Baltimore, Md.: Johns Hopkins University Press, 1956; Stobaeus. *Anthologium*, 5 vols. Ed. Curtis Wachsmuth and Otto Hense. Berlin, Ger.: Weidmann, 1958 [translation by DLB]; Van der Horst, Pieter W. *Chaeremon: Egyptian Priest and Stoic Philosopher. The Fragments Collected and Translated with Explanatory Notes*. Leiden, Holland: Brill, 1984; Ward, Roy Bowen. "Women in Roman Baths." *Harvard Theological Review* 85:2 (1992), 125–47; Wire, Antoinette Clark. *The Corinthian Women Prophets: A Reconstruction through Paul's Rhetoric*. Minneapolis, Minn.: Fortress, 1990; Von Arnim, Hans, ed. *Stoicorum Veterum Fragmenta*, 3 vols. Leipzig, Ger.: Teubner, 1903 [translation by DLB].

David L. Balch

ADDITIONAL READING

Ariès, Philippe. "St. Paul and the Flesh." In Philippe Ariès and André Béjin, eds., *Western Sexuality: Practice and Precept in Past and Present Times*. Trans. Anthony Forster. New York: Blackwell, 1985, 36–39; Babcock, William S. "Augustine's Interpretation of Romans (A.D. 394–396)." *Augustinian Studies* 10 (1979), 55–74; Balch, David L. "Romans 1:24–27, Science, and Homosexuality." *Currents in Theology and Mission* 25:6 (1998), 433–40; Balch, David L., ed. *Homosexuality, Science, and the "Plain Sense" of Scripture*. Grand Rapids, Mich.: Eerdmans, 2000; Baldwin, John W. "Consent and the Marital Debt: Five Discourses in Northern France around 1200." In Angeliki E. Laiou, ed., *Consent and Coercion to Sex and Marriage in Ancient and Medieval Societies*. Washington, D.C.: Dumbarton Oaks, 1993, 257–70; Barrett, C. K. *A Commentary on the First Epistle to the Corinthians*. London: Black, 1968; Boswell, John. "The Scriptures." In *Christianity, Social Tolerance, and Homosexuality: Gay People in Western Europe from the Beginning of the Christian Era to the Fourteenth Century*. Chicago, Ill.: University of Chicago Press, 1980, 91–117; Clarke, John R. *Roman Sex: 100 B.C.–A.D. 250*. New York: Harry N. Abrams, 2003; Fredriksen, Paula. "Paul and Augustine: Conversion Narratives, Orthodox Traditions, and the Retrospective Self." *Journal of Theological Studies* [n.s.] 37 (1986), 3–34; Gravrock, Mark. "Why Won't Paul Just Say No? Purity and Sex in 1 Corinthians 6." *Word and World* 14:4 (1996), 444–55; Gudorf, Christine E. "The Erosion of Sexual Dimorphism: Challenges to Religion and Religious Ethics." *Journal of the American Academy of Religion* 69:4 (2001), 863–91; Hallett, Judith P., and Marilyn B. Skinner, eds. *Roman Sexualities*. Princeton, N.J.: Princeton University Press, 1999; Hubbard, Thomas K. *Homosexuality in Greece and Rome: A Sourcebook of Basic Documents*. Berkeley: University of California Press, 2003; Jewett, Robert. *Paul's Anthropological Terms*. Leiden, Holland: Brill, 1971; Jordan, Mark D. *The Invention of Sodomy in Christian Theology*. Chicago, Ill.: University of Chicago Press, 1997; Jung, Patricia Beattie, and Ralph F. Smith. "The Bible and Heterosexism." In *Heterosexism: An Ethical Challenge*. Albany: State University of New York Press, 1993, 61–88; Kampen, Natalie B., ed. *Sexuality in Ancient Art*. New York: Cambridge University Press, 1996; Kierkegaard, Søren. (1844) *The Concept of Anxiety*. Trans. Howard V. Hong and Edna H. Hong. Princeton, N.J.: Princeton University Press, 1980; Koloski-Ostrow, Ann Olga, and Claire L. Lyons, eds. *Naked Truths: Women, Sexuality, and Gender in Classical Art and Archaeology*. London: Routledge, 1997; Miller, James. "The Practice of Romans 1:26: Homosexual or Heterosexual?" *Novum Testamentum* 37:1 (1995), 1–11; Murphy-O'Connor, Jerome. *1 Corinthians*. Wilmington, Del.: Michael Glazier, 1979; Richlin, Amy. *The Garden of Priapus: Sexuality and Aggression in Roman Humor*. New Haven, Conn.: Yale University Press, 1983. Rev. ed., New York: Oxford University Press, 1992; Robinson, J.A.T. *The Body: A Study in Pauline Theology*. London: SCM Press, 1952; Rudy, Kathy. *Sex and the Church: Gender, Homosexuality, and the Transformation of Christian Ethics*. Boston, Mass.: Beacon Press, 1997; Russell, Bertrand. "Christian Ethics." In *Marriage and Morals*. London: Allen and Unwin, 1929, 40–53; Sandmel, Samuel. *The Genius of Paul*. New York: Farrar, Straus, and Cuhady, 1958; Schmidt, Thomas E. "Romans 1:26–27 and Biblical Sexuality." In John Corvino, ed., *Same Sex: Debating the Ethics, Science, and Culture of Homosexuality*. Lanham, Md.: Rowman and Littlefield, 1997, 93–104; Smedes, Lewis B. *Love within Limits: A Realist's View of 1 Corinthians 13*. Grand Rapids, Mich.: Eerdmans, 1978; Smith, Mark. "Ancient Bisexuality and the Interpretation of Romans 1:26–27." *Journal of the American Academy of Religion* 64:2 (1996), 223–56; Spong, John Shelby. "The Man from Tarsus." In *Rescuing the Bible from Fundamentalism: A Bishop Rethinks the Meaning of Scripture*. San Francisco, Calif.: Harper, 1991, 91–106; Stewart, Andrew F. *Art, Desire, and the Body in Ancient Greece*. Cambridge: Cambridge University Press, 1997; Tang, Isabel. *Pornography: The Secret History of Civilization*. London: Macmillan, 1999; Watson, Francis. *Agape, Eros, Gender: Towards a Pauline Sexual Ethic*. Cambridge: Cambridge University Press, 2000; Westermarck, Edward. "The Ethics of Paul." In *Christianity and Morals*. New York: Macmillan, 1939, 102–29.

PEDOPHILIA. Pedophilia is sexual attraction some adults feel toward children that may lead to adult-child sex. The word is also used to refer to the practice of adult-child sex. In contemporary Western societies, the subject is highly contentious and fraught with strong feelings. The strength of the feelings is readily explained by concern for the welfare of children and for their healthy, unimpeded development. But it also reflects a set of stereotypes of pedophiles that for the most part are not borne out by the facts. These feelings are compounded by the distaste for and moral censure of **sexual perversion**. In contemporary Western societies, adult-child sex is both generally morally condemned and prohibited by **law**.

While there is considerable psychological and sociological literature about pedophilia, philosophers working in the philosophy of sex have given relatively little attention to the subject. As pedophilia is seen as a paradigmatic case of sexual perversion and is generally viewed with strong moral revulsion, it might have been expected to generate more philosophical interest. Yet only a handful of philosophers have discussed it in some detail (Ehman; Frye; Kershnar; Primoratz; Spiecker and Steutel). The subject has received extensive coverage in the media since the 1980s. But most publicized instances of pedophilia have been cases of (alleged) sexual interactions between adults and children within families or in educational or child-care institutions. These cases of pedophilia are compounded by **incest** or by violation of a relationship of care, trust, or authority. Here we are concerned only with pedophilia as such.

The contentious nature of the subject is reflected in the loaded terminology employed both by advocates of pedophilia and by its opponents. Its advocates tend to refer to pedophilia with the terms "cross-generational sex" or "intergenerational sex," which erase the distinction between sex involving adults belonging to different generations and sex involving an adult and a child. This terminology is misleading, because the former need not raise any moral worries, while the latter is generally considered gravely morally wrong. On the other hand, those who think that pedophilia is morally unacceptable tend to use terms such as "child molestation" or "child sexual abuse." This usage does not facilitate, but rather forecloses, rational discussion about the nature and moral and legal status of pedophilia, since it assumes that all sex between an adult and a child is necessarily molestation and abuse, that is, morally wrong and harmful to the child. Both types of terminology are best avoided. If the issue is not to be prejudged, it needs to be couched in neutral language, such as "adult-child sex" or simply "pedophilia."

"Pedophilia" has a narrow and a wide sense. In its wide sense it means sex between an adult and a minor and accordingly includes pederasty and ephebophilia. These are varieties of male **homosexuality** but differ from the type dominant in modern Western societies, in which both parties are adults. Pederasty is sexual attraction of adult males to boys in their mid-teens and sex with them. A pederast is attracted to the transient, androgynous quality that boys display in their mid-teens and lose by the end of puberty, when (in biological, although not in psychological and social terms) they reach manhood. An ephebophile, in contrast, is attracted to, and has sex with, postpubertal, sexually mature, highly virile youths.

In its narrow sense, "pedophilia" refers to sexual attraction of adults to prepubescent and pubescent children and sexual contact with them. Thus it includes pederasty but not ephebophilia; the end of puberty is the demarcation line. Obviously, given the differences in biological, psychological, and social development of prepubescent and pubescent children, on the one hand, and adolescents, on the other, even if ephebophilia gives rise to moral misgivings, they are not as strongly felt nor as widespread as those generated by pedophilia, narrowly understood. Our concern here is only with the latter.

In addition to terminological problems, discussions of pedophilia are often plagued by an array of factually inaccurate but widely accepted beliefs. (On these stereotypes of pedophilia, see Plummer, "Pedophilia"; Righton.) The pedophile is portrayed by the media and is imagined by the public to be a "dirty old man." He is envisaged as a stranger to the child who intrudes sexually on the child by means of force or deceit, the intrusion culminating in coitus. The experience the pedophile imposes on the child is assumed to be painful, frightening, and traumatic and to inflict serious and long-term psychological damage on the child. These stereotypes explain why pedophilia is "the most hated of all sexual variations" (Plummer, "Progress," 130). Yet, for the most part, they are not empirically confirmed. Most known pedophiles are indeed men. They are not, however, always old men but are spread over the entire age range. Typically, they are not strangers to the children involved. They are more likely to be family members or other adults from the immediate social surroundings of the children. The sex act is rarely forced on the child. The act committed is rarely sexual intercourse; the most characteristic activities are kissing, touching, and fondling. As for the overall character of the experience for the child and its long-term effects, these are highly contested by researchers and professionals as well as by advocates of pedophilia and those who seek to provide a rationale for its moral condemnation and legal prohibition.

According to the popular view of pedophilia, it is an unnatural or perverted sexual inclination and behavior. Nevertheless, in discussing its moral and legal standing, the topic of sexual perversion may be put aside. On some conceptions of sexual perversion, perverted acts are immoral, while other conceptions strip the term of its moral connotations. In the context of the traditional Judeo-Christian understanding of sex as geared to procreation, adult-child sex appears unnatural and perverted, and therefore also wrong, because it is not of the sort of sexuality that, under normal circumstances, can be procreative. But this understanding of sexual perversion is plagued by the oft-canvassed difficulties of ascribing a natural purpose or function to sex (Priest, 363–67). Moreover, most of those who hold pedophilia morally unacceptable do so for reasons that have nothing to do with its being nonprocreative.

For example, for **Roger Scruton** sexual perversion is any deviation from **sexual desire** that is directed at another human being as the embodied person he or she is. Because it fails to relate to the full personality of the other, perverted sexuality is "morally contaminated." This applies to the pedophile, whose sexual interest does not focus on the body of a mature person but rather on the body of "the prelude to the person" (Scruton, 295–98). However, as Scruton's critics have argued, his account of human sexuality is best presented as an ideal rather than a sexual norm. As a result, sexual inclination and behavior that falls short of this (or any other) ideal is not plausibly depicted as perverted nor fairly judged with the severity a moral conception of perversion calls for (Primoratz, 30–31, 54–55).

On the other hand, if sexual perversion is understood in nonmoral terms—as only a statistically abnormal sexual preference (Goldman, 284–87) or as deviation from prevailing sexual tastes (Margolis, "Perversion"; "Question," 297–300)—then the classification of pedophilia as a perversion is irrelevant to the question of its moral and legal standing. The same is true of the classification of pedophilia as a **paraphilia**, the concept that has replaced "sexual perversion" in contemporary psychiatry, precisely because it is free of the moral connotations usually associated with the latter. (On pedophilia as a "paraphilia," see the *Diagnostic and Statistical Manual* of the American Psychiatric Association, 527–28.)

There are several arguments advanced by advocates of pedophilia and meant to repeal or significantly circumscribe its moral condemnation and legal prohibition. One argument harks back to the "Greek love" of boys and similar phenomena in other cultures (see Eglinton). The argument ascribes great educational value to the relationship between an adult male and the boy he takes under his wing and steers from childhood immaturity and dependence to maturity and adult responsibilities. Because this relationship is deeply personal and is meant to initiate the boy into a range of adult practices, including adult sexuality, it also involves a sexual component. But the educational value of such a relationship may be doubted, in particular in contemporary Western societies. Whereas the educator's involvement with a young person is other-regarding, for the sake of the good of the young person, the involvement of the pederast is self-regarding, for he seeks to satisfy his own sexual desire (Spiecker and Steutel, 335). Be that as it may, this line of argument relates only to pederasty and is therefore of less interest than those arguments that apply to pedophilia in general.

Another line of argument focuses on child sexuality. Contemporary opposition to pedophilia is said to be based on the view of prepubescent children as asexual. This view, which leads to denying children any sexual experience and excluding them from all discourse about sex, is not mandated by the intrinsic nature of childhood, nor is it valid universally, for all societies and all historical periods. This view of childhood sexuality is, instead, a relatively recent development in Western society. Defenders of pedophilia draw on the work of Philippe Ariès on the history of childhood. Ariès claims that medieval and early modern Western societies had no "idea of childhood," that is, no conception of childhood as marked by a group of characteristics that set children apart from adults and enjoined their social segregation. On the contrary, children mingled freely with adults and took part in most areas of adult life. Nor were children sheltered from adult sexuality or denied sexual interests and activities of their own. It was only in the seventeenth and eighteenth centuries that the West "discovered" childhood as something different from adulthood, meaning that children were in need of separation from the social world of adults and of protection from many types of adult experience. In particular, children came to be seen as sexually innocent—lacking knowledge of and interest in sex—and in need of protection from exposure to adult sexuality (see Ariès, pt. I, chap. v).

Defenders of pedophilia point out that this view of childhood as different from adulthood in many important respects, and in particular as characterized by sexual "innocence," is at odds with what we have learned from **Sigmund Freud** (1856–1939) and his followers and from numerous empirical studies of human sexuality, including those conducted by Alfred Kinsey ([1894–1956]; see Ehman, "Adult-Child Sex"; O'Carroll). Those who oppose pedophilia may be captured by this dated notion of childhood innocence as well as by traditional morally derogatory approaches to sex: "[T]he [negative] attitude toward adult-child sex is the last unquestioned bastion of sexual puritanism" (Ehman, "Adult-Child Sex," 433). The dated notion of childhood as an asexual stage denies children experiences they seek and enjoy and choices they should have a right to make; it can be seen as another aspect of the oppression of children in our society. The view also hampers the normal sexual development of children: "Far from needing to be mature before having a sex life, an unthwarted sexual development helps lead to full sexual maturity" (O'Carroll, 154).

Perhaps some still adhere to the pre-Freudian notion of childhood as a sexually innocent stage in life and therefore think of pedophilia as deeply wrong because it prematurely initiates a child into sex, thus spoiling its natural, wholesome innocence. A variation of this view has been endorsed by Scruton. He does not claim that children *are* innocent, or at least not that they are entirely so. But he ascribes to adults a desire that children be innocent, which makes adults think of children as if they were innocent. Adults do not want children to be introduced into the world of sex before the "age of innocence" has expired and accordingly lay down a strict prohibition of adult-child sex (296–97). However, one need not subscribe to the view of children as asexual or, in Scruton's terms, as incapable of sexual desire, to reject pedophilia. Rejecting pedophilia is compatible with acknowledging childhood sexuality, the benefits of starting **sex education** early, and adopting a fairly permissive stand on the sexual play, exploration, and pleasure of children. There is an important distinction (which is obfuscated when "pedophilia" is replaced by terms such as "cross-generational" or "intergenerational sex") between sexual play and exploration among children and sexual interaction between children and adults. Opposition to the latter does not entail opposition to the former.

Advocates of pedophilia claim that, rather than being harmful to children, pedophilia is beneficial to them, or could be but for the unreasonably negative stance of parents and society. The widespread belief that pedophilia is harmful, and seriously so, to a child's psychological well-being and development is ascribed to stereotypes and flawed studies. Research on pedophilia tends to be based on clinical and legal data. But cases of adult-child sex in which the child needs medical attention and those that reach the courts are cases in which the child is likely to have been harmed. It is not surprising that research drawing on such cases confirms the view of pedophilia as harmful to children. The results of such research cannot be accepted as valid for the entire population of children who have been sexually involved with adults. This problem is compounded by the failure of pedophilia research to differentiate clearly, if at all, between cases in which the adult used force or put pressure on the child and cases in which no force or pressure was exerted. Yet it is likely that whatever harm is caused by adult-child sex is going to be caused in cases of the former type, while cases of the latter type may be harmless. Finally, research does not distinguish clearly, or at all, between the direct harm of pedophilia, that caused by the sexual encounter or relationship itself, and the indirect harm brought about by the harsh condemnation of pedophilia by society's morality and its laws and the drastic reaction of parents and others to the child's sexual involvement with an adult. If pedophilia is to be morally condemned and legally prohibited because it harms children, the argument should be based solely on direct harms. To prop up the argument against pedophilia by invoking indirect harms is to make it circular. For these reasons, defenders of pedophilia fault the vast majority of existing adult-child sex research. They also cite studies that lead to a different conclusion, that in cases of adult-child sexual involvement in which (1) the child had no negative feelings toward the adult to start with, (2) the adult did not use force or coercion, and (3) there was no trauma of discovery or a shocked response by parents or society, the relationship was evaluated as positive by the child and did not seem to have caused significant, long-term harm (see Burton; Tsai et al.).

Critics reply that many studies that defenders of pedophilia appeal to are also flawed. Since they are based solely on cases of ongoing adult-child relationships (see Sandfort), the results of these studies are not representative of the relevant child population. In an ongoing relationship that is not maintained by force or coercion, it is not surprising that the child should describe the relationship in favorable terms and should not show signs of being harmed by it. However, not all research that fails to support the claim that pedophilia is harmful to children is limited this way. A critical review of over forty studies of the effects of adult-child sexual encounters on children points out the methodological limitations of those studies and reaches the "somewhat muted" conclusion that the widespread belief that adult-child sex has long-term harmful consequences for the child is not borne out by evidence (Powell and Chalkley). The issue of harm can apparently not be settled either way at this stage and must await further empirical research.

Yet another line of argument in defense of pedophilia focuses on the force or coercion purportedly employed by pedophiles and the corresponding lack of **consent** or willingness on the part of the children. Advocates of pedophilia argue that force or coercion is not typically used by pedophiles and that the child often willingly participates in the relationship. Children are not incapable of making choices about sex, of consenting or expressing willingness or unwillingness to participate in sex acts with adults (Califia, 20). To be sure, the consent or willingness children express may fall short of the "informed consent" standard (commonly employed in medical contexts). But that standard is unrealistically high: Sexual choices and acts of many adults, too, do not measure up to it. How many adults actually know all they should know about the biological, psychological, and social aspects of sex and have a deep understanding of the nature and the entire range of consequences of their own sexual choices and acts? (See O'Carroll, 153.) Since nobody proposes to condemn all cases of sex between adults that do not satisfy the informed consent standard, and since the vast majority of sexual acts between adults and children are not imposed by force or coercion, but engaged in willingly by both parties, defenders of pedophilia argue that such acts should not be deemed wrong. The laws relating to pedophilia should be overhauled, too: Age-of-consent laws should be abolished, and problems arising in adult-child sex should be regulated mostly by civil, not criminal, law. (For a detailed proposal of law reform along these lines, see O'Carroll, chap. 6.)

In response, it has been argued by opponents of pedophilia that a child's willingness to engage in sexual acts with adults—which defenders of pedophilia propose as an alternative to consent—is, for several reasons, suspect. The fact that not all adults live up to the criterion of informed consent is not reason enough to conclude that it does not matter that children also fail to live up to it. Severely mentally challenged and psychotic adults aside, the sexual choices and acts of adults that are flawed according to a standard of informed consent are flawed contingently: An adult could have attained an appropriate level of knowledge of sex and a better understanding of his or her sexual options but has neglected to do so. But a child's position is different. Because of a child's limited experience and limited cognitive and emotional resources, a child's knowledge and understanding of sex are inevitably very limited. Unlike a negligent adult, a child does not happen to have, but is bound to have, little knowledge and a poor understanding of the physical, psychological, and social aspects of sex. While only some adults are at a disadvantage in this respect, all children are. Hence the willingness of a child to engage in sex with an adult cannot be enough for such sex to be considered morally acceptable.

There are further reasons for treating a child's willingness with caution. Advocates of pedophilia argue that the adult and the child can, and in many cases do, have a meaningful sexual relationship. They also claim that the relationship is often initiated by the child, not the adult, and that children act in seductive ways toward adults. But reports about such cases may indicate considerable misunderstanding brought about by a significant difference in the way the adult and the child understand the same interaction. Research on children who willingly participate in sexual contacts with adults suggests motivation for an interaction different from that of the adults. The child seeks sympathy, affection, and **love**, while the adult is seeking sex. The acts of the child are mere horseplay, or expressions of curiosity, but the adult construes them as (provocatively) sexual. In a study of boys participating in pedophile relationships with men, Michael Ingram concludes that "though there may well be a meaningful relationship between a loving man and an unhappy child, and . . . a sexual act takes place within the context of this relationship, nevertheless, the act is sexually meaningful only for the adult, not for the child" (184–85).

Further, a child's willingness to participate in a sexual interaction with an adult is not sufficiently voluntary, since it is not sufficiently free. The willingness is solicited and then granted against a background of radical inequality of physical, psychological, and social resourcefulness and power. This inequality is acknowledged and reinforced throughout the process of a child's upbringing. As a result, children tend to defer to adults and find it difficult to assert themselves against adults and to rebuff their advances. It might be objected that there is much inequality of power between adults, too, yet we do not take that as making their **sexual activity** insufficiently voluntary. But again, while only some adults have to manage their sexual lives in a position of gross inequality in relation to other adults, all children are in a position of greatly unequal power in relation to virtually all adults. Any willingness to participate in sex acts with adults expressed under these circumstances is seriously compromised.

While both philosophers (e.g., Primoratz) and psychologists (e.g., Finkelhor) have argued in favor of moral and legal prohibition of pedophilia along the lines sketched above, others have advanced alternative arguments. Robert Ehman, who once defended pedophilia (1984), no longer does so (2000). He still rejects the view that adult-child sex is illegitimate because a child cannot consent to it and the child's willingness to participate is seriously flawed. He agrees that the problem with pedophilia is that it is nonconsensual. But what matters, for Ehman, is not the actual consent of the child but the retrospective consent of the adult the child will become to the sexual interactions in which he or she is involved as a child. Adult-child sex is justified if the adult involved in the interaction has good reason to believe that when the child involved in it becomes an adult, he or she will retrospectively consent to that sexual encounter or relationship and will be justified in doing so because that consent will reflect his or her reasonable goals and values. If, when exercising mature judgment, the adult the child became finds the act or relationship unacceptable, that means he or she had been taken advantage of. Ehman's conclusion is that for the most part adults cannot make the case that children will give justified retrospective consent to adult-child sex when they come to consider it as mature persons. Therefore pedophilia is for the most part morally unacceptable ("What Really Is Wrong with Pedophilia?" 139).

Ehman, however, does not explain why for the most part adults cannot make the case that children will give justified retrospective consent. Indeed, it is not clear how such an argument is to be made. If the goals and values of the future mature person are sufficiently close to those of the present child, Ehman's proposed test of retrospective consent of the future mature person is in danger of collapsing into the test of consent of the actual immature person (a criterion that Ehman rejects). On the other hand, if the goals and values of the future adult are not of a piece with those of the child, but rather discontinuous with them, how can one predict what they are going to be?

A different argument in support of moral condemnation and legal prohibition of adult-child sex portrays it as exploitative. (On exploitation see Mappes; Wertheimer, *Exploitation*.) For Spiecker and Steutel, in sexual exploitation one party uses another in such a way that the sexual interaction is profitable for one but at the expense of the second, or the benefit for the second is disproportionately small. This outcome is made possible by the conditions in which the parties agree to the interaction: One takes advantage of the destitute circumstances or vulnerabilities of the other. Spiecker and Steutel argue that adult-child sex is always exploitative. The child either reaps no benefit or the benefit the child gets is disproportionately small relative to that acquired by the adult. This occurs because the adult takes advantage either of the child's psychological vulnerabilities or the child's wretched situation, as happens in sex tourism to Third World countries (336–38). There are two difficulties with this position. One might not agree that all interactions in which one party gains much more than the other should be categorized and morally condemned as exploitation (Wertheimer, *Consent*, 190–91, 219–20). And even if the adult in most cases gains much more from the sexual act or relationship than the child, should we grant that adult-child sex is morally legitimate in the atypical cases in which there is no disproportion in benefits gained?

In another contribution to the philosophical literature on the subject, Stephen Kershnar rejects all the main nonconsequentialist objections to adult-child sex: the argument that this sex is invariably exploitative, the argument that children cannot consent and that their willingness is deeply suspect, and the retrospective consent argument. Kershnar sees sex as on a par with activities such as gymnastics and sports. If adults may legitimately participate with children in these activities, provided the children are not harmed, even though children cannot give valid consent to these activities and their willingness is expressed under the same constraints as their willingness to have sex with adults, why should sex be any different? If sexual activity cannot be shown to be different, then the moral and legal standing of pedophilia depends solely on whether it is harmful to the children. On this question the jury is still out. Yet even those who accept this view may want to adopt a presumption against adult-child sex as the best or safest policy. We do not know at present that adult-child sex as a rule inflicts serious harm on children. But neither do we know that it does not. We need to take into account that the psychological vulnerability of children is bound to enhance greatly any serious harm that *might* be inflicted on them. Therefore the most prudent and morally appropriate choice would seem to be to maintain our society's moral rejection and legal prohibition of sexual involvement of adults with children.

In spite of its theoretical and practical importance, pedophilia has not received as much attention from philosophers as it deserves. The issues of its moral and legal standing are far from settled and await further philosophical and empirical investigation. In particular, the question of harm requires more, and more methodologically sophisticated, research.

See also Bestiality; Bisexuality; Consent; Greek Sexuality and Philosophy, Ancient; Herdt, Gilbert; Incest; Paraphilia; Perversion, Sexual; Rape; Scruton, Roger; Sexology

REFERENCES

American Psychiatric Association. *Diagnostic and Statistical Manual of Mental Disorders*, 4th ed. [DSM-IV] Washington, D.C.: Author, 1994; Ariès, Philippe. *Centuries of Childhood: A Social History of Family Life*. Trans. Robert Baldick. New York: Knopf, 1962; Burton, Lindy. *Vulnerable Children: Three Studies of Children in Conflict*. London: Routledge and Kegan Paul, 1968; Califia, Pat. "A Thorny Issue Splits a Movement." *Advocate* (30 October 1980), 17–24, 45; Eglinton, J. Z. [W. H. Breen] *Greek Love*. London: Neville Spearman, 1971; Ehman, Robert. "Adult-Child Sex." In Robert B. Baker and Frederick A. Elliston, eds., *Philosophy and Sex*, 2nd ed. Buffalo, N.Y.: Prometheus, 1984, 431–46; Ehman, Robert. "What Really Is Wrong with Pedophilia?" *Public Affairs Quarterly* 14:2 (2000), 129–41; Finkelhor, David. "What's Wrong with Sex between Adults and Children?" *American Journal of Orthopsychiatry* 49:4 (1979), 692–97; Frye, Marilyn. "Critique" [of Robert Ehman, "Adult-Child Sex"]. In Robert B. Baker and Frederick A. Elliston, eds., *Philosophy and Sex*, 2nd ed. Buffalo, N.Y.: Prometheus, 1984, 447–55; Goldman, Alan. "Plain Sex." *Philosophy and Public Affairs* 6:3 (1977), 267–87; Ingram, Michael. "Participating Victims: A Study of Sexual Offenses with Boys." In Larry L. Constantine and Floyd M. Martinson, eds., *Children and Sex: New Findings, New Perspectives*. Boston, Mass.: Little, Brown, 1981, 177–87; Kershnar, Stephen. "The Moral

Status of Harmless Adult-Child Sex." *Public Affairs Quarterly* 15:2 (2001), 111–32; Mappes, Thomas A. "Sexual Morality and the Concept of Using Another Person." In Thomas Mappes and Jane Zembaty, eds., *Social Ethics*, 4th ed. New York: McGraw-Hill, 1992, 203–16; Margolis, Joseph. "Perversion." In *Negativities: The Limits of Life*. Columbus, Ohio: Merrill, 1975, 119–30; Margolis, Joseph. "The Question of Homosexuality." In Robert B. Baker and Frederick A. Elliston, eds., *Philosophy and Sex*, 1st ed. Buffalo, N.Y.: Prometheus, 1975, 288–302; O'Carroll, Tom. *Paedophilia: The Radical Case*. London: Peter Owen, 1980; Plummer, Kenneth. " 'The Paedophile's' Progress: A View from Below." In Brian Taylor, ed., *Perspectives on Paedophilia*. London: Batsford, 1981, 113–32; Plummer, Kenneth. "Pedophilia: Constructing a Sociological Baseline." In Mark Cook and Kevin Howells, eds., *Adult Sexual Interest in Children*. London: Academic Press, 1981, 221–50; Powell, Graham E., and A. J. Chalkley. "The Effects of Paedophile Attention on the Child." In Brian Taylor, ed., *Perspectives on Paedophilia*. London: Batsford, 1981, 113–32; Priest, Graham. "Sexual Perversion." *Australasian Journal of Philosophy* 75:3 (1997), 360–71; Primoratz, Igor. *Ethics and Sex*. London: Routledge, 1999; Righton, Peter. "The Adult." In Brian Taylor, ed., *Perspectives on Paedophilia*. London: Batsford, 1981, 24–40; Sandfort, Theo. *The Sexual Aspect of Pedophile Relations*. Amsterdam, Holland: Pan/Spartacus, 1982; Scruton, Roger. *Sexual Desire: A Moral Philosophy of the Erotic*. New York: Free Press, 1986; Spiecker, Ben, and Steutel, Jan. "Paedophilia, Sexual Desire, and Perversity." *Journal of Moral Education* 26:3 (1997), 331–42; Tsai, Mavis, Shirley Feldman-Summers, and Margaret Edgar. "Childhood Molestation: Differential Impacts on Psychosexual Functioning." In Larry L. Constantine and Floyd M. Martinson, eds., *Children and Sex: New Findings, New Perspectives*. Boston, Mass.: Little, Brown, 1981, 201–16; Wertheimer, Alan. *Consent to Sexual Relations*. Cambridge: Cambridge University Press, 2003; Wertheimer, Alan. *Exploitation*. Princeton, N.J.: Princeton University Press, 1996.

Igor Primoratz

ADDITIONAL READING

Abel, Gene G., Suzann S. Lawry, Elisabeth Karlstrom, Candice A. Osborn, and Charles F. Gillespie. "Screening Tests for Pedophilia." *Criminal Justice and Behavior* 21:1 (1994), 115–27; Alcoff, Linda Martín. "Dangerous Pleasures: Foucault and the Politics of Pedophilia." In Susan J. Hekman, ed., *Feminist Interpretations of Michel Foucault*. University Park: Pennsylvania State University Press, 1996, 99–135. Reprinted in P&S3 (500–529); Archard, David. *Children: Rights and Childhood*. New York: Routledge, 1993; Archard, David. "Exploited Consent." *Journal of Social Philosophy* 25 (1994), 92–101. Reprinted in Leslie P. Francis, *Sexual Harassment as an Ethical Issue in Academic Life*. Lanham, Md.: Rowman and Littlefield, 2001, 212–18; Archard, David. "The Limits of Consensuality II: The Age of Sexual Consent." In *Sexual Consent*. Boulder, Colo.: Westview, 1998, 116–29; Bancroft, John. (1983) "Child Sexual Abuse, Paedophilia and Incest." In *Human Sexuality and Its Problems*, 2nd ed. Edinburgh, Scot.: Churchill Livingstone, 1989, 689–708; Beauvoir, Simone de. (1959) *Brigitte Bardot and the Lolita Syndrome*. Trans. Bernard Frechtman. New York: Reynal, 1960; Belliotti, Raymond. "The Sanctity of Contract and the Horror of Exploitation" and "Tier 3: Sexual Exploitation." In *Good Sex: Perspectives on Sexual Ethics*. Lawrence: University Press of Kansas, 1993, 86–108, 201–5; Benatar, David. "Two Views of Sexual Ethics: Promiscuity, Pedophilia, and Rape." *Public Affairs Quarterly* 16:3 (2002), 191–201; Berry, Jason. (1992) *Lead Us Not into Temptation*. Urbana: University of Illinois Press, 2000; Bullough, Vern L. "History in Adult Human Sexual Behavior with Children and Adolescents in Western Societies." In Jay R. Feierman, ed., *Pedophilia: Biosocial Dimensions*. New York: Springer-Verlag, 1990, 69–90; Burgess-Jackson, Keith. "Statutory Rape: A Philosophical Analysis." *Canadian Journal of Law and Jurisprudence* 8:1 (1995), 139–58. Reprinted in HS (463–82); Califia, Pat. "Feminism, Pedophilia, and Children's Rights." In *Public Sex: The Culture of Radical Sex*. Pittsburgh, Pa.: Cleis Press, 1994, 136–47; Denov, Myriam. "The Myth of Innocence: Sexual Scripts and the Recognition of Child Sexual Abuse by Female Perpetrators." *Journal of Sex Research* 40:3 (2003), 303–14; Dover, Kenneth. *Greek Homosexuality*. Cambridge, Mass.: Harvard University Press, 1978. *Updated and with a New*

Postscript, 1989; Ferguson, Ann. *Sexual Democracy: Women, Oppression, and Revolution*. Boulder, Colo.: Westview, 1991; Frye, Marilyn. "Critique" [of Robert Ehman, "Adult-Child Sex"]. In Robert B. Baker and Frederick A. Elliston, eds., *Philosophy and Sex*, 2nd ed. Buffalo, N.Y.: Prometheus, 1984, 447–55. Revised version, "Not-Knowing about Sex and Power." In *Willful Virgin: Essays in Feminism, 1976–1992*. Freedom, Calif.: Crossing Press, 1992, 39–50; Goldman, Alan. "Plain Sex." *Philosophy and Public Affairs* 6:3 (1977), 267–87. Reprinted in HS (103–23); POS1 (119–38); POS2 (73–92); POS3 (39–55); POS4 (39–55); Greer, Germaine. *The Boy*. London: Thames and Hudson, 2003; Howitt, Dennis. "Social Exclusion—Pedophile Style." In Robin Goodwin and Duncan Cramer, eds., *Inappropriate Relationships: The Unconventional, the Disapproved, and the Forbidden*. Mahwah, N.J.: Erlbaum, 2002, 221–43; Hughes, Donna M. "The Use of New Communications and Information Technologies for Sexual Exploitation of Women and Children." *Hastings Women's Law Journal* 13:1 (2002), 129–48; Jenkins, Philip. *Pedophiles and Priests: Anatomy of a Contemporary Crisis*. New York: Oxford University Press, 1996; Kelly, Liz. "What's in a Name? Defining Child Sexual Abuse." *Feminist Review*, no. 28 (Spring 1988), 65–73; Kipnis, Laura. "Fantasy in America: *The United States v. Daniel Thomas DePew*." In *Bound and Gagged: Pornography and the Politics of Fantasy in America*. New York: Grove Press, 1996, 3–63; Kitzinger, Jenny. "Defending Innocence: Ideologies of Childhood." *Feminist Review*, no. 28 (Spring 1988), 77–87; Levine, Judith. *Harmful to Minors: The Perils of Protecting Children from Sex*. Minneapolis: University of Minnesota Press, 2002; Mappes, Thomas A. (1985) "Sexual Morality and the Concept of Using Another Person." In Thomas A. Mappes and Jane S. Zembaty, eds., *Social Ethics*, 3rd ed. New York: McGraw-Hill, 1987, 248–62. 4th ed., 1992, 203–16. 5th ed., 1997, 163–76. 6th ed., 2002, 170–83. Reprinted in POS4 (207–23); Mohr, Richard D. "The Pedophilia of Everyday Life." *Art Issues*, no. 42 (March 1996), 28–31. Revised, expanded version in Natasha Hurley and Steven Bruhm, eds., *Curiouser: On the Queerness of Children*. Minneapolis: University of Minnesota Press, 2004, 17–30; Murray, Stephen O., and Will Roscoe, eds. *Islamic Homosexualities: Culture, History, and Literature*. New York: New York University Press, 1997; Nabokov, Vladimir. (1955) *Lolita*. New York: Berkley, 1977; Percy, William A. *Pederasty and Pedagogy in Archaic Greece*. Urbana: University of Illinois Press, 1996; Posner, Richard A., and Katharine B. Silbaugh. "Abuse of Position of Trust or Authority" and "Age of Consent." In *A Guide to America's Sex Laws*. Chicago, Ill.: University of Chicago Press, 1996, 111–28, 44–64; Prevost, Earle G. "Statutory Rape: A Growing Liberalization." *Southern Carolina Law Review* 18 (1966), 254–66; Primoratz, Igor. "Pedophilia." *Public Affairs Quarterly* 13:1 (1999), 99–110. Reprinted in *Ethics and Sex*. London: Routledge, 1999, 133–43; Sample, Ruth. *Exploitation: What It Is and Why It's Wrong*. Lanham, Md.: Rowman and Littlefield, 2003; Seidman, Steven. *Embattled Eros: Sexual Politics and Ethics in Contemporary America*. New York: Routledge, 1992; Shrage, Laurie. "Beyond Consent and Responsibility." In *Moral Dilemmas of Feminism: Prostitution, Adultery, and Abortion*. New York: Routledge, 1994, 51–54; Spiecker, Ben, and Steutel, Jan. "A Moral-Philosophical Perspective on Pedophilia and Incest." *Educational Philosophy and Theory* 32:3 (2000), 283–91; Taylor, Brian, ed. *Perspectives on Paedophilia*. London: Batsford, 1981; Tsang, Daniel, ed. *The Age Taboo: Gay Male Sexuality, Power, and Consent*. Boston, Mass.: Alyson, 1981; Weeks, Jeffrey. "Intergenerational Sex and Consent." In *Sexuality and Its Discontents: Meanings, Myths, and Modern Sexualities*. London: Routledge and Kegan Paul, 1985, 223–31; Werth, Barry. "Father's Helper: How the Church Used Psychiatry to Care for—and Protect—Abusive Priests." *The New Yorker* (9 June 2003), 61–67; Wertheimer, Alan. "Competence." In *Consent to Sexual Relations*. Cambridge, Mass.: Cambridge University Press, 2003, 215–31; Yates, Steven. "Making Pedophilia Acceptable: The Fruits of Government-Sponsored Tolerance." *Strike the Root* (24 May 2002). <www.strike-the-root.com/columns/Yates/yates1.html> [accessed 3 September 2004].

PERSONIFICATION, SEXUAL. A young married couple, according to a story that is almost certainly apocryphal, visited the Auguste Rodin (1840–1917) museum on Benjamin Franklin Parkway in Philadelphia. Both were dazzled by Rodin's sculpture of an uncompromising and noble, even if his hair was unkempt, Honoré de Balzac (1799–1850; see Sullivan's digital images). Later, at the wife's suggestion, they began referring to the husband's penis, whether flaccid or erect, as "Balzac." The practice of naming an erotic body part is "sexual personification." A nonsexual example of personification (if not also reification) would be worshiping an idol of gold, garnished with precious stones, and draped in silks and velvet, as if it were the Ultimate Itself. Personification can be understood, more generally, as raising something's ontological status, treating it as if it were higher in the Great Chain of Being, or thinking of it in terms of an ontological category superior to its own humble station. In this sense, sexual personification is the opposite of **sexual objectification**.

In objectification, one person X reduces (or attempts to reduce) the ontological status of another person Y. If X coerces or manipulates Y, so that some goal of X's is thereby attained, X has used Y, and has treated Y as a mere object, in the sense that X has ignored Y's personhood-defining features, Y's rational autonomy. X might not always actually reduce Y's status to that of an object, but at least X behaves toward Y as if Y were no more ontologically sophisticated than inanimate or a subhuman animal. In sexual objectification, X treats Y as a usable object, not fully as a person, in sexual contexts: say, prior to or while engaging in **sexual activity**. That sexual activity is by its nature objectifying is a notorious claim made by **Immanuel Kant** (1724–1804; *Lectures on Ethics*, Ak 27:384–85). For Kant, even when two adult persons freely **consent** to engage in sexual activity together, they are merely using each other. Further, they make objects not only of each other but also of themselves. But Kant does think that sexual activity carried out in a heterosexual **marriage** is morally permissible. An intriguing question in Kant scholarship is whether Kant permits objectification—otherwise morally wrong—in this special context or, instead, thought that marriage prevents sex from being objectifying.

Martha Nussbaum is one philosopher (among others) who concedes that there is some truth in the notion that sexual congress *per se* brings about the objectification of its participants. One of her proposals for how this objectification can be attenuated (but not eliminated) is for lovers or sexual partners to humanize (personify) their genitals by naming them:

> Giving a proper name to the genital organs of each is a way of signifying the special and individual way in which they desire one another. . . . It is a reminder that the genital organs of people are not really fungible, but have their own individual character, and are in effect parts of the person, if one will really look at them closely without shame. . . . We have to learn to call our genital organs by proper names—that would be at least the beginning of a properly complete human regard for one another. (401–2)

This suggestion is provocative, for it grants to **language**, through the illocution of christening and it various perlocutionary effects, the power to change the metaphysical and moral nature of our sexual activities. As in the writings of J. L. Austin (1911–1960), Nussbaum is telling us "how to do things with words." The suggestion also makes sense, for we can easily imagine that the couple that has named the man's penis "Balzac" has found a way to become closer to, more intimate with, each other. In using a private language that is unique to their relationship, they share a joke (and a pun) that they can laugh about for years to come. (On philosophical tangles in understanding "naming," see **Ludwig Wittgenstein** [1889–1951], e.g., §38, 18e–19e.)

Nussbaum's suggestion is not without its problems. She claims that giving names to the genitals reminds us that they "are not really fungible, but have their own individual character." Not being fungible (replaceable) and having individual character, though, are supposed to be what human beings are, *qua* persons. So Nussbaum is proposing that naming the genitals raises them so high in the ontological order of things that a part of a person, or a part of a person's body, comes to have something akin to the ontological status of the whole person. Nussbaum's argument, then, is that the objectification of the human being that essentially occurs in sexual congress, a sexual objectification that abnegates our nonfungibility and individuality, is attenuated by transforming our genitals into nonfungible and individualized persons—dignified persons with proper names—in their own right. Hence there are *four* persons in bed (not counting the parents of the lovers); the person-status of the penis and vagina (or penis-penis, vulva-vulva) is that which attenuates the objectification that exists in the congress of their possessors.

Nussbaum also claims that "giving a proper name to the genital organs of each [person] is a way of signifying the special and individual way in which they desire one another." Nussbaum is here speaking about sexual partners who know each other well, not about strangers who just met in a bar, about which it is inapposite to say that they have **sexual desire** for each other in a special way. Fungibility and nonindividuality reign in **casual sex**. Nussbaum is not claiming that strangers should interrupt their frenetic gropings to name their genitals, thereby attenuating the objectifying character of their sexual congress. For Nussbaum, the naming of the genitals, and what it signifies, derives from the specialness that has already been established in a relationship and helps these people attenuate the objectification of their sexual activity. If there is no background relationship, reducing objectification by naming the genitals cannot occur; casual sex remains, in this respect at least, unredeemed. Perhaps this is right, although more than a few thoughtful philosophers have begged to differ.

One could ask whether naming the genitals makes them nonfungible and individual, that is, whether naming them actually raises their status via personification. After all, naming my red-earred slider "Speedy" by itself does not make her nonfungible. One could also ask whether naming the genitals attenuates sexual objectification. Michael Kimmel, a sociologist who has written a great deal in the area of **men's feminism** and men's liberation, thinks that naming the genitals often contributes, instead, to sexual self-objectification:

> In locker rooms and playgrounds, men learn to detach their emotions from sexual expression. Detachment requires sexual self-objectification. . . . The penis is transformed from an organ of sexual pleasure into a "tool," an instrument by which the job is carried out, a thing, separate from the self. Men have developed a rather inventive assortment of nicknames for their penises, including the appropriation of real first names, like "John Thomas" and "Peter." ("Introduction," 9; see also *The Gendered Society*, 241)

Is it possible, when the couple speaks about the husband's penis as "Balzac," that what they are really doing, despite what is occurring phenomenologically, is objectifying him by identifying or equating him with his penis, or by making his penis such an important—and both independent and individual—"part" of him? If a man can "separate" his penis from the wholeness of his Being by naming it, treating it as a distinct personality that challenges and impugns, if not undermines and diminishes, his own personhood, then even the loving couple's "Balzac" joke might accomplish the same thing. Naming the genitals, if it humanizes them, may very well dehumanize the one whose genitals they are. Further, attempting to raise the ontological status of a mere material, fleshy thing acknowledges and confirms that this object *is* an object. Adam's assigning names to the lower creatures, doing the (impossible) job assigned him by the Lord, augmented—it did not attenuate—his objectification of and dominion over the animals. In the beginning was the Word and, along with it, a resplendent World, an object the Lord could feel proud of having created.

Kimmel mentions a locker-room name for the penis, "John Thomas," which is the name given to his penis by Oliver Mellors in D. H. Lawrence's (1885–1930) *Lady Chatterley's Lover*. Mellors is an estate's gardener and the paramour of his employer's wife, Constance Chatterley. Listen to the happy adulterous couple play their own "Balzac" game:

> "Do you know what I thought?" she said suddenly. "It suddenly came to me. You are the 'Knight of the Burning Pestle'!"
> "Ay! And you? Are you the Lady of the Red-Hot mortar?"
> "Yes!" she said. "Yes! You're Sir Pestle and I'm Lady Mortar."
> "All right, then I'm knighted. John Thomas is Sir John, to your Lady Jane." . . .
> "That's you in all your glory!" he said. "Lady Jane, at her wedding with John Thomas." . . .
> "This is John Thomas marryin' Lady Jane." (212–13)

All seems innocent enough. But Lawrence's novel does not provide a recipe for the attenuation of objectification by personifying the genitals. It may, in fact, portray the opposite. Consider this passage, in which Connie relentlessly, obsessively, talks about Mellors's penis as "He":

> "How strange!" she said slowly. "How strange he stands there! So big! and so dark and cock-sure! Is he like that?" . . .
> "So proud!" she murmured, uneasy. "And so lordly! Now I know why men are so overbearing! But he's lovely, *really*. Like another being!" . . .
> "And now he's tiny, and soft like a little bud of life!" she said, taking the soft small penis in her hand. "Isn't he somehow lovely! so on his own, so strange! And *so* innocent? And he comes so far into me! You must *never* insult him, you know. He's mine too. He's not only yours. He's mine! And so lovely and innocent! . . . And how lovely your hair is here! quite quite different."
> "That's John Thomas' hair, not mine!" he said.
> "John Thomas! John Thomas!" and she quickly kissed the soft penis, that was beginning to stir again.
> "Ay!" said the man, stretching his body almost painfully. "He's got his root in my soul, has that gentleman! An' sometimes I don' know what ter do wi' him. Ay, he's got a will of his own, an' its hard to suit him." . . .
> [T]he penis in slow soft undulations filled and surged and rose up, and grew hard, standing there hard and overweening, in its curious towering fashion. The woman too trembled a little as she watched.
> "There! Take him then! He's thine," said the man.
> And she quivered, and her own mind melted out. (196–97)

Despite the fact that Lady Chatterley and Mellors are far from strangers, the naming of the penis here does not quite "humanize" it, *pace* Nussbaum. Instead, Connie's referring to Mellors's penis as "he" seems to make (or keep) the organ an impersonal *tertium quid*, a pagan god, a golden lamb, an idol to be worshiped, the nucleus of a Gnostic, Tantric, or Satanic ritual. The Lawrentian penis *apparently* has a detached life and "will of its own."

And, being its own boss, the penis is autonomous, although perhaps not rationally so. (The autonomy of the penis greatly distressed **Saint Augustine** [354–430], who saw the post-lapsarian insolence of the penis as fitting punishment for the prelapsarian insolence of Adam. See *City of God*, 14.16.) But this personhood is fraudulent, as is the personhood of computers and the Animaniacs.

See also Adultery; Arts, Sex and the; Communication Model; Freud, Sigmund; Gnosticism; Hinduism; Humor; Love; MacKinnon, Catharine; Manichaeism; Objectification, Sexual; Pornography; Tantrism

REFERENCES

Augustine. (413–427) *The City of God*. Trans. Marcus Dods. New York: Modern Library, 1950; Austin, J. L. (1962) *How to Do Things with Words*, 2nd ed. Ed. J. O. Urmson and Marina Sbisá. Cambridge, Mass.: Harvard University Press, 1975; Kant, Immanuel. (ca. 1762–1794) *Lectures on Ethics*. Trans. Peter Heath. Ed. Peter Heath and J. B. Schneewind. Cambridge: Cambridge University Press, 1997; Kimmel, Michael S. *The Gendered Society*, 2nd ed. New York: Oxford University Press, 2004; Kimmel, Michael S. "Introduction: Guilty Pleasures—Pornography in Men's Lives." In Michael S. Kimmel, ed., *Men Confront Pornography*. New York: Crown Publishers, 1990, 1–22; Lawrence, D. H. (1928) *Lady Chatterley's Lover*. New York: New American Library, 1962; Nussbaum, Martha C. (1995) "Objectification." In Alan Soble, ed., *The Philosophy of Sex: Contemporary Readings*, 4th ed. Lanham, Md.: Rowman and Littlefield, 2002, 381–419; Sullivan, Mary Ann. "*Balzac*, Rodin Museum." [Digital images of the sculpture] <www.bluffton.edu/~sullivanm/rodin/balzac.html> [accessed 4 February 2005]; Wittgenstein, Ludwig. *Philosophical Investigations*. Trans. G.E.M. Anscombe. New York: Macmillan, 1953.

Alan Soble

ADDITIONAL READING

Cornog, Martha. "Language and Sex." In Vern L. Bullough and Bonnie Bullough, eds., *Human Sexuality: An Encyclopedia*. New York: Garland, 1994, 341–47; Cornog, Martha. "Sexual Body Parts: Preliminary Patterns and Implications." *Journal of Sex Research* 22:3 (1986), 393–98; Cornog, Martha. "Tom, Dick, and Hairy: Notes on Genital Pet Names." *Maledicta* 5:1–2 (1981), 31–40; Ferguson, Frances. "Connie, or the Lawrentian Woman." In *Pornography, the Theory: What Utilitarianism Did to Action*. Chicago, Ill.: University of Chicago Press, 2004, 125–45; Gramich, Katie. "Stripping Off the 'Civilized Body': Lawrence's *nostalgie de la boue* in *Lady Chatterley's Lover*." In Paul Poplawski, ed., *Writing the Body in D. H. Lawrence: Essays on Language, Representation, and Sexuality*. Westport, Conn.: Greenwood Press, 2001, 149–61; Lawrence, D. H. (1930) "A Propos of Lady Chatterley's Lover." In *Phoenix II: Uncollected, Unpublished, and Other Prose Works*. New York: Viking, 1959, 487–515; Nagel, Thomas. (1999) "Nussbaum on Sexual Injustice." In *Concealment and Exposure and Other Essays*. New York: Oxford University Press, 2002, 56–62; Nussbaum, Martha C. "Objectification." *Philosophy and Public Affairs* 24:4 (1995), 249–91. Reprinted in POS3 (283–321); POS4 (381–419). Reprinted, revised, in *Sex and Social Justice*. New York: Oxford University Press, 1999, 213–39; Soble, Alan. "Sexual Use and What to Do about It: Internalist and Externalist Sexual Ethics." *Essays in Philosophy* 2:2 (2001). <www.humboldt.edu/~essays/soble.html> [accessed 4 February 2005]. Reprinted, revised, in POS4 (225–58).

PERVERSION, SEXUAL. **Masturbation**, homosexual sex, anal sex, oral sex, voyeurism, exhibitionism, fetishism, sadism, masochism, transvestism, **bestiality**, necrophilia, coprophilia, and urophilia have all been thought perverse, but there is no philosophical or scientific consensus about the nature, origin, or even the genuine existence of sexual perversion. In analyzing sexual perversion, we need an account both of "perversion" and of "sexual," that is, of that which makes a sexual activity or sexual desire *sexual* to begin with (see Gray). And an account of what makes a sexual act perverted must be logically independent of the account of what makes it sexual. If what makes an act sexual (if what at least in part *defines* it as sexual) is that the act is procreative (reproductive), then acts that are not procreative might be perverted but not *sexually* perverted, since they are already eliminated from the class of sexual acts. So if one wants to argue that anal intercourse, say, is sexually perverted, one must not define the sexual in terms of the procreative form or function of an act.

"Perversion" ordinarily picks out aberrant sexual behavior. But the term is often used normatively, not purely descriptively, implying statistical abnormality and psychological disorder, deviance, or unnaturalness. In this usage, "unnatural" means more than merely unusual; it invokes a function or purpose for sexuality that some sexual acts violate. In this sense, sexual perversions are or involve sexual desires or acts that are "contrary" to nature. If so, understanding human nature and the nature of human sexuality is crucial to understanding sexual perversion. The pejorative content of the concept of sexual perversion raises many questions. The disapproval it expresses is often linked with disgust, but this does not necessarily have any moral implications (Ruse, 201; but cf. **Richard Posner**, 230 ff.). Further, deriving the immorality of sexual acts from their unnaturalness has always been a difficult task (see Ruddick, 95). To wit: "Perverted" is arguably distinct from "immoral," for immoral sex acts that are not perverted are possible (e.g., deceptive, adulterous heterosexual coitus) as are perverted yet morally permissible sex acts (loving, faithful **homosexuality**, or an innocuous fetish). Still, traditional views of sexual perversion, in particular Roman Catholic and Natural Law theories, identify perversion with unnaturalness and, from there, with immorality.

Medicopsychological use of "perversion" for unusual sexual activities dates only to the early nineteenth century, when regulating human sexual behavior increasingly became the province of medicine rather than theology and public morality (Conrad and Schneider; Davidson). Picking out reproduction as the purpose of sex and claiming that some sexuality is both unnatural and wrong occurs, however, much earlier. **Plato** (427–347 BCE) contends in his *Laws* that masturbation and male-male sexual activity are unnatural because they are neither procreative nor consistent with courage and self-control (bk. 8, 836 ff.). Roman law prohibited homosexual acts by 342, under Constantius II and Constans, and the use of the term "unnatural" in the Roman legal regulation of sexual behavior occurred as early by the sixth century. (Justinian's [527–565] laws included the death penalty for male homosexual activity.) Judaic sources condemned bestiality, masturbation, and homosexual acts as against nature, and early Church legislation forbid all nonreproductive forms of sex (Bullough and Bullough, 31). Both **Saint Augustine** (354–430; *Confessions*, bk. 3, chap. 8) and **Saint Thomas Aquinas** (1224/25–1274) condemned as sinful all sexual acts not open to procreation. Aquinas's *Summa theologiae* orders these unnatural acts from the least to the most sinful: masturbation, irregular heterosexual acts ("beastly and monstrous techniques" such as, presumably, anal intercourse), all homosexual acts, and bestiality (2a2ae, ques. 154, art. 12). Reliance on reproductive potential as the measure of naturalness and morality continues up to the eighteenth through twenty-first centuries, and not only in the Natural Law or Thomistic traditions. In his *Lectures on Ethics*, for example, **Immanuel Kant** (1724–1804) claimed that all sexual activity outside monogamous, heterosexual **marriage** is immoral, on the grounds that it violated the moral duty not to objectify ourselves or others. But Kant, no Catholic, nevertheless follows Aquinas's categorization and condemnation of contrary-to-nature sex acts, claiming that anyone who does them "no longer deserves to be a person" (170).

By the nineteenth century this moralizing tone takes a back seat to a "scientific" medicine that theorizes sexual perversions not as sins but as diseases in which the sexual instinct is diverted from its proper (reproductive) object. One early sexologist, Richard von Krafft-Ebing (1840–1902), claimed that "every expression [of the sexual instinct] that does not correspond with the purpose of nature—i.e., propagation—must be regarded as perverse" (79). He also noted the important distinction between perverse sexual acts that might be chosen (opportunistically) for reasons other than inclination and perversion as a feature of a person's psychology or personality (i.e., **sexual orientation**).

Most accounts of perversion before the twentieth century assume with little argument that reproduction is the natural function of sexual activity and that nonreproductive acts are therefore unnatural. One problem with this view is that reproduction cannot be the only function of human sexuality, except in the sense that all adaptive behaviors enhance reproduction (Wilson, 125–27). Just because reproduction sometimes results from sexual activity does not mean that this is its (sole) function; many things resulting from sex are not its purpose (gonorrhea). Further, pleasure is also an adaptive function of sex, insofar as sexual experiences help maintain the pair bond (see Masters and Johnson) and related social structures required for successful human reproduction. Pleasure thus is not contrary to the biological functions of sex but one of them. Consider, too, solitary masturbation, an act that many now acknowledge is a perfectly natural expression of human sexuality even though it is not procreative. A reproductive criterion of perversion includes too much.

Sigmund Freud (1856–1939) did not always avoid this difficulty. Even though he placed pleasure squarely at the center of sex, he kept adult male-female genital sex as a developmental ideal. The view of sexual perversion that results does not greatly differ from the traditional view: Roughly the same acts are classified as perverted. The innovation in Freud's *Three Essays on Sexuality* is his characterizing sex as libido, a drive for pleasure understood as the resolution of tension. Libido is expressed in an infant's or child's seeking pleasure as much as it is in adult sexuality. Freud posits for the child a developmental series of oral, anal, and genital libidinal satisfactions; at maturity, the desire for heterosexual intercourse is its natural outcome. For Freud perversions result from a failure to complete the "normal" sequence, so that variations appear in what might be employed to produce sexual pleasure, for example, satisfying the sexual urge by fondling a fetish material. His theory explains, advantageously, how these variations are *sexual* but lacks a fully cogent justification for calling them *perverted* (for discussion, see Neu). Later in the century some psychologists, psychiatrists, and psychoanalysts still thought that people with "perverse" sexualities were either damaged or immature, yet also maintained that perversion had no necessary moral import.

The claim that people who practice sexual perversions are psychologically defective has been vigorously disputed, especially regarding homosexuality (see, for example, Conrad and Schneider; Hooker; Margolis). The history of revisions to the American Psychiatric Association's *Diagnostic and Statistical Manual of Mental Disorders* (DSM) over the last half of the twentieth century is a good illustration. In 1952, DSM-I categorized deviant sexual practices, including homosexuality, as sociopathic personality disorders (38–39). In the early 1970s, after much rallying, petitioning, and debating, this judgment was reversed. DSM-III (1980; 266–82) relabeled sexual deviation with the more neutral term "**paraphilia**" and dropped homosexuality from this category (although ego-dystonic homosexuality was retained as a psychosexual disorder). Later editions of DSM (IV, 1994; IV-TR, 2000) define the paraphilias as conditions that "involve unusual objects, activities or situations and cause clinically significant distress or impairment in social, occupational, or other important areas of functioning" (DSM-IV, 493). This formulation may not provide any solid distinction between the merely unusual (or bizarre) and the genuinely psychologically disordered (see Kaplan, 18–21; Soble, "Paraphilia"). An interesting feature of the DSM is its reluctance to propose aetiologies for many sexual pathologies, including paraphilias. A noncommital stance is taken toward the virtues and vices of Freudian and other explanations of the origin of sexual deviance.

The philosophical literature on sexual perversion confirms the difficulty of distinguishing the merely uncommon from the perverted. **Thomas Nagel**'s "Sexual Perversion" inaugurated this discussion in 1969, arguing that perversion involves an unnatural psychological, not physiological, structure. Borrowing from Jean-Paul Sartre's (1905–1980) thoughts about interpersonal relations in *Being and Nothingness* (361–430), Nagel contends that in natural human sexual psychology there is a "reflexive mutual recognition" of desire and arousal (10). In psychologically natural sex, the partners are not only aroused by each other's bodies and touches but also by their awareness of each other's arousal and desire. On this account, the sexual perversions (bestiality, necrophilia, fetishism, **pedophilia**, voyeurism) are psychologically "truncated," or lack "**completeness**," since the requisite mental sophistication is absent. As a genuine modernist, Nagel refuses to draw any moral conclusions from these psychological observations and is, indeed, liberal in his moral, social, and political philosophy. (He denies that homosexuality is either unnatural/perverted or immoral.) But some philosophers argue that perversion has important moral implications. For **Roger Scruton**, human sexual desire is characterized by interpersonal intentionality, normally aiming at union with another person. Impersonal, **casual sex**, in focusing on the body instead of the person, is obscene, perverted, and morally condemnable (168), as is masturbation (319). Scruton draws on both Sartre (120–25) and Nagel, although he employs their insights in a decidedly conservative way.

Robert Solomon, who appreciates Nagel's lineage from Sartre, nonetheless offers an alternative way to understand perversion, through his **communication model**. For Solomon, sex is best understood as a **language** composed of bodily gestures that express interpersonal attitudes. This communication can founder through corruption either of structure or content. In **sadomasochism**, for example, reflexive mutual recognition may be present, but excessive attitudes of domination, aggression, fear, shame, and inferiority are expressed. Deceptive sexual interactions are also perverse, "the bodily equivalent of the lie" ("Sexual Paradigms," 345; see "Sex and Perversion").

Nagel's and Solomon's theories of perversion are contentious. For many people, sexual psychological completeness and communicating emotions sexually do constitute an ideal. But many others prefer anonymous sex, commercial sex, or solitary masturbation, and whether we or they should accept the claim that their preferences, or their sexuality, are defective is unclear. Nagel's and Solomon's views also have counterintuitive implications about which sexual practices are perverted. For example, sex in which the partners psychologically disconnect from each other from boredom or through private fantasies is likely perverted on Nagel's account. Masturbation is also problematic, since it is apparently incomplete and, on Solomon's view, is like "talking to oneself" (see Soble, *Investigations*, 71–78). But the ubiquity of masturbation makes suspicious any account of sexual perversion that raises doubts about it. Further, as Janice Moulton argues, communicative accounts of sex seem to privilege "novel sexual encounters" with relative strangers, since partners of long standing may not employ sex as frequently as other activities to express their emotions or attitudes toward each other.

Russell Vannoy's theory of sexual perversion (or "perversity") also shows the long reach of Sartre. Vannoy suggests that sexual perversions are "self-defeating in terms of their own goals" (360). One of his examples is sadism, which desires "absolute conquest" over the other. This desire is doomed to frustration, because the victim's death limits the suffering the sadist can impose, while absolute conquest is foiled by the continued life of the victim. Another example is the pedophile who desires both sex from and innocence in his "partner" (361–63). This complex desire is doomed, and hence the pedophile is perverted, because having sex with the child destroys innocence, while maintaining the innocence prevents the occurrence of sex. One counterintuitive consequence of Vannoy's theory is that the sadist who desires and gets only his victim's suffering is not perverted, by desiring something less than absolute conquest (perhaps precisely to protect his arousal and satisfaction). Nor is the pedophile perverted if he values the violation of innocence instead of innocence. Vannoy could reply that this sadist and pedophile are not the genuine articles; but that move saves his theory by *ad hoc* and probably inaccurate definitions of these sexual types.

However, an advantage of Vannoy's theory is that, unlike the procreative, completeness, and communicative accounts of sexuality, it does not rely on positing any essential goal to sex beyond arousal and pleasure. Alan Goldman has argued that conceptually attaching extra goals to sex overlooks sex's intrinsic value and generates false views of perversion. In the best analysis of human sexuality, sexual desire is "desire for contact with another person's body and for the pleasure which such contact produces," and sexual acts are those that "tend" to satisfy the desire for contact and pleasure (268). For Goldman, no extraneous purpose is even partially definitive of the sexual. If there is any perverted sex, it is not a contravention of an extraneous purpose, but of something intrinsic to sexual desire or activity. Perversions are unusual sexual practices that deviate from "the *form of the desire*" (284). An example might be fetishism, which often involves a desire for sexual pleasure produced not by contact with a human body but an inanimate material. But the example hints at something wrong in Goldman's account. It apparently entails that there is no *sexual* perversion, for a desire with a deviant form, such as a desire to fondle panties, is not a sexual desire on Goldman's definition to begin with, and acts that tend to satisfy *this* desire cannot be sexual acts. Further, if sexual desire requires desiring bodily contact with a person, then some masturbation is not sexual. Goldman does say that masturbation is sexual if it substitutes for "the real thing" (a revealing phrase). Much masturbation, however, is not meant to replace other activities but is valued for its own sake, and this masturbation, on Goldman's view, does not (which is odd) count as sexual.

For Goldman, "sexual perversion" is purely descriptive, since it only picks out statistically unusual sexualities. Robert Gray also attempts to give a descriptive account of sexual perversion, claiming it must be understood in terms of the "natural adaptive function of sexual activity" (197). Because sexual activities are those and only those acts that "give rise to sexual pleasure," a sexual perversion would be an act that produced pleasure but was inconsistent with the evolutionarily adaptive function(s) of sexuality. A complete account of the sexual, in Gray's terms, would also explain why (or when) certain pleasures are sexual and others not. Still, he avoids the Natural Law view that natural sex is always potentially procreative and, in opposition to the traditional view, Gray thinks sex done solely for pleasure is not perverse (if pleasure is adaptive). Even supposing that one function of sex is reproduction, success in raising new generations requires the maintenance of "fairly stable male-female reproductive pairs" and "well organized, stable societies." Thus, any sexual activity that contributes to (or does not interfere with) either dimension of reproduction in this broad sense might avoid the label "perverse." Which acts are perversions is also culturally relative, if adaptiveness depends on cultural context. If so, homosexuality would not be perverted in overpopulated societies that require large decreases in procreation to survive. Homosexuality might avoid being perverted on Gray's account also because it produces pleasure, and people who experience sexual pleasure more effectively contribute to projects that keep society going. As Gray rightly admits, determining what is "normal" and "perverted" (adaptive and nonadaptive) becomes, on his account, a task for the empirical scientist (197). Whether evolutionary biology will ever settle such disputes about sexuality is anyone's guess. There is not even consensus over why *some* human females experience orgasm, when orgasm is inessential to a woman's reproductive success (see Hrdy).

Donald Levy is one philosopher who has attempted to maintain, outside the context of Catholicism, a significant link between perversion and morality. Levy views the perverted as a subcategory of the unnatural, *defining* unnatural acts as those that bring about an unjustifiable denial of a basic human good. (Right here Levy welds together the natural and the moral.) The basic goods are those general goods that are desired whatever else is specifically desired, so they are goods needed for realizing any other goods (see John Rawls [1921–2002], 396). For Levy, these goods are "life, health, control of one's bodily and psychic functions, and the capacity for knowledge and love" (199; see Finnis's alternative formulation, chap. 4, sec. 2). Denial of basic goods can be justified only "for the sake of another basic human good" (200). Pleasure, for Levy, is not a basic human good, so acts that reduce basic human goods merely for sexual pleasure are *unnatural* (even bizarre, monstrous) and hence sexual perversions. Levy's theory is plausible for sex acts in which harm to others occurs and the harmfulness and sexuality are difficult to distinguish (for example, sexual murder). However, constructing a list of basic human goods is a problematic enterprise. Levy's including the capacity for **love** as a *basic* human good is not obviously right. Yet it grounds Levy's judgment that pedophilia, bestiality, and necrophilia are perverted, for he claims that these activities undermine the capacity for love.

The apparent failure of attempts to analyze the perverted in a fully satisfactory fashion supports the claim of some philosophers that we should reject the concept altogether. Michael Slote, for example, argues that the concept of perversion is empty because sense cannot be made of "unnatural" desires or practices—anything in the world is, by being there, natural. "Perverted," then, can express only disgust and horror, not describe something real (262). Slote's view echos the **Marquis de Sade** (1740–1814), who promoted sexual libertinism on the grounds that no sexual impulses or practices occur outside nature, and so none are immoral. But Slote does not follow Sade's claim that everything natural is moral. Igor Primoratz agrees that the concept of perversion should be discarded (*Ethics*, 63–66), precisely because it "is plagued by considerable inconsistency and confusion" ("Perversion," 345). Philosophical accounts do not fare much better than our confused everyday discourse. Furthermore, we need not retain the categories of natural and unnatural sex to "get on with saying whatever needs to be said about human sexuality" (345). Graham Priest, too, insists that we eliminate the concept of sexual perversion, arguing it makes sense only in the context of a largely abandoned teleological interpretation of the universe, like the one developed by **Aristotle** (384–322 BCE) or even Aquinas, which sees everything as having a purpose. Whether Priest is right that teleology has been substantially abandoned, left in the trash can of the history of philosophy and social/cultural thought, is debatable, and to that extent his repudiation of "sexual perversion" stumbles. (For more on teleology and sexual perversion, see Baltzly; Humber; Levinson.)

Regardless, "sexual perversion" certainly has had its social and political uses. **Michel Foucault** (1926–1984) argued that, through the invention of medical and criminal categories like sexual perversion, sexuality became an object of knowledge and hence of domination. Individuals internalize the social and political norms of sexuality, and their oppression is increased through self-regulation. Some feminists adopt this argument in some form, claiming that our society uses the derogatory label "sexually perverted" (regarding homosexuality and other deviant sexualities) to enforce "compulsory heterosexuality" (and female submission to male sexuality) by intimidation, shame, and embarrassment (the *locus classicus* is Rich's essay). Therefore "sex radicals" embrace perversion, maintaining that this can subvert sexual oppression by weakening one of its tools. Other feminists argue that forms of sexuality like pedophilia, sadism, and masochism must be rejected because they reproduce rather than undermine hierarchical or patriarchal power relations (see Califia; LeMoncheck; Linden et al.; Samois).

See also Activity, Sexual; Addiction, Sexual; Animal Sexuality; Bestiality; Bisexuality; Catholicism, History of; Completeness, Sexual; Evolution; Existentialism; Foucault, Michel; Homosexuality and Science; Incest; Kolnai, Aurel; Lacan, Jacques; Nagel, Thomas; Natural Law (New); Orientation, Sexual; Paraphilia; Pedophilia; Psychology, Evolutionary; Psychology, Twentieth- and Twenty-First-Century; Queer Theory; Sadomasochism; Schopenhauer, Arthur; Sexology; Sherfey, Mary Jane

REFERENCES

American Psychiatric Association. *Diagnostic and Statistical Manual of Mental Disorders*, 1st ed. [DSM-I] Washington, D.C.: Author, 1952; American Psychiatric Association. *Diagnostic and Statistical Manual of Mental Disorders*, 3rd ed. [DSM-III] Washington, D.C.: Author, 1980; American Psychiatric Association. *Diagnostic and Statistical Manual of Mental Disorders*, rev. 3rd ed. [DSM-III-R] Washington, D.C.: Author, 1987; American Psychiatric Association. *Diagnostic and Statistical Manual of Mental Disorders*, 4th ed. [DSM-IV] Washington, D.C.: Author, 1994; American Psychiatric Association. *Diagnostic and Statistical Manual of Mental Disorders*, text revision of the 4th ed. [DSM-IV-TR] Washington, D.C.: Author, 2000; Augustine. (397) *Confessions*. Trans. F. J. Sheed. Indianapolis, Ind.: Hackett, 1993; Baltzly, Dirk. "Peripatetic Perversions: A Neo-Aristotelean Account of the Nature of Sexual Perversion." *The Monist* 85:1 (2003), 3–29; Bullough, Vern L., and Bonnie Bullough. *Sin, Sickness, and Sanity: A History of Sexual Attitudes*. New York: Garland, 1977; Califia, Pat. "Feminism and Sadomasochism." *Heresies* no. 12 ["Sex Issue"] 3:4 (1981), 30–34; Conrad, Peter, and Joseph W. Schneider. *Deviance and Medicalization: From Badness to Sickness*. St. Louis, Mo.: Mosby, 1980; Davidson, Arnold. "Conceptual History and Conceptions of Perversions." In Robert B. Baker, Kathleen Wininger, and Frederick A. Elliston, eds., *Philosophy and Sex*, 3rd ed. Amherst, N.Y.: Prometheus, 1998, 476–86; Finnis, John. *Natural Law and Natural Rights*. Oxford, U.K.: Clarendon Press, 1980; Foucault, Michel. (1976) *The History of Sexuality*, vol. 1: *An Introduction*. Trans. Robert Hurley. New York: Random House, 1978; Freud, Sigmund. (1905) *Three Essays on the Theory of Sexuality*. In *The Standard Edition of the Complete Psychological Works of Sigmund Freud*, vol. 7. Trans. James Strachey. London: Hogarth Press, 1953–1974, 125–245; Goldman, Alan. "Plain Sex." *Philosophy and Public Affairs* 6:3 (1977), 267–87; Gray, Robert. "Sex and Sexual Perversion." *Journal of Philosophy* 75:4 (1978), 189–99; Hooker, Evelyn. "The Adjustment of the Male Overt Homosexual." *Journal of Projective Techniques* 21:1 (1957), 18–31; Hrdy, Sarah Blaffer. "The Evolution of Human Sexuality: The Latest Word and the Last." *Quarterly Review of Biology* 54:3 (1979), 309–14; Humber, James. "Sexual Perversion and Human Nature." *Philosophy Research Archives* 13 (1987–1988), 331–50; Kant, Immanuel. (ca. 1780) *Lectures on Ethics*. Trans. Louis Infield. Indianapolis, Ind.: Hackett, 1963; Kaplan, Louise. *Female Perversions: The Temptations of Emma Bovary*. New York: Anchor Books, 1991; Krafft-Ebing, Richard von. (1886) *Psychopathia Sexualis: With Especial Reference to the Antipathic Sexual Instinct*, 12th rev. ed. Trans. F. J. Rebman. Brooklyn, N.Y.: Physicians and Surgeons Book Company, 1934; LeMoncheck, Linda. *Loose Women, Lecherous Men: A Feminist Philosophy of Sex*. New York: Oxford University Press,

1997; Levinson, Jerrold. "Sexual Perversity." *The Monist* 86:1 (2003), 30–54; Levy, Donald. "Perversion and the Unnatural as Moral Categories." *Ethics* 90:2 (1980), 191–202; Linden, Robin Ruth, Darlene R. Pagano, Diana E. H. Russell, and Susan Leigh Star, eds. *Against Sadomasochism: A Radical Feminist Analysis*. San Francisco, Calif.: Frog in the Well, 1982; Margolis, Joseph. "The Question of Homosexuality." In Robert B. Baker and Frederick A. Elliston, eds., *Philosophy and Sex*, 1st ed. Buffalo, N.Y.: Prometheus, 1975, 289–302; Masters, William H., and Virginia E. Johnson. *The Pleasure Bond: A New Look at Sexuality and Commitment*. Boston, Mass.: Little, Brown, 1974; Moulton, Janice. "Sexual Behavior: Another Position." *Journal of Philosophy* 73:16 (1976), 537–46; Nagel, Thomas. "Sexual Perversion." *Journal of Philosophy* 66:1 (1969), 5–17; Neu, Jerome. "Freud and Perversion." In Earl E. Shelp, ed., *Sexuality and Medicine*, vol. 1: *Conceptual Roots*. Dordrecht, Holland: Reidel, 1987, 153–84; Plato. (ca. 355–347 BCE) *Laws*. Trans. Trevor J. Saunders. In John Cooper, ed., and D. S. Hutchinson, assoc. ed., *Plato: Complete Works*. Indianapolis, Ind.: Hackett, 1997, 1318–1616; Posner, Richard. *Sex and Reason*. Cambridge, Mass.: Harvard University Press, 1992; Priest, Graham. "Sexual Perversion." *Australasian Journal of Philosophy* 75:3 (1997), 360–72; Primoratz, Igor. *Ethics and Sex*. London: Routledge, 1999; Primoratz, Igor. "Sexual Perversion." *American Philosophical Quarterly* 34:2 (1997), 245–58; Rawls, John. *A Theory of Justice*. Cambridge, Mass.: Harvard University Press, 1971; Rich, Adrienne. "Compulsory Heterosexuality and Lesbian Existence." *Signs* 5:4 (1980), 631–60; Ruddick, Sara. (1971) "Better Sex." In Robert B. Baker and Frederick A. Elliston, eds., *Philosophy and Sex*, 1st ed. Buffalo, N.Y.: Prometheus, 1975, 83–104; Ruse, Michael. *Homosexuality: A Philosophical Inquiry*. New York: Blackwell, 1988; Samois Collective, eds. (1981) *Coming to Power: Writings and Graphics on Lesbian S/M*, rev. eds. Boston, Mass.: Alyson, 1982, 1987; Sartre, Jean-Paul. (1943) *Being and Nothingness*. Trans. Hazel Barnes. New York: Washington Square Press, 1956; Scruton, Roger. *Sexual Desire: A Moral Philosophy of the Erotic*. New York: Free Press, 1986; Slote, Michael. "Inapplicable Concepts and Sexual Perversion." In Robert B. Baker and Frederick A. Elliston, eds., *Philosophy and Sex*, 1st ed. Buffalo, N.Y.: Prometheus, 1975, 261–67; Soble, Alan. "Paraphilia and Distress in DSM-IV." In Jennifer Radden, ed., *The Philosophy of Psychiatry: A Companion*. New York: Oxford University Press, 2004, 54–63; Soble, Alan. *Sexual Investigations*. New York: New York University Press, 1996; Solomon, Robert. "Sex and Perversion." In Robert B. Baker and Frederick A. Elliston, eds., *Philosophy and Sex*, 1st ed. Buffalo, N.Y.: Prometheus, 1975, 268–87; Solomon, Robert. "Sexual Paradigms." *Journal of Philosophy* 71:11 (1974), 336–45; Thomas Aquinas. (1265–1273) *Summa theologiae*, 60 vols. Cambridge, U.K.: Blackfriars, 1964–1976; Vannoy, Russell. "The Structure of Sexual Perversity." In Alan Soble, ed., *Sex, Love, and Friendship*. Amsterdam, Holland: Rodopi, 1997, 359–73; Wilson, Edward O. *On Human Nature*. New York: Bantam, 1979.

Sarah Hoffman

ADDITIONAL READING

Allen, Clifford. "Perversions, Sexual." In Albert Ellis and Albert Abarbanel, eds., *The Encyclopedia of Sexual Behavior*. New York: Jason Aronson, 1973, 802–11; Allen, Clifford. (1940, 1949) *The Sexual Perversions and Abnormalities: A Study in the Psychology of Paraphilia*. Westport, Conn.: Greenwood Press, 1979; American Psychiatric Association. *Diagnostic and Statistical Manual of Mental Disorders*, 2nd ed. Washington, D.C.: Author, 1968; American Psychiatric Association. "Sexual and Gender Identity Disorders." In *Diagnostic and Statistical Manual of Mental Disorders*, 4th ed. [DSM-IV] Washington, D.C.: Author, 1994, 493–538; Bergner, Raymond M. "Money's 'Lovemap' Account of the Paraphilias: A Critique and Reformulation." *American Journal of Psychotherapy* 42:2 (1988), 254–59; Bloch, Iwan. "Pathology." In *Odoratus Sexualis: A Scientific and Literary Study of Sexual Scents and Erotic Perfumes*. New York: Panurge Press, 1934. Reprint, New York: AMS Press, 1976, 85–153; Boss, Medard. *Meaning and Content of Sexual Perversions: A Daseinanalytic Approach to the Psychopathology of the Phenomenon of Love*. Trans. Liese Lewis Abel. New York: Grune and Stratton, 1949; Califia, Pat. "Feminism and Sadomasochism." *Heresies* no. 12 ["Sex Issue"] 3:4 (1981), 30–34. Reprinted in *CoEvolution Quarterly* 33 (Spring 1982), 33–40; and

Stevi Jackson and Sue Scott, eds., *Feminism and Sexuality: A Reader*. New York: Columbia University Press, 1996, 230–37; Chauncey, George, Jr. (1983) "From Sexual Inversion to Homosexuality: The Changing Medical Conceptualization of Female Deviance." In Kathy Peiss and Christina Simmons, eds., *Passion and Power: Sexuality in History*. Philadelphia, Pa.: Temple University Press, 1989, 87–117; Davidson, Arnold I. "Sex and the Emergence of Sexuality." *Critical Inquiry* 14:1 (1987), 16–48; Davidson, Arnold I. "Styles of Reasoning, Conceptual History, and the Emergence of Psychiatry." In Peter Galison and David J. Strump, eds., *The Disunity of Science: Boundaries, Contexts, and Power*. Stanford, Calif.: Stanford University Press, 1996, 75–100. Reprinted, edited and abridged, as "Conceptual History and Conceptions of Perversions," in P&S2 (476–86); De Lauretis, Teresa. *The Practice of Love: Lesbian Sexuality and Perverse Desire*. Bloomington: Indiana University Press, 1994; de Sousa, Ronald. "Norms and the Normal." In Richard Wollheim, ed., *Freud: A Collection of Critical Essays*. Garden City, N.Y.: Anchor Books, 1974, 196–221; de Sousa, Ronald. "Perversion and Death." *The Monist* 86:1 (2003), 90–114; Denis, Lara. "Kant on the Wrongness of 'Unnatural' Sex." *History of Philosophy Quarterly* 16:2 (1999), 225–48; Ellis, Havelock. (1897–1928) *Studies in the Psychology of Sex*. New York: Random House, 1936; Ferguson, Frances. "Emma, or Happiness (or Sex Work)." In *Pornography, the Theory: What Utilitarianism Did to Action*. Chicago, Ill.: University of Chicago Press, 2004, 96–124; Finnis, John. "Natural Law and Unnatural Acts." *Heythrop Journal* 11 (1970), 365–87. Reprinted in HS (5–28); Fogel, Gerald I., and Wayne A. Myers, eds. *Perversions and Near-Perversions in Clinical Practice: New Psychoanalytic Perspectives*. New Haven, Conn.: Yale University Press, 1991; Foucault, Michel. (1976/1984/1984) *The History of Sexuality*. Vol. 1: *An Introduction*. Trans. Robert Hurley. New York: Vintage, 1978. Vol. 2: *The Use of Pleasure*. Trans. Robert Hurley. New York: Pantheon, 1985. Vol. 3: *The Care of the Self*. Trans. Robert Hurley. New York: Vintage, 1986; Frenkel, F. E. "Sex-Crime and Its Socio-Historical Background." *Journal of the History of Ideas* 25:3 (1964), 333–52; Gamman, Lorraine, and Merja Makinen. *Female Fetishism: A New Look*. London: Lawrence and Wishart, 1994. New York: New York University Press, 1995; Gates, Katharine. *Deviant Desires: Incredibly Strange Sex*. New York: Juno Books, 2000. Web site, <www.deviantdesires.com> [accessed 28 October 2004]; Goldberg, Arnold. *The Problem of Perversion: The View from Self Psychology*. New Haven, Conn.: Yale University Press, 1995; Goldman, Alan. "Plain Sex." *Philosophy and Public Affairs* 6:3 (1977), 267–87. Reprinted in HS (103–23); POS1 (119–38); POS2 (73–92); POS3 (39–55); POS4 (39–55); Gray, Robert. "Sex and Sexual Perversion." *Journal of Philosophy* 75:4 (1978), 189–99. Reprinted in POS1 (158–68); POS3 (57–66); POS4 (57–66); Groneman, Carol. *Nymphomania: A History*. New York: Norton, 2000; Grosz, Elizabeth. *Space, Time, and Perversion: Essays on the Politics of Bodies*. New York: Routledge, 1995; Hooker, Evelyn. "The Adjustment of the Male Overt Homosexual." *Journal of Projective Techniques* 21:1 (1957), 18–31. Reprinted in Hendrik Ruitenbeek, ed., *The Problem of Homosexuality in Modern Society*. New York: Dutton, 1963, 141–61; Hopkins, Patrick D. "Rethinking Sadomasochism: Feminism, Interpretation, and Simulation." *Hypatia* 9:1 (1994), 116–41. Reprinted in POS3 (189–214); Hopkins, Patrick D. "Simulation and the Reproduction of Injustice: A Reply." *Hypatia* 10:2 (1995), 162–70; Humber, James. "Sexual Perversion and Human Nature." *Philosophy Research Archives* 13 (1987–1988), 331–50. Reprinted in HS (153–72); Irvine, Janice. "Reinventing Perversion: Sex Addiction and Cultural Anxieties." *Journal of the History of Sexuality* 5:3 (1995), 429–50; Kadish, Mortimer R. "The Possibility of Perversion." *Philosophical Forum* 19:1 (1987), 34–53. Reprinted in POS2 (93–116); Kant, Immanuel. (ca. 1780) "Duties towards the Body in Respect of Sexual Impulse." In *Lectures on Ethics*. Trans. Louis Infield (1930). Indianapolis, Ind.: Hackett, 1963, 162–71. Reprinted in POS4 (199–205); STW (140–45); Kaplan, Louise J. "Women Masquerading as Women." In Gerald I. Fogel and Wayne A. Myers, eds., *Perversions and Near-Perversions in Clinical Practice: New Psychoanalytic Perspectives*. New Haven, Conn.: Yale University Press, 1991, 127–52; Ketchum, Sara Ann. "The Good, the Bad, and the Perverted: Sexual Paradigms Revisited." In Alan Soble, ed., *The Philosophy of Sex: Contemporary Readings*, 1st ed. Totowa, N.J.: Rowman and Littlefield, 1980, 139–57; Kupfer, Joseph. "Sexual Perversion and the Good." *The Personalist* 59:1 (1978), 70–77; Lee, J. Roger. "Sadomasochism: An Ethical Analysis." In Robert Stewart, ed., *Philosophical Perspectives on Sex and Love*. New York:

Oxford University Press, 1995, 125–37; Levy, Donald. "Perversion and the Unnatural as Moral Categories." *Ethics* 90:2 (1980), 191–202. Reprinted, revised, in POS1 (169–89); Lorand, Sandor, and Michael Balint. *Perversions: Psychodynamics and Therapy*. New York: Random House, 1956; Lotringer, Sylvère. *Overexposed: Treating Sexual Perversion in America*. New York: Pantheon, 1988; Margolis, Joseph. "Perversion." In *Negativities: The Limits of Life*. Columbus, Ohio: Merrill, 1975, 119–30; Merck, Mandy. *Perversions: Deviant Readings*. New York: Virago, 1993; Moll, Albert. (1931) *Perversions of the Sex Instinct*. New York: AMS Press, 1976; Money, John. *Lovemaps: Clinical Concepts of Sexual/Erotic Health and Pathology, Paraphilia, and Gender Transposition in Childhood, Adolescence, and Maturity*. New York: Irvington, 1986. Paperback reprint, Buffalo, N.Y.: Prometheus, 1988; Money, John. "Paraphilias." In John Money and Herman Musaph, eds., *Handbook of Sexology*. Amsterdam, Holland: Excerpta Medica, 1977, 917–28; Money, John. "Paraphilias: Phyletic Origins of Erotosexual Dysfunction." *International Journal of Mental Health* 10:2–3 (1981), 75–109; Moulton, Janice. "Sexual Behavior: Another Position." *Journal of Philosophy* 73:16 (1976), 537–46. Reprinted in HS (91–100); POS1 (110–18); POS2 (63–71); POS3 (31–38); POS4 (31–38); Nagel, Thomas, "Sexual Perversion." *Journal of Philosophy* 66:1 (1969), 5–17. Reprinted in P&S1 (247–60); POS1 (76–88). Reprinted, revised, in Thomas Nagel, *Mortal Questions*. Cambridge: Cambridge University Press, 1979, 39–52; Eugene F. Rogers, Jr., ed., *Theology and Sexuality: Classic and Contemporary Readings*. Oxford, U.K.: Blackwell, 2002, 125–36; and POS2 (39–51); POS3 (9–20); POS4 (9–20); STW (105–12); Neu, Jerome. "Freud and Perversion." In Earl E. Shelp, ed., *Sexuality and Medicine*, vol. 1. Dordrecht, Holland: Reidel, 1987, 153–84. Reprinted in Jerome Neu, ed., *The Cambridge Companion to Freud*. Cambridge: Cambridge University Press, 1991, 175–208; *A Tear Is an Intellectual Thing: The Meanings of Emotion*. New York: Oxford University Press, 2002, 144–65; STW (87–104); Neu, Jerome. "What's Wrong with Incest?" *Inquiry* 19:1 (1979), 27–39. Reprinted in *A Tear Is an Intellectual Thing: The Meanings of Emotion*. New York: Oxford University Press, 2002, 166–76; Nobus, Danny. "Over My Dead Body: On the Histories and Cultures of Necrophilia." In Robin Goodwin and Duncan Cramer, eds., *Inappropriate Relationships: The Unconventional, the Disapproved, and the Forbidden*. Mahwah, N.J.: Erlbaum, 2002, 171–89; Posner, Richard. "The Biology of 'Deviant' Sex." In *Sex and Reason*. Cambridge, Mass.: Harvard University Press, 1992, 98–108; Posner, Richard A., and Katharine B. Silbaugh. "Bestiality," "Necrophilia," and "Voyeurism." In *A Guide to America's Sex Laws*. Chicago, Ill.: University of Chicago Press, 1996, 207–12, 213–16, 233–37, respectively; Rich, Adrienne. "Compulsory Heterosexuality and Lesbian Existence." *Signs* 5:4 (1980), 631–60. Reprinted in *Blood, Bread, and Poetry: Selected Prose 1979–1985*. New York: Norton, 1986, 23–75; and Henry Abelove, Michèle Aina Barale, and David M. Halperin, eds., *The Lesbian and Gay Studies Reader*. New York: Routledge, 1993, 227–54; Rosen, Ismond. (1964, 1979) *Sexual Deviation*, 3rd ed. New York: Oxford University Press, 1996 (earlier editions titled *The Pathology and Treatment of Sexual Deviation: A Methodological Approach*); Rothenberg, Molly Anne, Dennis Foster, and Slavoj Žižek, eds. *Perversion and the Social Relation*. Durham, N.C.: Duke University Press, 2003; Ruddick, Sara. "On Sexual Morality." In James Rachels, ed., *Moral Problems: A Collection of Philosophical Essays*, 2nd ed. New York: Harper and Row, 1971, 16–34. Reprinted, revised, as "Better Sex," in Robert B. Baker and Frederick A. Elliston, eds., *Philosophy and Sex*, 1st ed. Buffalo, N.Y.: Prometheus, 1975, 83–104; P&S2 (280–99); Sade, The Marquis de. *The Complete Justine, Philosophy in the Bedroom, and Other Writings*. Trans. Richard Seaver and Austryn Wainhouse. New York: Grove Press, 1965; Samois Collective, eds. *Coming to Power: Writings and Graphics on Lesbian S/M*, 1st ed. Palo Alto, Calif.: Up Press, 1981. Revised eds., Boston, Mass.: Alyson, 1982, 1987; Shaffer, Jerome. "Sexual Desire." *Journal of Philosophy* 75:4 (1978), 175–89. Reprinted in SLF (1–12); Silverstein, Charles. "The Ethical and Moral Implications of Sexual Classification: A Commentary." *Journal of Homosexuality* 9:4 (1984), 29–38; Slote, Michael. "Inapplicable Concepts and Sexual Perversion." *Philosophical Studies* 28 (October 1975), 265–71. Reprinted in P&S1 (261–67); Soble, Alan. "Kant and Sexual Perversion." *The Monist* 86:1 (2003), 55–89; Solomon, Robert. "Sexual Paradigms." *Journal of Philosophy* 71:11 (1974), 336–45. Reprinted in HS (81–90); POS1 (89–98); POS2 (53–62); POS3 (21–29); POS4 (21–29); Spiecker, Ben, and Jan Steutel. "Paedophilia, Sexual Desire and Perversity."

Journal of Moral Education 26:3 (1997), 331–42; Steele, Valerie. *Fetish: Fashion, Sex and Power.* New York: Oxford University Press, 1996; Stoller, Robert. *Observing the Erotic Imagination.* New Haven, Conn.: Yale University Press, 1985; Stoller, Robert. *Pain and Passion: A Psychoanalyst Explores the World of S&M.* New York: Plenum, 1991; Stoller, Robert. *Perversion: The Erotic Form of Hatred.* New York: Random House, 1975; Stoller, Robert. "The Samuel Novey Lecture. Does Sexual Perversion Exist?" *Johns Hopkins Medical Journal* 134 (1974), 43–57; Vadas, Melinda. "Reply to Patrick Hopkins." *Hypatia* 10:2 (1995), 159–61. Reprinted in POS3 (215–17); Vannoy, Russell. "The Structure of Sexual Perversity." *Philosophy and Theology* 2:5 [disk supp. no. 1] (1988), 30–44. Reprinted in *Philosophy and Theology* 12:2 (2000), 255–73; and, with "Postscript" (1997; 371–72), in SLF (359–73); Welldon, Estela V. "Female Perversion and Hysteria." *British Journal of Psychotherapy* 11:3 (1995), 406–14; Wilder, Hugh. "The Language of Sex and the Sex of Language." In Alan Soble, ed., *The Philosophy of Sex: Contemporary Readings*, 1st ed. Totowa, N.J.: Rowman and Littlefield, 1980, 99–109. Reprinted in SLF (23–31); Williams, Christopher. "Perverted Attractions." *The Monist* 86:1 (2003), 115–40.

PHENOMENOLOGY. Phenomenology is the philosophical inquiry into the essential structures of pure experience. As such, it studies the act of experiencing, the object experienced, and the systematic correlations between them. When investigating **love**, for example, the phenomenologist reflects separately on the act of loving, the object loved (which might be a person or an idea, such as wisdom), and the relationship between them. Similarly, when investigating **sexual desire** for another person's body, the phenomenologist describes, analyzes, and correlates the act of desiring and the body as desired. These emotional acts and their objects are studied in relation to other kinds of acts and objects. The ultimate goal is to disclose the essential structures of all experience. In carrying out this project, the phenomenologist explains, for example, how affective experiences necessarily differ from cognitive experiences and how the objects of perception relate to the objects of imagination and understanding.

"Phenomenology" is also used in the general sense of any investigation into human experience. This general meaning differs in two crucial respects from the idea of phenomenology as a *philosophical* inquiry: Philosophical phenomenology concerns *pure* experience and aims at disclosing its *essential* features. This is how Edmund Husserl (1859–1938), the founder of the phenomenological movement, defined the inquiry, and this is how it was understood by Husserl's early followers (and critics), such as **Martin Heidegger** (1889–1976), Edith Stein (1891–1942), Eugen Fink (1905–1975), and Maurice Merleau-Ponty (1908–1961).

By "purity" Husserl means that the phenomenologist suspends all existential judgments in the description and analysis of experience. The phenomenologist must not base inquiries on any prior thesis about being or existence, because the aim is to grasp the object as it appears to the experiencing subject, thus disclosing the different modes and meanings of being. For example, the desired body is not posited as a biomechanical system or as a cultural construct but studied as it is given to the desiring person. Similarly, the act of desiring is not assumed to be a psychic state or an electrochemical process but is described as it is lived through. This process of purifying experience of existential theses is called *phenomenological* or *transcendental reduction*. In addition to this methodological step, the phenomenologist must also proceed from particular experiences to their possible variations. This step is necessary, because the aim is not a theory of any particular set of experiences but discovering the essential features of different types of experience and, ultimately, of all experience. The methodological step of proceeding from particular experiences to their variations is called *eidetic reduction*; it consists of the activity of varying particular experiences freely in the imagination.

Husserl's classical phenomenology contributed two starting points for subsequent phenomenological and postphenomenological accounts of sexual relations. First, he developed a powerful methodological and conceptual framework for the study of *living bodies* (*Leib*) as they are given in perception, affection, and sensation. Second, he provided a basic account of the *self-other relation* and its role in the constitution of objectivity. Both dimensions of Husserl's classical phenomenology greatly influenced his followers, not only Heidegger and Merleau-Ponty but also **Emmanuel Levinas** (1906–1995), Jean-Paul Sartre (1905–1980), and Simone de Beauvoir (1908–1986). The phenomenological account of embodiment also became central for later thinkers critically working on the phenomenological inheritance, such as **Michel Foucault** (1926–1984), Jacques Derrida (1930–2004), Luce Irigaray, and Julia Kristeva.

Husserl first introduced the concept of the living body (*Leib*) in his lectures in 1907 on objectivity and spatiality, *Ding und Raum* (*Thing and Space*). In the years 1912 to 1928, he worked on a thorough phenomenological explication of the phenomena of nature, animality, and spirituality. The result of these investigations, the second volume of *Ideen zu einer reinen Phänomenologie und phänomenologischen Philosophie* (*Ideas Pertaining to a Pure Phenomenology and to a Phenomenological Philosophy*), remained unpublished until 1952 but was known to Husserl's students and followers in manuscript form. The volume includes a detailed analysis of the different modes in which bodies are given to us in sensation, affection, and cognition. The second volume of *Ideen* and the later work *Die Krisis der europäischen Wissenschaften und die transzendentale Phänomenologie* (*The Crisis of European Sciences and Transcendental Phenomenology*) together constitute the conceptual source for existential-phenomenological studies of embodiment and sexuality.

Husserl's analysis of embodiment begins with the fact that we have two different kinds of material things given in our experience. We perceive mere *material things* (*Körper*), that is, pieces of inert matter, and we experience living bodies (*Leib*), that is, the bodies of animals and humans—the bodies of other people as well as our own. Having made this basic distinction, Husserl points out that we can relate to living bodies in two fundamentally different ways. On the one hand, we can take the attitude of the natural scientist and abstract all meaning, value, and purpose from the bodies that we study. Their position and movement therefore appear to us as the mere effects of external and internal causes. We can then try to explain and predict their behavior by subsuming them under general laws. On the other hand, we also relate to living bodies as meaningful, purposive agents—as *persons*, in Husserl's terminology. In this case, our own activity and interest are not in causally explaining or predicting the behavior of others but in responding to their movements and gestures. Transcendental and eidetic reduction allow us to study the characteristics of these two attitudes toward the living body, the scientific and the purposive, and the living body as it appears within each perspective.

In Husserl's analysis, living bodies are fundamentally distinguished from mere material, physical things by three features. First, living bodies are given to us as *fields of sensations*. Feelings of touch, contact, pressure, movement, tension, temperature, and pleasure and pain are localized on the surface of the body and in its different organs. Second, living bodies appear as immediate "starting points" of *spontaneous movement*. The body of an animal is the only thing the animal is able to move immediately, without moving something else first, and conversely, the animal needs its own body to move all other things. Third, living bodies function as *fixed points* in perceptions of direction, distance, and movement.

Other material things appear in relation to living bodies; they are near or far away, above or below, on the right-hand side or the left- of a living body. But living bodies, for Husserl, also take part in causal relations: They cause movements and react to external and internal changes. Thus they function as members in the nexus of causes and effects, and in this respect they are similar to material things.

On Husserl's account, then, the identification of the living body as a *living* body depends on its teleological features. He observes that the natural scientist works on the hypothesis that *all* features of this type can be explained as features of complex physical systems. The natural scientist posits a world of chemical and physical entities and processes "behind" the world of living bodies. This assumption about the primacy of the physical is challenged by Husserl, who argues that the natural scientific attitude and its physical world are secondary, dependent on something more profound. Indeed, they are based on the *personalistic attitude* in which we do not explain or predict the behavior of bodies but in which we express ourselves in our bodies and address other bodies. Originally, in perception, affection, and sensation, we see and hear living bodies as full of meaning. The body as an object of the biological and psychological sciences is actually something that can be "achieved" only by abstracting from these more profound objects of experience.

As long as we retain this personalistic attitude, living bodies are given to us as *expressive* wholes. The body's expressivity has two aspects. First, a living body appears as an expression of a conscious life: sensations, feelings, perceptions, desires, and cognitions. Second, the expressive relation holds also between the different organs, movements, and sections of the material body. Thus the body forms a unity that cannot be divided into discrete parts or pieces. It is an expressive whole, and its movements and organs contribute to the formation of its style. Bodies are, in this sense, similar to works of art, paintings, and novels: They can be classified as belonging to different *types*, but they cannot be conceived as interchangeable and substitutable for each other.

Thus, Husserl's contribution to the phenomenology of embodiment is twofold. First, he developed the distinction between the living body and the physical thing and the distinction between the two different attitudes we can take toward bodies: the natural scientific and the personalistic. Second, he argued that the natural scientific attitude and its physical objects are secondary, dependent on the primary personalistic attitude and its expressive objects. Husserl's distinctions and arguments influenced the later phenomenological discussion of sexuality and sexual differences. The concepts of *body scheme*, *body image*, and *sexual scheme* have their basis in Husserl's classical phenomenological investigations into expressive wholes.

Husserl's published works do not include any analysis of sexuality. In *Krisis*, he points out, however, that among the transcendental problems of origins and development there is "the problem of the sexes" (*Krisis*, 192; *Crisis*, 187–88). Husserl does not explore this topic but leaves it for future phenomenological research. Husserl's manuscripts on intersubjectivity contain working notes and fragmentary discussions about drives, reproduction, love, parenthood, and motherhood. Among these is a text, "Universale Teleologie" (written in 1933), which contains a sketch for an analysis of the sex drive (*Geschlechttrieb*). Husserl's concern here is to study the relations between procreation (*Zeugung*), development (*Entwicklung*), temporality, and sociality. To understand the basis of the temporality of social relations, he reflects on procreation and the attraction between males and females.

No comprehensive analyses of sexuality were provided by the near followers of Husserl, either. However, two important endeavors in this direction occurred in French phenomenology in the 1940s. There was, for one, Beauvoir. Influenced by Husserl and his existentialist followers, Beauvoir used the phenomenology of embodiment as the foundation for her feminist analysis of sexual relations in *Le deuxième sexe* (*The Second Sex*). Relying on phenomenology's conceptual and methodological framework, she argued that the issue of sexual difference is not only practical and political but involves all levels of human spirituality, from the arts and religion to science and metaphysics. Later philosophical inquiries into sexuality and sexual difference have often neglected the Husserlian aspects of Beauvoir's arguments. Only in the 1990s and beyond did scholars such as Debra Bergoffen, Jo-Ann Pilardi, Kristana Arp, Eleanore Holveck, and Sara Heinämaa finally demonstrate that Beauvoir's thought has roots in Husserl's discussions of persons and their bodies.

There was also, at the time, Maurice Merleau-Ponty, who developed a rich account of the sexuality of expressive living bodies in *Phénoménologie de la perception* (*Phenomenology of Perception*). Merleau-Ponty has been seen as an important early figure by many theorists of sex and sexuality, even though his interpretations of human behavior have also been criticized as androcentric and heterosexist. Thinkers as diverse as Irigaray, Martin Dillon, David Levin, Judith Butler, Iris Marion Young, and Elizabeth Grosz all base their discussions of sexual bodies partly on Merleau-Ponty's insights. In *Phénoménologie*, Merleau-Ponty uses the Husserlian concepts of "person" and "style" to account for the different aspects of human sexuality. He argues (in the fashion of Husserl) that causal explanations of sexual acts, sexual orientations, and sexual identities, even if useful and effective for certain purposes, cannot grasp the essence of sexuality but instead presupposes a prior understanding of it.

Merleau-Ponty's thesis holds for biological, physiological, psychological, sociological, anthropological, and historical explanations of the domain of human sexuality. The task of the philosopher is to investigate their common basis, that is, their shared presuppositions about the meaning of sexuality. This central line of Merleau-Ponty's argument adheres to the transcendental phenomenology that Husserl explicated: "To predict, or to recognize the objective forms of the composition of physical or chemical bodies and to predict accordingly—all this explains nothing but is in need of explanation. The only true way to explain something is to make it transcendentally understandable. Everything objective demands to be understood" (*Crisis*, 189). For Merleau-Ponty, sexuality belongs primarily to persons, to their living bodies, and not to natural objects or cultural artifacts:

> In so far as behavior is a form, in which "visual" and "tactile contents," sensibility and motility, appear only as inseparable moments, it remains inaccessible to causal thought and is capable of being apprehended only by another kind of thought, that which grasps it object as it comes into being and as it appears to the person experiencing it, with the atmosphere of meaning surrounding it, and which tries to infiltrate into that atmosphere in order to discover, behind scattered facts and symptoms, the subject's whole being. (*Phénoménologie*, 139–40; *Phenomenology*, 120)

The methodological claim is that sexual behavior, **sexual orientation**, and sexual identity must be investigated from the point of view of the experiencing subject. The philosophical question is not only, or primarily, how sexually aroused individuals relate to the object of their attraction, when studied from a third-person perspective. Rather, we must ask how the attractive other appears to the person who lives in desire. (This claim is also made, more recently, by British analytic philosopher **Roger Scruton** in *Sexual Desire*.) We must study how bodies are given to persons living through the different modes of sexual experience, from excitement and arousal to love and desire, from passionate affection to insensibility and indifference. Instead of explanatory causes, we need to track down the motivational relations between different levels of experience. From living bodies, sexual meaning disperses to other kinds of objects, both artificial and natural. So clothing and food, plants and animals, and material elements can have sexual significance.

In *Phénoménologie*, Merleau-Ponty studies two specific cases: a man who has lost his ability to see any sexual significance in the world, and a girl who has ceased to speak and eat because her love was forbidden. Merleau-Ponty argues that when studying these behaviors, we should not proceed by subsuming them under general laws about human or animal behavior. We must, instead, insert the behaviors into the totality of the person's life. Only as moments in a comprehensive totality can particular behaviors and experiences be compared with other modes. Sexuality is not a separate level of human life (a discrete "animal" or "primitive" level) but is inseparably intertwined with other modes of experience, including motility, perception, and cognition. "The genital life is geared to the whole life of the subject" (*Phénoménologie*, 185; *Phenomenology*, 158). In this way, a person's sexuality is an expression of his or her *manner* of relating to the world and its different objects. A person's erotic and sexual relations implement the very same *style* as his or her other actions and affections, intellectual, cognitive, perceptual, and emotional. We can even say that sexuality "condenses" a person's manner of relating to others. This should not be misunderstood along the lines of Freudian reductionism: Sexuality is not more primary or more basic than other modes of experience and behavior. It develops in a relation of mutual expression with them all (*Phénoménologie*, 186–87; *Phenomenology*, 160).

The concepts of manner and style make possible descriptions of both individual variations in sexuality and general types. We can speak about unique sexual styles of individual persons, about a general human type, as well as a masculine type and a feminine type (*Phénoménologie*, 182; *Phenomenology*, 156). We can also describe culturally or historically specific variations in sexuality and study them as modifications of the form that we find in our own life. The phenomenological framework is normative in the sense that it takes the self to be transcendentally primary: It claims that alien forms of sexual behavior and interaction can be recognized as sexual only on the basis of prior experience of one's *own* sexuality. Merleau-Ponty states this explicitly when he reflects on the relation between philosophy and anthropology in the late essay "Le philosophe et la sociologie" ("The Philosopher and Sociology"). He argues that a list of different erotic organizations of the body is only "an invitation to imagine, on the basis of our experience of the body, other techniques of the body. The technique which happens to be actualized in us can never be reduced to simply one among all possible techniques; for it is against this privileged experience, where we learn to know the body as a structuring principle, that we glimpse the other possibilities no matter how different from it they may be" (*Signes*, 126–27; *Signs*, 101).

See also Existentialism; Feminism, French; Fichte, Johann Gottlieb; Heidegger, Martin; Kolnai, Aurel; Poststructuralism; Scruton, Roger; Sexuality, Dimensions of

REFERENCES

Arp, Kristana. *The Bonds of Freedom: Simone de Beauvoir's Existentialist Ethics*. Chicago, Ill.: Open Court, 2001; Beauvoir, Simone de. (1949) *Le deuxième sexe I: Les faits et les mythes*. Paris: Gallimard, 1993. *The Second Sex*. (1953) Trans. Howard M. Parshley. Harmondsworth, U.K.: Penguin, 1987; Beauvoir, Simone de. (1949) *Le deuxième sexe II: L'expérience vécue*. Paris: Gallimard, 1991. *The Second Sex*. (1953) Trans. Howard M. Parshley. Harmondsworth, U.K.: Penguin, 1987; Bergoffen, Debra B. *The Philosophy of Simone de Beauvoir: Gendered Phenomenologies, Erotic*

Generosities. Albany: State University of New York Press, 1997; Butler, Judith. "Performative Acts and Gender Constitution: An Essay in Phenomenology and Feminist Theory." In Sue-Ellen Case, ed., *Performing Feminism: Feminist Critical Theory and Theatre*. Baltimore, Md.: Johns Hopkins University Press, 1990; Dillon, M. C. "Sex, Time, and Love: Erotic Temporality." *Journal of Phenomenological Psychology* 18:1 (1987), 33–48; Grosz, Elizabeth. *Volatile Bodies: Toward a Corporeal Feminism*. Bloomington: Indiana University Press, 1994; Heinämaa, Sara. "Simone de Beauvoir's Phenomenology of Sexual Difference." *Hypatia* 14:4 (1999), 114–32; Heinämaa, Sara. *Toward a Phenomenology of Sexual Difference: Husserl, Merleau-Ponty, Beauvoir*. Lanham, Md.: Rowman and Littlefield, 2003; Holveck, Eleanore. *Simone de Beauvoir's Philosophy of Lived Experience: Literature and Metaphysics*. Lanham, N.J.: Rowman and Littlefield, 2002; Husserl, Edmund. *Ding und Raum: Vorlesungen 1907. Husserliana XVI*. Ed. Ulrich Claesges. The Hague: Martinus Nijhoff, 1973. *Thing and Space: Lectures of 1907*. Trans. Richard Rojceicz. In *Collected Works*, vol. 7. Dordrecht, Holland: Kluwer, 1998; Husserl, Edmund. (1931) *Ideen zu einer reinen Phänomenologie und phänomenologischen Philosophie. Zweites Buch: Phänomenologische Untersuchungen zur Konstitution. Husserliana IV*. Ed. Marly Bimel. The Hague: Martinus Nijhoff, 1952. *Ideas Pertaining to a Pure Phenomenology and to a Phenomenological Philosophy. Second Book: Studies in the Phenomenology of Constitution* (1989). Trans. Richard Rojcewicz and André Schuwer. In *Collected Works*, vol. 3. Dordrecht, Holland: Kluwer, 1993; Husserl, Edmund. (1936–1937) *Die Krisis der europäischen Wissenschaften und die transzendentale Phänomenologie: Eine Einleitung in die phänomenologische Philosophie. Husserliana VI*. Ed. Walter Biemel. The Hague: Martinus Nijhoff, 1954. *The Crisis of European Sciences and Transcendental Phenomenology: An Introduction to Phenomenological Philosophy* (1970). Trans. David Carr. Evanston, Ill.: Northwestern University Press, 1988; Husserl, Edmund. "Universale Teleologie." In *Zur Phänomenologie der Intersubjektivität: Texte aus dem Nachlass. Dritter Teil: 1929–35. Husserliana XV*. Ed. Iso Kern. The Hague: Martinus Nijhoff, 1973, 593–97. "Universal Teleology" (1969). Trans. Marly Biemel. In Peter McCormick and Frederick A. Elliston, eds., *Husserl: Shorter Works*. Notre Dame: University of Notre Dame Press, 1981, 335–37; Irigaray, Luce. *Éthique la différence sexuelle*. Paris: Minuit, 1984. *An Ethics of Sexual Difference*. Trans. Carolyn Burke and Gillian C. Gill. Ithaca, N.Y.: Cornell University Press, 1993; Levin, David. *The Opening of Vision: Nihilism and the Postmodern Situation*. New York: Routledge, 1988; Merleau-Ponty, Maurice. (1945) *Phénoménologie de la perception*. Paris: Gallimard, 1993. *Phenomenology of Perception*. (1962) Trans. Colin Smith. New York: Routledge and Kegan Paul, 1995; Merleau-Ponty, Maurice. (1960) "Le philosophe et la sociologie." In *Signes*. Paris: Gallimard, 1998, 123–42. "The Philosopher and Sociology" (1964). In *Signs*. Trans. Richard C. McCleary. Evanston, Ill.: Northwestern University Press, 1987, 98–113; Pilardi, Jo-Ann. *Simone de Beauvoir: Writing the Self. Philosophy Becomes Autobiography*. Westport, Conn.: Praeger, 1999; Scruton, Roger. *Sexual Desire: A Moral Philosophy of the Erotic*. New York: Free Press, 1986; Young, Iris Marion. *Throwing Like a Girl and Other Essays in Feminist Philosophy and Social Theory*. Bloomington: Indiana University Press, 1990.

Sara Heinämaa

ADDITIONAL READING

Anderson, Clelia Smyth, and Yolanda Estes. "The Myth of the Happy Hooker: Kantian Moral Reflections on a Phenomenology of Prostitution." In Stanley G. French, Wanda Teays, and Laura M. Purdy, eds., *Violence against Women: Philosophical Perspectives*. Ithaca, N.Y.: Cornell University Press, 1998, 152–58; Bartky, Sandra Lee. *Femininity and Domination: Studies in the Phenomenology of Oppression*. New York: Routledge, 1990; Beauvoir, Simone de. (1959) *Brigitte Bardot and the Lolita Syndrome*. Trans. Bernard Frechtman. New York: Reynal, 1960; Beauvoir, Simone de. (1951–1952) "Must We Burn Sade?" Trans. Annette Michelson. In Austryn Wainhouse and Richard Seaver, comps., *The Marquis de Sade: The 120 Days of Sodom and Other Writings*. New York: Grove Press, 1966, 3–64; Beauvoir, Simone de. *Pour une morale de l'ambiguïté*. Paris: Gallimard, 1947. *The Ethics of Ambiguity*. Trans. Bernard Frechtman. Secaucus, N.J.: Citadel Press/Philosophical

Library, 1948; Bogart, John H. "Commodification and Phenomenology: Evading Consent in Theory Regarding Rape." *Legal Theory* 2:3 (1996), 253–64; Cohen, Richard. "Merleau-Ponty, the Flesh, and Foucault." *Philosophy Today* 28 (Winter 1984), 329–38; Derrida, Jacques. *La voix et le phénomène: Introduction au problème du signe dans la phénoménologie de Husserl.* Paris: Quadrige/PUF, 1967. *Speech and Phenomenon and Other Essays on Husserl's Theory of Signs.* Trans. David Allison and Newton Garver. Evanston, Ill.: Northwestern University Press, 1973; Dillon, Martin C. *Beyond Romance.* New York: State University of New York Press, 2001; Dillon, Martin C. "Erotic Desire." *Research in Phenomenology* 15 (1985), 145–63; Dillon, Martin C. "Merleau-Ponty on Existential Sexuality: A Critique." *Journal of Phenomenological Psychology* 11:1 (1980), 67–81; Dillon, Martin C. "Sex, Time, and Love: Erotic Temporality." *Journal of Phenomenological Psychology* 18:1 (1987), 33–48. Reprinted in SLF (313–25); Dillon, Martin C. "Toward a Phenomenology of Love and Sexuality: An Inquiry into the Limits of the Human Situation as They Condition Loving." *Soundings* 63:4 (1980), 341–60; Fink, Eugen. (1930–1933) *VI. Cartesianische Meditation: Teile 1–2. Husserliana: Dokumente, Band II/1-2.* Ed. Guy van Kerckhoven, H. Ebeling, and J. Holl. Dordrecht, Holland: Kluwer, 1988. *The Sixth Cartesian Meditation: The Idea of a Transcendental Theory of Method.* Trans. Ronald Bruzina. Bloomington: Indiana University Press, 1995; Fisher, Linda, and Lester Embree, eds. *Feminist Phenomenology. Contributions to Phenomenology*, vol. 40. Dordrecht, Holland: Kluwer, 2000; Foucault, Michel. (1966) *Les mots et les choses: archéologie des sciences humaines.* Paris: Gallimard, 1990. *The Order of Things: An Archaeology of the Human Sciences.* Trans. Alan Sheridan. New York: Vintage, 1970; Gier, Nicholas F. *Wittgenstein and Phenomenology: A Comparative Study of the Later Wittgenstein, Husserl, Heidegger, and Merleau-Ponty.* Albany: State University of New York Press, 1981; Heidegger, Martin. (1927) *Sein und Zeit.* Tübingen, Ger.: Max Niemeyer, 1993. *Being and Time.* Trans. John Macquarrie and Edward Robinson. Oxford, U.K.: Blackwell, 1992; Heinämaa, Sara. "On Luce Irigaray's Inquiries into Intersubjectivity: Between the Feminine Body and Its Other." In Maria Cimitile and Elaine Miller, ed., *Returning to Irigaray.* Albany: State University of New York Press, 2005; Heinämaa, Sara. "Woman—Nature, Product, Style? Rethinking the Foundations of Feminist Philosophy of Science." In Lynn Hankinson Nelson and Jack Nelson, eds., *Feminism, Science, and the Philosophy of Science.* Dordrecht, Holland: Kluwer, 1997, 289–308; Hunter, C. K. "The Problem of Fichte's Phenomenology of Love." *Idealistic Studies* 6:2 (1976), 178–90; Husserl, Edmund. (1913) *Ideen zu einer reinen Phänomenologie und phänomenologischen Philosophie. Erstes Buch: Allgemeine Einführung in die reine Phänomenologie. Husserliana III.* Ed. Walter Biemel. The Hague: Martinus Nijhoff, 1950. *Ideas Pertaining to a Pure Phenomenology and to a Phenomenological Philosophy. First Book: General Introduction to a Pure Phenomenology.* Trans. Fred Kersten. *Collected Works*, vol. 2. The Hague: Martinus Nijhoff, 1982; Husserl, Edmund. "Universal Teleology." Trans. Paul Piccone. *Telos*, no. 4 (Fall 1969), 176–80; Irigaray, Luce. (1984) "The Invisible of the Flesh: A Reading of Merleau-Ponty, *The Visible and the Invisible*, 'The Intertwining—The Chiasm.'" In *An Ethics of Sexual Difference.* Trans. Carolyn Burke and Gillian C. Gill. Ithaca, N.Y.: Cornell University Press, 1993, 154–84; Irigaray, Luce. *J'aime à toi: Esquisse d'une félicité dans l'histoire.* Paris: Grasset, 1992. *I Love to You: Sketch for a Felicity within History.* Trans. Alison Martin. New York: Routledge, 1996; Kosok, Michael. "The Phenomenology of Fucking." *Telos*, no. 8 (1971), 64–76; Krell, David. "Merleau-Ponty on 'Eros' and 'Logos.'" *Man and World* 7 (1974), 37–51; Kristeva, Julia. *La révolution du langage poétique.* Paris: Éditions du Seuil, 1974. *Revolution in Poetic Language.* Trans. Margaret Waller. New York: Columbia University Press, 1984; Levinas, Emmanuel. (1947) *Le temps et l'autre.* Paris: Quadrige/PUF, 1994. *Time and Other.* Trans. R. A. Cohen. Pittsburgh, Pa.: Duquesne University Press, 1987; O'Brien, Wendy, and Lester Embree, eds. *The Existential Phenomenology of Simone de Beauvoir. Contributions to Phenomenology*, vol. 43. Dordrecht, Holland: Kluwer, 2001; Sartre, Jean-Paul. "La transcendance de l'ego: Esquisse d'une decription phénoménologique." *Recherches Philosophiques* 6 (1936–1937). *The Transcendence of the Ego: An Existentialist Theory of Consciousness.* Trans. Forrest Williams and Robert Kirkpatrick. New York: Hill and Wang, 1960; Schwartz, Michael Alan, and Osborne P. Wiggins. "Understanding and Interpretation in Psychiatry." In Jennifer Radden, ed., *The Philosophy of Psychiatry: A Companion.* New York: Oxford University Press, 2004, 351–63; Solomon, Robert

C. (1981) *Love: Emotion, Myth, and Metaphor*. Buffalo, N.Y.: Prometheus, 1990; Stein, Edith. *Zum Problem der Einfühlung*. Halle, Ger.: Buchdrucheri des Weisenhauses, 1917. Reprinted, Munich, Ger.: Kaffke, 1980. *On the Problem of Empathy* (1964). Trans. Waltraut Stein. In *The Collected Works of Edith Stein*, vol. 3. Washington, D.C.: Institute of Carmelite Studies, 1989; Stoller, Sylvia, and Helmuth Vetter, ed. *Phänomenologie und Geschlechterdifferenz*. [*Phenomenology and Sexual Difference*] Vienna, Austria: Universitätsverlag, 1997; Welton, Donn, ed. *The Body: Classic and Contemporary Readings*. Oxford, U.K.: Blackwell, 1999; Zahavi, Dan. *Husserl's Phenomenology*. Stanford, Calif.: Stanford University Press, 2003; Zimmerman, Michael E. "Ontical Craving versus Ontological Desire." In Babette Babich, ed., *From Phenomenology to Thought, Errancy, and Desire: Essays in Honor of William Richardson, S.J.* Dordrecht, Holland: Kluwer, 1995, 501–23.

PHILOSOPHY OF SEX, OVERVIEW OF. The philosophy of sex, like the philosophy of science, art, law, or medicine (and so forth), is the study of the concepts, propositions, and arguments surrounding its central protagonist, which is in this case "sex." The breadth of the philosophy of sex is demonstrated by the variety of topics it investigates: **abortion, contraception, acquaintance rape, pornography, sexual harassment,** and **objectification,** to name a few. The philosophy of sex begins with a picture of a privileged pattern of relationship, in which two adult heterosexuals **love** each other, are faithful to each other within a formal **marriage,** and look forward to procreation and family. Philosophy of sex, as the Socratic scrutiny (perhaps best displayed in **Plato**'s [427–347 BCE] *Republic*) of our sexual practices and beliefs, challenges, or at least raises pointed questions about, this privileged pattern by exploring the possible virtues, and not only the possible vices, of group sex, **adultery, prostitution, incest, pedophilia, homosexuality, bestiality, masturbation, sadomasochism,** and promiscuous, **casual sex** with anonymous strangers. Doing so provides the same illumination about sex that is provided when the philosophies of science, art, and law probe the privileged pictures in their own domains. We usually find out that what we have been in the habit of believing is (partially) wrong or not well grounded in reason or experience, or we uncover better reasons why what we have been in the habit of believing is in fact right. If neither, we go to a flick.

It has been contended that the philosophy of X is, without exception, less exciting and satisfying than X itself. True enough, **sexual activity** can be and often is exciting and satisfying, and it is exciting and satisfying in ways that no purely intellectual endeavor could be. The body is the locale of the lived, experiential, phenomenological "bottom," we might say. But comparing the philosophy of X with X is unfair. Many people make lots of money doing *law*, for example, while very few people make any money to brag about doing the *philosophy* of law. (You would have to be an H.L.A. Hart [1907–1992] or a Joel Feinberg [1926–2004].) Yet that does not mean that the philosophy of law brings no joy of any kind to those who study it. If you ever abort your coupling *in medias res*, not merely to answer the insistent telephone or change the crying baby's diaper but to ask yourself and your partner, "What, now, is *really* going on here?" (a candidate scene for a Woody Allen movie), you might be surprised how *interesting* the question and its multifarious answers are. Much of the philosophy of sex yields this intellectual excitement, and if the issues are pursued with determination, satisfaction sometimes results and, as a bonus, you do not even have to be in bed while doing it. You could easily be in the kitchen, sneaking that cold, left-over slice of pizza. Further, the philosophy of sex, unlike the philosophy of *anything else*, can be libidinally satisfying, that is, can provide precisely the joys of sex, at least some of them (see **Sigmund Freud** [1856–1939], "Infantile Genital Organization"). Thinking about sex, rethinking your thoughts about sex, writing down your thoughts about sex, and revising your writings about sex (especially if you are tapping away on that sexy, brand-spanking-new laptop you had been eyeballing for months)—all this thinking and writing about sex *is* sex. True, it may be one-person (masturbatory) sex, but that it *is* sex follows from more general principles. Paramours know well that talking about sex, like **flirting** and dancing, can be as delicious as foreplay, and *is* foreplay (except when it is unwanted sex talk, in which case it transubstantiates into sexual harassment). No matter how long and deeply you think and write about the law, by contrast, you will never actually be *doing* law and never actually bank that six-figure income. Nor does meditating about torts and contracts seem suited to tapping into any erotic undercurrent.

The practitioners of the philosophy of sex focus, as do other philosophers, on conceptual, metaphysical, normative, and historical questions, although it is not always possible to keep these four areas absolutely distinct. For example, conceptual and normative matters in the philosophy of sex, as they are in the philosophy of law, are often intertwined with each other.

The Concepts of Sex. *Conceptual philosophy of sex* analyzes the central notions that apply to sex, which include **sexual desire**, sexual activity, sexual pleasure, sexual arousal, sexual satisfaction, and others. In part, "analyzing" a notion means trying to *define* a term, going beyond often misleading, vague, or incomplete dictionary definitions. From another perspective, analyzing a notion means trying to discover the *essence* of the thing being spoken about (an essential feature is one without which it would not be what it is) and figuring out what features of that thing *make it* what it is or account for its being what it is. For example, what is it about a feeling that makes it a *sexual* sensation instead of some other kind of feeling? We can ask similar questions about the other core concepts: What features of a desire (activity, arousal, etc.) make it a sexual desire and not a different type of desire? And what would have to be subtracted or removed from the desire for it no longer to *be* a sexual desire? What makes an act sexual? A touch on the arm might be a friendly pat, an assault, or part of a sexual exchange; the physical features alone—that fingers, pieces of epidermis, come in contact with another piece of epidermis, the other person's arm—do not distinguish a friendly, consoling pat from a sexual event or a request for attention. One way of making the point is to say that the arm-touch is ambiguous (or, having many meanings, it exhibits "polysemicity"): It could be any of these, and the touch by itself does not pick out one and only one. Another way of making the point is to say that in itself the arm-touch means *nothing* at all, instead of anything and everything; it is not that it has ambiguous meaning, but rather no meaning, and will not have any meaning until other features or factors are brought onto the scene or taken into account. (Of course, analysis does not have to be carried out in terms of necessary and sufficient conditions. We can look also or instead at *family resemblances*—or the lack of resemblance—among sexual phenomena and between sexual phenomena and other human experiences and activities. See Hamilton.)

There are two other sorts of conceptual question. First, what are the logical links among all these central notions? It is one thing to be able to say, with some precision, what sexual desire and sexual activity are. It is quite another thing to take note of, if not emphasize, that in analyzing sexual desire or sexual activity one is mentioning (or invoking) one or more of the other central notions. Then we should ask: Must this be so? Must the analysis of this particular sexual concept rest or depend on the analysis of some other sexual concept, or could we analyze it independently of that other concept? For instance, it has been proposed that "sexual act" be analyzed as all and only those acts that produce sexual pleasure (see

Gray, 61). In this case, it is suggested that the act's feature of producing sexual pleasure *makes* the act sexual; and in the absence of yielding sexual pleasure, the act is not or would not be a sexual act but some other kind of act (if it is still an act).

On Gray's analysis, "sexual activity" logically depends on "sexual pleasure." This means that we cannot say, which we *might* have wanted to say (in the analysis of sexual pleasure), that sexual pleasure is exactly that pleasure produced by sexual acts. Further, if "sexual act" depends on "sexual pleasure," we do not know how to identify sexual acts until or unless we can, in turn, identify sexual pleasures and distinguish them from other bodily pleasures (not an easy task, and we are prohibited from ever appealing to "sexual act"). So one conceptual question that arises here, if "sexual pleasure" turns out to be intractable, is whether a coherent analysis of sexual activity can be devised that does not, *pace* Gray, mention sexual pleasure. Is not an answer to that question sufficiently valuable and fascinating to warrant pursuing it even at the cost of *coitus interruptus*? But make sure, in this quest, to heed the advice of **Søren Kierkegaard** (1813–1855): "[H]e who would end with the inexplicable had best begin with it and say not a word more, so as not to become an object of suspicion" (50).

Defining "sexual act" is not an idle, "academic" question or puzzle. It also has practical significance. Precise definitions of "sexual act" (and the other sexual concepts) are needed for social scientific studies of sexual behavior (How often do people engage in sex? What do they get out of it, or want to get out of it?) and for arriving at moral judgments or enacting legislation about child sexual abuse, harassment, **rape**, adultery, and other things. Mentioning these sexual phenomena brings us to yet another type of conceptual question in the philosophy of sex, questions that involve "derivative" sexual concepts. These questions have to do not with what makes an act, desire, or feeling sexual but with what makes it the type of sexual act, desire, or feeling it is. How should "rape" be defined? (See, for example, Bogart.) What are the differences, if any, between obtaining sex through physical force and obtaining it by offering money? Does one, but not the other, undermine **consent**? Is one, but not the other, coercive? Understanding these derivative sexual concepts presupposes an understanding of the core concepts, but they are also the subject of analysis in their own right. Defining or finding the essential features of rape, date rape, incest, harassment, **sexual addiction**, **jealousy**, flirting, **seduction**, **sexual orientation**, **sexual perversion**, **fantasy**, prostitution, pornography, masturbation, objectification, sadomasochism (and a host of other phenomena) is no elementary matter and occupies the time and energy of a platoon of analytic philosophers of sex.

The Metaphysics of Sex. *Metaphysical philosophy of sex* deals with ontological, epistemological, theological, and anthropological matters. What is the place of sexuality in human nature, or how does it fit in with the rest of our nature? Is it an important part? Some say it is on a par with the cranium although somewhat less important than the patellae. What are the relationships between sexuality, emotion, and cognition? Is sex a brute, instinctual drive, a thoughtless reflex (men *are* panting dogs; see **Catharine MacKinnon**, *Only Words*, 21), or is it decisively informed by beliefs, attitudes, and visions of the *summum bonum* or *summum malum*? Some men, we have been told by Freud, cannot perform sexually with a woman unless they mentally attribute "sluthood" (as opposed to "Maryhood") to their partner; simply being in the presence of a willing, attractive, young female is apparently not biology enough ("On the Universal Tendency to Debasement"). The astute philosophical historian Paul Robinson expresses this dilemma well (xi):

> David Halperin [a classical scholar and proponent of social constructionism] says somewhere, "There is no orgasm without ideology." I know what he

> means and even agree, up to a point: every sexual act has an imaginative dimension; it exists in the mind as well as the flesh, and thus it engages our socially constructed ideas about gender, desire, the self, and even politics. . . . But sex is never just ideological; it is also a rudely physical, indeed animal, need for the pleasure we get doing particular things with particular parts of our bodies. This is as true for intellectuals as it is for anyone else. Sex is an often humbling experience for intellectuals [including philosophers and historians of sex] precisely because it reminds them, so unconditionally, of the extent to which they are not pure Geist.

Here we encounter a rudimentary version of the theory that sex is as much, even if not totally, a matter of the brain as it is of the loins. No wonder "Sex in the Head" is such a popular title (see Cameron; Morgan; Nussbaum.) *Or*, we could equivalently make the point, it is as much about the loins, although not totally, as it is about the brain (like the seesaw with essentialism on one side and **social constructionism** on the other).

Indeed, the relationship between the stirrings of the loins and the stirrings of the soul is not, for us (postlapsarian creatures that we are), one to one. For Adam and Eve, as perfect as humans could be, there was complete harmony between the desire of the mind or soul and the activity of the groin: Genital tingles and arousal, erection and lubrication, occurred *if and only if* the mind, still in charge of such matters (see the homunculi in *Everything You Wanted to Know about Sex*), decided it was time to engage in coitus and to procreate—at least in **Saint Augustine**'s (354–430) version of the story (*City of God*, bk. 14, chap. 24). But after the Fall, as part of the punishment meted out by God, all bets are off: Desire rages without any groinly response (the fate primarily of the elderly), and groinly activity bubbles forth while the mind tries in vain to control and subdue the disobedient body parts (the fate primarily of the young). Michel Montaigne (1533–1592) observed this disparity well:

> People are right to notice the unruly liberty of this member [the penis], obtruding so importunately when we have no use for it [say, on the *bema*], and failing so importunately when we have the most use for it [with the star of our dreams], and struggling for mastery so imperiously with our will, refusing with so much pride and obstinacy our solicitations, both mental and manual. (72)

Augustine, too, made much of the disparity, even suggesting that as punishment it was exquisitely fitting (*City of God*, 14.15, 14.16; *On Marriage and Concupiscence*, bk. 1, chap. 7).

Metaphysical philosophy of sex also raises the *in medias res* question: What, after all, is the meaning or significance of sex for the person, the family, the downstairs neighbor, the species, the *entire cosmos*? What is sex all about, anyway? That sexual desire is a crude, hormone-driven instinct implanted by a God or Nature red in tooth and claw acting in the service of the species, and that it has a profound spiritual dimension as the human's contribution to the ongoing work of creation, working together with God or Nature as friends do in pursuing a common goal, are but two—and not necessarily incompatible—views. Perhaps, as many have said, the significance of sexuality is little different from that of eating, breathing, bleeding, belching, perspiring, passing gas, and defecating. It (meaning tumescence, engorgement, ejaculation, orgasm) is merely another physiological process with which we, as minds trapped in a hunk of flesh, have to come to grips, or at least partially repress our knowledge of. But maybe instead, or in addition, as some hope, our sexual natures are partly constitutive of our moral personalities and identities. The meaning and importance of sex has been a perennially popular topic among the religiously inclined, and to get a glimpse of the variety of divinely inspired metaphysics that have recommended themselves to eminently rational people, one should delve into **Islam**, **Tantrism**, **Buddhism**, **Jainism**, **Hinduism**, and the Judeo-Christian religions, including Branch Davidianism. (Murray Davis presents, in his bravely titled *Smut*, an engaging account of "Jehovanist," "Naturalist," and "Gnostic" metaphysics of sex. *Rosemary's Baby* is also enlightening.) This is not to imply that Benthamitic hedonistic utilitarianism is not also a theological metaphysics of the sexual, albeit dressed up in (or stripped down to) its secular lingerie.

Sometimes the metaphysics of sex is absolutely darling, as in Joycelyn Elders's (once the surgeon general of the United States, canned by Bill Clinton) splendid defense of, in effect, thinking and writing about sex, or doing the philosophy of sex: "Masturbation, practiced consciously or unconsciously, cultivates in us a humble elegance—an awareness that we are part of a larger natural system, the passions and rhythms of which live on in us." But the metaphysical answers are not always comforting or spiritually uplifting. What you might stumble across while munching postcoitally on that pizza in the kitchen might induce you to put down that treat, at least momentarily. From Christianity, as we are reminded time and again by **Bertrand Russell** (1872–1970) and other advanced thinkers (e.g., **Albert Ellis** [1913–]; contrast MacKinnon, *Toward*, 132 ff.), we inherited a powerful sex-negativity, for which there is, it must be admitted, some evidence. Consider the chilling words of the traditional whipping boy Augustine:

> A man turns to good use the evil of concupiscence . . . when he bridles and restrains its rage . . . and never relaxes his hold upon it except when intent on offspring, and then controls and applies it to the carnal generation of children . . . not to the subjection of the spirit to the flesh in a sordid servitude. (*On Marriage and Concupiscence*, 1.9)

> What friend of wisdom and holy joys, who, being married . . . would not prefer, if this were possible, to beget children without this lust, so that in this function of begetting offspring the members created for this purpose should not be stimulated by the heat of lust, but should be actuated by his volition, in the same way as his other members [for example, his arms] serve him for their respective ends? (*City of God*, 14.16)

Augustine was not the only scholar in the history of philosophy who bemoaned the sexual impulse and wished it could be eradicated. Secular philosopher **Immanuel Kant** (1724–1804), famous for his brilliant transcendental deductions, equally feared the body: "Inclinations [including the sexual] . . . , as sources of needs, are so far from having an absolute value to make them desirable for their own sake that it must rather be the universal wish of every rational being to be wholly free from them" (Ak 4:428). The twentieth century, too, knows its own purveyors of doom. "A metaphysical illusion resid[es] in the heart of sexual desire," **Roger Scruton** informs us (95), warning us that sexuality is full of tricks and deception. Sexual passion misleads us: It makes us seem to be ontologically greater or more than we are, transcendental selves (gods, even) rather than mere material beings like ants (130). Plato, in the *Symposium*, had also warned us about deceptive desire: What we think we seek (the hottie or honey across the room) is not *really* what we want; our *eros* for bodies is, underneath it all, *eros* for timeless Truth and unadulterated **Beauty** (*Symp.*, 206 ff.). Plato at least puts a positive spin (in his own mind) on the deception, but not **Arthur Schopenhauer** (1788–1860): The beauty of the object of sexual desire is Nature's way of tricking a man (a male) into thinking that satisfaction of his erotic love for his beloved is for his own individual good. To the contrary, sexuality benefits only the species, for the sake of which Nature manipulates and makes mere use of the male, who, after the delightful but brief event, finds his resources committed to the next generation instead of his stamp collection (vol. 2, 538–40). Schopenhauer's cruel cynicism is at least a refreshing antidote to the banal philosophical sentimentality that regards sexual activity as "metaphysical exploration, knowing the body and person of another as a map or microcosm of the very deepest reality, a clue to its nature and purpose" (so opines Harvard University's acclaimed Robert Nozick [1938–2002], 67).

Values and Sex. Normative philosophy of sex explores the bewildering questions of **sexual ethics.** In what circumstances is it morally permissible (or wrong, obligatory, supererogatory) to engage in sexual activity or experience sexual pleasure? With whom? For what purpose? With which body parts or orifices? For how long? What about the Super Bowl? The historically central answers come from **Aristotle**'s (384–322 BCE) **virtue ethics, Thomas Aquinas**'s (1224/25–1274) Natural Law theory, the ethics of respect devised by the deontological Kant, and the utilitarianism (or **liberalism**) of John Stuart Mill (1806–1873). These ethical positions can be and have been applied (casuistically) to a wide variety of sexual subjects. Normative philosophy of sex also addresses legal, social, and political issues. Should society steer people in the direction of heterosexuality, marriage, and family? Both **feminism** and **Marxism**, let alone conservative social and political philosophy, have applied themselves to this question. Is it within the proper province of the law to regulate sexual conduct by, say, prohibiting prostitution, gay and lesbian sex, or pornography? The U.S. Supreme Court has issued rulings about these matters. (See **Law, Sex and the; Privacy.**)

Normative philosophy of sex includes nonethical value questions as well. What is good sex? What is its contribution to the good life? Indeed, there are five different questions that may be asked about sexual acts, only three of which are normative, while the others are often confused with the normative. First, we can inquire about the morality of the act. Second, we can examine its nonmoral quality: Does it provide pleasure (nonmoral goodness) or is the act tedious, boring, and unenjoyable (nonmoral badness)? Third is the pragmatic evaluation of sexual acts, similar to but broader than the evaluation of its nonmoral quality. Some sexual acts are medically and psychologically safe or have desired consequences (for example, revenge); others are medically or psychologically unsafe or have undesired consequences (for example, vulnerability to blackmail). These pragmatic factors may have or generate moral or nonmoral value or disvalue. Fourth, we can ask about the legality of a sexual act: Is it legally permissible or prohibited? This varies by jurisdiction, and although there are some strong social and historical connections between law and morality, they are conceptually distinct (see Kramer). Finally, sexual acts can be evaluated as biologically or psychologically natural or unnatural ("perverted"). For some people that an act is a sexual perversion necessarily makes it immoral, but that is, arguably, a subtle mistake. Sexual ethics is a topic that many writers and parents find compelling, although some make sure the dishes are done first.

The Historical Frontier. Finally, there is the *history of the philosophy of sex,* in which philosophers carefully explicate the writings of significant philosophical figures from the past, attempting to fashion into a coherent whole what may look like an inconsistent or loosely structured set of widely scattered propositions, or trying to provide a useful guide to the thought of various thinkers to find out what, if anything, we might learn either about the times in which they wrote or about our own time. (For paradigm cases of the history of philosophy of sex, see Denis's two essays on Kant.) We can use the philosophy of the past as a mirror or a lamp to see ourselves in a new light or more clearly—as long as we get the exegesis and the translations right. There are still plenty of puzzles waiting to be worked on in the philosophy of sex of Plato, Aristotle, Augustine, **David Hume** (1711–1776), Kant, Russell, and Annie Sprinkle. Another sort of project in the history of the philosophy of sex is tracing an idea, theme, argument, or problem through a series of thinkers, showing in which ways the theme stays the same and in which ways it gets modified along the way, until it emerges into the present age. One can, for example, follow the idea of sexual desire—its nature, effects, causes, dynamics, and value—from Plato and the other ancients through **René Descartes** (1596–1650), Hume, Kant, and **G.W.F. Hegel** (1770–1831) to Jean-Paul Sartre (1905–1980) and Jerome Shaffer. (Keith Thomas has written an absorbing essay on the double standard.) It is not farfetched to say that of all four areas in the philosophy of sex, it is the history of the philosophy of sex that is the least developed and deserves the most attention. In the humble prophetic estimate of one Serbian philosopher, Ladislaw Windboitel (1644–1701), we have by now heard enough, if not too much, from ethicists prompting us about what we should or should not do; from analysts defining exactly what it is that we are doing when we do what we should or should not do; and from metaphysicians telling us scary or cheery "just so" bedtime stories about what we are really doing when we do what we should or should not do.

Despite falling occasionally into flippancy and insufferability, philosophers of sex do take their scholarly work seriously. In an essay on **Friedrich Nietzsche** (1844–1900) and *eros* published in 2000, Fordham University philosopher Babette Babich issued some complaints about late-twentieth-century philosophy of sex. At the beginning of her essay she wrote, "Although in what follows I address the question of erotic love (that is: the domain of sexuality), it is important to emphasise that I will offer as oblique an approach to the issue of eros and sex as any other philosophical discussion. In philosophic reviews of the erotic (particularly analytic treatments)[1] abstraction invariably ablates the wings of the god" (159). In note 1, Babich shares her gut feelings about the philosophy of sex:

> For examples of this fatal banality, consider Roger Scruton's chillingly asexual, monotononic [*sic*] account or accounts by Robert C. Solomon or Alan Soble, or indeed Irving Singer's three volume treatment, or, in German, the tome by the one-man encyclopedia, Hermann Schmitz, or else Niklaus Luhmann's patently oxymoronic "codification" of *Love as Passion*. That these authors are male, that men are (in fact and despite the mythologization of male desire to the contrary) typically uninterested in the ideal of eros and even less interested in the nature of the erotic (which is always all about the Other) but write utterly incidental books (none of the aforenamed specialises in the subject: their books are extras, written on the fly, for fun, impotent efforts delivering nothing of philosophic relevance on a necessarily dyadic topic), all this is doubtless part but not the whole of the monological drabness of such philosophic studies of love.

It is not obviously true, however, that the male scholars mentioned here wrote their books "on the fly, for fun" and that none "specializes" in the philosophy of sex, at least regarding the American scholars **Irving Singer** and Robert Solomon. And if Scruton meant his book to be an exercise in fun, he failed miserably—*Sexual Desire* is erudition front to back. What is *bewitching* about this commentary on the practitioners of the philosophy of sex is the metaphorical sexual criticism contained in the phrase "impotent efforts delivering nothing." Male philosophers of sex are shooting blanks, and because they lack viable sperm they "deliver nothing," achieving no Platonic procreation of ideas. Further, being impotent, they cannot even sport an erection, in which case no *penetrating* analysis will be forthcoming from them.

It may be difficult to decide, then, why (or whether) the philosophy of sex should be chastised: because it is not nearly as exciting as sexual activity itself; because, if it is erotically satisfying, it is satisfying in an autoerotic or masturbatory way; or because it causes, results from, or constitutes an embarrassing **sexual dysfunction**.

See also Activity, Sexual; Beauty; Desire, Sexual; Ethics, Sexual; Feminism, French; Humor; Indian Erotology; Lacan, Jacques; Masturbation; Philosophy of sex, Teaching the; Sexuality, Dimensions of; Wittgenstein, Ludwig

REFERENCES

Augustine. (413–427) *The City of God*. Trans. Marcus Dods. New York: Modern Library, 1993; Augustine. (418?–421) *On Marriage and Concupiscence*. In Marcus Dods, ed., *The Works of Aurelius Augustine, Bishop of Hippo*, vol. 12. Trans. Peter Holmes. Edinburgh, Scot.: T. and T. Clark, 1874, 93–202; Babich, Babette E. "Nietzsche and Eros between the Devil and God's Deep Blue Sea: The Problem of the Artist as Actor—Jew—Woman." *Continental Philosophy Review* 33 (April 2000), 159–88. <www.fordham.edu/philosophy/lc/babich/Babich.Erotic-Valence-of-Art.kluwer.htm> [accessed 15 February 2005]; Bogart, John H. "On the Nature of Rape." *Public Affairs Quarterly* 5:2 (1991), 117–36; Cameron, J. M. "Sex in the Head." *New York Review of Books* (13 May 1976), 19–27; Davis, Murray. *Smut: Erotic Reality/ Obscene Ideology*. Chicago, Ill.: University of Chicago Press, 1983; Denis, Lara. "From Friendship to Marriage: Revising Kant." *Philosophy and Phenomenological Research* 63:1 (2001), 1–28; Denis, Lara. "Kant on the Wrongness of 'Unnatural' Sex." *History of Philosophy Quarterly* 16:2 (1999), 225–48; Elders, M. Joycelyn. "The Dreaded M Word[:] It's Not a Four-Letter Word." *Nerve* (26 June 1997). <www.nerve.com/dispatches/elders/mword/> [accessed 2 February 2005]; Freud, Sigmund. (1923) "The Infantile Genital Organization." In *The Standard Edition of the Complete Psychological Works of Sigmund Freud*, vol. 19. Trans. James Strachey. London: Hogarth Press, 1953–1974, 140–45; Freud, Sigmund. (1912) "On the Universal Tendency to Debasement in the Sphere of Love." In *The Standard Edition of the Complete Psychological Works of Sigmund Freud*, vol. 11. Trans. James Strachey. London: Hogarth Press, 1953–1974, 179–90; Gray, Robert. "Sex and Sexual Perversion." In Alan Soble, ed., *The Philosophy of Sex: Contemporary Readings*, 4th ed. Totowa, N.J.: Rowman and Littlefield, 2002, 57–66; Hamilton, Christopher. "Sex." In *Living Philosophy: Reflections on Life, Meaning and Morality*. Edinburgh, Scot.: Edinburgh University Press, 2001, 125–41; Kant, Immanuel. (1785) *Groundwork of the Metaphysic of Morals*. Trans. H. J. Paton. New York: Harper Torchbooks, 1964; Kierkegaard, Søren. (1845) *Stages on Life's Way*. Trans. Walter Lowrie. Princeton, N.J.: Princeton University Press, 1945; Kramer, Matthew H. *Where Law and Morality Meet*. New York: Oxford University Press, 2004; MacKinnon, Catharine A. *Only Words*. Cambridge, Mass.: Harvard University Press, 1993; MacKinnon, Catharine A. "Sexuality." In *Toward a Feminist Theory of the State*. Cambridge, Mass.: Harvard University Press, 1989, 126–54; Montaigne, Michel. (1580–1595) "Of the Power of the Imagination." In *The Complete Essays of Montaigne*. Trans. Donald M. Frame. Stanford, Calif.: Stanford University Press, 1958, 68–76; Morgan, Seiriol. "Sex in the Head." *Journal of Applied Philosophy* 20:1 (2003), 1–16; Nozick, Robert. "Sexuality." In *The Examined Life*. New York: Simon and Schuster, 1989, 61–67; Nussbaum, Martha. "Sex in the Head." *New York Review of Books* (18 December 1986), 49–52; Plato. (ca. 375–370 BCE) *Republic*. Trans. G.M.A. Grube. Indianapolis, Ind.: Hackett, 1992; Plato. (ca. 380 BCE) *Symposium*. Trans. Michael Joyce. In Edith Hamilton and Huntington Cairns, eds., *The Collected Dialogues of Plato*. Princeton, N.J.: Princeton University Press, 1961, 526–74; Robinson, Paul. *Gay Lives: Homosexual Autobiography from John Addington Symonds to Paul Monette*. Chicago, Ill.: University of Chicago Press, 1999; Russell, Bertrand. *Marriage and*

Morals. London: George Allen and Unwin, 1929; Schopenhauer, Arthur. (1818, 1844, 1859) *The World as Will and Representation*, 2 vols. Trans. E.F.J. Payne. Indian Hills, Colo.: Falcon's Wing Press, 1958; Scruton, Roger. *Sexual Desire: A Moral Philosophy of the Erotic.* New York: Free Press, 1986; Shaffer, Jerome. "Sexual Desire." *Journal of Philosophy* 75:4 (1978), 175–89; Singer, Irving. (1973) *The Goals of Human Sexuality.* New York: Schocken, 1974; Singer, Irving. *The Nature of Love.* Vol. 1: *Plato to Luther*, 2nd ed. Chicago, Ill.: University of Chicago Press, 1984. Vol. 2: *Courtly and Romantic*, 1984. Vol. 3: *The Modern World*, 1987; Solomon, Robert C. "Sexual Paradigms." *Journal of Philosophy* 71:11 (1974), 336–45; Solomon, Robert C., and Kathleen M. Higgins, eds. *The Philosophy of (Erotic) Love.* Lawrence: University Press of Kansas, 1991; Sprinkle, Annie. (Web site) <www.anniesprinkle.org> [accessed 15 February 2005]; Thomas, Keith. "The Double Standard." *Journal of the History of Ideas* 20:2 (1959), 195–216.

Alan Soble

ADDITIONAL READING

Appiah, Kwame Anthony. "Telling It Like It Is." [Review of *Sexual Investigations*, by Alan Soble] *Times Literary Supplement* (20 June 1997), 5; Augustine. (413–427) *The City of God.* Trans. John Healey. Ed. R.V.G. Tasker. London: J. M. Dent and Sons, 1947; Baker, Robert. "The Clinician as Sexual Philosopher." In Earl E. Shelp, ed., *Sexuality and Medicine*, vol. 2: *Ethical Viewpoints in Transition.* Dordrecht, Holland: Reidel, 1987, 87–109; Belliotti, Raymond. "Sex." In Peter Singer, ed., *A Companion to Ethics.* Oxford, U.K.: Blackwell, 1991, 315–26; Bersani, Leo. "Is the Rectum a Grave?" *October*, no. 43 (Winter 1987), 197–222; Bogart, John H. "On the Nature of Rape." *Public Affairs Quarterly* 5:2 (1991), 117–36. Reprinted in STW (168–80); Friedman, David M. *A Mind of Its Own: A Cultural History of the Penis.* New York: Free Press, 2001; Gray, Robert. "Sex and Sexual Perversion." *Journal of Philosophy* 75:4 (1978), 189–99. Reprinted in POS1 (158–68); POS3 (57–66); POS4 (57–66); Hall, Ronald L. *The Human Embrace: The Love of Philosophy and the Philosophy of Love. Kierkegaard, Cavell, Nussbaum.* University Park: Pennsylvania State University Press, 2000; Hawkes, Gail. *Sex and Pleasure in Western Culture.* Malden, Mass.: Polity, 2004; Kalnins, Mara, ed. *D. H. Lawrence: Centenary Essays.* Bristol, Avon, U.K.: Bristol Classical Press, 1986; Krell, David Farrell. "Pitch: Genitality/Excrementality from Hegel to Crazy Jane." *Boundary 2* 12:2 (1984), 113–41; Polhemus, Robert M. *Erotic Faith: Being in Love from Jane Austen to D. H. Lawrence.* Chicago, Ill.: University of Chicago Press, 1990; Rhees, Rush. "Sexuality" (1962–1963), "The Tree of Nebuchadnezzar" (1971–1972), and "Chastity" (1963). In *Moral Questions.* Ed. D. Z. Phillips. New York: St. Martin's Press, 1999, 139–50, 151–58, 159–63; Schopenhauer, Arthur. (1818, 1844, 1859) "The Metaphysics of Sexual Love." In *The World as Will and Representation*, 2 vols. Trans. E.F.J. Payne. Indian Hills, Colo.: Falcon's Wing Press, 1958, chap. 44, bk. 4 supp.; Shaffer, Jerome A. "Sexual Desire." *Journal of Philosophy* 75:4 (1978), 175–89. Reprinted in SLF (1–12); Soble, Alan. "The Fundamentals of the Philosophy of Sex." In Alan Soble, ed., *The Philosophy of Sex: Contemporary Readings*, 4th ed. Lanham, Md.: Rowman and Littlefield, 2002, xvii–xlii; Soble, Alan. (1977) "Introduction." In Alan Soble, ed., *Sex, Love, and Friendship.* Amsterdam, Holland: Rodopi, 1997, xli–lii; Soble, Alan. "Philosophy of Sexuality." In James Fieser, ed., *The Internet Encyclopedia of Philosophy* (2000). <www.iep.utm.edu/s/sexualit.htm> [accessed 18 January 2005]; Soble, Alan. "Sexuality, Philosophy of." In Edward Craig, ed., *Routledge Encyclopedia of Philosophy*, vol. 8. London: Routledge, 1998, 717–30; Soble, Alan. "Sexuality and Sexual Ethics." In Lawrence C. Becker and Charlotte B. Becker, eds., *Encyclopedia of Ethics*, 1st ed., vol. 2. New York: Garland, 1992, 1141–47. Reprinted, revised, in *Encyclopedia of Ethics*, 2nd ed., vol. 3. New York: Routledge, 2001, 1570–77; Solomon, Robert C. "Heterosex." In Earl E. Shelp, ed., *Sexuality and Medicine*, vol. 1: *Conceptual Roots.* Dordrecht, Holland: Reidel, 1987, 205–24; Solomon, Robert C. "Sex, Contraception, and Conceptions of Sex." In S. F. Spicker, W. B. Bondeson, and H. T. Engelhardt, eds., *The Contraceptive Ethos.* Dordrecht, Holland: Reidel, 1987, 223–40. Reprinted in G. Lee Bowie, Meredith W. Michaels, and Kathleen Higgins, eds., *Thirteen Questions in Ethics*, 2nd ed. Fort Worth, Tex.: Harcourt, Brace, Jovanovich, 1992, 95–107; Solomon, Robert C. "Sexual Paradigms."

Journal of Philosophy 71:11 (1974), 336–45. Reprinted in HS (81–90); POS1 (89–98); POS2 (53–62); POS3 (21–29); POS4 (21–29); Spender, Stephen, ed. *D. H. Lawrence: Novelist, Poet, Prophet.* New York: Harper and Row, 1973; Tuana, Nancy, and Laurie Shrage. "Sexuality." In Hugh LaFollette, ed., *The Oxford Handbook of Practical Ethics.* Oxford, U.K.: Oxford University Press, 2003, 15–41; Vannoy, Russell C. "Philosophy and Sex." In Vern L. Bullough and Bonnie Bullough, eds., *Human Sexuality: An Encyclopedia.* New York: Garland, 1994, 442–49.

PHILOSOPHY OF SEX, TEACHING THE. If the philosophy of sexuality is a relatively new field of reflection and scholarly research, *teaching* the philosophy of sex—especially to young undergraduates—has an even briefer history. On both counts, of course, **Plato** (427–347 BCE) is the exception.

Speculation about sexuality began with the ancients, for example, Hippocrates (460–380 BCE) and **Aristotle** (384–322 BCE), but genuine scientific **sexology** did not take root until the late nineteenth and early twentieth centuries. (Some major figures were Richard von Krafft-Ebing [1840–1902], **Havelock Ellis** [1859–1939], and **Sigmund Freud** [1856–1939].) In Europe, Magnus Hirschfeld's Institut für Sexualwissenschaft (Institute for Sexual Science; 1919–1933) was a leading force in the 1920s, and in mid-century America the studies of Alfred Kinsey (1894–1956) and his colleagues at Indiana University made a huge splash. These forays into the science of sex had spin-off effects in the arts, social sciences, and the humanities. Mid-twentieth-century courses in the anthropology, sociology, and psychology of sex (perhaps spurred by **Margaret Mead**'s [1901–1978] investigations) eventually brought on the academic development of **feminism** and, much later, the appearance of **queer theory**. The emergence of philosophical writing on sexuality and related issues (gender, **sexual orientation**, **love**, **marriage**) in the late 1960s and early 1970s led to the first college and university courses in the philosophy of sex (in whole or in part) in the late 1970s and beyond. Incrementally, academia has grown more receptive to these courses. Still, courses in the philosophy of sex are hardly as common as courses in general applied ethics or more standard philosophical areas such as logic and epistemology. Not every college or university has a philosophical course on sex, not even universities with graduate programs in philosophy.

If an institution's catalog does not already include a course in the philosophy of sex, a motivated instructor may propose it to the department and send it through a formal curriculum review process. Sometimes plugging into an already approved course is easier and quicker. (I once subtitled, as "Sex and Sexuality," a special topics section of Contemporary Moral Conflicts.) If one cannot countenance teaching *only* the philosophy of sex in an introduction to a metaphysics and epistemology course, one might devote some segment of the course to these topics. Or one could focus the course on questions in the philosophy of sex as a means of teaching the basic concepts and theories of metaphysics and epistemology. (The textbook assembled by Feder et al. was designed for this purpose, so that philosophers wanting to teach sex, love, epistemology, metaphysics, ethics, and political theory could both have their cake and eat it.)

Teaching the philosophy of sex presents instructors with unique opportunities and challenges. My own experience (others have had these, too) includes some extremely satisfying moments as well as some that were heartbreakingly painful or even frightening. Both the "ups" and "downs" are due in large part to the unusual and inevitably controversial subject matter: Students are discussing *sex* in the classroom. And they will be doing so probably for the first time in front of their peers (let alone a professor), so they are excited yet also nervous. Although many are unabashedly full of questions, recognizing the opportunity to explore an aspect of life about which they are naturally curious, others struggle to overcome shyness or reticence about talking about sex (especially women in a mixed-sex class).

Philosophers, despite the interesting nature and significance of sexuality, have historically tended to ignore it (see Alexander). Philosophers (many of whom, like theologians, remained bachelors) have usually focused on the *mind* and its ideas, concepts, and rationality, as opposed to the *body* with its "animalistic" instincts and urges. But many exceptions do exist, including the theologians **Saint Augustine** (354–430) and **Saint Thomas Aquinas** (1224/25–1274), as well as such prominent figures as **David Hume** (1711–1776), **Immanuel Kant** (1724–1804), **Søren Kierkegaard** (1813–1855), Jean-Paul Sartre (1905–1980), and others (see below). Since the late 1960s, however, the area has blossomed (for two ample bibliographies, see Vitek's, in Baker and Elliston, 2nd ed., 471–521; Soble, *Philosophy of Sex*, 483–500). Contemporary philosophers have come to appreciate that sex, for a multitude of reasons, *is* worthy of philosophical reflection (see Garry). Sex is important in most human lives (it often leads to **marriage** and children, about which careful value decisions must be made). We have strong biological drives for sex, and we must reflect on how, why, when, and with whom to act on these urges. Sex is the source of a unique and profound type of pleasure that is widely regarded as a central component of happiness or human fulfillment (but also denied to have that status by the Stoics and, to name one Christian theologian, Clement of Alexandria [ca. 150–215 CE], as well as the **New Natural Law** philosophers). Sex is a powerful way of connecting with another human being and communicating a wide variety of emotions (indeed, it is used to express attitudes as disparate as love and dominance). Sex-role and gender-role expectations are among the most significant social forces shaping our lives, and with which we must come to grips in understanding our identities. And sexual interaction has significant consequences: not only pregnancy, but also contracting sexually transmitted diseases, damaging **friendship**s and other intimate relationships, and being liable to criminal prosecution.

Sexuality therefore raises a rich panoply of issues and questions ripe for philosophical examination. While each person has questions about the proper role of sex in his or her life, we rarely have venues in which we can openly and *thoughtfully* explore these topics. The bookstores, of course, are stocked with sexual self-help books, and television programs from the *Dr. Phil* and *Jerry Springer* shows to *Friends*, *Queer as Folk*, and *Sex in the City* deal with sexuality *ad nauseum*. But the distinctive purpose of a philosophy of sex course is to uncover nonsense, develop clear concepts, sort out plausible theories, and even arrive occasionally at some truth, all of which is not only intrinsically interesting but pragmatically valuable.

The course, then, should teach the skills and tools of philosophy. For example, one can teach the importance of careful definition and the tool of conceptual analysis by asking students to write, in class, a paragraph in which they define "sex" or "**sexual activity**." Many will quickly propose the paradigm case of male-female genital intercourse, but then with guidance (ideally Socratic: Ask them what *they* think about the interactions of Bill Clinton and Monica Lewinsky) will discover the defects of that definition. (For helpful discussions of the difficulty of defining "sex," see the entertaining essay by Greta Christina; Frye; Soble, *Sexual Investigations*, chap. 2.) This in-class exercise can lead to a conversation, both enjoyable and instructive, about the foundational questions: What is sex and what is not? How should we understand the related ideas of **sexual desire** and sexual pleasure? Where does **sexual perversion** fit into all this? Does sex have an inherent meaning or purpose, or do we decide what meaning and value it has in our lives?

A philosophy of sex course can be organized in a variety of ways: *historically*, *topically*, or *theoretically*.

A historical approach centered around "the great philosophers" is possible, and several textbooks could be profitably used in such a course (e.g., Solomon and Higgins; Trevas et al.; Verene; **Irving Singer**'s trilogy). Aristotle, **René Descartes** (1596–1650), Hume, **G.W.F. Hegel** (1770–1831), and other philosophers occasionally discuss sex, and deserve some attention, but the most noteworthy efforts in the history of philosophy include Plato's dialogues (*Symposium*, *Lysis*, *Phaedrus*, *Laws*, *Republic*), Aquinas's exposition of Natural Law in *Summa theologiae* and *Summa contra gentiles*, and the writings of Michel Montaigne (1533–1592), **Jean-Jacques Rousseau** (1712–1778), **Johann Gottlieb Fichte** (1762–1814), Kant, the utilitarians Jeremy Bentham (1748–1832) and John Stuart Mill (1806–1873), and **Arthur Schopenhauer** (1788–1860). Moreover, in the late eighteenth century we encounter the radical thought of the sexual libertine **Marquis de Sade** (1740–1814), and in the late nineteenth we find the nearly equally notorious writings of **Friedrich Nietzsche** (1844–1900). The twentieth century begins with England's Lord **Bertrand Russell** (1872–1970), followed by Wilhelm Reich (1897–1957), Herbert Marcuse (1898–1979), and others of the **Freudian Left**, Sartre, and the postmodernist, social constructionist **Michel Foucault** (1926–1984). To recognize women's voices in this history, works by at least Mary Wollstonecraft (1759–1797), Harriet Taylor (1807–1858), Simone de Beauvoir (1908–1986) and more recent French feminists (e.g., Luce Irigaray), Carole Pateman, **Catharine MacKinnon**, **Andrea Dworkin** (1946–2005), Judith Butler, Claudia Card, Sandra Bartky, and others should be included.

The breadth of the philosophy of sex is easily demonstrated by the variety of topics it investigates. This variety suggests that a philosophy of sex course could be organized by topic(s). The teacher could, for example, discuss some manageable set of these sexual activities, practices, or phenomena: **masturbation**, premarital sex, promiscuity, **causal sex**, forms of marriage, **flirting**, **adultery**, **jealousy**, group sex, pederasty, **pedophilia**, perversion, **sadomasochism**, **homosexuality**, **bisexuality**, transexualism, **abortion**, **contraception**, **rape**, **incest**, **seduction**, **sexual harassment**, **sexual objectification**, **prostitution**, **cybersex**, **sexual addiction**, **pornography**—and more. A number of edited collections or anthology textbooks could be used in such courses, since they include essays on at least some of these activities or practices (Baker et al.; Jackson and Scott; Primoratz, *Human Sexuality*; Soble, *Philosophy of Sex*; Stewart). Courses that wanted to concentrate on or include issues surrounding gays and lesbians also have edited collections available (Baird and Baird; Beemyn and Eliason; Corvino; Jay; Murphy; and Mohr's classic *Gays/Justice*, which includes his "Gay Basics"). For more advanced students and especially for seminars, focusing on several monographs instead of edited collections might be pedagogically more valuable. (Consider the competent treatments by Belliotti, Card, Gudorf, Halwani, LeMoncheck, **Richard Posner**, Primoratz [*Ethics and Sex*], Russell, **Roger Scruton**, Vannoy, and **Karol Wojtyła** [Pope John Paul II; 1920–2005].)

Finally, one could organize a course in the philosophy of sex by theoretical emphasis. I mean by this that the course would be divided into three segments, each of which treated a distinct philosophical approach to sexuality: the conceptual, the metaphysical and epistemological, and the normative (Soble, "Sexuality"). It is unknown whether most courses in the philosophy of sexuality currently taught are organized historically, topically, or theoretically. All three have their advantages and disadvantages.

It has been observed that

> the philosophy of sex begins with a picture of a privileged pattern of relationship, in which two adult heterosexuals love each other, are faithful to each other within a formal marriage, and look forward to procreation and family. Philosophy of sex, as the Socratic scrutiny of our sexual practices, beliefs and concepts, challenges this privileged pattern by exploring the virtues, and not only the vices, of adultery, prostitution, homosexuality, group sex, bestiality, masturbation, sadomasochism, incest, pedophilia and casual sex with anonymous strangers. (Soble, "Sexuality," 718)

If this is intrinsic to the philosophy of sex *qua* philosophy, it would make (nearly) any course in the philosophy of sex a target for persons who, for one reason or another, prefer that such matters not be discussed in colleges and universities (especially if they are not private institutions). Some are offended by any public discussion of "taboo" topics; others object to using public money to support courses and faculty who teach about sex; some take offense at the inclusion of particular topics (e.g., homosexuality, pedophilia); while others object to (what they assume are) the normative views or values that professors in these courses espouse or at least raise as serious possibilities (e.g., the permissibility of adultery). Instructors should be prepared for and expect that students, faculty, administrators, and others might make all sorts of assumptions about them because they teach the philosophy of sex.

Ponder this cautionary tale. In the early 1990s, while still a graduate student, I began to teach, one section of "Contemporary Moral Conflicts" each semester, a standard applied ethics course in which students are introduced to the usual range of social and moral issues. In one section, which I subtitled "Sex and Sexuality," we concentrated on theories of **sexual ethics** and explored their application to various topics in sexual morality. In the last third of the course homosexuality and gay/lesbian issues were the focus of discussion. The third time I taught this course, I learned that the president of my community college had been confronted in the halls of the state legislature by the chair of the education committee, who was brandishing a copy of my course syllabus. I can only speculate how my little course came to the attention of this legislator 400 miles away. I was, of course, suddenly concerned about the course, the college, and my own job security. I met with my chair and with the president who, to her credit, defended the course to the legislator in terms of academic rigor and freedom. But imagine my nervousness the night the president visited one of my classes to examine what we were up to. She found that all was well, the controversy died away, and I continue to teach the course each semester. The chance that an instructor will be confronted by objections and be compelled to endure controversy likely varies by school and state. One cannot, however, rely on easy assumptions. My college is progressive, gay-friendly, and located in a notoriously liberal city near Los Angeles, yet we were still scrutinized and questioned.

It is important to have clearly thought out the pedagogical philosophy for a course in the philosophy of sex, including the rationale for teaching exactly the topics you are teaching and a justification for reading lists and methods of presenting the material. Making sure the course is philosophically and academically rigorous (in part manifested by a detailed syllabus) is excellent protection against critics. It is also wise to impress on students the importance of treating the subject matter with the seriousness it deserves. Students may sometimes need to be reminded that the course is not an opportunity to practice their comedy routines, to seek dates, or to work out their psychosexual dramas.

They should also be advised that candid discussion—and criticism—of sexual values does not thereby mean that they have permission to engage in sex. Moreover, even though class discussion should be frank and open, the **language** and manner of discourse should also be polite, civil, and respectful. To be sure, a sense of **humor** is indispensable, to provide relief from the otherwise serious atmosphere (see Greenblatt, however). But instructors should be vigilant about their own and students' choice of language, examples, and jokes. It would not take much to run afoul of sexual harassment policies (Dershowitz, 251–53; Patai, 87–92; Strossen, 26–29) or even just to make some students uncomfortable.

One question instructors must confront is whether and to what extent to reveal to the class their own sexual identity, orientation, or facts from their sexual history. When I first meet my sexuality class I come out to them as a gay man (which I *do not* do in other classes). This fact about me is part of the narrative I offer about how the sexuality course came to exist, and given that gay and lesbian issues figures prominently in the course, it is arguable that my students deserve to know it ("full disclosure"). Similarly, one should soberly consider whether to share one's experiences when discussing adultery, premarital sex, abortion, and so forth. Opening up to students can be risky and make the teacher vulnerable, but the points or lessons the teacher is trying to get across can emerge more powerfully and memorably. Further, it can enhance the classroom atmosphere in virtue of personalizing and hence deepening the connection between the instructor and some sympathetic or empathetic students. But the professor should be prepared for one welcome or unwelcome effect: The more open you are with students in the classroom, the more likely that a few will drop in during office hours to share some astonishing facts about themselves (see Robinson).

See also Activity, Sexual; Communication Model; Desire, Sexual; Ethics, Sexual; Harassment, Sexual; Language; Love; Philosophy of Sex, Overview of; Sex Education; Sexuality, Dimensions of

REFERENCES

Alexander, W. M. "Philosophers Have Avoided Sex." *Diogenes* 72 (Winter 1970), 56–74; Baird, Robert M., and M. Katherine Baird, eds. *Homosexuality: Debating the Issues.* Amherst, N.Y.: Prometheus, 1995; Baker, Robert B., and Frederick A. Elliston, eds. (1975) *Philosophy and Sex*, 2nd ed. Buffalo, N.Y.: Prometheus, 1984; Baker, Robert B., Kathleen J. Wininger, and Frederick A. Elliston, eds. *Philosophy and Sex*, 3rd ed. Amherst, N.Y.: Prometheus, 1998; Beemyn, Brett, and Mickey Eliason, eds. *Queer Studies: A Lesbian, Gay, Bisexual, and Transgender Anthology.* New York: New York University Press, 1996; Belliotti, Raymond. *Good Sex: Perspectives on Sexual Ethics.* Lawrence: University Press of Kansas, 1993; Card, Claudia. *Lesbian Choices.* New York: Columbia University Press, 1995; Christina, Greta. "Are We Having Sex Now or What?" In David Steinberg, ed., *The Erotic Impulse: Honoring the Sensual Self.* New York: Jeremy P. Tarcher, 1992, 24–29; Corvino, John, ed. *Same Sex: Debating the Ethics, Science, and Culture of Homosexuality.* Lanham, Md.: Rowman and Littlefield, 1997; Dershowitz, Alan M. "The Talmud as Sexual Harassment." In *The Abuse Excuse and Other Cop-outs, Sob Stories, and Evasions of Responsibility.* Boston, Mass.: Little, Brown, 1994, 251–53; Feder, Ellen K., Karmen MacKendrick, and Sybol S. Cook, eds. *A Passion for Wisdom: Readings in Western Philosophy on Love and Desire.* Upper Saddle River, N.J.: Prentice Hall, 2004; Frye, Marilyn. (1990) "Lesbian 'Sex.'" In *Willful Virgin: Essays in Feminism 1976–1992.* Freedom, Calif.: Crossing Press, 1992, 109–19; Garry, Ann. "Why Are Love and Sex Philosophically Interesting?" *Metaphilosophy* 11:2 (1980), 165–77; Greenblatt, Stephen. "Me, Myself, and I." [Review of *Solitary Sex: A Cultural History of Masturbation*, by Thomas W. Laqueur] *New York Review of Books* (8 April 2004), 32–36; Gudorf, Christine E. *Body, Sex, and Pleasure: Reconstructing Christian Sexual Ethics.* Cleveland, Ohio: Pilgrim Press, 1994; Halwani, Raja. *Virtuous*

Liaisons: Care, Love, Sex, and Virtue Ethics. Chicago, Ill.: Open Court, 2003; Jackson, Stevi, and Sue Scott, eds. *Feminism and Sexuality: A Reader*. New York: Columbia University Press, 1996; Jay, Karla, ed. *Lesbian Erotics*. New York: New York University Press, 1995; LeMoncheck, Linda. *Loose Women, Lecherous Men: A Feminist Philosophy of Sex*. New York: Oxford University Press, 1997; Mohr, Richard D. *Gays/Justice: A Study of Ethics, Society, and Law*. New York: Columbia University Press, 1988; Murphy, Timothy F., ed. *Gay Ethics. Controversies in Outing, Civil Rights, and Sexual Science*. New York: Haworth Press, 1994; Patai, Daphne. *Heterophobia: Sexual Harassment and the Future of Feminism*. Lanham, Md.: Rowman and Littlefield, 1998; Posner, Richard. *Sex and Reason*. Cambridge, Mass.: Harvard University Press, 1992; Primoratz, Igor. *Ethics and Sex*. London: Routledge, 1999; Primoratz, Igor, ed. *Human Sexuality*. Aldershot, U.K.: Ashgate, 1997; Robinson, Paul. " 'Dear Paul': An Exchange between Student and Teacher." In *Opera, Sex, and Other Vital Matters*. Chicago, Ill.: University of Chicago Press, 2002, 219–37; Russell, Bertrand. *Marriage and Morals*. London: George Allen and Unwin, 1929; Scruton, Roger. *Sexual Desire: A Moral Philosophy of the Erotic*. New York: Free Press, 1986; Singer, Irving. *The Nature of Love*. Vol. 1: *Plato to Luther*, 2nd ed. Chicago, Ill.: University of Chicago Press, 1984. Vol. 2: *Courtly and Romantic*, 1984. Vol. 3: *The Modern World*, 1987; Soble, Alan. *Sexual Investigations*. New York: New York University Press, 1996; Soble, Alan. "Sexuality, Philosophy of." In Edward Craig, ed., *Routledge Encyclopedia of Philosophy*, vol. 8. London: Routledge, 1998, 717–30; Soble, Alan, ed. (1980) *The Philosophy of Sex: Contemporary Readings*, 4th ed. Lanham, Md.: Rowman and Littlefield, 2002; Solomon, Robert C., and Kathleen M. Higgins, eds. *The Philosophy of (Erotic) Love*. Lawrence: University Press of Kansas, 1991; Stewart, Robert M., ed. *Philosophical Perspectives on Sex and Love*. New York: Oxford University Press, 1995; Strossen, Nadine. *Defending Pornography: Free Speech, Sex, and the Fight for Women's Rights*. New York: Scribner's, 1995; Trevas, Robert, Arthur Zucker, and Donald Borchert, eds. *Philosophy of Sex and Love: A Reader*. Upper Saddle River, N.J.: Prentice Hall, 1997; Vannoy, Russell. *Sex without Love: A Philosophical Exploration*. Buffalo, N.Y.: Prometheus, 1980; Verene, Donald, ed. (1972) *Sexual Love and Western Morality: A Philosophical Anthology*, 2nd ed. Boston, Mass.: Jones and Bartlett, 1995; Wojtyła, Karol (Pope John Paul II). *Love and Responsibility*. New York: Farrar, Straus and Giroux, 1981.

James S. Stramel

ADDITIONAL READING

Abelove, Henry, Michèle Aina Barale, and David M. Halperin, eds. *The Lesbian and Gay Studies Reader*. New York: Routledge, 1993; Alexander, W. M. "Philosophers Have Avoided Sex." *Diogenes* 72 (Winter 1970), 56–74. Reprinted in POS2 (3–19); Appiah, Kwame Anthony. "Telling It Like It Is." [Review of *Sexual Investigations*, by Alan Soble] *Times Literary Supplement* (20 June 1997), 5; Archard, David. "How Should We Teach Sex?" *Journal of the Philosophy of Education* 32:3 (1998), 437–49; Archard, David. Review of *The Philosophy of Sex: Contemporary Readings*, 4th ed., ed. Alan Soble. *Journal of Applied Philosophy* 21:1 (2004), 93–97; Atkinson, Ronald. *Sexual Morality*. London: Hutchinson, 1965; Bartky, Sandra. *Femininity and Domination: Studies in the Phenomenology of Oppression*. New York: Routledge, 1990; Beauvoir, Simone de. (1949) *The Second Sex*. Trans. Howard M. Parshley. New York: Bantam, 1961; Becker, Lawrence C., and Charlotte B. Becker, eds. *Encyclopedia of Ethics*, 1st ed., 2 vols. New York: Garland, 1992. 2nd ed., 3 vols. New York: Routledge, 2001; Belliotti, Raymond. "Sex." In Peter Singer, ed., *A Companion to Ethics*. Oxford, U.K.: Blackwell, 1991, 315–26; Bloodsworth, Mary K. "Teachers." In Timothy F. Murphy, ed., *Reader's Guide to Lesbian and Gay Studies*. Chicago, Ill.: Fitzroy Dearborn, 2000, 578–80; Boonin, David, and Graham Oddie, eds. "What's Wrong with Sex?" Part 2 of *What's Wrong? Applied Ethicists and Their Critics*. New York: Oxford University Press, 2005, 165–277; Brundage, James A. *Law, Sex, and Christian Society in Medieval Europe*. Chicago, Ill.: University of Chicago Press, 1987; Bullough, Vern L., and Bonnie Bullough, eds. *Human Sexuality: An Encyclopedia*. New York: Garland, 1994; Burgess-Jackson, Keith. Review of *Ethics and Sex*, by Igor Primoratz. *Journal of Applied Philosophy* 17:3 (2000), 307–10; Butler, Judith. *Bodies That Matter: On the Discursive Limits of "Sex."* New

York: Routledge, 1993; Cagle, Randy. Review of *The Philosophy of Sex: Contemporary Readings*, 4th ed., ed. Alan Soble. *Essays in Philosophy* 4:2 (2003). <www.humboldt.edu/~essays/caglerev.html> [accessed 11 January 2005]; Calhoun, Cheshire. Review of *Sexual Investigations*, by Alan Soble. *Ethics* 109:4 (1999), 928–31; Christina, Greta. "Are We Having Sex Now or What?" In David Steinberg, ed., *The Erotic Impulse: Honoring the Sensual Self*. New York: Jeremy P. Tarcher, 1992, 24–29. Reprinted in POS3 (3–8); POS4 (3–8); de Sousa, Ronald, and Kathryn Pauly Morgan. "Philosophy, Sex, and Feminism." <www.chass.utoronto.ca/~sousa/sexphil.html> [accessed 14 October 2004]; Devine, Philip E., and Celia Wolf-Devine, eds. *Sex and Gender: A Spectrum of Views*. Belmont, Calif.: Wadsworth, 2003; Diorio, Joseph A. "Sex, Love, and Justice: A Problem in Moral Education." *Educational Theory* 31:3–4 (1982), 225–35. Reprinted in Alan Soble, ed., *Eros, Agape, and Philia: Readings in the Philosophy of Love*. New York: Paragon House, 1989, 273–88; Ellis, Albert, and Albert Abarbanel, eds. *The Encyclopedia of Sexual Behavior*, 2 vols. New York: Hawthorn Books, 1961; Farley, Margaret A. "Sexual Ethics." In Warren Reich, ed., *Encyclopedia of Bioethics*, vol. 4. New York: Free Press, 1978, 1575–89. Rev. ed., vol. 5. New York: Simon Schuster Macmillan, 1995, 2363–75; Frueh, Joanna. "Fuck Theory." In *Erotic Faculties*. Berkeley: University of California Press, 1996, 43–50; Frye, Marilyn. "Lesbian 'Sex.' " In Jeffner Allen, ed., *Lesbian Philosophies and Cultures*. Albany: State University of New York Press, 1990, 305–15. Reprinted in *Willful Virgin: Essays in Feminism 1976–1992*. Freedom, Calif.: Crossing Press, 1992, 109–19; and Anne Minas, ed., *Gender Basics: Feminist Perspectives on Women and Men*, 1st ed. Belmont, Calif.: Wadsworth, 1993, 328–33; Gallop, Jane. *Feminist Accused of Sexual Harassment*. Durham, N.C.: Duke University Press, 1997; Garber, Linda, ed. *Tilting the Tower: Lesbians, Teaching, Queer Subjects*. New York: Routledge, 1994; Garry, Ann. "Why Are Love and Sex Philosophically Interesting?" *Metaphilosophy* 11:2 (1980), 165–77. Reprinted in POS2 (21–36); SLF (39–50); Gilbert, Paul. *Human Relationships: A Philosophical Introduction*. Oxford, U.K.: Blackwell, 1991; Gruen, Lori, and George F. Panichas, eds. *Sex, Morality, and the Law*. New York: Routledge, 1997; Gudorf, Christine E. "On Teaching Christian Sexual Ethics." In Larry L. Rasmussen, ed., *The Annual of the Society of Christian Ethics*. Dallas, Tex.: Society of Christian Ethics, 1983, 265–67; Harding, Sandra. "Why Sex and Love Are Really Interesting." In Alan Soble, ed., *Sex, Love, and Friendship*. Amsterdam, Holland: Rodopi, 1997, 53–59; Hunter, J.F.M. *Thinking about Sex and Love*. New York: St. Martin's Press, 1980; Irigaray, Luce. (1974) *Speculum of the Other Woman*. Trans. Gillian C. Gill. Ithaca, N.Y.: Cornell University Press, 1985; Irigaray, Luce. (1977) *This Sex Which Is Not One*. Trans. Catherine Porter, with Carolyn Burke. Ithaca, N.Y.: Cornell University Press, 1985. Reprinted in Claudia Zanardi, ed., *Essential Papers on the Psychology of Women*. New York: New York University Press, 1990, 344–51; Jenness, Valerie. "Feminism, Sexual Harassment, and the Atypical Case." [Review of *Feminist Accused of Sexual Harassment*, by Jane Gallop] In Barry M. Dank and Roberto Refinetti, eds., *Sex Work and Sex Workers*. New Brunswick, N.J.: Transaction Publishers, 1999, 191–200; Kissen, Rita M., ed. *Getting Ready for Benjamin: Preparing Teachers for Sexual Diversity in the Classroom*. Lanham, Md.: Rowman and Littlefield, 2002; Marietta, Don E., Jr. *Philosophy of Sexuality*. Armonk, N.Y.: M. E. Sharpe, 1997; Minas, Anne, ed. *Gender Basics: Feminist Perspectives on Women and Men*, 1st ed. Belmont, Calif.: Wadsworth, 1993. 2nd ed., 2000; Mohr, Richard D. "Gay Studies in the Big Ten: A Survival's Manual." In *Gays/Justice: A Study of Ethics, Society, and Law*. New York: Columbia University Press, 1988, 277–92; Montaigne, Michel. (1595) *The Essays of Michel de Montaigne*. Ed. and trans. M. A. Screech. London: Penguin, 1991; Nye, Robert A., ed. *Sexuality*. Oxford, U.K.: Oxford University Press, 1999; Patai, Daphne. *Heterophobia: Sexual Harassment and the Future of Feminism*. Lanham, Md.: Rowman and Littlefield, 1998; Patai, Daphne. "Women on Top." [Review essay] *Academic Questions* 16:2 (2003), 70–82; Patai, Daphne, and Noretta Koertge. *Professing Feminism: Cautionary Tales from the Strange World of Women's Studies*. New York: Basic Books, 1994. *Professing Feminism: Education and Indoctrination in Women's Studies*, new and expanded ed. Lanham, Md.: Lexington, 2003; Pateman, Carole. *The Disorder of Women: Democracy, Feminism, and Political Theory*. Cambridge: Cambridge University Press, 1989, 71–89; Penn, Donna, and Janice Irvine. "Gay/Lesbian/Queer Studies." *Contemporary Sociology* 24:3 (1995), 328–30; Peterson, Patricia. Review of *The Philosophy of Sex: Contemporary*

Readings, 4th ed., ed. Alan Soble. *Sexualities* 6:3–4 (2003), 504–6; Pierce, Christine. "Review Essay: Philosophy." *Signs* 1:2 (1975), 487–503; Posner, Richard. *Sex and Reason*. Cambridge, Mass.: Harvard University Press, 1992; Purdy, Laura M. Review of *The Philosophy of Sex: Contemporary Readings*, 1st ed., ed. Alan Soble. *Philosophical Investigations* 4:4 (1981), 68–70; Raymond, Diane. "Homosexuality and Feminism: Some Suggestions for Teaching." *Teaching Philosophy* 6:4 (1983), 355–65; Robson, Ruthann. "Pedagogy, Jurisprudence, and Finger-Fucking: Lesbian Sex in a Law School Classroom." In Karla Jay, ed., *Lesbian Erotics*. New York: New York University Press, 1995, 28–39; Rossi, Alice, ed. *Essays on Sex Equality: John Stuart Mill and Harriet Taylor Mill*. Chicago, Ill.: University of Chicago Press, 1970; Rubin, Gayle S. "Thinking Sex: Notes for a Radical Theory of the Politics of Sexuality." In Carole S. Vance, ed., *Pleasure and Danger: Exploring Female Sexuality*. London: Routledge and Kegan Paul, 1984, 267–319. Reprinted in Henry Abelove, Michèle Aina Barale, and David Halperin, eds., *The Lesbian and Gay Studies Reader*. New York: Routledge, 1993, 3–44; and Peter M. Nardi and Beth E. Schneider, eds., *Social Perspectives in Lesbian and Gay Studies*. New York: Routledge, 1998, 100–133; Sears, James T., ed. *Sexuality and the Curriculum: The Politics and Practices of Sexuality Education*. New York: Teachers College Press, Columbia University, 1992; Shelp, Earl E., ed. *Sexuality and Medicine*, Vol. 1: *Conceptual Roots*. Vol. 2: *Ethical Viewpoints in Transition*. Dordrecht, Holland: Reidel, 1987; Singer, Irving. *The Pursuit of Love*. Baltimore, Md.: Johns Hopkins University Press, 1994; Singer, Irving. *Sex: A Philosophical Primer*. Lanham, Md.: Rowman and Littlefield, 2001. Expanded ed., Lanham, Md.: Rowman and Littlefield, 2004; Soble, Alan. (1976) "Introduction." In Alan Soble, ed., *Sex, Love, and Friendship*. Amsterdam, Holland: Rodopi, 1997, xli–lii; Soble, Alan. "Philosophy of Sexuality." In James Fieser, ed., *The Internet Encyclopedia of Philosophy* (2000). <www.iep.utm.edu/s/sexualit.htm> [accessed 18 January 2005]; Soble, Alan. Review of *Ethics and Sex*, by Igor Primoratz. *Ethics* 111:2 (2001), 455; Soble, Alan. Review of *Philosophy and Sex*, 2nd ed., ed. Robert B. Baker and Frederick A. Elliston. *Teaching Philosophy* 8:3 (1985), 250–51; Soble, Alan. "Sexuality and Sexual Ethics." In Lawrence C. Becker and Charlotte B. Becker, eds., *Encyclopedia of Ethics*, 1st ed., vol. 2. New York: Garland, 1141–47. Reprinted, revised, in Lawrence C. Becker and Charlotte B. Becker, eds., *Encyclopedia of Ethics*, 2nd ed., vol. 3. New York: Routledge, 2001, 1570–77; Soble, Alan. "Sitting in Kant's Classroom." In "Kant and Sexual Perversion," *The Monist* 86:1 (2003), 55–89, at 79–81 (sec. 4). <www.uno.edu/~asoble/pages/kmonist.htm> [accessed 5 June 2004]; Soble, Alan, ed. *Eros, Agape, and Philia: Readings in the Philosophy of Love*. New York: Paragon House, 1989. Reprinted, corrected, 1999; Soble, Alan, ed. *The Philosophy of Sex: Contemporary Readings*, 1st ed. Totowa, N.J.: Rowman and Littlefield, 1980. 2nd ed., Savage, Md.: 1991. 3rd ed., Lanham, Md.: 1997. 4th ed., Lanham, Md.: 2002; Tuana, Nancy, and Laurie Shrage. "Sexuality." In Hugh LaFollette, ed., *The Oxford Handbook of Practical Ethics*. Oxford, U.K.: Oxford University Press, 2003, 15–41; Vitek, William. "Bibliography." In Robert B. Baker and Frederick A. Elliston, eds., *Philosophy and Sex*, 2nd ed. Buffalo, N.Y.: Prometheus, 1984, 471–521; Wilson, John. *Logic and Sexual Morality*. Baltimore, Md.: Penguin, 1956; Wollstonecraft, Mary. (1792) *A Vindication of the Rights of Women*. Buffalo, N.Y.: Prometheus, 1989.

PLATO (427–347 BCE). Plato is better known for his scorn for carnality than for his professed **love** of sex. His dialogues, however, are so replete with observations and prescriptions about human coupling that they prove a rich mine for the philosophy of sex. Plato's philosophy of sexuality, even at its most practical, is firmly rooted in his philosophical psychology and theory of reality. On these topics, as on most, Plato changed his mind, sharing with his readers his genuine intellectual struggles.

Plato's creative life as a philosopher and activist spanned approximately fifty years, during which time he established and taught at the Academy in Athens, one of the first institutions of higher learning (and where **Aristotle** [384–322 BCE] was a student). He traveled widely, engaged in mathematical research, got entangled in Sicilian politics, and produced a body of philosophical writings that would become central to the Western canon. Plato employed the dialogue form, in particular, to frame with innovative precision the fundamental problems with which philosophers continue to struggle and in so doing advanced the genre of philosophical writing.

Plato deals with some surprisingly modern sexual issues: the power of sexuality in the human psyche, the relation between love and sex, and the ethics of nonconsensual sex, **seduction**, extramarital sex, **pornography**, and genetic engineering. Considering the number of years over which Plato wrote, it is not surprising that many of his ideas change, including his ideas on the role of sexuality in the human psyche. For example, Plato never abandons the value of a well-lived philosophical life, but he does come to change his notion of what makes life well lived and who is capable of managing his or her own life. In the early *Apology*, Plato envisions an Athens where education gives all citizens the ability to make reasonable decisions; in his last dialogue, *Laws*, he designs a city where the benighted, intemperate majority requires wiser leaders to impose laws about even the most personal matters, including the details of one's sex life (8.835e–837a, 838a–841e).

One reason for Plato's abiding interest in sex is that it is bound to the themes of power and autonomy, issues that never lose their urgency for Plato. He connects power and autonomy to sexuality in two ways. First, he explicates the role of power dynamics in interpersonal, sexual relationships. This is a central concern in the dialogues *Charmides*, *Symposium*, *Phaedrus*, and *Republic*. Second, in examining the human psyche and the sources of human motivation, Plato investigates the influence (in some cases absolute sovereignty) that **sexual desire** and pleasure can have on a person's actions and life plans. When one reads *Republic*, *Symposium*, *Protagoras*, *Phaedrus*, and *Laws*, one cannot help but see anew the extent to which sexual pleasure can govern human life and how Plato draws on sexual topics to illuminate human psychology and history. Sexuality, therefore, is enmeshed with one of Plato's deepest concerns, how a human can attain freedom, which he believes is necessary for a happy life. At various points, most notably in *Republic* (for example, 403a–b), he argues that given the intensity of sexual (and other) pleasures, some people must sacrifice (political, civil) liberty to have freedom (autonomy; self-governance) and thus happiness.

Plato's philosophy of sex goes beyond his philosophy of love, but they clearly intersect, particularly on the point of desire. Plato devotes three dialogues to love: *Lysis*, which focuses on *philia*, and *Symposium* and *Phaedrus*, which deal with *eros* and are relevant to his philosophy of sex. Greek has three words translatable into English as "love": *eros* (sexual passion), *agape* (admiration; later New Testament usage, "divine love"), and *philia* (**friendship**, familial love). Plato engages in a linguistic analysis of *philia* in *Republic* (5.474c–475c), speaking first of the "love of young men," which here means "appreciation." This is different from erotic attachment to some particular man, in that *philia* is more like, say, the love of red wine, be it a good Cabernet or Merlot, appreciating the different virtues of each. When one feels passion for a particular vintage from a particular vineyard and find it like no other, one moves into erotic territory. This, Plato indicates, starts with *philia* for red wine generally. As Plato puts it (*Rep.* 475b), "*philia* of X" implies an appetite (*epithumia*) for all X, so that a wine lover feels *philia* for all kinds of wine. To have a favorite X, one must like the sort of being that X is. Historian James Davidson, perhaps hyperbolically, likens the "-philia" suffix to the English "-oholic" (159), so that a "chocoholic" would be someone who enjoys all kinds of chocolate and whose life would feel incomplete without it.

With regard to the difference between *philia* and *eros*, it must be noted that *philia* can refer to love of an individual—someone who is one's friend, parent, sibling, or other close family member. It would be odd to use *eros* to describe, say, filial affection (*Symposium* 199d; see Rosen, 211–15). As Arthur Adkins (1929–1996) says about *philia* between individuals, it "encompasses all cooperative relationships" (232) and it, unlike *eros*, is "not overcome by passion" (230). *Eros* applies to one's relation to a lover or object of libidinal desire. Still, one might feel *philia* for a class of things the individual members of which provide libidinal release. For example, a foot fetishist might be a friend (in the sense of *philia*) to women's feet in general, which would be different from feeling desire (*eros*) for a particular lover's feet. *Philia*, arguably, ranges over a broader semantic field. Plato's discussion of *philia* in *Lysis* deals with a relation of friendship between individuals. For Plato's idea of *eros* and its relation to *aphrodisia*, one must look elsewhere.

Like many other Athenians with money and a distinguished pedigree, especially those fascinated by Socrates (469–399 BCE), Plato questions the social mores and political foundation of the Athenian democracy. Unlike most of them, however, Plato the author challenges the underlying ethical and metaphysical assumptions of his broader culture, as he develops his theory of Forms and sophisticated philosophical psychology. He began writing dialogues probably after the execution of Socrates. Scholars cannot conclusively establish their exact dates, for various reasons (see W.K.C. Guthrie [1906–1981], 41–56). While many find it helpful to classify Plato's works in terms of early, middle, and late dialogues (Benson, 4–6), others have suggested problems with this approach (Cooper, xi–xviii).

In looking at Plato's philosophy of sexual passion, however, one can find three distinct attitudes in three groups of dialogues. The Socratic, early, dialogues depict rationality as always the master of lust; the middle dialogues, the so-to-speak "Platonist" dialogues, draw sexual passion as endangering rationality and human integrity; the third group offers an ideal in which sexual passion can be compatible with a well-lived rational life. His last dialogue, *Laws*, arguably stands alone, as a fourth, draconian approach, in response to the ethos of free love (8.840e) that he perceives as prevalent. There he argues that *only* biologically reproductive sexual acts should be permitted and that citizens should be conditioned to fear the power of lust. It seems that *Laws* offers a Natural Law argument against **homosexuality** (like that of **Thomas Aquinas** [1224/25–1274]), though some forcefully challenge this interpretation (Nussbaum, "Platonic Love," esp. 1623–40; but see Rist). This scholarly matter became the center of a bitter legal case concerning gay rights in the state of Colorado (Clark, 1–6).

Regardless, *Laws* clearly reflects Plato's observations on his own culture. Like the *Laws*, many of his dialogues, from early to late, allude to the Athenian ethos of homoeroticism and the Greek tradition of viewing *aphrodisia* as an exquisite, brutal force. About the Hellenic view of sexuality, the myth of Aphrodite speaks clearly. Aphrodite, the goddess of sexual desire and animal magnetism, mother of Eros, is primal, beautiful, and capricious. Born of the foam (*aphros*) that seeped from her father's severed genitals after they were thrown into the sea, Aphrodite was instrumental in starting the Trojan War and causing much other mayhem. She was associated with the sea, which the Greeks knew to be both necessary for life and potentially deadly (Thornton, 49–67). The word *aphrodisia*, **Michel Foucault** (1926–1984) reminds us (35–52), is untranslatable, referring to sexual activities and the associated pleasures. Plato shares the Greek awe of sexuality. In the early pages of the *Republic*, Socrates relates Cephalus's story about Sophocles (1.329c), who in his old age was asked by a friend, "How's your sex life (*pros tàphrodísia*), Sophocles? Are you still able to be with a woman?" Sophocles says that he is not and now he feels free of "a wild and savage despot." This idea of the libido as tyrannical encapsulates the cultural view of Aphrodite. Aphrodite is, for the Greeks, a force to be reckoned with. This is a central motif of Plato's *Republic*.

The Athenians, particularly citizen males, of the fifth and fourth centuries BCE enjoyed varied sex lives, but they were neither utterly unbridled nor oblivious to the dangerous consequences of crossing certain boundaries. Plato, in the fourth century BCE, wrote dialogues set in the fifth century, when male partnerships were more celebrated, at least in visual documents (Shapiro, 71–72). Many assume that all Greek males were homosexual, but this is misleading. Homoeroticism was prevalent in Spartan culture, and most citizen males in fifth-century Athens had some homoerotic experiences as a normal part of their adolescence and early adulthood before going on to marry, have children, and gratify heterosexual appetites with a variety of partners, be they wives, slaves, paid escorts, mistresses, or brothel workers (Cantarella, 48–51; Davidson, 73–112; Keuls, 156–65). Relationships between males, particularly in the more affluent classes, had a defined structure, with one partner being the lover (*erastēs*), the other being the beloved (*erōmenos*). The situation was asymmetrical in two ways. First, the lover pursued, courted, and tried to seduce, while the beloved, usually after an appropriate period of demurring, would grant (or refuse) his favors. Second, the lover expressed sexual ardor and pleasure, whereas the beloved would be more subtle. If the beloved was aroused, etiquette would forbid him to show it, even in consummating desire.

To consummate desire did not have to include penetrating and being penetrated. It is controversial whether a lover's penetrating the beloved was considered deviant, but ancient authors make it clear that for a man to seek out being penetrated was considered shameful (Davidson, 167–82; Thornton, 99–102). Scholars disagree about the reason. Foucault argues that to enjoy penetration was equivalent to enjoying being subordinate in a power relation. Davidson, criticizing Foucault, argues that penetration and power structures are not at stake. Rather, the defining trait is what the Greeks perceived as the "insatiability" of the male "pathic" or *kinaidos* (175–77), which this male was believed to share accidentally with the female. Thus, Davidson says that a *kinaidos* could be "a virgin" and still be *kinaidos*: It is his perceived lack of self-control, not whether he has actually been entered, that earns him his social status. Thornton, in contrast to both, sees the issue as feminization and the politically dangerous licentiousness that the Greeks associated with female desire. The Greeks viewed the *kinaidos* as imposing a distortion on the Greek "heterosexual paradigm" in which female desire, however lascivious, has a procreative purpose (101–10).

Men who enjoyed the "pathic" role *were* seen as soft and feminine and thus on the brink of being out of control. The feminine, to the typical Athenian male, was lascivious, soft, feral, and closer to nature than to the political order. The beloved needed to maintain his self-possession to further his growing political respectability and esteem in the community. Adult males who enjoyed the "pathic" role (*kinaidoi*) were looked upon with contempt (Poole, 117–200). Aristophanes made them the butt of his comedies, especially if they were politicians (Thornton, 107–8). Thus, it becomes a moral issue of just how much a lover should expect from a beloved, a moral issue always in the background of Plato's *Symposium* (e.g., 184a–185b, 216d–219d) and *Phaedrus* (231–234c, 238e–241c, 255a–256b), the two dialogues explicitly centered on *eros*. The beloved, especially once he develops more visible secondary sex characteristics (Thornton, 107), hovers perilously close to shame. Presumably, a sincere lover would want to spare his beloved this unhappiness, as Plato insinuates in *Phaedrus*.

Why, then, would a young man submit? Generally, the allure of a lover was based on his (perceived or real) experience, political savvy, and knowledge. The relationship, ideally, would be mutually beneficial in that the lover would have the pleasure of sensuality and gallantry, while the beloved would be improved by his intimacy with a partner of greater wisdom and sophistication. Plato, particularly in the *Symposium* and *Phaedrus*, objects to the moral implications of the customary structure of the lover/beloved relationship. In the *Symposium*, he tacitly implies that the power dynamics involve a lack of autonomy that impedes the personal and intellectual development of both partners. One should aspire to be emotionally independent, thus making such relationships impossible. This emerges from the dramatic elements of the dialogue, especially the episode starring Alcibiades (Nussbaum, *Fragility*, 181–99).

In his probably later *Phaedrus*, Plato does not proscribe erotic relationships but offers a different ideal of a relationship based on mutual attraction (255d–e), in which the partners embark on a joint pursuit of philosophical understanding. Their mutual respect, further strengthened by their growing enlightenment, guarantees that they will not be enemies after erotic intoxication wears off (256d). On the traditional model, when the lover has been gratified or the beloved grows beyond him, the two may become alienated, even enemies. A jealous lover could impede rather than encourage the beloved's accomplishment or development, a possibility that Plato brings up early in the *Phaedrus*. In the best of situations, the traditional Athenian relationship would be formative for both men and lead to a long friendship. This was not incompatible with later (or concurrent) **sexual activity** with women. In both *Symposium* and (especially) *Phaedrus*, Plato critiques the conventions surrounding the Athenian male relationships, while exploring deeper issues about the power dynamics in sexual and affectionate relationships. Plato's *Republic*, a defense of metaphysical and political Platonism, is also an extended argument on how to avoid being enslaved by one's sexuality and by other people, lovers and friends alike.

Plato's early dialogues are those that draw a sympathetic portrait of Socrates and defend a philosophical system associated with the historical Socrates. Those relevant to Plato's philosophy of sex are *Charmides*, *Gorgias*, *Protagoras*, *Menexenus*, and the probably authentic *Alcibiades* (Cooper, ix). At first glance, the Socratic Plato's view of sexuality seems paradoxical. The character of Socrates displays a robust sexuality and appreciates the sexual allure of beautiful boys. He enjoys flirting and seems well acquainted with courtship rituals. Yet the *Charmides* is devoted to self-control. Socrates feels weak in the knees, "on fire," when accidentally glimpsing inside the robe of the stunning young Charmides (155d–e). Socrates compares himself to a young deer who should beware of gazing at a lion, lest he become the lion's feast. However, even ignited by the accidental glimpse of Charmides's naked body, he proceeds in his level-headed way to lead a philosophical discussion about the virtue of self-control, a virtue that the historical Charmides (died ca. 403 BCE) would eventually reject.

Socrates realizes that *aphrodisia* appear to dominate most people. Plato's Socrates, defying the observations of *hoi polloi*, argues that passion never dominates reason. Socrates sexually desires Charmides, but he is more strongly attracted to a stable, honorable life. A dalliance with Charmides might interfere with his continuing to have that life. Socrates does not view his own self-control as psychologically inconsistent with his sexual appetite, because his self-control, as he sees it, emerges from a greater desire to protect his rationally conceived interests. This theory, known as "Socratic intellectualism," posits that the intellect is the only source of motivation for choice and action, which entails that we never choose badly from weakness of will (*akrasia*) but only from ignorance. Thus, according to Socrates, one never chooses to do wrong knowingly. Suppose that *A*, overcome by lust, wants to have sex with B, but A believes that sex with B is wrong. According to Socrates, A's belief guarantees that A will not have sex with B. Weakness of will never occurs, for we never act against our beliefs about what we ought to do and what is in our interests. Because this tenet contradicts many of our observations of human nature, it is called a "Socratic paradox."

Plato's Socrates argues that this contradiction is only apparent and defends his view in the *Protagoras* (352d–358c). Socrates avers that our actions, however irrationally motivated they may appear, are based on a rational calculation of our own interests. Thus, if I want X and believe that X is harmful, I will not pursue X. Once people understand the nature of the good and see that X does not fall in that category, they will not choose X. Thus, Socrates claims, apparent cases of weakness of will are in fact failures of judgment. To explain, Socrates draws an analogy between acting and perceiving (356c–357e). If A succumbs to desire for B, A sees the anticipated pleasure more clearly than the pain and inconvenience that might come later. This is analogous to seeing a small, nearby object as larger, more prominent, than a large object that is far away. Just as illusion occurs in sense perception, it occurs in perceiving the future results of our choices. With sense perception, we learn how to judge relative sizes of visual objects. Therefore, one should learn how to calculate the value of chosen outcomes, and doing that requires cultivated judgmental powers and knowledge of good and evil. Socrates would thus say that it is never sexual passion that masters one's beliefs about what is good (as we sometimes think). Instead, one wrongly believes that gratifying a given desire would be good. These false beliefs come from misunderstanding oneself and the nature of the good. We easily become deluded by the temporal immediacy of the anticipated pleasures, and these delusions overshadow our vague awareness of the devastation that will likely ensue. The seeming triumph of lust over intellect, then, is actually a matter of ignorance.

Plato eventually rejects Socratic intellectualism in the middle dialogues *Phaedo*, *Republic*, and *Symposium*. In *Phaedo*, the scene of Socrates's death, Socrates speaks of the burden of the body. According to Plato's new metaphysics of the person, the body and soul are separate entities; the soul is tethered to the base physical world by the senses and passions. The body's needs and persistent desires distract the soul from its important task of contemplating reality (the "Forms"), which requires transcending the appetitive and epistemic limitations of the body. The Platonist Plato views the flesh as problematic and carnal desire as an unfortunate condition of human life (Santas, 73–74). Plato espouses a view of reality as transcendent, nonphysical, and good. He also puts forth a "degrees of reality" theory: The further something is from absolute reality, the lesser value it has. For Plato, then, the physical body is morally inferior to the mind. In separating the self from nature, Plato thereby denies the role of sexuality in personal identity.

In the *Republic*, however, Plato advances an argument that depends on his observations about human happiness instead of his metaphysics. Rejecting his earlier, Socratic beliefs, Plato argues that the intellect is not the only source of human motivation; passions and appetites also motivate our choices and actions (4.435b–441c). Psychic conflict does occur, and sometimes reason is defeated by the passions and appetites (for acquiring money, eating to excess, sexual pleasure). At the core of the *Republic*, which is an extended argument about the relation between human happiness and justice, is Plato's famous analogy between the state and the individual, both of which have three parts (2.368c–369b, 4.435b–445a). To represent the ideal human life, he delineates the ideal society. The ideal Platonic life— the happiest, truly free life—is the philosophical life of contemplation. The best city is one ruled by people ("guardians") living this life of rationality, who are free of carnal desires, greed, and excessive passions.

Plato therefore recommends strict principles of breeding to reproduce the best possible specimens, among the guardians at any rate. He discourages love between those who are sexually attracted to one another, because he wants both to dissolve the family with its attendant loyalties and to ensure that citizens will be free of infatuations and sexual madness. John Lucas remarks that Plato has two problems in the *Republic*: "sons and . . . lovers" (231). Plato would welcome twenty-first-century advances in genetic engineering, provided that decisions are made only by moral authorities, elite members of the highest intellectual group. Thus, he advocates state control over the sexual activities of citizens during their peak fertility years (ages twenty to forty for a woman; twenty-five to fifty-five for a man) and over the care of infants. He envisions breeding pens staffed by male and female nurses, where children will be segregated according to their natural endowments. Mothers should breast-feed different babies day to day; his plan requires that parents not bond with any child, let alone know who their child is. The concept of parenthood, however, persists: A man should consider as his own any child born to a woman within the right time. This is necessary to prevent vertical **incest**—incest between parent and child or between grandparent and grandchild (see 457c–462e). Vertical incest, for Plato, is eugenically maladaptive. Incest between siblings is sometimes permissible; indeed, it can occur only randomly, without the knowledge of the siblings that it occurs, precisely because they do not know who their parents are. Children born to parents beyond their peak fertility years are cast out of the city. Plato implies (461c) that **abortion** is preferable.

Plato considers incest impermissible not only for reasons of political or genetic utility. He advances moral objections to it as well. In the *Republic* (bk. 9, 571c), he describes having sex with one's mother as coming from desires of the self's bestial part. He seems to acknowledge that the incest taboo, among others, separates human from beast. In *Laws*, he objects more forcefully to incest (838a–d), rejecting both vertical and horizontal incest. The Athenian Stranger points out that *A*'s being attracted to *B* does not entail that *A* sexually desires *B*, when, for instance, *A* knows that *B* is *A*'s sibling. In deviant cases, some feel and even act on incestuous desires, which can be a powerful motif in tragedy or ridiculous in comedy. (Even, according to **Sigmund Freud** [1856–1939], a significant part of human psychology; see his "Oedipus Complex" in, for one place, *Ego and Id*, chap. 3.) Treating the incest taboo as universal and deeply rooted in the human soul, Plato presents a Natural Law argument in the *Laws* (bk. 8) to support a prohibition against nonreproductive sex. He argues that it is a natural law that all sex acts done other than for procreation are evil and that incest rarely produces good offspring, from which it follows that incest is wrong. In the *Republic*, Plato claims that incest is eugenically dubious but denies that procreation is the only purpose of sex. His concern there is primarily with the integrity of the human psyche and therefore personal happiness.

In the *Republic*, Plato divides the psyche into three parts: appetite, spirit, and reason (or intellect). Each has its own set of desires and pleasures, and each is a source of motivation. Thus, belief is not sufficient for choice, because spirit or appetite may defeat reason. Sexual appetites, he notes, overcome rational judgment in most people (a claim validated by history). In general, the appetites are hard to tame, and some people are naturally inclined to be dominated by them. Plato describes this part of the psyche as a many-headed beast, with heads both tame and ferocious. In a well-balanced psyche, the beast has only heads that are necessary and tame, a challenging goal for moral educators. The sexual appetite, which Plato describes as the most intense and maddening (bk. 3, 403a–d), is a necessary appetite (for continuing the species). Plato realizes that sexual pleasure can strongly motivate people, even members of the upper stratum of his meritocracy. Hence, as a reward, valorous and brilliant men could be affectionate with any women they desired and father as many children as possible (468c). Presumably Plato would acknowledge sexual inducements for females, given that guardian women perform the same roles as male guardians and that sexual differences are irrelevant to character.

Each person has a certain quantity of psychic energy, which in the *Symposium* he terms *eros*. Plato, as if anticipating Freud's idea of sublimation, claims energy can be channeled from one part to another. One can thus deprive the appetite of energy by giving more to reason or spirit (by, for example, studying logic or through political ambition, respectively). Someone with a truly robust intellect, Plato optimistically thinks, will be armed against the violence of lust and other appetites. As he analyzes in *Republic* the three parts of the psyche, in the *Symposium* he analyzes *eros*, the force suffusing all parts of the soul. *Symposium* depicts a ritualized cocktail party, a long-established Athenian custom, given by the playwright Agathon in honor of his victory at the tragic poetry festival. After dinner and ritual libations, each guest gives a speech in praise of the god Eros, whom all but Socrates see as the god of personal erotic love. Phaedrus, the first speaker, views Eros as bringing an earthshaking emotion, so strong that the lover is willing to die for the beloved. Eros inspires us to be noble so that we will be praised and admired by the ones we desire. Phaedrus's *eros* makes one abnegate the self. In contrast, another speaker, the comic poet Aristophanes, claims that *eros* or sexual desire is the drive for personal completion or wholeness through a union with another person. This view, despite what some general readers of the *Symposium* assume, is not Plato's. As for Plato's account, Plato's Socrates, who credits his knowledge to a wise woman, Diotima, disdains romantic love, the ideal expressed in both these speeches (178a–180b; see Dandekar; Gould). Diotima teaches Socrates that Eros is not desire for the "half" or "whole" unless the half or whole is good (*kalos*; 205e).

In his *Symposium*, Plato presents Eros as the force that impels us toward a self-actualizing wholeness, through a continual quest for knowledge, which leads ultimately to psychic procreation. Presupposing the *Republic*'s degrees-of-reality theory, Socrates depicts this process as an "Ascent" from the world of sensible particulars to the more abstract world of collections of them, to the Forms, and finally to the governing Form, **Beauty**. Erotic attraction to an individual is really attraction to the beauty one perceives in the individual (see Vlastos). As one becomes more Platonically enlightened, one sees that the same beauty exists in many individuals, so erotic attraction to many individuals is a sign of increasing emotional maturity. One then replaces erotic feelings for the body with erotic feelings for the soul and, continuing the Ascent, one arrives at the exemplar of Beauty, "Absolute Beauty," the Form of Beauty itself. The crucial step, for Plato, is moving beyond a sexual, affective attachment to a single person, precisely the form of *eros* honored by the other party participants. The Platonic lover, embodied in the character of Socrates, is free of attachments to particular persons, even, for example, the pleading Alcibiades. Just as sexual attraction leads to the desire to procreate physical progeny, *eros* for Beauty leads to the desire to procreate intellectually. Sexual activity and philosophical contemplation are motivated by the same psychic force, but one is done at sea level, the other at the top of Mt. Olympus. But Plato (unlike his Christian successors) does not dismiss sexuality, as one might think. To channel *eros* into sexual relationships, for Plato, is important: It helps a person gain self-knowledge through knowledge of other selves, and it makes the young lover appreciate something *as* beautiful, the first step toward understanding Beauty itself.

The *Phaedrus* presents a more sympathetic view of *eros* for a single individual that is compatible with, even necessary for, the philosophical life. Plato's employs a metaphor in which the soul is a charioteer (reason) driving two horses: a white horse, representing passions (honor, dignity, pride), and a black horse, representing appetite. In the finest sort of love relationship, the driver, seeing the desired person, becomes filled with warmth. The black horse takes command of the chariot, lunging toward the beloved, despite the futile struggle of the mortified white horse. Plato describes with breathtaking vivacity (253e–254e) the experience of sexual attraction and the internecine conflict that erotic arousal provokes. Only the beloved's dismay can stop the black horse in its tracks. But the beloved, also enduring an internal war between desire and shame, comes to feel what Plato calls "counter-love," a weaker, narcissistic type of desire. The pair experiences mutual longing to consummate their desire and to be together. The couple that succumbs share a noble love, but not so noble as the love between those who resist. The text is ambiguous (255e–256e) as to whether the better couple enjoys some physical affection short of complete gratification or do achieve gratification (refraining from penetration). In either case, Plato in the *Phaedrus* rejects the ideal detachment of the *Republic* and *Symposium*. Moreover, he acknowledges that under certain circumstances a primal sexual attraction between two people can lead to an emotional connection that enhances their lives.

An overview of Plato's writings shows that he became increasingly pessimistic about the human ability to master desire. In the Socratic works he exhibits the belief that humans can master lust and thus their own fates. In *Republic* and *Symposium* he believes that only some people can be trained to control their sexuality, and this achievement requires keeping it apart from love. In *Phaedrus*, Plato is more tolerant of sexuality, recognizing its role in love relationships based on mutual respect. But traveling from *Phaedrus* to *Laws* is like finding a harsh winter on the heels of a sultry Indian summer. For Plato expresses in the *Laws* utter antipathy toward sexual intimacy and love, which he had included as components of the good life in *Phaedrus*.

See also Aristotle; Beauty; Bisexuality; Chinese Philosophy; Desire, Sexual; Firestone, Shulamith; Greek Sexuality and Philosophy, Ancient; Homosexuality, Ethics of; Homosexuality and Science; Love; Marriage; Military, Sex and the; Natural Law (New); Reproductive Technology; Singer, Irving; Social Constructionism; Utopianism

REFERENCES

Adkins, Arthur W. H. "The 'Speech of Lysias' in Plato's *Phaedrus*." In Robert B. Louden and Paul Schollmeier, eds., *The Greeks and Us: Essays in Honor of Arthur W. H. Adkins*. Chicago, Ill.: University of Chicago Press, 1996, 224–40; Benson, Hugh H., ed. *Essays on the Philosophy of Socrates*. Oxford, U.K.: Oxford University Press, 1992; Cantarella, Eva. (1981) *Pandora's Daughters: The Role and Status of Women in Greek and Roman Antiquity*. Trans. Mauren K. Fant. Baltimore, Md.: Johns Hopkins University Press, 1987; Clark, Randall Baldwin. "Platonic Love in a Colorado Courtroom: Martha Nussbaum, John Finnis, and Plato's *Laws* in Evans v. Romer." *Yale Journal of Law and the Humanities* 12:1 (2000), 1–38; Cooper, John, ed., and D. S. Hutchinson, assoc. ed. *Plato: Complete Works*. Indianapolis, Ind.: Hackett, 1997; Dandekar, Natalie. "Eros, Romantic Illusion, and Political Opportunism (*Symposium* 178–180)." In Alan Soble, ed., *Sex, Love, and Friendship*. Amsterdam, Holland: Rodopi, 1997, 558–69; Davidson, James. *Courtesans and Fishcakes: The Consuming Passions of Classical Athens*. New York: St. Martin's Press, 1998; Gould, Carol S. "Romantic and Philosophical Views of Eros in Plato's *Symposium*." In Alan Soble, ed., *Sex, Love, and Friendship*. Amsterdam, Holland: Rodopi, 1997, 570–77; Guthrie, W.K.C. *History of Greek Philosophy*, vol. 4: *Plato: The Man and His Dialogues, Earlier Period*. Cambridge: Cambridge University Press, 1975; Foucault, Michel. (1984) *The History of Sexuality*, vol. 2: *The Use of Pleasure*. Trans. Robert Hurley. New York: Vintage, 1985; Freud, Sigmund. (1923) *The Ego and the Id*. In *The Standard

Edition of the Complete Psychological Works of Sigmund Freud, vol. 19. Trans. and ed. James Strachey. London: Hogarth Press, 1953–1974, 12–68; Keuls, Eva. *The Reign of the Phallus: Sexual Politics in Ancient Athens*. New York: Harper and Row, 1985; Lucas, John. "Plato's Philosophy of Sex." In E. M. Craink, ed., *"Owls to Athens": Essays on Classical Subjects Presented to Sir Kenneth Dover*. Oxford, U.K.: Oxford University Press, 1990, 223–31; Nussbaum, Martha C. *The Fragility of Goodness: Luck and Ethics in Greek Tragedy and Philosophy*. Cambridge: Cambridge University Press, 1986; Nussbaum, Martha C. "Platonic Love and Colorado Law: The Relevance of Ancient Greek Norms to Modern Sexual Controversies." *Virginia Law Review* 80:7 (1994), 1515–1651 (includes "Appendix 4: Dover and Nussbaum Respond to Finnis," coauthored with Kenneth J. Dover, 1641–51); Plato. (ca. 385 BCE) *Alcibiades*. Trans. D. S. Hutchinson. In Cooper, 557–95; Plato. (ca. 390 BCE) *Apology*. Trans. G.M.A. Grube. In Cooper, 17–36; Plato. (ca. 389 BCE) *Charmides*. Trans. Rosamond Kent Sprague. In Cooper, 639–63; Plato. (ca. 381 BCE) *Gorgias*. Trans. Donald J. Zeyl. In Cooper, 791–869; Plato. (ca. 355–347 BCE) *Laws*. Trans. Trevor J. Saunders. In Cooper, 1318–1616; Plato. (ca. 392 BCE) *Lysis*. Trans. Stanley Lombardo. In Cooper, 687–707; Plato. (ca. 380 BCE) *Menexenus*. Trans. Paul Ryan. In Cooper, 950–64; Plato. (ca. 378 BCE) *Phaedo*. Trans. G.M.A. Grube. In Cooper, 49–100; Plato. (ca. 365 BCE) *Phaedrus*. Trans. Alexander Nehamas and Paul Woodruff. In Cooper, 506–56; Plato. (ca. 386 BCE) *Protagoras*. Trans. Stanley Lombardo and Karen Bell. In Cooper, 746–90; Plato. (ca. 375–370 BCE) *Republic*. Trans. G.M.A. Grube; rev. C.D.C. Reeve. In Cooper, 971–1223; Plato. (ca. 380 BCE) *Symposium*. Trans. Alexander Nehamas and Paul Woodruff. In Cooper, 457–505; Poole, William. "Male Homosexuality in Euripides." In Anton Powell, ed., *Euripides, Women, and Sexuality*. New York: Routledge, 1990, 108–50; Rist, John M. "Plato and Professor Nussbaum on Acts 'Contrary to Nature.' " In Mark Joyal, ed., *Studies in Plato and the Platonic Tradition: Essays Presented to John Whittaker*. Aldershot, U.K.: Ashgate, 1997, 65–79; Rosen, Stanley. (1968) *Plato's Symposium*, 2nd ed. New Haven, Conn.: Yale University Press, 1987; Santas, Gerasimos. *Plato and Freud: Two Theories of Love*. Oxford, U.K.: Blackwell, 1988; Shapiro, H. A. "Eros in Love: Pederasty and Pornography in Greece." In Amy Richlin, ed., *Pornography and Representation in Greece and Rome*. Oxford, U.K.: Oxford University Press, 1992, 53–72; Thornton, Bruce S. *Eros: The Myth of Ancient Greek Sexuality*. Boulder, Colo.: Westview, 1997; Vlastos, Gregory. "The Individual as an Object of Love in Plato" and "Appendix II: Sex in Platonic Love." In *Platonic Studies*. Princeton, N.J.: Princeton University Press, 1973, 3–34, 38–42.

Carol Steinberg Gould

ADDITIONAL READING

Allen, Christine Garside. "Plato on Women." *Feminist Studies* 2:2–3 (1975), 1–8; Amir, Lydia. "Plato's Theory of Love: Rationality as Passion." *Practical Philosophy* 4:3 (2001), 6–14. <members.aol.com/PracticalPhilo/Volume4Articles/PlatoTheoryOfLove.htm> [accessed 27 September 2004]; Anton, John. "The Secret of Plato's *Symposium*." *Southern Journal of Philosophy* 12 (1974), 277–93; Bergmann, Martin S. *The Anatomy of Loving: The Story of Man's Quest to Know What Love Is*. New York: Columbia University Press, 1987; Blackburn, Simon. "Two Problems from Plato." In *Lust*. New York: Oxford University Press/New York Public Library, 2004, 29–39; Buchan, Morag. *Women in Plato's Political Theory*. New York: Routledge, 1999; Cantarella, Eva. (1988) *Bisexuality in the Ancient World*. Trans. Cormac Ó Cuilleanáin. New Haven, Conn.: Yale University Press, 1992; Carson, Anne. "Putting Her in Her Place: Woman, Dirt, and Desire." In David Halperin, John J. Winkler, and Froma Zeitlin, eds., *Before Sexuality: The Construction of Erotic Experience in the Ancient Greek World*. Princeton, N.J.: Princeton University Press, 1990, 135–70; Daise, Benjamin. *Kierkegaard's Socratic Art*. Macon, Ga.: Mercer University Press, 1999; Dickason, Anne. "Anatomy Is Destiny: The Role of Biology in Plato's Views of Women." *Philosophical Forum* 5:1–2 (1973–1974), 45–53; Dover, Kenneth J. "The Date of Plato's *Symposium*." *Phronesis* 10:1 (1965), 2–20; Dover, Kenneth J. "Eros and Nomos (Plato, *Symposium* 182A–185C)." *Bulletin of the Institute of Classical Studies* (London) 11 (1964), 31–42; Dover, Kenneth J. (1978) *Greek Homosexuality*. Updated with a new postscript. Cambridge, Mass.: Harvard University Press, 1989; Ferrari, G.R.F.

Listening to the Cicadas: A Study of Plato's Phaedrus. Cambridge: Cambridge University Press, 1987; Ferrari, G.R.F. "Platonic Love." In Richard Kraut, ed., *The Cambridge Companion to Plato.* Cambridge: Cambridge University Press, 1992, 248–76; Finnis, John. "'Shameless Acts' in Colorado: Abuse of Scholarship in Constitutional Cases." *Academic Questions* 7:4 (1994), 10–41; Gelven, Michael. "Eros and Projection: Plato and Heidegger." *Southwestern Journal of Philosophy* 4 (1973), 125–36; George, Robert P. "'Shameless Acts' Revisited: Some Questions for Martha Nussbaum." *Academic Questions* 9:1 (1995–1996), 24–42; Gooch, Paul. "A Mind to Love: Friends and Lovers in Ancient Greek Philosophy." In David Goicoechea, ed., *The Nature and Pursuit of Love: The Philosophy of Irving Singer.* Amherst, N.Y.: Prometheus, 1995, 83–97; Gould, Thomas. *Platonic Love.* London: Routledge and Kegan Paul, 1963; Griffin, Jasper. "The Love That Dared to Speak Its Name." [Review of *Bisexuality in the Ancient World,* by Eva Cantarella] *New York Review of Books* (22 October 1992), 30–32; Griswold, Charles L. *Self-Knowledge in Plato's Phaedrus.* New Haven, Conn.: Yale University Press, 1986. Reprinted, University Park: Pennsylvania State University Press, 1996; Guthrie, W.K.C. (1969) "Attitude to Sex and Love." In *Socrates.* Cambridge: Cambridge University Press, 1971, 70–78; Halperin, David. "Why Is Diotima a Woman? Platonic *Erōs* and the Figuration of Gender." In David Halperin, John J. Winkler, and Froma I. Zeitlin, eds., *Before Sexuality: The Construction of Erotic Experience in the Ancient Greek World.* Princeton, N.J.: Princeton University Press, 1990, 257–308. Also in *One Hundred Years of Homosexuality: And Other Essays on Greek Love.* New York: Routledge, 1990, 113–51; Irwin, Terence. *Plato's Moral Theory: The Early and Middle Dialogues.* Oxford, U.K.: Clarendon Press, 1977; Kosman, L. A. "Platonic Love." In W. H. Werkmeister, ed., *Facets of Plato's Philosophy.* Amsterdam, Holland: Van Gorcum, 1976, 53–69. Reprinted in Alan Soble, ed., *Eros, Agape, and Philia: Readings in the Philosophy of Love.* New York: Paragon House, 1989, 149–63; Kraut, Richard, ed. *The Cambridge Companion to Plato.* Cambridge: Cambridge University Press, 1992; Louden, Robert B., and Paul Schollmeier, eds. *The Greeks and Us: Essays in Honor of Arthur W. H. Adkins.* Chicago, Ill.: University of Chicago Press, 1996; Lucas, John. "Plato's Philosophy of Sex." In E. M. Craink, ed., *"Owls to Athens": Essays on Classical Subjects Presented to Sir Kenneth Dover.* Oxford, U.K.: Oxford University Press, 1990, 223–31. <users.ox.ac.uk/~jrlucas/libeqsor/platsex.html> [accessed 14 October 2004]; Mendelsohn, Daniel. "The Stand: Expert Witnesses and Ancient Mysteries in a Colorado Courtroom." *Lingua Franca* (September–October 1996), 34–46; Mirandola, Giovanni Pico Della. (1651) *A Platonick Discourse upon Love.* Ed. Edmund G. Gardner. Boston, Mass.: Merrymount Press, 1914; Moravcsik, J.M.E. "Reason and Eros in the 'Ascent'-Passage of the *Symposium.*" In John P. Anton, ed., with George L. Kustas, *Essays in Ancient Greek Philosophy.* Albany: State University of New York Press, 1971, 285–302; Morgan, Douglas N. *Love: Plato, the Bible, and Freud.* Englewood Cliffs, N.J.: Prentice-Hall, 1964; Nehamas, Alexander. *Virtues of Authenticity: Essays on Plato and Socrates.* Princeton, N.J.: Princeton University Press, 1999; Neu, Jerome. "Plato's Homoerotic *Symposium.*" In Robert C. Solomon and Kathleen M. Higgins, eds., *The Philosophy of (Erotic) Love.* Lawrence: University Press of Kansas, 1991, 317–35. Reprinted in *A Tear Is an Intellectual Thing: The Meanings of Emotion.* New York: Oxford University Press, 2000, 130–43; Nussbaum, Martha C. "*Eros* and Ethical Norms: Philosophers Respond to a Cultural Dilemma." In Martha C. Nussbaum and Juha Sihvola, eds., *The Sleep of Reason: Erotic Experience and Sexual Ethics in Ancient Greece and Rome.* Chicago, Ill.: University of Chicago Press, 2002, 55–94; Nussbaum, Martha C. "Platonic Love and Colorado Law: The Relevance of Ancient Greek Norms to Modern Sexual Controversies." *Virginia Law Review* 80:7 (1994), 1515–1651. Shorter versions reprinted in *Sex and Social Justice.* New York: Oxford University Press, 1999, 299–331; and Robert B. Louden and Paul Schollmeier, eds., *The Greeks and Us: Essays in Honor of Arthur W. H. Adkins.* Chicago, Ill.: University of Chicago Press, 1996, 168–218; Nussbaum, Martha C. "The Speech of Alcibiades: A Reading of the *Symposium.*" In *The Fragility of Goodness: Luck and Ethics in Greek Tragedy and Philosophy.* Cambridge: Cambridge University Press, 1986, 165–99. Revised from "The Speech of Alcibiades: A Reading of Plato's *Symposium.*" *Philosophy and Literature* 3:2 (1979), 131–72; Nussbaum, Martha C., and Juha Sihvola, eds. *The Sleep of Reason: Erotic Experience and Sexual Ethics in Ancient Greece and Rome.* Chicago, Ill.: University of Chicago Press, 2002; Okin, Susan Moller. (1977)

"Philosopher Queens and Private Wives: Plato on Women and the Family." In Mary Lyndon Shanley and Carole Pateman, eds., *Feminist Interpretations and Political Theory*. University Park: Pennsylvania State University Press, 1991, 11–31; Okin, Susan Moller. "Plato." In *Women in Western Political Thought*. Princeton, N.J.: Princeton University Press, 1979, 15–50; Osborne, Catherine. *Eros Unveiled: Plato and the God of Love*. Oxford, U.K.: Oxford University Press, 1994; Pender, E. E. "Spiritual Pregnancy in Plato's *Symposium*." *Classical Quarterly* 42:1 (1992), 72–86; Peters, F. E. "érōs: desire, love." In *Greek Philosophical Terms: A Historical Lexicon*. New York: New York University Press, 1967, 62–66; Popper, Karl R. (1945) *The Open Society and Its Enemies*, vol. 1: *The Spell of Plato*, 5th ed. Princeton, N.J.: Princeton University Press, 1966; Posner, Richard A. "Response" [to Martha C. Nussbaum, "Platonic Love and Colorado Law"]. In Robert B. Louden and Paul Schollmeier, eds., *The Greeks and Us: Essays in Honor of Arthur W. H. Adkins*. Chicago, Ill.: University of Chicago Press, 1996, 218–23; Price, A. W. *Love and Friendship in Plato and Aristotle*. Oxford, U.K.: Oxford University Press, 1994; Price, A. W. "Martha Nussbaum's *Symposium*." *Ancient Philosophy* 11 (1991), 285–99; Price, A. W. "Plato, Zeno, and the Object of Love." In Martha C. Nussbaum and Juha Sihvola, eds., *The Sleep of Reason: Erotic Experience and Sexual Ethics in Ancient Greece and Rome*. Chicago, Ill.: University of Chicago Press, 2002, 170–99; Reeve, C.D.C. "Plato on Eros and Friendship." In Edward Zalta, ed., *Stanford Encyclopedia of Philosophy*. <plato.stanford.edu/entries/plato-friendship> [accessed 2 February 2005]; Reeve, C.D.C. *Women in the Academy: Dialogues on Themes from Plato's* Republic. Indianapolis, Ind.: Hackett, 2001; Rosen, Stanley. (1968) "A Digression on Incest." In *Plato's Symposium*, 2nd ed. New Haven, Conn.: Yale University Press, 1987, 211–15; Roy, J[ames]. "An Alternative Sexual Morality for Classical Athenians." *Greece and Rome* 44:1 (1997), 11–22; Saxonhouse, Arlene W. "Eros and the Female in Greek Political Thought: An Interpretation of Plato's *Symposium*." *Political Theory* 12:1 (1984), 5–27; Saxonhouse, Arlene W. "The Philosopher and the Female in the Political Thought of Plato." *Political Theory* 4:2 (1976), 195–212. Reprinted in Nancy Tuana, ed., *Feminist Interpretations of Plato*. University Park: Pennsylvania State University Press, 1994, 67–85; Schott, Robin May. (1988) "Philosophical Origins of Ascetic Philosophy: Plato's Views of Women and Eros." In *Cognition and Eros: A Critique of the Kantian Paradigm*. University Park: Pennsylvania State University Press, 1993, 3–17; Singer, Irving. (1966) "Platonic Eros." In *The Nature of Love*, vol. 1: *Plato to Luther*, 2nd ed. Chicago, Ill.: University of Chicago Press, 1984, 47–87; Soble, Alan. "Love Is Not Beautiful: *Symposium* 200e–20lc." *Apeiron* 19:1 (1985), 43–52; Soble, Alan. " 'Something Stupid' about *Eros*." Presentation at Tulane University (20 September 2002). <www.uno.edu/~asoble/pages/TULANE.HTM> [accessed 8 October 2004]; Soble, Alan. "Union, Autonomy, and Concern." In Roger Lamb, ed., *Love Analyzed*. Boulder, Colo.: Westview, 1997, 65–92; Soble, Alan, ed. *Eros, Agape, and Philia: Readings in the Philosophy of Love*. St. Paul, Minn.: Paragon House, 1989. Corrected reprint, 1999; Thorp, John. "The Social Construction of Homosexuality." *Phoenix* 46:1 (1992), 54–65. <www.fordham.edu/halsall/med/thorp.html> [accessed 14 October 2004]; Tuana, Nancy, ed. *Feminist Interpretations of Plato*. University Park: Pennsylvania State University Press, 1994; Vlastos, Gregory. "The Individual as an Object of Love in Plato." In *Platonic Studies*. Princeton, N.J.: Princeton University Press, 1973, 3–34. Reprinted in Alan Soble, ed., *Eros, Agape, and Philia: Readings in the Philosophy of Love*. New York: Paragon House, 1989, 96–124. Also, "Appendix II: Sex in Platonic Love," 38–42 (in Soble, 124–28); Walcot, Peter. "Plato's Mother and Other Terrible Women." *Greece and Rome* 34:1 (1987), 12–31; Ward, Julie K., ed. *Feminism and Ancient Philosophy*. New York: Routledge, 1996; Winkler, John J. *The Constraints of Desire: The Anthropology of Sex and Desire in Ancient Greece*. New York: Routledge, 1990; Wood, Robert E. "Recollection and Two Banquets: Plato's and Kierkegaard's." In Robert L. Perkins, ed., *International Kierkegaard Commentary: Stages on Life's Way*. Macon, Ga.: Mercer University Press, 2000, 49–68.

PORNOGRAPHY. Prior to the nineteenth century, the term "pornography" had a very different connotation than it does today. Derived from the Greek *pornographos*, it referred to writing about prostitutes, and much ancient pornography was merely descriptive. Not until the middle of the 1800s did "pornography" gain its normative gloss. Terms such as "obscene," "unchaste," and "lascivious" became associated with it, and the representation of sexual subject matters became a cause for concern. Yet what counts as obscene or lascivious has changed as aesthetic tastes changed, and the emerging social concern yielded interesting questions about just what to do about pornographic material (Kendrick, chap. 1).

U.S. Law. In the United States, a series of tests were developed to determine whether material was pornographic (or obscene) and thus subject to censorship. The first test, the *Hicklin* test, came from English common law as set forth in *Regina v. Hicklin* (1868). In this test, material that corrupted the minds of those susceptible to it was deemed pornographic. If a particularly sensitive individual found any part of a work offensive, it was subject to censorship. This standard, Felix Frankfurter (1882–1965) commented, reduced "the adult population . . . to reading only what is fit for children" (*Butler v. Michigan*, 1957). The *Hicklin* test was found to be too restrictive and was refined by the U.S. Supreme Court over the next century. In 1933, the susceptible individual was replaced by the "reasonable person," and the intention of the work was also deemed an important component in determining whether the work was pornography warranting censorship (see *U.S. v. One Book Called "Ulysses"*). In a pair of cases in 1957 (*Roth v. U.S.*; *Alberts v. California*), the *Hicklin* test was explicitly "rejected as unconstitutionally restrictive of the freedoms of speech and press." In place of the *Hicklin* test, the Court in *Roth* established a new standard for censoring materials: "whether to the average person, applying contemporary community standards, the dominant theme of the material taken as a whole appeals to prurient interest."

As a result of what was perceived to be a strengthening of First Amendment freedoms as well as the so-called sexual revolution, sexually explicit material proliferated during the 1960s. Many found this increase in pornography problematic, including Richard M. Nixon (1913–1994), who made it an issue in his 1968 presidential campaign. In 1973, with three Nixon appointees on the bench, the Supreme Court developed a new standard to attempt to stem the pornographic tide (O'Brien, 386–87). In *Miller v. California* (1973), Justice Warren Burger (1907–1995), writing for the majority, established the test that is still in place today. To determine that a work may be censored, courts must look for the coalescence of three elements:

> (a) whether "the average person, applying contemporary community standards" would find that the work, taken as a whole appeals to the prurient interest; (b) whether the work depicts or describes in a patently offensive way, sexual conduct specifically defined by the applicable state law; (c) whether the work, taken as a whole, lacks serious literary, artistic, political, or scientific value.

The Supreme Court was not unanimous in this ruling, however. The dissent, led by Justice William J. Brennan, Jr. (1906–1997), expressed significant concerns about a standard to be applied based on the subjective tastes and aversions of the judges. As he wrote, "[W]hat shocks me may be sustenance for my neighbor. What causes one person to boil up in rage over one pamphlet or movie may reflect only his neurosis, not shared by others" (*Miller*). Because the definition of obscenity or pornography had not been specified with sufficient clarity, the dissent worried that it would be impossible to provide fair notice to persons who may wish to create or distribute sexually explicit material. We all may "know it when we see it," but that does not serve as enough of a warning for those who may face legal challenges after the fact.

Debates about the definition of pornography faded in the late twentieth century as the industry in sexually explicit material burgeoned. For the most part, producers of pornography no longer work in dingy garages, and consumers no longer have to tiptoe over bodily fluids as they sneak into X-rated theaters. Scenes that would have undoubtedly failed the *Hicklin* test are regularly displayed on prime-time network television. Sexually explicit materials designed to arouse are available in upscale hotels, on cable television, and are readily accessible on the Internet. Former "smut dealers," like Larry Flynt, are now ensconced in multimillion-dollar office buildings. Aesthetic tastes and contemporary community standards appear to have changed.

Social Harm. For some, this apparent change in community standards that encourages, or at least tolerates, the growing availability of pornography is a source of anger and alarm. Many conservatives argue that the widespread production and distribution of pornographic materials represent significant decay in public morality and traditional values. Pornography, insofar as it promotes "infantile, masturbatory" sexuality, interferes with intimacy between married couples, undermines the view that sex is primarily for reproduction, condones sex outside of **marriage**, and corrupts citizens through its displays of indecent, offensive sexual behavior. A society that tolerates pornography promotes moral disease and the debasement of its citizens. This corruption detracts from a high quality of public life and, according to some conservatives, leads to all sorts of social ills, from increased high school dropout rates to terrorism. (For a representative essay making the conservative case, see Walter Berns; for critical discussion, see Fred Berger [1937–1986].)

Two assumptions about the nature of pornographic representations underlie these conservative claims, assumptions that when illuminated can help determine what, if anything, society should do about pornography. One assumption is based on a theory of representation that suggests that pornographic images capture the sentiments of the community. Pornography might be thought of as a moral barometer, revealing the state and character of social sensibilities. Insofar as the demand for pornographic material has grown, it could be argued that the decency and civility of the populace have declined. More people, with greater frequency, are choosing to spend their time watching pornography rather than pursuing activities that enhance themselves, others, and their communities. The increased demand for and use of pornography represents an increase in social isolation, self-indulgence, and degenerate desires. However, even if this is accurate, censoring pornography is not an obvious answer to ending the alleged social decay. Indeed, if increases in the consumption of pornography merely track a decrease in traditional values, its elimination will not necessarily enhance those values. Pornography may be a symptom of decay rather than being its cause.

The second assumption is that pornography is indeed a cause of the debasement of moral character and social ills. Instead of reflecting what is latent in popular sentiment, pornography creates perverted citizens. The widespread availability of pornography generates both an appetite for decadent and demeaning forms of sexuality and the malformed human relations that the satisfaction of such **sexual desire** requires. This view suggests that there are good, healthy forms of sexual interaction, generally those that occur between a married man and woman for the purposes of reproduction and maintaining tight familial bonds. This desirable form of sexual interest and expression helps to stabilize social relations and serves as an important ground for the inculcation of traditional community values. Pornography undermines this process, contributing to the breakdown of the family and the social problems that allegedly follow from this collapse. If a society is justified in maintaining social stability and preventing social decay, the production and distribution of pornography should not be tolerated.

While preserving social stability is a justification for state action, such as censoring pornography, there are two problems with doing so. The first is empirical. Pornography might contribute to a breakdown in traditional values, just as violent video games might contribute to a breakdown in social stability. But the evidence has not established a causal connection. Second, and more important, given that the facts are not in, there are competing social values that have long been part of social tradition and **law** that weigh against censoring pornography: values like freedom of choice, **privacy**, and being able to determine for oneself what interests one wants to pursue. As long as no harm is being done to another, there is a strong presumption against social interference with how individuals pursue what they take to be a good life.

That certain activities cause harm can serve as a justification for societal action, even state intervention, but only if that harm can be identified as affecting a particular victim or victims. Harm to society, or community values, or public life, in the form of words or images that offend because they are indecent, crude, banal, or even repugnant, is not a strong enough reason to interfere with individual liberty. A society that values freedom must allow citizens to make what some consider to be mistakes, even if those mistakes involve their own debasement. If the people engaged in the production, distribution, and consumption of pornography are consenting adults, individuals are free to argue that these activities are perverted or corrupt, but the state is not justified in substituting its judgment of what is worthy of pursuit for the judgments of those engaged in the production or consumption of pornography. According to this classical liberal view, censorship, in the absence of harm to specifiable individuals, is not justified.

Individual Harm. The question now becomes whether the production and consumption of pornography harm specific individuals. Some proponents of censoring pornography argue that it does, that women in particular are harmed by pornography in a variety of ways. They are harmed, for example, in the production of pornography. The most noted case of this sort of harm has been described by Linda (Lovelace) Marchiano, who claims she was abducted, drugged, and assaulted during the production of *Deep Throat* (see her book *Ordeal*). If a woman is forced to engage in **sexual activity** without her **consent**, she is being sexually assaulted, which is obviously a harm to that woman. As the demand for pornography grew, some pornographers produced more extreme versions and have developed what is called "gonzo" porn. Gonzo porn is unscripted: The participants do not know what will happen to them during the making of the film or video. Some women report that they are hit, choked, or otherwise physically injured in gonzo productions. They are typically penetrated in multiple orifices by multiple people, often simultaneously. When women are physically and/or sexually harmed in the production of pornography (or in any other context, for that matter), state action is justified in preventing the harm and punishing the perpetrators. However, there is a complication: If a woman agrees to participate in a gonzo production, knowing that she may be injured, has she consented to the harm that may befall her? Many people in the course of seeking thrills and/or money apparently consent to undertake risks that may lead to harm, possibly even death. Extreme sports, reality television, and war are a few examples. Perhaps when a person consents to engage in potentially harmful activities, the state should allow that choice to be made, however misguided it may in fact be. Some might argue that the state should not engage in parentalistic action as long as the individual making the potentially harmful choice is in a good position to deliberate about her actions.

Children, for example, are generally thought not to be able to engage in the appropriate forms of deliberation; hence parentalism by the state is warranted to protect young people (and, indirectly, others) from their own bad decisions. Using children in the making of pornography is unlawful, so most of those producing pornography are extremely cautious about verifying the age of participants, generally weeding out those under the age of eighteen. However, women who have just turned eighteen often "star" in pornographic movies and appear in magazines. *Hustler*'s video series "Barely Legal" is one of the most popular, comprising at least sixteen volumes, and has earned over $10 million. An interesting problem about the notion of adult consent arises here. Is a young woman on her eighteenth birthday in a better position to deliberate about her actions than she had been two days earlier? (A similar question arises about the distinction between illegal pedophiliac sexual acts and acts conducted with someone barely an "adult.") Many young women who are over the legal age of consent are unable to deliberate clearly about the possible harms, both physical and psychological, that they may suffer by participating in pornography. Many of these women do not have other options for making money. While it may be a stretch to say that their decisions are coerced, in some cases it would be hard to argue that their choices were fully or even substantially free. ("You don't have women in your freely-consenting model waking up one morning and saying, 'Today is the day on which I make a free choice. Today is the day in which I'm going to decide whether I want to be a brain surgeon, or whether I want to go and find a man and spread my legs for a camera' "; **Catharine MacKinnon**, in MacKinnon and **Andrea Dworkin** [1946–2005], *In Harm's Way,* 392–93.)

Even if we assume that individuals who participate in pornography freely choose to do so and knowingly accept the potential risk of the harms that may accompany their participation, there is another argument that pornography causes harm. Some critics of pornography claim that women are raped, battered, harassed, and subject to other forms of violence by men who consume pornography and, further, that women as a group are harmed due to the climate of violence against women that pornography engenders. Social scientific studies on sexual arousal, attitudes toward women, and self-reported likelihood to **rape** after viewing pornography are often cited in support of the claim that exposure to pornography causes violence against women. (For some of this literature and discussion, see Christensen; Donnerstein et al.; Malamuth and Donnerstein; Russell; Wheeler; Zillmann and Bryant.)

While it may be true that violent crimes committed against women are perpetrated by men who consume pornography, the claim that it is the consumption of pornography by these men that causes violence against women is debatable and difficult to establish. Perhaps pornography leads men to act out their violent fantasies on real women; perhaps pornography creates those fantasies; perhaps pornography desensitizes men to violence against women. But perhaps pornography acts as a release for violence that would otherwise be perpetrated on women. Or pornography might even be causally inert. While some social scientific studies suggest that there is a causal link between exposure to pornography and violence against women, other studies suggest the opposite and still others are inconclusive. If there were a strong causal connection between the availability of pornography and violence against women, we might expect a higher incidence of violence against women in places where pornography is widely available and, conversely, we might expect a lower incidence of violence against women where pornography is banned. This correlation does not exist, however. Utah ranks the lowest in availability of pornography in the United States and ranks twenty-fifth in the number of (reported) rapes. New

Hampshire ranks ninth in availability of pornography and forty-fourth in the number of rapes (Strossen, 254).

Whether or not pornography harms women by creating and sustaining a culture of violence against women, there are additional harms cited by those who criticize pornography that may warrant its elimination. These harms are not primarily physical but emotional. Pornography, it has been argued, creates the belief that women like being degraded, that they enjoy being treated as objects for men's pleasure, and that they desire to be penetrated by various body parts and objects in all their orifices. When men view women this way, women's dignity and actual desires are ignored and their sexual activity is reduced to satisfying men. (For discussion, see Hill; Jarvie.)

Degradation may indeed be an element of most, if not all, pornographic representations. However, it could be argued that it is not simply women who are degraded but men and the viewers of pornography as well (see Brod). In much "girl-girl" pornography, whether produced by men or by lesbians, those being degraded are most often the absent men. Female pleasure is portrayed in the absence of the penis, and the (admittedly simplistic) dialogue predicates this pleasure on the superfluousness of men. Or consider a pornographic film such as *Café Flesh* (1984; dir. Stephen Sayadian), set in a post–World War III world in which 99 percent of the population is unable to engage in sex due to radiation-induced genetic mutations. The 1 percent who can have sex are forced to perform sexual acts in a cabaret for the gratification of the majority who cannot. The nasty master of ceremonies, between performances, chastises and ridicules those watching; the lack of subtlety makes it hard not to conclude that the viewers of the film, not merely the audience in the film, are being mocked and degraded.

Subordination. In the early 1980s, antipornography feminists Catharine MacKinnon and Andrea Dworkin altered the nature of the debate by claiming that the production, distribution, and consumption of pornography silenced and subordinated women (see MacKinnon, *Feminism Unmodified*, 156, 193–95; *Only Words*, 6–7, 40–41, 72–73; *Toward a Feminist Theory*, 205, 247). Their arguments did not rest on pornography's having objectionable sexual content that is destructive of social values; nor did they rely on establishing that pornography causes harm. Instead, they asserted that pornography denied women equality because it silences and subordinates them. Pornography, by undermining women's social and political status, thus constitutes a form of gender discrimination.

Subordination occurs when an individual (or group) is placed in a position of inferior worth or lesser status by another individual (or group) who has the authority to place him or her (them) in such a position and, further, this placement is unjust, discriminatory, or otherwise morally objectionable. If the owner of a small business writes in an job advertisement "Only white people need apply," she could be considered to be performing a subordinating act insofar as it objectionably denies nonwhites access to a job to which white people have access. The case is more persuasive if the government does the same thing: In this situation, a group with authority is diminishing or denying the political status of another group. Having authority is crucial. If I, a university professor, write an editorial discouraging nonwhite people from working, I have not acted with authority in denying nonwhite people work. I may succeed in performing an annoying, offensive, or obnoxious act in publishing racist words, but I have not succeeded in performing a subordinating act. Is pornography subordinating in this way? According to MacKinnon, it is:

> [P]ornography institutionalizes the sexuality of male supremacy, which fuses the erotization of dominance and submission with the social construction of

male and female. Gender is sexual. Pornography constitutes the meaning of that sexuality. Men treat women as who they see women as being. Pornography constructs who that is. Men's power over women means that the way men see women defines who women can be. Pornography is that way. (*Feminism Unmodified*, 148)

Pornography sexualizes gender inequality and inferiority. It constructs women as having less worth than men, it discriminates against women, and it denies them the equal status they deserve (see MacKinnon's model antipornography ordinance, *Women's Lives*, 493n.22 [to 497]).

But does pornography have the authority that is required for it to subordinate women? (See Hornsby; Jacobson; Langton; Soble.) Many sexually explicit videos, images, and texts produced and distributed by the pornography industry are aimed at gay men and lesbians. These products do not follow the heterosexual pattern of subordination that some feminist critics decry. Another sector of the pornography industry is composed of materials produced by and for women, some claiming to be feminists, and most of these cannot be described as sexualizing gender inequality. Another large section of the industry consists of comical videos and cartoons (for example, Japanese manga), media that are not likely to be taken as representing reality. To possess the authority to subordinate, one must participate in a specific set of practices and conventions in an appropriate way. Subordinating acts require a very special set of conventions. Not just any person will be recognized as having the power or authority to perform such acts. Arguing that pornographers have such power is not easy.

It might be claimed that young people learn about sex and gender subordination through pornography, and they enact what pornography teaches them. Rather than pornographers trying to assert authority, it may simply be that such authority is actually granted, albeit mistakenly, by young people and others who do not know any better. Pornography can be said to have authority insofar as young women do become subordinate and young men do come to view subordination as erotic. Whether the existence of pornography that portrays women as sexually subordinate causes women to be sexually subordinated is difficult to answer, a difficulty heightened in a culture in which sexist messages and institutions are ubiquitous and there are numerous sources from which young people can learn (mistaken ideas) about sex, gender, and sexuality.

Perhaps pornography does not subordinate women in ways that warrant its elimination. But does it silence women in ways that deny women full participation in social and political life? Pornography might condition women to believe that they deserve their inferior status and discriminatory treatment. It might thus create an illusion that makes women reluctant even to claim they are being treated in morally objectionable or reprehensible ways. It is true that some women do not recognize discrimination as such, but some women—for example, those who argue for the elimination of pornography—do. Perhaps the claim that pornography silences women means that women have less power to persuade others that discrimination occurs. If pornography disables women so that they cannot make the meaning of their words and arguments clear—if an act of saying "no" to sex cannot be perceived as an act of refusal (Langton, "Speech Acts")—then pornography does silence women and denies them equal participation in both private (sexual) and public (legal) matters. Again, there are certainly cases in which a woman's attempt at convincing others about the detrimental effects of pornography, about her own pain and abuse, about her actual subordination, or about her desire not to engage in sex, is unsuccessful. But her failure is likely a result of her inability to articulate a strong argument, rather than a result of pornography's silencing effect. Socialization undoubtedly contributes to women's inability to make strong arguments, particularly in male-dominated contexts, but whether pornography is the cause of this socialization, or how much of a cause, will vary considerably from context to context.

The claim that pornography silences women and denies them full participation in social life is belied by the fact that there are many women involved in the pornography industry who are making pornography their way and profiting considerably. Some of the women in the business consider themselves feminists. Nina Hartley suggests that her work in the pornography industry as a performer in over a hundred videos was physically and psychologically safe, satisfying for her, and provided an opportunity to celebrate positive female sexuality. Other feminists who are not directly involved in the production of pornography also support it for a variety of reasons—it can be educational, it can alter sexual stereotypes of both men and women, and it can be pleasurable for women (see Assiter and Carol; Caught Looking, Inc.). Given the size of the industry and that pornographic representations take a variety of forms and satisfy a variety of desires, general claims about the industry and its effects on particular women or women as a group are difficult to sustain.

The increasing availability and demand for pornography in the late twentieth century had two related consequences. The first was the mainstreaming of pornography. As is true of any industry, those engaged in the production of pornography are concerned about protecting and increasing their profits. To some extent this can be accomplished by self-imposed restrictions on what is depicted, avoiding the more extreme or offensive types of pornography. The second consequence of increased demand is the other side of the coin. Some in the business realized that what was once thought of as excessive or extreme was becoming more commonplace. They speculated that part of the allure of pornography is crossing certain lines and entering the zone of the taboo, so there will be a demand for more extreme, more taboo-breaking materials. They seem to have been right; gonzo productions that push the boundaries are a booming part of the industry.

See also Arts, Sex and the; Consent; Cybersex; Dworkin, Andrea; Feminism, Liberal; Greek Sexuality and Philosophy, Ancient; Harassment, Sexual; Language; Law, Sex and the; Liberalism; MacKinnon, Catharine; Objectification, Sexual; Pedophilia; Privacy; Prostitution; Rape; Rimmer, Robert; Sex Work

REFERENCES

Alberts v. California. 354 U.S. 476 (1957); Assiter, Alison, and Carol Avedon, eds. *Bad Girls and Dirty Pictures.* London: Pluto Press, 1993; Berger, Fred R. "Pornography, Sex, and Censorship." *Social Theory and Practice* 4:2 (1977), 183–209; Berns, Walter. "Pornography vs. Democracy: The Case for Censorship." *The Public Interest*, no. 22 (Winter 1971), 3–24; Brod, Harry. "Pornography and the Alienation of Male Sexuality." *Social Theory and Practice* 14:3 (1988), 265–84; *Butler v. Michigan.* 352 U.S. 389 (1957); Caught Looking, Inc., eds. *Caught Looking: Feminism, Pornography, and Censorship.* East Haven, Conn.: Long River Books, 1992; Christensen, F[errel] M. "The Alleged Link between Pornography and Violence." In J. J. Krivacska and John Money, eds., *The Handbook of Forensic Sexology: Biomedical and Criminological Perspectives.* Amherst, N.Y.: Prometheus, 1994, 422–48; Donnerstein, Edward, Daniel Linz, and Steven Penrod. *The Question of Pornography.* New York: Free Press, 1987; Hartley, Nina. "Confessions of a Feminist Porno Star." In Frédérique Delacoste and Priscilla Alexander, eds., *Sex Work: Writings by Women in the Sex Industry*, 1st ed. Pittsburgh, Pa.: Cleis Press, 1987, 142–44; Hill, Judith M. "Pornography and Degradation." *Hypatia* 2:2 (1987), 39–54; Hornsby, Jennifer. "Disempowered Speech." *Philosophical Topics* 23:2 (1995), 127–47; Hornsby, Jennifer. "Speech Acts and Pornography." *Women's Philosophical*

Review, no. 10 (November 1993), 38–45; Jacobson, Daniel. "Freedom of Speech Acts? A Response to Langton." *Philosophy and Public Affairs* 24:1 (1995), 64–79; Jarvie, Ian C. "Pornography and/as Degradation." *International Journal of Law and Psychiatry* 14 (1991), 13–27; Kendrick, Walter. *The Secret Museum: Pornography in Modern Culture*. New York: Viking, 1987; Langton, Rae. "Speech Acts and Unspeakable Acts." *Philosophy and Public Affairs* 22:4 (1993), 293–330; Langton, Rae. "Subordination, Silence, and Pornography's Authority." In R. C. Post, ed., *Censorship and Silencing: Practices of Cultural Regulation*. Los Angeles, Calif.: Getty Research Institute, 1998, 261–83; Lovelace, Linda. *Ordeal*. London: W. H. Allen, 1981; MacKinnon, Catharine A. *Feminism Unmodified: Discourses on Life and Law*. Cambridge, Mass.: Harvard University Press, 1987; MacKinnon, Catharine A. *Only Words*. Cambridge, Mass.: Harvard University Press, 1993; MacKinnon, Catharine A. *Toward a Feminist Theory of the State*. Cambridge, Mass.: Harvard University Press, 1989; MacKinnon, Catharine A. *Women's Lives, Men's Laws*. Cambridge, Mass.: Harvard University Press, 2005; MacKinnon, Catharine A., and Andrea Dworkin, eds. *In Harm's Way: The Pornography Civil Rights Hearings*. Cambridge, Mass.: Harvard University Press, 1997; Malamuth, Neil M., and Edward Donnerstein, eds. *Pornography and Sexual Aggression*. Orlando, Fla.: Academic Press, 1984; *Miller v. California*. 413 U.S. 15 (1973); O'Brien, David. *Constitutional Law and Politics*, vol. 2: *Civil Rights and Civil Liberties*. New York: Norton, 1991; *Regina v. Hicklin*. L. R. 3 Q.B. 360 (1868); *Roth v. U.S.* 354 U.S. 476 (1957); Russell, Diana E. H. "Pornography and Rape: A Causal Model." *Political Psychology* 9:1 (1988), 41–73. Revised version in Diana E. H. Russell, ed., *Making Violence Sexy: Feminist Views on Pornography*. New York: Teachers College Press, 1993, 120–50; Russell, Diana E. H. "Pornography and Violence: What Does the New Research Say?" In Laura Lederer, ed., *Take Back the Night: Women on Pornography*. New York: Morrow, 1980, 218–38; Soble, Alan. "Bad Apples: Feminist Politics and Feminist Scholarship." *Philosophy of the Social Sciences* 29:3 (1999), 354–88; Strossen, Nadine. *Defending Pornography: Free Speech, Sex, and the Fight for Women's Rights*. New York: Scribner's, 1995; *U.S. v. One Book Called "Ulysses."* 5 F. Supp. 182, 183–84 (S.D.N.Y.) (1933); Wheeler, Hollis. "Pornography and Rape: A Feminist Perspective." In Ann Wolbert Burgess, ed., *Rape and Sexual Assault: A Research Handbook*. New York: Garland, 1985, 374–91; Zillmann, Dolf, and Jennings Bryant, eds. *Pornography: Research Advances and Policy Considerations*. Hillsdale, N.J.: Erlbaum, 1989.

Lori Gruen

ADDITIONAL READING

Abramson, Paul R., and Haruo Hayashi. "Pornography in Japan: Cross-Cultural and Theoretical Considerations." In Neil M. Malamuth and Edward Donnerstein, eds., *Pornography and Sexual Aggression*. Orlando, Fla.: Academic Press, 1984, 173–83; Adam, Alison. "Cyberstalking and Internet Pornography: Gender and the Gaze." *Ethics and Information Technology* 4:2 (2002), 133–42; Adler, Amy. "The Perverse Law of Child Pornography." *Columbia Law Review* 101 (March 2001), 209–73. <www.ipce.info/library_3/files/adler.htm> and <cyber.law.harvard.edu/ilaw/Speech/Adler_full.html> [accessed 16 February 2005]; *American Booksellers Association, Inc. v. Hudnut*. 771 F.2d 323 (1985); Antoniou, Laura. "Defending Pornography (for Real This Time)." *Harvard Gay and Lesbian Review* (Summer 1995), 21–22; *Ashcroft v. Free Speech Coalition*. 122 S.Ct. 1389 (2002); Atlas, James. "The Loose Canon: Why Higher Learning Has Embraced Pornography." *The New Yorker* (29 March 1999), 60–65; Atwood, Margaret. "Atwood on Pornography." *Chatelaine* (Toronto) 56:9 (September 1983), 61, 118, 126; Baird, Robert M., and Stuart E. Rosenbaum, eds. *Pornography: Private Right or Public Menace?* Buffalo, N.Y.: Prometheus, 1991. Revised ed., 1998; Baldwin, Margaret. "The Sexuality of Inequality: The Minneapolis Pornography Ordinance." *Law and Inequality: A Journal of Theory and Practice* 2:2 (1984), 629–53; Benjamin, Jessica. "Sympathy for the Devil: Notes on Sexuality and Aggression, with Special Reference to Pornography." In *Like Subjects, Love Objects: Essays on Recognition and Sexual Difference*. New Haven, Conn.: Yale University Press, 1995, 175–215; Berger, Fred R. "Pornography, Feminism, and Censorship." In Robert B. Baker and Frederick A. Elliston, eds., *Philosophy and Sex*, 2nd ed. Buffalo, N.Y., 1984, 327–51; Berger, Fred R.

"Pornography, Sex, and Censorship." *Social Theory and Practice* 4:2 (1977), 183–209. Reprinted in POS1 (322–47); Berns, Walter. "Dirty Words." *The Public Interest*, no. 114 (Winter 1994), 119–25; Brod, Harry. "Pornography and the Alienation of Male Sexuality." *Social Theory and Practice* 14:3 (1988), 265–84. Reprinted in Michael S. Kimmel and Michael A. Messner, eds., *Men's Lives*, 3rd ed. Needham Heights, Mass.: Allyn and Bacon, 1995, 393–404; Larry May, Robert Strikwerda, and Patrick D. Hopkins, eds., *Rethinking Masculinity: Philosophical Explorations in Light of Feminism*, 2nd ed. Lanham, Md.: Rowman and Littlefield, 1996, 237–53; POS2 (281–99); Bullough, Vern L. "Research and Archival Value of Erotica/Pornography." In Martha Cornog, ed., *Libraries, Erotica, and Pornography*. Phoenix, Ariz.: Oryx, 1991, 99–105; Burger, John R. *One-Handed Histories: The Eroto-Politics of Gay Male Video Pornography*. New York: Haworth Press, 1995; Burstyn, Varda, ed. *Women against Censorship*. Vancouver, Can.: Douglas and McIntyre, 1985; Butterworth, Dianne. "Wanking in Cyberspace: The Development of Computer Porn." In Stevi Jackson and Sue Scott, eds., *Feminism and Sexuality: A Reader*. New York: Columbia University Press, 1996, 314–20; Carol, Avedon. *Nudes, Prudes, and Attitudes: Pornography and Censorship*. Cheltenham, U.K.: New Clarion Press, 1994; Carse, Alisa L. "Pornography: An Uncivil Liberty?" *Hypatia* 10:1 (1995), 156–82; Carter, Angela. *The Sadeian Woman and the Ideology of Pornography*. New York: Pantheon Books, 1978; Cavalier, Robert J. "Feminism and Pornography: A Dialogical Perspective." <caae.phil.cmu.edu/Cavalier/Forum/pornography/background/CMC_article.html> [accessed 6 June 2005]; Chiu, Monica. *Filthy Fictions: Asian American Literature by Women*. Lanham, Md.: AltaMira, 2004; Christensen, F[errel] M. "Cultural and Ideological Bias in Pornography Research." *Philosophy of the Social Sciences* 20:3 (1990), 351–75; Christensen, F[errel] M. *Pornography: The Other Side*. New York: Praeger, 1990; Cohen, Joshua. "Freedom, Equality, Pornography." In Austin Sarat and Thomas R. Kearns, eds., *Justice and Injustice in Law and Legal Theory*. Ann Arbor: University of Michigan Press, 1996, 99–137; Cornell, Drucilla. *The Imaginary Domain: Abortion, Pornography, and Sexual Harassment*. New York: Routledge, 1995; Cornell, Drucilla, ed. *Feminism and Pornography*. New York: Oxford University Press, 2000; Cornog, Martha, ed. *Libraries, Erotica, and Pornography*. Phoenix, Ariz.: Oryx, 1991; Dollimore, Jonathan. *Sex, Literature and Censorship*. Cambridge, U.K.: Polity Press, 2005; Dworkin, Andrea. "Against the Male Flood: Censorship, Pornography, and Equality." In Patricia Smith, ed., *Feminist Jurisprudence*. New York: Oxford University Press, 1993, 449–66; Dworkin, Andrea. *Life and Death: Unapologetic Writings on the Continuing War against Women*. New York: Free Press, 1997; Dworkin, Andrea. *Pornography: Men Possessing Women*. New York: Perigee, 1981; Dworkin, Andrea. "Why So-Called Radical Men Love and Need Pornography." In Laura Lederer, ed., *Take Back the Night*. New York: Morrow, 1980, 148–54; Dworkin, Andrea, and Catharine A. MacKinnon. *Pornography and Civil Rights: A New Day for Women's Equality*. Minneapolis, Minn.: Organizing Against Pornography, 1988; Dworkin, Ronald. "Is There a Right to Pornography?" *Oxford Journal of Legal Studies* 1:2 (1981), 177–212. Reprinted in Susan Dwyer, ed., *The Problem of Pornography*. Belmont, Calif.: Wadsworth, 1995, 77–90; Dworkin, Ronald. "Liberty and Pornography." *New York Review of Books* (21 October 1993), 12–15. Reprinted in Susan Dwyer, ed., *The Problem of Pornography*. Belmont, Calif.: Wadsworth, 1995, 113–21; Dworkin, Ronald. "Women and Pornography." *New York Review of Books* (21 October 1993), 36–42; [reply to letter] *New York Review of Books* (3 March 1994), 48–49; Dwyer, Susan. "Enter Here—At Your Own Risk: The Moral Dangers of Cyberporn." In Robert J. Cavalier, ed., *The Impact of the Internet on Our Moral Lives*. Albany: State University of New York Press, 2005, 69–94; Dwyer, Susan, ed. *The Problem of Pornography*. Belmont, Calif.: Wadsworth, 1995; Dyzenhaus, David. "John Stuart Mill and the Harm of Pornography." *Ethics* 102:3 (1992), 534–51; Easton, Susan M. "Pornography." In Ruth Chadwick, ed., *Encyclopedia of Applied Ethics*, vol. 3. San Diego, Calif.: Academic Press, 1998, 605–14; Easton, Susan M. *The Problem of Pornography: Regulation and the Right to Free Speech*. London: Routledge, 1994; Elshtain, Jean Bethke. "The New Porn Wars." *The New Republic* (25 June 1984), 19; Estlund, David M. "MacKinnon." [Reply to Catharine A. MacKinnon, "Pornography Left and Right" (q.v.)] In David M. Estlund and Martha C. Nussbaum, eds., *Sex, Preference, and Family: Essays on Law and Nature*. New York: Oxford University Press, 1997, 164–68; Estlund, David M. "The Visit and the Video: Publication and the Line between Sex and Speech." In David M.

Estlund and Martha C. Nussbaum, eds., *Sex, Preference, and Family: Essays on Law and Nature.* New York: Oxford University Press, 1997, 126–47; Ferguson, Frances. "Pornography: The Theory." *Critical Inquiry* 21:3 (1995), 670–95; Ferguson, Frances. *Pornography, the Theory: What Utilitarianism Did to Action.* Chicago, Ill.: University of Chicago Press, 2004; *Final Report of the Attorney General's [Meese] Commission on Pornography.* Nashville, Tenn.: Rutledge Hill Press, 1986. Washington, D.C.: U.S. Government Printing Office, 1986; Garb, Sarah H. "Sex for Money Is Sex for Money: The Illegality of Pornographic Film as Prostitution." *Law and Inequality* 13:2 (1995), 281–301; Garry, Ann. "Pornography and Respect for Women." *Social Theory and Practice* 4:4 (1978), 395–421. Reprinted in Sharon Bishop and Marjorie Weinzweig, eds., *Philosophy and Women.* Belmont, Calif.: Wadsworth, 1979, 128–39; P&S2 (312–26); Garry, Ann. "Sex, Lies, and Pornography." In Hugh LaFollette, ed., *Ethics in Practice: An Anthology*, 2nd ed. Malden, Mass.: Blackwell, 2002, 344–55; Gastil, Raymond D. "The Moral Right of the Majority to Restrict Obscenity and Pornography through Law." *Ethics* 86:3 (1976), 231–40; Gibson, Pamela Church, and Roma Gibson, eds. *Dirty Looks: Women, Pornography, Power.* London: British Film Institute (BFI), 1993; Glenmullen, Joseph. *The Pornographer's Grief and Other Tales of Human Sexuality.* New York: HarperCollins, 1993; Goldhill, Simon. "The Erotic Experience of Looking: Cultural Conflict and the Gaze in Empire Culture." In Martha C. Nussbaum and Juha Sihvola, eds., *The Sleep of Reason: Erotic Experience and Sexual Ethics in Ancient Greece and Rome.* Chicago, Ill.: University of Chicago Press, 2002, 374–99; Grazia, Edward de. *Girls Lean Back Everywhere: The Law of Obscenity and the Assault on Genius.* New York: Random House, 1992; Griffin, Susan. *Pornography and Silence: Culture's Revenge against Nature.* New York: Harper and Row, 1979; Gruen, Lori. "Pornography and Censorship." In R. G. Frey and Christopher Heath Wellman, eds., *A Companion to Applied Ethics.* Oxford, U.K.: Blackwell, 2002, 154–66; Gubar, Susan, and Joan Hoff, eds. *For Adult Users Only: The Dilemma of Violent Pornography.* Bloomington: Indiana University Press, 1989; Gurstein, Rochelle. *The Repeal of Reticence: A History of America's Cultural and Legal Struggles over Free Speech, Obscenity, Sexual Liberation, and Modern Art.* New York: Hill and Wang, 1996; Hill, Judith M. "Pornography and Degradation." *Hypatia* 2:2 (1987), 39–54. Reprinted in Robert M. Baird and Stuart E. Rosenbaum, eds., *Pornography: Private Right or Public Menace?*, rev. ed. Amherst, N.Y.: Prometheus, 1998, 100–113; Hoffman, Eric. "Feminism, Pornography, and Law." *University of Pennsylvania Law Review* 133:2 (1985), 497–534; Hornsby, Jennifer. "Speech Acts and Pornography." *Women's Philosophical Review*, no. 10 (November 1993), 38–45. Reprinted, revised, with Postscript (231–32), in Susan Dwyer, ed., *The Problem of Pornography.* Belmont, Calif.: Wadsworth, 1995, 220–32; Hunter, Nan D., and Sylvia A. Law. "Brief *Amici Curiae* of Feminist Anticensorship Task Force et al., in *American Booksellers Association v. Hudnut*." In Patricia Smith, ed., *Feminist Jurisprudence.* New York: Oxford University Press, 1993, 467–81; Itzin, Catherine, ed. *Pornography: Women, Violence and Civil Liberties.* Oxford, U.K.: Oxford University Press, 1992; Juffer, Jane. *At Home with Pornography: Women, Sex, and Everyday Life.* New York: New York University Press, 1998; Kaite, Berkeley. *Pornography and Difference.* Bloomington: Indiana University Press, 1995; Kappeler, Susanne. *The Pornography of Representation.* Minneapolis: University of Minnesota Press, 1986; Kimmel, Michael S. "Introduction: Guilty Pleasures—Pornography in Men's Lives." In Michael S. Kimmel, ed., *Men Confront Pornography.* New York: Crown, 1990, 1–22; Kimmel, Michael S., ed. *Men Confront Pornography.* New York: Crown, 1990; Kipnis, Laura. *Bound and Gagged: Pornography and the Politics of Fantasy in America.* New York: Grove Press, 1996; Kipnis, Laura. "(Male) Desire and (Female) Disgust: Reading *Hustler*." In Lawrence Grossberg, Cary Nelson, and Paula A. Treichler, eds., *Cultural Studies.* New York: Routledge, 1992, 373–91. Reprinted in Robert J. Corber and Stephen Valocchi, eds., *Queer Studies: An Interdisciplinary Reader.* Malden, Mass.: Blackwell, 2003, 102–18; Kittay, Eva Feder. "Pornography and the Erotics of Domination." In Carol C. Gould, ed., *Beyond Domination: New Perspectives on Women and Philosophy.* Totowa, N.J.: Rowman and Allanheld, 1984, 145–74; Koppelman, Andrew. "Racist Speech and Pornography." *Antidiscrimination Law and Social Equality.* New Haven, Conn.: Yale University Press, 1996, 220–65; Langton, Rae. "Love and Solipsism." In Roger E. Lamb, ed., *Love Analyzed.* Boulder, Colo.: Westview, 1997, 123–52; Langton, Rae. "Pornography, Speech Acts, and

Silence." In Hugh LaFollette, ed., *Ethics in Practice: An Anthology.* Cambridge, Mass.: Blackwell, 1997, 338–49; Langton, Rae. "Sexual Solipsism." *Philosophical Topics* 23:2 (1995), 149–87; Langton, Rae. "Speech Acts and Unspeakable Acts." *Philosophy and Public Affairs* 22:4 (1993), 293–330. Reprinted in Susan Dwyer, ed., *The Problem of Pornography.* Belmont, Calif.: Wadsworth, 1985, 203–19; Langton, Rae. "Whose Right? Ronald Dworkin, Women, and Pornographers." *Philosophy and Public Affairs* 19:4 (1990), 311–59. Reprinted in Susan Dwyer, ed., *The Problem of Pornography.* Belmont, Calif.: Wadsworth, 1995, 91–112; Lapham, Lewis H., Al Goldstein, Midge Decter, Erica Jong, Susan Brownmiller, Jean Bethke Elshtain, and Aryeh Neier. "The Place of Pornography: Packaging Eros for a Violent Age." [Panel discussion] *Harper's Magazine* (November 1984), 31–45. See "Letters." *Harper's Magazine* (February 1985), 4–6, 73–76; Lawrence, D. H. (1930) "A Propos of Lady Chatterley's Lover." In *Phoenix II: Uncollected, Unpublished, and Other Prose Works.* New York: Viking, 1959, 487–515; Lawrence, D. H. (1929) "Pornography and Obscenity." In *Sex, Literature, and Censorship.* Ed. Harry T. Moore. New York: Twayne, 1953, 69–88; Lederer, Laura, ed. *Take Back the Night: Women on Pornography.* New York: Morrow, 1980; Leiber, Justin. "Pornography, Art, and the Origins of Consciousness." In Alan Soble, ed., *Sex, Love, and Friendship.* Amsterdam, Holland: Rodopi, 1997, 601–7; LeMoncheck, Linda. "I Only Do It for the Money: Pornography, Prostitution, and the Business of Sex." In *Loose Women, Lecherous Men: A Feminist Philosophy of Sex.* New York: Oxford University Press, 1997, 110–54; Levy, Neil. "Virtual Child Pornography: The Eroticization of Inequality." *Ethics and Information Technology* 4:4 (2002), 319–23; Loftus, David. *Watching Sex: How Men Really Respond to Pornography.* Berkeley, Calif.: Thunder's Mouth Press, 2002; Longino, Helen. "Pornography, Oppression, and Freedom: A Closer Look." In Laura Lederer, ed., *Take Back the Night: Women on Pornography.* New York: Morrow, 1990, 40–54. Reprinted in Susan Dwyer, ed., *The Problem of Pornography.* Belmont, Calif.: Wadsworth, 1995, 34–47; Lord, M. G. "Pornutopia: How Feminist Scholars Learned to Love Dirty Pictures." *Lingua Franca* 7:4 (1997), 40–48; Lynn, Barry W. " 'Civil Rights' Ordinances and the Attorney General's Commission: New Developments in Pornography Regulation." *Harvard Civil Rights–Civil Liberties Law Review* 21:1 (1986), 27–125; MacKinnon, Catharine A. "Pornography as Sex Inequality." [Part 2, section B] In *Women's Lives, Men's Laws.* Cambridge, Mass.: Harvard University Press, 2005, 297–372; MacKinnon, Catharine A. "Pornography Left and Right." [Review of *Sex and Reason*, by Richard A. Posner, and *Girls Lean Back Everywhere: The Law of Obscenity and the Assault on Genius*, by Edward de Grazia] In David M. Estlund and Martha C. Nussbaum, eds., *Sex, Preference, and Family: Essays on Law and Nature.* New York: Oxford University Press, 1997, 102–25; MacKinnon, Catharine A. "Preface." In Jeffrey Moussaieff Masson, *A Dark Science: Women, Sexuality, and Psychiatry in the Nineteenth Century.* New York: Farrar, Straus and Giroux, 1986, xi–xxii. Reprinted as "Sex, Lies, and Psychotherapy," in *Women's Lives, Men's Laws.* Cambridge, Mass.: Harvard University Press, 2005, 251–58; MacKinnon, Catharine A. "Sexuality, Pornography, and Method: 'Pleasure under Patriarchy.' " *Ethics* 99 (January 1989), 314–46; MacKinnon, Catharine A. "Vindication and Resistance: A Response to the Carnegie Mellon Study of Pornography in Cyberspace." *Georgetown Law Journal* 83:4 (June 1995), 1959–67; Marcus, Steven. (1966) *The Other Victorians: A Study of Sexuality and Pornography in Mid-Nineteenth-Century England.* New York: Bantam, 1977; Mason-Grant, Joan. *Pornography Embodied: From Speech to Sexual Practice.* Lanham, Md.: Rowman and Littlefield, 2004; May, Larry. "Pornography and Pollution." In *Masculinity and Morality.* Ithaca, N.Y.: Cornell University Press, 1998, 58–78; McCormack, Thelma. "If Pornography Is the Theory, Is Inequality the Practice?" *Philosophy of the Social Sciences* 23:3 (1993), 298–326; McNair, Brian. *Mediated Sex: Pornography and Postmodern Culture.* London: Arnold, 1996; McNair, Brian. " 'Not Some Kind of Kinky Porno Flick': The Return of Porno-Fear?" *Bridge*, no. 11 (August–September 2004), 16–19; McNair, Brian. *Striptease Culture: Sex, Media and the Democratisation of Desire.* London: Routledge, 2002; Morgan, Robin. "Theory and Practice: Pornography and Rape." In *Going Too Far: The Personal Chronicle of a Feminist.* New York: Random House, 1977, 163–69; Nalezinski, Alix. "Acceptable and Unacceptable Levels of Risk: The Case of Pornography." *Social Theory and Practice* 22:1 (1996), 83–104; Parent, W. A. "A Second Look at Pornography and the Subordination of Women." *Journal of Philosophy* 87:4 (1990), 205–11; Penley, Constance. "Crackers and

Whackers: The White Trashing of Porn." In Matt Wray and Annalee Newitz, eds., *White Trash: Race and Class in America*. New York: Routledge, 1977, 89–112. Reprinted in Linda Williams, ed., *Porn Studies*. Durham, N.C.: Duke University Press, 2004, 309–31; Posner, Richard A. "Obsession." [Review of *Only Words*, by Catharine A. MacKinnon] *The New Republic* (18 October 1993), 31–36; Posner, Richard A., and Katharine B. Silbaugh. "Possession of Obscene Materials." In *A Guide to America's Sex Laws*. Chicago, Ill.: University of Chicago Press, 1996, 188–206; Rea, Michael C. "What Is Pornography?" *Noûs* 35:1 (2001), 118–45; Read, Daphne. "(De)Constructing Pornography: Feminisms in Conflict." In Kathy Peiss and Christina Simmons, eds., *Passion and Power: Sexuality in History*. Philadelphia, Pa.: Temple University Press, 1989, 277–92; Reeve, C.D.C. "Violence, Pornography, and Sadomasochism." In *Love's Confusions*. Cambridge, Mass.: Harvard University Press, 2005, 125–45; Reisman, Judith A. *Images of Children, Crime, and Violence in Playboy, Penthouse, and Hustler: The Role of Pornography and Media Violence in Family Violence, Sexual Abuse and Exploitation, and Juvenile Delinquency*. Arlington, Va.: Institute for Media Education, 1989; Richlin, Amy, ed. *Pornography and Representation in Greece and Rome*. New York: Oxford University Press, 1992; Rimm, Marty. "Marketing Pornography on the Information Superhighway: A Survey of 917,410 Images, Descriptions, Short Stories, and Animations Downloaded 8.5 Million Times by Consumers in Over 2000 Cities in Forty Countries, Provinces, and Territories." *Georgetown Law Journal* 83 (1995), 1849–1934; Russell, Diana E. H. *Against Pornography: The Evidence of Harm*. Berkeley, Calif.: Russell Publications, 1993; Russell, Diana E. H. *Dangerous Relationships: Pornography, Misogyny, and Rape*. Thousand Oaks, Calif.: Sage, 1998; Russell, Diana E. H. (1982) *Rape in Marriage*, rev. ed. Bloomington: Indiana University Press, 1990; Russell, Diana E. H., ed. *Making Violence Sexy: Feminist Views on Pornography*. New York: Teachers College Press, 1993; Scoccia, Danny. "Can Liberals Support a Ban on Violent Pornography?" *Ethics* 106:4 (1996), 776–99; Segal, Lynne, and Mary McIntosh, eds. *Sex Exposed: Sexuality and the Pornography Debate*. New Brunswick, N.J.: Rutgers University Press, 1993; Shattuck, Roger. *Forbidden Knowledge: From Prometheus to Pornography*. San Diego, Calif.: Harcourt Brace, 1996; Shrage, Laurie. "Feminist Perspectives on Sex Markets." In Edward Zalta, ed., *The Stanford Encyclopedia of Philosophy* (18 February 2004). <plato.stanford.edu/entries/feminist-sex-markets/> [accessed 24 August 2004]; Skipper, Robert. "Mill and Pornography." *Ethics* 103:4 (1993), 726–30; Snitow, Ann Barr. "Mass Market Romance: Pornography for Women Is Different." *Radical History Review* 20 (Spring–Summer 1979), 141–61. Reprinted in Kathy Peiss and Christina Simmons, eds., *Passion and Power: Sexuality in History*. Philadelphia, Pa.: Temple University Press, 1989, 259–76; Soble, Alan. "The Mainstream Has Always Been Pornographic." *Bridge*, no. 12 (October–November 2004), 33–36; Soble, Alan. "Pornography." In *Sexual Investigations*. New York: New York University Press, 1996, 214–49; Soble, Alan. *Pornography, Sex, and Feminism*. Amherst, N.Y.: Prometheus, 2002; Soble, Alan. "Pornography and the Social Sciences." *Social Epistemology* 2:2 (1988), 135–44. Reprinted in POS2 (317–31); POS4 (421–34); Soble, Alan. "Pornography: Defamation and the Endorsement of Degradation." *Social Theory and Practice* 11:1 (1985), 61–87. Reprinted, abridged, in Robert M. Baird and Stuart E. Rosenblum, eds., *Pornography: Private Right or Public Menace?* Buffalo, N.Y.: Prometheus, 1991, 96–107. 2nd ed., 1998, 134–45; and Steven Satris, ed., *Taking Sides: Clashing Views on Controversial Moral Issues*, 5th ed. Guilford, Conn.: Dushkin, 1996, 198–205. 6th ed., 1998, 200–207; Soble, Alan. *Pornography: Marxism, Feminism, and the Future of Sexuality*. New Haven, Conn.: Yale University Press, 1986; Soble, Alan. Review of *The Pornography of Representation*, by Susanne Kappeler. *Philosophy of the Social Sciences* 19:1 (1989), 128–31; Stark, Cynthia A. "Is Pornography an Action? The Causal vs. the Conceptual View of Pornography's Harm." *Social Theory and Practice* 23:2 (1997), 277–306; Steinem, Gloria. (1977–1978) "Erotica vs. Pornography." In *Outrageous Acts and Everyday Rebellions*. New York: Holt, Rinehart and Winston, 1983, 219–30; Steiner, George. "Night Words: High Pornography and Human Privacy." *Encounter* 25:4 (1965), 14–19. Reprinted in *Language and Silence: Essays on Language, Literature, and the Inhuman*. New York: Atheneum, 1967, 68–77; Stoltenberg, John. *Refusing to Be a Man: Essays on Sex and Justice*. Portland, Ore.: Breitenbush Books, 1989; Stoltenberg, John. *What Makes Pornography "Sexy"?* Minneapolis, Minn.: Milkweed, 1994; Strossen, Nadine. *Defending Pornography: Free*

Speech, Sex, and the Fight for Women's Rights. New York: Scribner's, 1995; Tisdale, Sallie. "Talk Dirty to Me." *Harper's Magazine* (February 1992), 37–46. Reprinted in POS3 (271–81); POS4 (369–79); Tisdale, Sallie. *Talk Dirty to Me: An Intimate Philosophy of Sex*. New York: Doubleday, 1994; Tong, Rosemarie. "Brief Encounter." *Women's Review of Books* 3:8 (1986), 7–9; Tong, Rosemarie. "Feminism, Pornography, and Censorship." *Social Theory and Practice* 8 (1982), 1–17; Tong, Rosemarie. "Women, Pornography, and the Law." *Academe* 73:5 (1987), 14–22. Reprinted in POS2 (301–16); Tucker, Scott. "Gender, Fucking, and Utopia: An Essay in Response to John Stoltenberg's *Refusing to Be a Man*." *Social Text*, no. 27 (1990), 3–34; Turley, Donna. "The Feminist Debate on Pornography: An Unorthodox Interpretation." *Socialist Review* 16:3–4 (1986), 81–96; Vadas, Melinda. "A First Look at the Pornography/Civil Rights Ordinance: Could Pornography Be the Subordination of Women?" *Journal of Philosophy* 84:9 (1987), 487–511; Vadas, Melinda. "The Pornography/Civil Rights Ordinance v. The BOG: And the Winner Is . . . ?" *Hypatia* 7:3 (1992), 94–109; Vernon, Richard. "John Stuart Mill and Pornography: Beyond the Harm Principle." *Ethics* 106 (April 1996), 621–32; Ward, David. "Should Pornography Be Censored?" In James A. Gould, ed., *Classic Philosophical Questions*. New York: Prentice Hall, 1995, 504–12; Weinstein, James. *Hate Speech, Pornography, and the Radical Attack on Free Speech Doctrine*. Boulder, Colo.: Westview, 1999; Weisberg, D. Kelly, ed. "Pornography." Section of *Applications of Feminist Legal Theory to Women's Lives: Sex, Violence, Work, and Reproduction*. Philadelphia, Pa.: Temple University Press, 1996, 5–183; Weitzer, Richard, ed. *Selling Sex: Pornography, Prostitution, and the Sex Industry*. London: Routledge, 2000; West, Caroline. "Pornography and Censorship." In Edward N. Zalta, ed., *Stanford Encyclopedia of Philosophy*. (2004) <plato.stanford.edu/entries/pornography-censorship/> [accessed 18 January 2005]; Wicclair, Mark R. "Feminism, Pornography, and Censorship." In Thomas A. Mappes and Jane S. Zembaty, eds., *Social Ethics: Morality and Social Policy*, 4th ed. New York: McGraw-Hill, 1992, 282–88; Williams, Bernard, ed. *Report on the Commission on Obscenity and Film Censorship*. Cambridge: Cambridge University Press, 1981; Williams, Linda. *Hard Core: Power, Pleasure, and the "Frenzy of the Visible."* Berkeley: University of California Press, 1989; Williams, Linda. "Second Thoughts on *Hard Core*: American Obscenity Law and the Scapegoating of Deviance." In Pamela Church Gibson and Roma Gibson, eds., *Dirty Looks: Women, Pornography, Power*. London: British Film Institute (BFI), 1993, 46–61; Williams, Linda. "Sexual Politics: Strange Bedfellows." *In These Times* (29 October–4 November 1986), 18–20; Williams, Linda. "Skin Flicks on the Racial Border: Pornography, Exploitation, and Interracial Lust." In Linda Williams, ed., *Porn Studies*. Durham, N.C.: Duke University Press, 2004, 271–308; Williams, Linda, ed. *Porn Studies*. Durham, N.C.: Duke University Press, 2004; Zillmann, Dolf, and Jennings Bryant. "Pornography's Impact on Sexual Satisfaction." *Journal of Applied Social Psychology* 18:5 (1988), 438–53.

POSNER, RICHARD (1939–). Richard Allen Posner has undertaken many bold projects. One of them, primarily carried out in his massive *Sex and Reason*, relies on the "dismal science" of economics to investigate the passionate realm of human sexuality. Posner proposes that economics can illuminate sexual issues from **abortion** and **adultery** to virginity and voyeurism.

A prolific writer, Posner has, in each year since the 1970s, authored on average one book, several scholarly articles, and upwards of a hundred judicial opinions. He graduated first in his class at Harvard Law School (1962) and since 1969 has taught at the University of Chicago Law School. Posner has also served, since 1981, as judge on the 7th Circuit U.S. Court of Appeals. With William M. Landes, he cofounded the "law and economics" movement and has applied economics to an array of subjects. His writings are extensively researched, extremely intelligent, aggressively unconventional, widely read, and strongly criticized.

A standard humanist criticism of economics is that it knows the price of everything but the value of nothing. Posner reverses this criticism: Philosophy might think it knows the value of things, but it does not know their cost. Since moral philosophy, on his view, produces incisive critiques but is incapable of providing convincing proofs about substantive moral matters such as abortion and infanticide (*Overcoming*, 467), academic moral theory is useless (*Problematics*, 3–90). The science of economics, on the other hand, works with facts and yields testable hypotheses (*Problems*, 348–52). Still, instead of employing, say, statistics or mathematical arguments, as would an empirical economist, Posner theorizes about nonmarket areas of life with the help of economic concepts: "search costs," "competition," "substitution," "satisfaction-theory of value," "taxes," "trade-offs," "externalities" (*Overcoming*, 336, 558). For example, Posner describes **rape** as "sex theft" because by performing this act a "man obtains sexual gratification without having to negotiate for it in the 'market'" (*Overcoming*, 341; *Sex*, 182–83, 386–87). Posner, however, is not always careful with his economic concepts. At times "benefit" and "cost" seem to refer to almost the entire range of good and evil, while at other times they seem to refer narrowly to what can be measured.

Posner rejects any moralism that presumes sexuality in general is sinful (see Nussbaum, "Only Grey," 1701). His ideological enemy seems to be a deontological ethics in which sexual activities such as **masturbation** or **prostitution** are *prima facie* wrong. His own approach—typical for an economist—is akin to utilitarianism in that it aims at maximizing personal satisfaction (*Sex*, 386). In Posner's anthropology, we are, broadly, *homo economicus*: The human self has a set of desires that reason chooses among and tries to satisfy. Posner has been criticized on the grounds that this notion of the human person fails to account for the complexity of human life, including its history and commitments (see Bartlett; Robson).

Posner's "basic assumption," as an economist, is that "people are rational maximizers of their satisfactions—*all* people . . . in *all* of their [chosen] activities" (*Problems*, 353). Both judges and the prostitutes they send to jail are motivated to provide their respective services not out of public interest but to fulfill their own personal satisfactions ("Economic Analysis," 1313). Since, for Posner, rationality does not require conscious decision making, animals can also be rational ("Economic Approach," 173; *Problems*, 354). To be rational in Posner's sense is simply to suit the means to the ends. In this instrumental rationality, one does not reflect on the intrinsic nature of the ends or the means, only caring that they are *effective* means (*Problems*, 354). Posner's account of reason, as opposed to other accounts, thereby strips human reason of an ability to appreciate what is intrinsically valuable (see **Roger Scruton**, 49).

Posner sides with **social constructionism** in holding that there are no "essences" such as those posited by, for example, Natural Law ethics. Sexual norms are merely whatever rules societies devise in response to their material and historical circumstances (*Overcoming*, 572–78; *Problematics*, 19–21; *Sex*, 213–15). But Posner disagrees with other aspects of social constructionism: Its proponents are disinterested in "facts," and they imply (to his mind) that human life can be remade just by changes in thinking (*Overcoming*, 572–78; see *Sex*, 23, 29–30). Posner plumps instead for a libertarian pragmatism that pushes for change while recognizing that biological facts and entrenched cultural traditions constitute givens that people can alter only somewhat. For example, Posner defends a piecemeal, go-slow approach to instituting **same-sex marriage** ("Should There Be").

Posner holds that a person's sexual drive is a given and that cultural shifts only modify the forms and costs of satisfying that drive. He suggests, for example, that scarcity of women in a locale or society likely results in greater pederasty (*Overcoming*, 574; *Sex*, 100,

147–48). Similarly, he claims that the sexual revolution of the 1960s was a only a matter of "changing prices" due to the availability of abortion and oral **contraception** rather than the effect of, for example, a shift in ethical factors (Philipson and Posner, "Sexual Behaviour," 99). In reply, several critics of Posner have replied that the human spirit not only chooses among sexual practices but also shapes the very meaning of human **sexual activity** in a way that cannot be captured by cost/benefit analyses (see Hadfield, "Not the 'Radical' Feminist Critique," 543–45; Halley, 193–207; Nussbaum, "Only Grey," 1716–26).

On the basis of his anthropology, Posner tends to describe sexual activity in terms of the self-interested pursuit by the body of what satisfies it. When, for example, the "search costs" of finding a female are "infinite," as in the all-male environment of a prison, heterosexuals turn to same-sex sexual activity as the best available sex ("Economic Approach," 179–83; *Sex*, 121). Critics object that, even if Posner succeeds in explaining why some people "deviate" from normal practice, his economic analyses cannot determine whether the deviations are morally good or bad (Nussbaum, "Only Grey," 1698–1700). Posner rejects this criticism by arguing that, like other human activities such as driving a car, sexual activity has, in itself, no particular moral quality ("Radical," 525). Sexual activity is like eating: People may buy and consume expensive gourmet food, but they do not do anything wrong when they eat hamburgers (*Sex*, 182). Posner concludes that "no good reason to deter premarital sex" exists; such activity is in general a "harmless search for pleasure" (*Sex*, 330).

Sexuality is, of course, distinct in its own ways. Posner turns to sociobiology to delineate three ends or purposes of sexuality that are set down not by human reason but by our evolutionary heritage (*Sex*, 111–12). The first end is procreation, which tends to be the end that Posner stresses the most. Sexual activity produces babies, and any theory that ignores this obvious biological fact is inadequate. Second, sexual activity produces pleasure. Third, sexual activity promotes sociability; people engage in a sexual "trade" or exchange that is mutually beneficial (Philipson and Posner, *Private*, 5–6). Sex, like other human activities for *homo economicus*, is an exercise in mutual back-scratching. People get their sexual itches scratched in exchange for goods or services sought by their sexual partners. Martha Nussbaum laments that Posner's view of sex lacks romanticism. Sex as he depicts it is "sex without the soul" ("Only Grey," 1717). Posner usually thinks of sexuality not as involving union with an attractive or loved person but as a pressure that needs release in some outlet (Nussbaum, "Venus," 39). One is reminded here of the hydraulic model sometimes attributed to **Sigmund Freud** (1856–1939).

Posner also appeals to sociobiology to explain differences between men's and women's sexuality (in a way hotly contested by Hadfield in "Flirting with Science"). Posner offers the standard evolutionary argument that because male and female investments in procreation are widely different, they have innately different sexual strategies (*Overcoming*, 338, 353; *Sex*, 90–92). Writing chiefly from an androcentric perspective (see Ertman; Fineman), Posner holds that men generally have a stronger sex drive than women and seek a greater variety of outlets, which leads to adultery, opportunistic **homosexuality**, and a "prostitution industry" (*Overcoming*, 353; *Sex*, 91–92, 179–80). The more females men impregnate, the more offspring they will have. Women, who can get pregnant relatively infrequently, are as a result more selective with whom they mate and are generally not promiscuous (*Sex*, 90–91). Within **marriage**, women offer sex as "payment for services" (*Overcoming*, 353–54) and as an inducement to keep men from straying. (See *Sex*, 88–98, for the evolutionary biology of sexuality on which Posner draws. For supporting arguments, see Symons; for criticism, Hrdy.)

The institution of marriage, according to Posner (*Sex*, 5), has gone through two strikingly different stages. In the first stage, which Posner locates in ancient times, wives were "breeders," not emotional partners. In the second stage, beginning approximately with the rise of Christianity, women assumed the role of companion and were co-responsible for the family economy. Western civilization, in his view, is moving toward a third stage because women can now be independent due to the changed nature of work, the reduction of child mortality, the advent of labor-saving devices, and the rise of **reproductive technology** (*Overcoming*, 329–30). The institution of marriage, consequently, is becoming simply one option among many. Indeed, it is likely that in the future more people will prefer temporary forms of contractual or uncommitted cohabitation ("Radical," 522; Sanoff).

With the help of economics, Posner tries to show that sex discrimination laws have not helped women but have likely harmed them. The "price" to employers of restructuring the workplace to avoid prosecution or to enhance women's self-esteem has been so high that employers resist hiring women or have had to limit everyone's pay increases ("Economic Analysis"). Posner favors surrogate pregnancy, where one woman "rents" her womb, since the surrogate is compensated and everyone, including the prospective child, is better off (*Overcoming*, 333). Posner compares the benefits of infanticide, particularly of females, to that of thinning trees in a forest (*Sex*, 143–44, 216). He points out the economic advantages of "baby-selling," arguing (among other reasons) that there is too little commodification of such goods (*Sex*, 405–16). He writes that marriage is not fundamentally different from prostitution (*Sex*, 131). Obviously, Posner does not shy away from the implications of his theory. His views, however, seem outrageous to his critics: "The result is about as unreasonable as a discussion of sex could be" (Scruton, 47). Posner's counterintuitive conclusions derive from the unusual approach he takes. His task, as he sees it, is to expose what is left when the "acid bath" of economics is applied to an area of human life that is so often encrusted that one cannot see what is really at stake.

It is clear from the text and abundant notes in *Sex and Reason* that Posner has read more widely than most specialists in the area of sexuality. He has boldly applied economics to sex. Kept within bounds, his approach is novel and illuminating. But, to his critics, what he offers is not true to the full life and dignity of the human person.

See also Animal Sexuality; Bestiality; Consequentialism; Ethics, Sexual; Evolution; Greek Sexuality and Philosophy, Ancient; Law, Sex and the; Privacy; Psychology, Evolutionary; Rimmer, Robert; Sherfey, Mary Jane; Social Constructionism

REFERENCES

Bartlett, Katharine T. "Rumpelstiltskin." *Connecticut Law Review* 25:2 (1993), 473–90; Ertman, Martha M. "Denying the Secret of Joy: A Critique of Posner's Theory of Sexuality." *Stanford Law Review* 45:5 (1993), 1485–1524; Fineman, Martha Albertson. "The Hermeneutics of Reason: A Commentary on *Sex and Reason*." *Connecticut Law Review* 25:2 (1993), 503–13; Hadfield, Gillian K. "Flirting with Science: Richard Posner on the Bioeconomics of Sexual Man." *Harvard Law Review* 106:2 (1992), 479–503; Hadfield, Gillian K. "Not the 'Radical' Feminist Critique of *Sex and Reason*." *Connecticut Law Review* 25:2 (1993), 533–46; Halley, Janet E. "The Sexual Economist and Legal Regulation of the Sexual Orientations." In David M. Estlund and Martha C. Nussbaum, eds., *Sex, Preference, and Family: Essays on Law and Nature*. New York: Oxford University Press, 1997, 192–207; Hrdy, Sarah Blaffer. *The Woman That Never Evolved*. Cambridge, Mass.: Harvard University Press, 1981; Nussbaum, Martha C. " 'Only Grey Matter'? Richard Posner's Cost-Benefit Analysis of Sex." *University of Chicago Law Review* 59:4 (1992), 1689–1734; Nussbaum, Martha C. "Venus in Robes." *The New Republic* (20 April 1992), 36–41; Philipson, Tomas J., and Richard A. Posner. *Private Choices and Public Health: The AIDS Epidemic in an Economic Perspective*.

Cambridge, Mass.: Harvard University Press, 1993; Philipson, Tomas J., and Richard A. Posner. "Sexual Behaviour, Disease and Fertility Risk." *Risk Decision and Policy* 1:1 (1996), 91–104; Posner, Richard A. "An Economic Analysis of Sex Discrimination Laws." *University of Chicago Law Review* 56:4 (1989), 1311–35; Posner, Richard A. "The Economic Approach to Homosexuality." In David M. Estlund and Martha C. Nussbaum, eds., *Sex, Preference, and Family: Essays on Law and Nature.* New York: Oxford University Press, 1997, 173–91; Posner, Richard A. *Overcoming Law.* Cambridge, Mass.: Harvard University Press, 1995; Posner, Richard A. *The Problematics of Moral and Legal Theory.* Cambridge, Mass.: Harvard University Press, 1999; Posner, Richard A. *The Problems of Jurisprudence.* Cambridge, Mass.: Harvard University Press, 1990; Posner, Richard A. "The Radical Feminist Critique of *Sex and Reason.*" *Connecticut Law Review* 25:2 (1993), 515–31; Posner, Richard A. *Sex and Reason.* Cambridge, Mass.: Harvard University Press, 1992; Posner, Richard A. "Should There Be Homosexual Marriage? And If So, Who Should Decide?" *Michigan Law Review* 95:6 (1997), 1578–87; Robson, Ruthann. "Posner's Lesbians: Neither Sexy Nor Reasonable." *Connecticut Law Review* 25:2 (1993), 491–502; Sanoff, A. P. "The Economics of Sex." [Interview with Richard Posner] *U.S. News and World Report* (4 May 1992), 61; Scruton, Roger. "Sex For Sale." *National Review* (8 June 1992), 47–49; Symons, Donald. *The Evolution of Human Sexuality.* Oxford, U.K.: Oxford University Press, 1979.

Edward Collins Vacek

ADDITIONAL READING

Becker, Gary S., and Richard A. Posner. "Cross-Cultural Differences in Family and Sexual Life: An Economic Analysis." *Rationality and Society* 5:4 (1993), 421–31; Belliotti, Raymond A. *Good Sex: Perspectives on Sexual Ethics.* Lawrence: University Press of Kansas, 1993; Chamallas, Martha. "The Backlash against Feminist Legal Theory." In Anita M. Superson and Ann E. Cudd, eds., *Theorizing Backlash: Philosophical Reflections on the Resistance to Feminism.* Lanham, Md.: Rowman and Littlefield, 2002, 67–86; Decter, Midge. "Marriage as a Trade: Bridging the Private/Private Distinction." *Harvard Civil Rights—Civil Liberties Law Review* 36:1 (2001), 79–132; Decter, Midge. "Sex and Reason?" *The Public Interest*, no. 107 (Spring 1992), 113–18; Eskridge, William N., Jr. "A Social Constructionist Critique of Posner's *Sex and Reason*: Steps toward a Gaylegal Agenda." *Yale Law Journal* 102:1 (1992), 333–86; Gagnon, John H. "The Dismal Science and Sex." *American Journal of Sociology* 99:4 (1994), 1078–82; Hrdy, Sarah Blaffer. "The Evolution of Human Sexuality: The Latest Word and the Last." *Quarterly Review of Biology* 54:3 (1979), 309–14; Kristol, Elizabeth. "*Sex and Reason.*" *American Spectator* 25:5 (May 1992), 68–73; Kurtz, Steve. "Sex, Economics, and Other Legal Matters: An Interview with Richard A. Posner." *Reason* 32:11 (2001), 36–43; Landes, William M., and Richard A. Posner. *The Economic Structure of Intellectual Property Law.* Cambridge, Mass.: Harvard University Press, 2003; Landes, William M., and Richard A. Posner. *The Economic Structure of Tort Law.* Cambridge, Mass.: Harvard University Press, 1987; MacKinnon, Catharine A. "Pornography Left and Right." [Review of *Sex and Reason*, by Richard A. Posner, and *Girls Lean Back Everywhere: The Law of Obscenity and the Assault on Genius*, by Edward de Grazia] In David M. Estlund and Martha C. Nussbaum, eds., *Sex, Preference, and Family: Essays on Law and Nature.* New York: Oxford University Press, 1997, 102–25; Philipson, Tomas J., and Richard A. Posner. *Private Choices and Public Health: The AIDS Epidemic in an Economic Perspective.* Cambridge, Mass.: Harvard University Press, 1993; Posner, Richard A. "Emotion versus Emotionalism in Law." In Susan A. Bandes, ed., *The Passions of Law.* New York: New York University Press, 1999, 309–29; Posner, Richard A. "Obsession." [Review of *Only Words*, by Catharine A. MacKinnon] *The New Republic* (18 October 1993), 31–36; Posner, Richard A. "Publications, Presentations, and Works in Progress." <www.law.uchicago.edu/faculty/posner-r/publications.html> [accessed 30 May 2004]; Posner, Richard A. "Response" [to Martha C. Nussbaum, "Platonic Love and Colorado Law"]. In Robert B. Louden and Paul Schollmeier, eds., *The Greeks and Us: Essays in Honor of Arthur W. H. Adkins.* Chicago, Ill.: University of Chicago Press, 1996, 218–23; Posner, Richard A., and Katharine B. Silbaugh. *A Guide to America's Sex Laws.* Chicago, Ill.: University of

Chicago Press, 1996; Scruton, Roger. "Gay Reservations." In Michael Leahy and Dan Cohn-Sherbok, eds., *The Liberation Debate: Rights at Issue*. London: Routledge, 1996, 108–24; Scruton, Roger. *Sexual Desire: A Moral Philosophy of the Erotic*. New York: Free Press, 1986; West, Robin. "Authority, Autonomy, and Choice: The Role of Consent in the Moral and Political Visions of Franz Kafka and Richard Posner." *Harvard Law Review* 99:2 (1985), 384–428; Zelder, Martin. "Incompletely Reasoned *Sex*: A Review of Posner's Somewhat Misleading Guide to the Economic Analysis of Sex and Family Law." *Michigan Law Review* 91:6 (1993), 1584–1608.

POSTSTRUCTURALISM. Poststructuralism, a distinctly French phenomenon, arose in the early 1960s and is linked with the more widespread phenomenon of postmodernism. Both are critical of modernity and modernization. However, where postmodernism frequently gets its vitality from the modern periods of art, and concerns itself with new forms and arts (as well as technologies, corporealities, and sexualities) that will follow the modern period, poststructuralism raises questions about the meaning of modernity, modernization, subjectivity, and sexuality. From poststructuralism have emerged several well-known, connected critiques of Western thought: that it is "logocentric," claiming privilege for certain rational, universalistic modes of **language** and discourse, and that it is "phallogocentric," bestowing privilege on male (that is, virile and logical) perspectives.

The relationship between poststructuralism and postmodernism is complex. One link is the postmodernist critique of modern philosophy (see Rorty), frequently understood as a denial of objective truth, which bears affinities with poststructuralism's critique of modern science's claim to provide the truth about desire and sex. A second is the recurrent theme in postmodern art of the use of fragments and disorderly assemblages—*bricolage*—as principles of presentation that relate to the past not as something to move beyond but as something to mine, draw from, and build on. Poststructuralism, too, is concerned with fragmentation and disorder in modern society.

The relationship between postmodernism and poststructuralism is exhibited by Jean-François Lyotard (1924–1998), a poststructuralist who established his reputation in *The Postmodern Condition*, which includes the essay "Answering the Question: What Is Postmodernism?" (71–82) and contains the widely quoted line about postmodernism/poststructuralism: "Let us wage a war on totality; let us be witnesses to the unpresentable; let us activate the differences and save the honor of the name" (82). In these words lie many of the themes of poststructuralism. It is concerned with the limits of language, speech, knowledge, intelligibility; with what cannot be said in a certain language or régime of discourse, and what is said obliquely; with what can and cannot be presented, known, or made familiar; and with resistance to established forms of discourse, academic disciplines, institutions, and state powers. All these factors and forces are understood to shape subjectivity through what **Michel Foucault** (1926–1984) called *subjectivation* ("Genealogy of Ethics," 264). The emphasis on resistance to the shaping of subjectivity and on the transformation of subjectivity brings ethics and politics to the foreground, yet poststructuralism is also significantly concerned with aesthetics and the separation between the sciences and the arts and humanities. Lyotard's "war on totality" is waged against any pretense of establishing (say, in the manner of **G.W.F. Hegel** [1770–1831]) a comprehensive, universal system (an overarching "metanarrative"; see *Postmodern Condition*, 34, 37), as well as against dividing thought and practice, nature and culture, into separate domains. Sexuality enters in the caesura of subjectivation, that is, in relation to questions about "propriety." One might understand much of modern thought, including that of **Sigmund Freud** (1856–1939) and

Karl Marx (1818–1883), as searching for a new sexual propriety, for our time and for the future, in the name of human liberation. Sexuality, though, remains ensnared in the traps of propriety, correctness, and conformism, against the promise and allure of polymorphous perversity, multiplicity, and variability.

Two other determinants of the modern world against which poststructuralism offers critique are the "hard" sciences (physics, chemistry, biology), which to many seem to have nothing to do with human sexuality, and the human sciences (anthropology, economics, history, psychology, sociology), which have everything to do with human sexuality, yet assert that their practices of knowledge are authoritative. Thus questions about science and the authority of knowledge are the background of poststructuralism's approach to sexuality, construed broadly to include intimate behaviors, all types of desire, and gender differences. In this context, **Friedrich Nietzsche** (1844–1900) and **Martin Heidegger** (1889–1976) are two additional figures who criticize modernity and from whom poststructuralism draws strength. Nietzsche and Heidegger criticize not only the practices and reflections of modernity but also the assumptions of modernity that define its origin. For both, major transformations in sensibility and thought occurred in ancient Greece and again with the rise of modern science (viz., rationalization and secularization), transformations that need to be minutely examined. These transformations involved sexual, intimate, and private practices; human corporeality; and the differences and relations between men and women.

The major figures of poststructuralism are Gilles Deleuze (1925–1995), Félix Guattari (1930–1992), Jacques Derrida (1930–2004), Foucault, and Lyotard. From the 1960s on, many other French writers influenced and were influenced by poststructuralism: Louis Althusser (1918–1990), Antonin Artaud (1896–1948), Alain Badiou, Étienne Balibar, Roland Barthes (1915–1980), **Georges Bataille** (1897–1962), Jean Baudrillard, Maurice Blanchot, Pierre Bourdieu (1930–2002), Michel de Certeau (1925–1986), Pierre Klossowski (1905–2001), **Jacques Lacan** (1901–1981), Philippe Lacoue-Labarthes, **Emmanuel Levinas** (1906–1995), Claude Lévi-Strauss, Maurice Merleau-Ponty (1908–1961), Jean-Luc Nancy, Jean-Paul Sartre (1905–1980), as well as the authors called the "French feminists": Simone de Beauvoir (1908–1986), Hélène Cixous, Luce Irigaray, Julia Kristeva, and Monique Wittig (1935–2003). Other European writers have been influenced by poststructuralism (Giorgio Agamben, Rosi Braidotti, Slavoj Žižek), as have some American feminists (Judith Butler, Jane Gallop, Elizabeth Grosz, Donna Haraway).

All these writers addressed sexuality in interesting ways, often in the shadow of the **Marquis de Sade** (1740–1814). Thus, to investigate poststructuralist philosophy of sexuality is to discuss a wide phenomenon taking place in France and the rest of Europe in relation to Freud's work on sexuality and to the ongoing critique of the Christian (Augustinian, Thomistic) view of bodies and sexual practices, both of which have important links with Sade. For Foucault,

> Sade attains the end of Classical discourse and thought. He holds sway precisely upon their frontier. After him, violence, life and death, desire, and sexuality will extend, below the level of representation, an immense expanse of shade which we are now attempting to recover, as far as we can, in our discourse, in our freedom, in our thought. But our thought is so brief, our freedom so enslaved, our discourse so repetitive, that we must face the fact that expanse of shade below is really a bottomless sea. (*Order of Things*, 211)

To grasp the poststructuralist phenomenon in its force and vitality, it is helpful to focus on the years 1972–1974, during which three major works were written, all responsive to

Sade, through Klossowski and Bataille, and emerging from close affinities with Nietzsche and Heidegger: Deleuze and Guattari's *Anti-Oedipus*, Wittig's *The Lesbian Body*, and Lyotard's *Libidinal Economy*. The character of each of their perspectives on sexuality can be illustrated with these representatively dramatic passages:

> It is at work everywhere, functioning smoothly at times, at other times in fits and starts. It breathes, it heats, it eats. It shits and fucks. What a mistake to have ever said *the* id. Everywhere *it* is machines—real ones, not figurative ones; machines driving other machines, machines being driven by other machines, with all the necessary couplings and connections. (Deleuze and Guattari, *Anti-Oedipus*, 1)

> M/y kneecaps appear at m/y knees from which shreds of flesh fall. M/y armpits are musty. M/y breasts are eaten away. *I* have a hole in m/y throat. The smell that escapes from m/e is noisome. You do not stop your nostrils. You do not exclaim with fright when at a given moment m/y putrescent and half-liquid body touches the length of your bare back. (Wittig, *Lesbian*, 20)

> Open the so-called body and spread out all its surfaces: not only the skin with each of its folds, wrinkles, scars, with its great velvety planes, and contiguous to that, the scalp and its mane of hair, the tender pubic fur, nipples, nails, hard transparent skin under the heel, the light frills of the eyelids, set with lashes—but open and spread, expose the labia majora, so also the labia minora with their blue network bathed in mucus, dilate the diaphragm of the anal sphincter, longitudinally cut and flatten out the black conduit of the rectum, then the colon, the caecum, now a ribbon with this surface all striated and polluted with shit; . . . armed with scalpels and tweezers, dismantle and lay out the bundles and bodies of the encephalon; and then the whole network of veins and arteries, intact, . . . take them apart and put them end to end with all the layers of nerve tissue which surround the aqueous humours and the cavernous body of the penis, and extract the great muscles, the great dorsal nets, spread them out like smooth sleeping dolphins. (Lyotard, *Libidinal*, 1)

It is hardly possible to overlook that these works constitute an event in rethinking bodies and sexualities, linking the materiality of bodies with the excessiveness of desire. They follow, and owe their existence to, Bataille. Sartre's related view of sexuality in *Being and Nothingness* (1943) as one of the primary expressions of the ego's freedom and individuality, Beauvoir's much more social and gender-sensitive reading of sexual identification and freedom in *The Second Sex* (1949), and Merleau-Ponty's view of the body and sex in *Phenomenology of Perception* (1945) were also pivotal influences.

With Sade and Nietzsche in the background, read as challenging with desire the entire machinery of modern reason and social order, poststructuralism draws three crucial themes from Heidegger's *Being and Time* (1927): the importance of questioning to human life and to Being itself; the importance of *thrownness*, being thrown into the world temporally and corporeally; and the opening in which language is the house of Being, emphasizing the opening of Being to meaning. It follows that eros, desire, and sexuality are recurrent questions that pervade every moment and interstice of life. The being of the human cannot be separated from the Being into which it is thrown: It is thrown in body, materially; it is thrown through words and images; and it is thrown among other bodies and humans. Sexuality is one of these throwings, and it exists in the mode of questioning. Irigaray says this of sexuality as difference, opening up another question in relation to desire:

> Sexual difference represents one of the questions or the question that is to be thought in our age. According to Heidegger, each age has one thought to think. One only. Sexual difference is probably the thought of our time. The thing of our time that, thought, will bring us "salvation" [«salut»]. (Irigaray, *Ethics*, 5; translation by Ross)

In this way there lie in sexuality questions concerning the meaning of being and being human: first, in a critique of the forms of knowledge that would claim to know this meaning, especially the social sciences; second, in a critique of the institutional forms that would seek to control what it is to be human by regulating sexuality and personal life, relations between men and women, and forms of reproduction and population control; and, third, in the alternatives and possibilities for sexuality and desire that are to be thought and lived in response to the control and reduction of desire that institutions of knowledge and social practice impose on us. The question of the "post" here in poststructuralism is a question of alternatives, which emerges in the context of Freudian and Marxist aspirations to social and human liberation that turn on sexual freedom. Sexuality is one of the most intensely controlled and articulated aspects of human life; yet it is also claimed to be a source of liberation. It is both abundantly regulated and yet one of the most unregulated possibilities of excess. Between these poles lies a caesura, a gap or interruption in intelligible sexual patterns. Poststructuralism can be understood as seeking to reveal these forms without necessarily proposing their superiority.

Derrida's principle from *The Politics of Friendship* can thus be read to express both the caesura and another set of questions for sexuality and **love**: "At the centre of the principle, always, the One does violence to itself, and guards itself against the other" (*Politics*, ix). The importance of the other, human or otherwise, now comes into play: the one (every one) guards itself against the other (every other) by doing violence to itself. This may pertain to philosophy and science and all forms of knowledge and rationality. It may pertain to language and all social practices. It may pertain to sexuality, love, and desire in relation to violence and **perversion**. Derrida proposes it here (and in "Plato's Pharmacy," *Dissemination*, 61–171) in relation to **friendship**, which we may presume is neither sexual nor erotic. Yet the guarding is visible. *Philia* and *eros* are both translated as *love*, and love cannot be restricted except through the violence and guarding of which Derrida speaks. *Anti-Oedipus*, *Lesbian Body*, and *Libidinal Economy* all occupy this space of guarding and violence in which the transformation of life takes place in relation to a love and desire that exceed any given practice.

Sade, Nietzsche, and Bataille present the field of desire as excessive, infinite, multiple, transgressive, perverse, beyond determination, and they do so while critiquing social institutions and forms of knowledge as setting boundaries for and restricting desire. Bataille's distinction between restricted and general economy, the familiar economy of desire versus the extravagant economy of desire that exceeds all bounds (*Accursed Share*, vol. 1, 19–41; vol. 2, 89–184), returns throughout this literature in different forms. Marx and Freud may be read as presenting far-reaching critiques of modern institutions—industrial capitalism and sexual repression—while exhibiting ambiguity as to what might follow, from such a critique, as the liberatory alternative of the future. Marx and Friedrich Engels (1820–1895), in *The Communist Manifesto* (72), emphatically speak of ending **prostitution**. But their critique seems, to Lyotard, to lead to a conventional family structure with equality between men and women, as if to reinstate or even reinvigorate conventional, if not idealized bourgeois, constraints on desire (see *Libidinal*, 95–154). The question of limits, which is always inherent in the excess and transgression of desire, can be addressed to propose other sets of social possibilities less restrictive of desire and/or to acknowledge that such social violence and guarding are inherent in language, society, and intelligibility.

One of the most irresistible themes in Nietzsche (*Zarathustra*, 406–8), continued into Bataille (*Accursed Share*), is that this condition need not be a cause for despair but a time for exuberance, laughter, and affirmation. Thus poststructuralism may be an intense critique of the social institutions and practices that restrict desire and channel sexuality and subjectivity as well as an affirmative relation to new forms of sexuality, desire, and subjectivity, without proposing institutions and practices that themselves restrict desire. It is because *every* institution or practice does violence to itself and guards itself against the other (other institutions, other sexes, other sexualities) that the excessiveness of desire is realized in the moment, in the transgressive event itself, rather than in a durable set of social institutions. Poststructuralism (and even postmodernism in this sense) is the emergent, transformative, and affirmative moment of the appearance of new sexualities. To rewrite Derrida: Sexuality, desire, and love all remain "to come" [*a-venir*]—never present, in the sense of always coming. In Nancy's words, "Love arrives, it comes, or else it is not love. But it is thus that it endlessly goes elsewhere than to 'me' who would receive it: its coming is only a departure for the other, its departure only the coming of the other" ("Shattered Love," 98; in *Inoperative Community*, 82–109). This coming, or coming and going, is not a human or social phenomenon but lies at the heart of the world. The "crossing—the coming-and-going, the comings-and-goings of love—is constitutive of the occurrence. This takes place before the face and signification. Or rather, this takes place on another level: *at the heart of being*" (105).

If these are shared understandings of sexuality, desire, and love among poststructuralists and their contemporaries, how these writers express them are frequently quite different in ways that evince more than differences of position and thematic emphases. The question here is whether the form of expression is *itself* an object of desire, to designate what Barthes calls the fully erotic "pleasure of the text." Writing and speaking are themselves objects and signs of desire (with or without Freudian sublimation). Language is erotically imbued with desire. Barthes's words, too, are erotic. "[T]he pleasure of the text is not sure: nothing can say that this same text will please us a second time: it's a friable pleasure, crumbled by mood, habit, circumstance; it's a precarious pleasure" (*Pleasure of the Text*, 83). This is just what sex is like. Language and thought, being erotic, contribute to the joy that pervades sexual experiences.

In *S/Z*, Barthes presents a *tour de force* reading of Honoré de Balzac's (1799–1850) short story *Sarrasin*, as if it were a series of codings distinguishing "readerly" from "writerly" texts, texts that can be read as they are presented and texts that are produced by the reader. Barthes evokes the theme of indeterminate desire and sexuality in this structuralist setting. The title's "*S/Z*" represents the desire of Sarrasin (in the masculine) for the male La Zambinella, a castrato who appears in an opera as a woman (in the feminine). Barthes links the coding of Balzac's text with the coding of gender, the indeterminateness of a text with the indeterminateness of gender, the plurality of writerly readings with a plurality of sexualities. Sexuality itself is always a coded text, to be framed within socially established codes, or produced and transformed plurally and transgressively. Sexuality occupies the caesura of the "/" and the mirrors of *S* and *Z*.

This theme of indeterminateness and multiplicity of sexual and corporeal identity runs through nineteenth- and twentieth-century European writing, including Klossowski and Foucault, the former's paintings and the latter's *Herculine Barbin*, which offers a study of indeterminate gender and its social and personal costs, while Klossowski's works explored the multiplicities and ambiguities of sexual identity, sexed bodies, and sexual practices. These works continue to echo Sade and Nietzsche as well as such well-known works as Wolfgang Amadeus Mozart's (1756–1791) operas *Così Fan Tutte* (1790) and *Don Giovanni* (1787) and **Søren Kierkegaard**'s (1813–1855) *Either/Or*.

The most influential poststructuralist work on sexuality is the first volume of Foucault's *History of Sexuality*. Together with *The Birth of the Clinic*, it criticizes the medicalization and institutionalization of sexuality as part of the modern concern (*bio-power*) with the ordering and control of populations. Sexual identity and subjectivity are inscribed on the body through techniques of power; power gives its rule to sex; the body is marked by institutional practices and discourses, including academic disciplines that lay claim to knowledge of bodies and sex. Foucault proposes that knowledge, subjectivity, and power are the axes of his work and that sex and sexuality are central sites where these axes meet. There is no pure biology of sex and no knowledge of sex that can be separated from what is said and named as sex. (For this reason, Foucault is often associated with **social constructionism**. See Stein.)

Althusser speaks of this Foucauldian naming as *interpellation* (*Lenin*, 109–19), where we are named and called, and identified in our identity and our materiality by this calling and naming. Thus we are constituted in our subjectivities through specific discursive practices. Bourdieu offers a related theory of "social capital" (89) in which certain practices—giving gifts, for example—function to promote social hierarchies. In every case, naming and calling play multiple roles, some canceling or obscuring the others. Sex and sexuality are therefore frequently oppressive but are also scenes of the transformation of subjectivities. What is required is microanalysis of the concrete, specific relations in which they are embedded. In the last two volumes of *History of Sexuality*, Foucault explores the way individual practices and self-organized techniques are productive in the formation and support of subjectivities. In effect, through local arts and the construction of habits pertaining to their bodies, selves are able to create alternative sexualities and sexual identifications.

Holding views similar to Foucault's, Deleuze and Guattari, in the two most extravagant books of their collaboration, engage in an extensive critique of capitalism and modern sexuality that they call "schizoanalysis." *Anti-Oedipus* and *A Thousand Plateaus* are both subtitled *Capitalism and Schizophrenia*. Both are a critique of capitalism's reduction of desire to certain institutional and disciplinary forms (restricted economy) and the much wider capacity of capitalism to manipulate, transform, and create new sexualities and new desires (general economy) organized around capitalist consumption. Freud and Marx are major sources of this critique (which converge in the work of Herbert Marcuse [1898–1979]), yet both are criticized, not only here but throughout poststructuralism, for participating in the reduction of desire and the formation of sexualities according to forms of knowledge imposed on them.

> Hence, instead of participating in an undertaking that will bring about genuine liberation, psychoanalysis is taking part in the work of bourgeois repression at its most far-reaching level, that is to say, keeping European humanity harnessed to the yoke of daddy-mommy and *making no effort to do away with this problem once and for all*. (*Anti-Oedipus*, 50)

On the side of liberation, including multiple sexual liberations (identifications, practices, bodily transformations), they speak of becomings that remain minoritarian and imperceptible and that do not coalesce around majoritarian (stable, dominant, hegemonic) identities. Becomings are the transformation of human identities through practices of knowledge and subjectivation where the processes of formation and transformation are more imperative than the subjectivities and sexualities produced. There is a becoming-woman, becoming-sexual, becoming-sexed, becoming-another-identity with another desire/sexuality, in which the social, human, and sexual identities we know do not occupy privileged positions (see *Thousand*, 275). They emphasize releasing, transforming identities in the unfolding of the multiplicities of sexuality, for which imagination is required.

One of the most striking expressions of this imagination is Lyotard's *Libidinal Economy*. From within an intense and playful critique of Freud and Marx, Lyotard imagines an economy of desire, corporeality, and sexuality composed of pure excess—if that really is imaginable. Freud creates the possibilities in the modern world of conceiving of sexuality and desire—the libido—as pervasive of humanity and thereby of the world that humanity constructs for itself. Marx creates the realization that everything modern is economic, where economy, desire, and production are inseparable. Lyotard criticizes Freud for the restriction of desire to the Oedipal structure—that is, to a restricted economy—when Freud so clearly opens the possibility of a general economy of desire; and he mocks Marx for his prudish and almost obsessive concern for familiar, equal sexual relations between men and women and his constant worry about prostitution, in the midst of an otherwise radical critique of capitalism that suggests an entirely different set of postcapitalist sexualities.

Like *Anti-Oedipus* and *Lesbian Body*, Lyotard's *Libidinal Economy* is notable not only for what it says about sexuality but for the kind of writing it proffers: desirous, pleasurable, sexual, perverse.

> Our danger, we libidinal economists, lies in building a new morality with this consolation, of proclaiming and broadcasting that the libidinal band *is good*, that the circulation of affects *is joyful*, that the anonymity and the incompossibility of figures *are great and free*, that all pain is reactionary and conceals the poison of a formation issuing from the great Zero—what I have just said. But it is not an ethics, this or another, that is required. Perhaps we need an *ars vitae*, young man, but then one in which we would be the artists and not the propagators, the adventurers and not the theoreticians, the hypothesizers and not the censors. (11)

> If mimesis gives you an erection, gentlemen, who are we to object? This is rather what interests us. Capital is also mimetic, commodities producing commodities, that is to say, being exchanged for commodities, the same commuted into the same according to an immanent standard. (249)

> What would be interesting would be to stay put, but quietly seize every chance to function as good intensity-conducting bodies. No need for declarations, manifestos, organizations, provocations, no need for *exemplary actions*. Set dissimulation to work on behalf of intensities. Invulnerable conspiracy, headless, homeless, with neither programme nor project, deploying a thousand cancerous tensors in the bodies of signs. We invent nothing, that's it, yes, yes, yes, yes. (262)

We invent nothing, do not imagine a better economy, sexuality, libido, pleasure, but seize every chance of intensification—not fulfillment—of desire. Desire is already everywhere, together with signs and commodities. That's it! Desire, commodities, art, and language are already everywhere. As sex! As art and theater! The interplay of language with desire is art, is sex, is capitalist economy. The affirmation and intensification of this relation is libidinal economy.

Finally, we may turn to Derrida, who seldom speaks directly on love and sex but often sidles up to them obliquely. One place is in several essays on the word *Geschlecht*, a term for sexual and social identity. He reads Heidegger as insisting on corporeality yet denying sexual difference ("Geschlecht"; "*Geschlecht* II"; "Heidegger's Ear"). Another place where Derrida addresses sex and love is in *The Post Card*, which may be read as a series of love letters from Derrida to Freud. At times the love is flagrant; for example, right at the beginning, on the first day:

3 June 1977

and when I call you my love, my love is it you I am calling or my love? You, my love, is it you I thereby name, is it to you that I address myself? . . .
when I call you my love, is it that I am calling you, yourself, or is it that I am telling my love? and when I tell you my love is it that I am declaring my love to you or indeed that I am telling *you*, yourself, my love, and that you are my love. I want so much to tell you. (8)

The key here is the calling and sending. To love is to send, to write is to love. Love comes and goes in the sending and the calling. It takes place in language, and if it is not altogether language, nothing can separate it from the speaking and the messaging. Here what Derrida calls *iterability* is the condition of meaning: To utter, to mean, in any way (and true love is surely meant, sex is sent and received) is to be public, to be able to be said again, repeated, the same meaning uttered at another time and place. In speaking we say words that have a repeatable meaning. Yet in the sending and calling repetition is transformation. There can be no guarantees of iterable meanings. There can be no guarantees of love or sexual ecstasy. More truthfully, perhaps, as he suggests in *Politics of Friendship* (217–19), to want to speak truly, to offer one's love, to seek sexual joy, to engage in intimacy, is always to want not to do so, to want to deceive and postpone. Sex and love are language, sending, calling, showing, revealing. Even in their most hidden moments they are sending and showing.

The consequence is that boundaries are set up to be shattered, including boundaries between love and friendship, sexuality and asexuality, subjectivity and objectivity, thought and corporeality, intimacy and perversity, things and desires, eroticism and **pornography**. Desire pervades everything as language, as if desire were language, and language is pervaded by desire: sexual, erotic, sexed, asexual, acquisitive, and nonacquisitive desire. The critique of pornography as the same thing over and over again and as reinforcing the same stereotypes time and time again is transformed by iterability, where whatever it is meant to be and do it cannot control what it becomes and does.

Love is everything, sex is everything, language is everything, everything appears; and in this appearance vanishes only to reappear in another form. Sex is both one of the most visible forms of being human, being animal, being corporeal, and is one of the most oblique ways of thinking, desiring, feeling. It attaches itself to anything and everything, as sex and as desire, above all as identification and identities. Who we are, we humans, is sexual, but that is no identification of humanity; it is not humanistic. To the contrary, it is an endless set of questions, and still more.

See also Arts, Sex and the; Bataille, Georges; Desire, Sexual; Existentialism; Feminism, French; Foucault, Michel; Freud, Sigmund; Freudian Left, The; Intersexuality; Kierkegaard, Søren; Kolnai, Aurel; Lacan, Jacques; Levinas, Emmanuel; Marxism; Money, John; Nietzsche, Friedrich; Phenomenology; Sade, Marquis de; Social Constructionism

REFERENCES

Althusser, Louis. (1965) *Lenin and Philosophy, and Other Essays.* Trans. Ben Brewster. New York: Monthly Review Press, 1971; Barthes, Roland. (1973) *The Pleasure of the Text.* Trans. Richard Miller. New York: Noonday Press, 1975; Barthes, Roland. (1970) *S/Z: An Essay.* Trans. Richard Miller. New York: Hill and Wang, 1974; Bataille, Georges. (1967, 1976) *The Accursed Share: An Essay on General Economy,* 2 vols. Trans. Richard Hurley. New York: Zone Books, 1988, 1993. Translation of *La Part maudite, L'Histoire de l'érotisme,* and *La Souveraineté (Consumption* [1]; *The History of Eroticism* [2]; and *Sovereignty* [3]), in Georges Bataille, *Oeuvres Complètes.* Paris: Gallimard, 1976; Beauvoir, Simone de. (1949) *The Second Sex.* Trans. Howard M. Parshley. New York: Vintage, 1989; Bourdieu, Pierre. (1972) *Outline of a Theory of Practice.* Trans. Richard Nice. Cambridge: Cambridge University Press, 1977; Deleuze, Gilles, and Félix Guattari. (1972) *Anti-Oedipus: Capitalism and Schizophrenia.* Trans. Robert Hurley, Mark Seem, and Helen R. Lane. Minneapolis: University of Minnesota Press, 1983; Deleuze, Gilles, and Félix Guattari. (1980) *A Thousand Plateaus: Capitalism and Schizophrenia.* Trans. Brian Massumi. Minneapolis: University of Minnesota Press, 1987; Derrida, Jacques. (1972) *Dissemination.* Trans. Barbara Johnson. Chicago, Ill.: University of Chicago Press, 1981; Derrida, Jacques. (1983) "Geschlecht: Sexual Difference, Ontological Difference." *Research in Phenomenology* 13 (1983), 65–83; Derrida, Jacques. "*Geschlecht* II: Heidegger's Hand." Trans. John P. Leavey, Jr. In John Sallis, ed., *Deconstruction in Philosophy: The Texts of Jacques Derrida.* Chicago, Ill.: University of Chicago Press, 1987, 161–96; Derrida, Jacques. "Heidegger's Ear: Philopolemology (*Geschlecht* IV)." In John Sallis, ed., *Reading Heidegger.* Bloomington: Indiana University Press, 1993, 163–218; Derrida, Jacques. (1994) *The Politics of Friendship.* Trans. George Collins. London: Verso, 1997; Derrida, Jacques. (1980) *The Post Card: From Socrates to Freud and Beyond.* Trans. Alan Bass. Chicago, Ill.: University of Chicago Press, 1987; Foucault, Michel. (1963) *The Birth of the Clinic: An Archaeology of Medical Perception.* Trans. A. M. Sheridan-Smith. New York: Vintage, 1975; Foucault, Michel. (1978) *Herculine Barbin: Being the Recently Discovered Memoirs of a Nineteenth-Century French Hermaphrodite.* Trans. Richard McDougall. New York: Pantheon Books, 1980; Foucault, Michel. (1976/1984/1984) *The History of Sexuality.* Vol. 1: *An Introduction.* Trans. Robert Hurley. New York: Vintage, 1978. Vol. 2: *The Use of Pleasure.* Trans. Robert Hurley. New York: Pantheon, 1985. Vol. 3: *The Care of the Self.* Trans. Robert Hurley. New York: Vintage, 1986; Foucault, Michel. (1994) "On the Genealogy of Ethics: An Overview of Work in Progress." In *The Essential Works of Michel Foucault, 1954–1984,* vol. 1: *Ethics: Subjectivity and Truth.* Ed. Paul Rabinow. Trans. Robert Hurley and others. New York: New Press, 1997, 281–301; Foucault, Michel. (1966) *The Order of Things: An Archaeology of the Human Sciences.* New York: Vintage, 1973; Heidegger, Martin. (1927) *Being and Time: A Translation of Sein und Zeit.* Trans. John Macquarrie and Edward Robinson. New York: Harper and Row, 1962; Irigaray, Luce. (1984) *An Ethics of Sexual Difference.* Trans. Carolyn Burke and Gillian C. Gill. Ithaca, N.Y.: Cornell University Press, 1993; Kierkegaard, Søren. (1843) *Either/Or,* 2 vols. Trans. Howard V. Hong and Edna H. Hong. Princeton, N.J.: Princeton University Press, 1987; Lyotard, Jean-François. (1974) *Libidinal Economy.* Trans. Iain Hamilton Grant. Bloomington: Indiana University Press, 1993; Lyotard, Jean-François. (1979) *The Postmodern Condition: A Report on Knowledge.* Trans. Geoffrey Bennington and Brian Massumi. Minneapolis: University of Minnesota Press, 1984; Marx, Karl, and Friedrich Engels. (1848) *The Communist Manifesto.* Ed. Martin Malia. New York: Penguin Putnam, 1998; Merleau-Ponty, Maurice. (1945) *Phenomenology of Perception.* Trans. Colin Smith. London: Routledge and Kegan Paul, 1962; Nancy, Jean-Luc. (1986) *The Inoperative Community.* Trans. P. Connor, L. Garbus, M. Holland, and S. Sawhney. Minneapolis: University of Minnesota Press, 1991; Nietzsche, Friedrich. (1883/1892) *Thus Spoke Zarathustra.* Trans. Walter Kaufmann. *The Portable Nietzsche.* New York: Viking, 1954, 121–439; Rorty, Richard. *Philosophy and the Mirror of Nature*. Princeton, N.J.: Princeton University Press, 1979; Stein, Edward, ed. *Forms of Desire: Sexual Orientation and the Social Constructionist Controversy*, 1st pnt. New York: Garland, 1990. 2nd pnt., New York: Routledge, 1992; Wittig, Monique. (1973) *The Lesbian Body*. Trans. David Le Vay. Boston, Mass.: Beacon Press, 1973.

Stephen David Ross

ADDITIONAL READING

Agamben, Giorgio. (2002) *The Open: Man and Animal*. Trans. Kevin Attell. Stanford, Calif.: Stanford University Press, 2004; Althusser, Louis. *Althusser: A Critical Reader*. Ed. Gregory Elliott. Oxford, U.K.: Oxford University Press, 1994; Althusser, Louis. (1965) *For Marx*. Trans. Ben Brewster. New York: Verso, 1996; Althusser, Louis. *Writings on Psychoanalysis: Freud and Lacan*. New York: Columbia University Press, 1996; Althusser, Louis, and Étienne Balibar. (1965) *Reading Capital*. Trans. Ben Brewster. London: NLB, 1970; Artaud, Antonin. *Watchfiends and Rack Screams: Works from the Final Period*. Trans. Clayton Eshleman, with Bernard Bador. Boston, Mass.: Exact Change, 1995; Badiou, Alain. (1993) *Ethics: An Essay on the Understanding of Evil*. Trans. Peter Hallward. London: Verso, 2001; Balibar, Étienne. (1993) *The Philosophy of Marx*. Trans. Chris Turner. London: Verso, 1995; Barthes, Roland. (1977) *A Lover's Discourse: Fragments*. Trans. Richard Howard. New York: Hill and Wang, 1978; Barthes, Roland. (1971) *Sade, Fourier, Loyola*. Trans. Richard Miller. New York: Hill and Wang, 1976; Bataille, Georges. *The Bataille Reader*. Ed. Fred Botting and Scott Wilson. Oxford, U.K.: Blackwell, 1997; Bataille, Georges. (1957) *Erotism: Death and Sensuality*. Trans. Mary Dalwood. New York: City Lights Books, 1991; Bataille, Georges. (1961) *The Tears of Eros*. Trans. Peter Connor. San Francisco, Calif.: City Lights Books, 1989; Baudrillard, Jean. (1977) *Forget Foucault*. Trans. Nicole Dufresne. New York: Semiotext(e), 1987; Baudrillard, Jean. *Selected Writings*. Ed. Mark Poster. Trans. Jacques Mourrain and others. Stanford, Calif.: Stanford University Press, 2001; Blanchot, Maurice. (1949) *Lautréamont and Sade*. Trans. Stuart Kendall and Michelle Kendall. Stanford, Calif.: Stanford University Press, 2004; Bourdieu, Pierre. *The Field of Cultural Production: Essays on Art and Literature*. Ed. Randal Johnson. New York: Columbia University Press, 1993; Braidotti, Rosi. *Patterns of Dissonance: A Study of Women and Contemporary Philosophy*. Trans. Elizabeth Guild. New York: Routledge, 1991; Butler, Judith. *The Judith Butler Reader*. Ed. Sara Salih, with Judith Butler. Oxford, U.K.: Blackwell, 2004; Certeau, Michel de. *The Certeau Reader*. Ed. Graham Ward. Oxford, U.K.: Blackwell, 2000; Cixous, Hélène, and Jacques Derrida. *Veils*. Trans. Geoffrey Bennington. Stanford, Calif.: Stanford University Press, 2001; Cornell, Drucilla. *Beyond Accommodation: Ethical Feminism, Deconstruction, and the Law*. New York: Routledge, 1991; Cornell, Drucilla. *The Imaginary Domain: Abortion, Pornography and Sexual Harassment*. New York: Routledge, 1995; Cornell, Drucilla. *The Philosophy of the Limit*. New York: Routledge, 1992; Cornell, Drucilla. *Transformations: Recollective Imagination and Sexual Difference*. New York: Routledge, 1993; Cornell, Drucilla, Michel Rosenfeld, and David Gray Carlson, eds. *Deconstruction and the Possibility of Justice*. New York: Routledge, Chapman, and Hall, 1992; Deleuze, Gilles. (1968) *Difference and Repetition*. Trans. Paul Patton. New York: Columbia University Press, 1994; Deleuze, Gilles. (1969) *The Logic of Sense*. Trans. Mark Lester, with Charles Stivale. New York: Columbia University Press, 1990; Deleuze, Gilles. (1974) "Preface to Hocquenghem's *L'Après-Mai des faunes*." In *Desert Islands and Other Texts 1953–1974*. Trans. Michael Taormina. Los Angeles, Calif.: Semiotext(e), 2004, 284–88; Derrida, Jacques. (1983) "*Geschlecht*: Sexual Difference and Ontological Difference." In Nancy J. Holland and Patricia Huntington, eds., *Feminist Interpretations of Martin Heidegger*. University Park: Pennsylvania State University Press, 2001, 53–72. Originally published as "*Geschlecht*: Sexual Difference, Ontological Difference." *Research in Phenomenology* 13 (1983), 65–83; Derrida, Jacques. (1967) *Of Grammatology*. Trans. Gayatri Chakravorty Spivak. Baltimore, Md.: Johns Hopkins University Press, 1974; Derrida, Jacques. "The Politics of Friendship." Trans. Gabriel Motzkin. *Journal of Philosophy* 85:11 (1988), 632–44; Foucault, Michel. *The Essential Foucault*. Ed. Paul Rabinow and Nikolas Rose. New York: New Press, 2003; Gallop, Jane. *Intersections, a Reading of Sade with Bataille, Blanchot, and*

Klossowski. Lincoln: University of Nebraska Press, 1981; Grosz, Elizabeth. *Jacques Lacan: A Feminist Introduction*. London: Routledge, 1990; Grosz, Elizabeth. *Sexual Subversions: Three French Feminists*. Winchester, Mass.: Unwin Hyman, 1989; Grosz, Elizabeth. *Space, Time, and Perversion: Essays on the Politics of Bodies*. New York: Routledge, 1995; Grosz, Elizabeth. *Volatile Bodies: Toward a Corporeal Feminism*. Bloomington: Indiana University Press, 1994; Haraway, Donna. *The Haraway Reader*. New York: Routledge, 2004; Holland, Nancy J., ed. *Feminist Interpretations of Jacques Derrida*. University Park: Pennsylvania State University Press, 1997; Hoy, David Couzens. *Critical Resistance: From Poststructuralism to Post-Critique*. Cambridge, Mass.: MIT Press, 2004; Klossowski, Pierre. (1969) *Nietzsche and the Vicious Circle*. Trans. Daniel W. Smith. Chicago, Ill.: University of Chicago Press, 1997; Klossowski, Pierre, and Maurice Blanchot. *The Decadence of the Nude*. Ed. Sarah Wilson. London: Black Dog Publishing, 2002; Kroker, Arthur, and Marilouise Kroker, eds. *The Last Sex: Feminism and Outlaw Bodies*. New York: St. Martin's Press, 1993; Lacoue-Labarthe, Philippe. (1979) *The Subject of Philosophy*. Trans. Thomas Trezise, Hugh J. Silverman, Gary M. Cole, Timothy D. Bent, Karen McPherson, and Claudette Sartiliot. Minneapolis: University of Minnesota Press, 1993; Lévi-Strauss, Claude. "The Family." In Harry L. Shapiro, ed., *Man, Culture, and Society*. New York: Oxford University Press, 1960, 261–85; Lingis, Alphonso. *Foreign Bodies*. New York: Routledge, 1994; Lyotard, Jean-François. *The Lyotard Reader*. Ed. Andrew Benjamin. Oxford, U.K.: Blackwell, 1989; MacKinnon, Catharine A. "Points against Postmodernism." *Chicago-Kent Law Review* 75:3 (2000), 687–712; May, Todd. "Poststructuralism." In Ruth Chadwick, ed., *Encyclopedia of Applied Ethics*, vol. 3. San Diego, Calif.: Academic Press, 1998, 615–23; Miller, D. A. *Bringing Out Roland Barthes*. Berkeley: University of California Press, 1992; Minot, Leslie Ann. "Barthes, Roland." In Timothy F. Murphy, ed., *Reader's Guide to Lesbian and Gay Studies*. Chicago, Ill.: Fitzroy Dearborn, 2000, 77–78; Nancy, Jean-Luc. *The Muses*. Trans. Peggy Kamuf. Stanford, Calif.: Stanford University Press, 1996; Neu, Jerome. "Lévi-Strauss on Shamanism." *Man: The Journal of the Royal Anthropological Institute* [n.s.] 10 (1975), 285–92; Nicholson, Linda J., ed. *Feminism/Postmodernism*. New York: Routledge, 1990; Rorty, Richard. *Consequences of Pragmatism*. Minneapolis: University of Minnesota Press, 1982; Rorty, Richard. *Contingency, Irony, and Solidarity*. New York: Cambridge University Press, 1989; Rorty, Richard. *Objectivity, Relativism, and Truth*. New York: Cambridge University Press, 1991; Ross, Stephen David. "The Limits of Sexuality." *Philosophy and Social Criticism* 9:3–4 (1984), 321–36. Reprinted in POS2 (259–75); Simon, William. *Postmodern Sexualities*. New York: Routledge, 1996; Smyth, John Vignaux. *A Question of Eros: Irony in Sterne, Kierkegaard, and Barthes*. Tallahassee: Florida State University Press, 1986; Žižek, Slavoj. *The Metastases of Enjoyment: Six Essays on Woman and Causality*. London: Verso, 1994; Žižek, Slavoj. *The Plague of Fantasies*. London: Verso, 1997.

PRIVACY. The central question in the philosophical investigation of privacy is whether a single moral right to privacy exists that underlies the various specific moral and legal rights that go by that name or whether the "right to privacy" is merely an ambiguous label that we attach confusingly to a number of distinct rights. More precisely, the central question is whether what is generally referred to as the right to privacy is unified by a common, theoretically illuminating, justification while being significantly distinct from other rights.

Because claims involving the right to privacy are most often made in discussions about the law, including moral criticisms of the law and proposals for its change, fully understanding the philosophical literature about privacy requires basic familiarity with the roles that "privacy" and related terms play in the law.

The longest established legal use of the term is within the law of torts. That use has its roots in Samuel D. Warren (1852–1910) and Louis D. Brandeis's (1856–1941) article "The Right to Privacy" (1890), which argued that the law ought to recognize explicitly and protect the right named in its title. As is standard when such extensions of the law are advocated in legal literature, the argument was based on analyzing a number of earlier judicial opinions and showing that they could be construed as already protecting that right, even though they had not recognized it explicitly. The argument was accepted by numerous courts, and protection of the right to privacy eventually became a well-established element of the law of torts in the United States. William L. Prosser (1898–1972) observed that Warren and Brandeis's article "has come to be regarded as the outstanding example of the influence of legal periodicals upon the American law" (383).

Prosser's own article ("Privacy") ended up having almost as much influence. He argued that what the courts had been labeling as invasions of privacy was not a single tort but rather four distinct torts. Although Prosser's view received some criticism, most theoreticians and the courts eventually agreed with his position. In the law of torts, it is now standard to treat "invasion of privacy" as merely a common name for four distinct torts, which the *Restatement (Second) of Torts* (§§652B–652E) defines as follows:

> [1] intentionally intrud[ing], physically or otherwise, upon the solitude or seclusion of another or his private affairs or concerns, . . . if the intrusion would be highly offensive to a reasonable person[;]
>
> [2] appropriat[ing] to [one's] own use or benefit the name or likeness of another[;]
>
> [3] giv[ing] publicity to a matter concerning the private life of another . . . if the matter publicized is of a kind that (a) would be highly offensive to a reasonable person, and (b) is not of legitimate concern to the public[;]
>
> [4] giv[ing] publicity to a matter concerning another that places the other before the public in a false light . . . , if (a) the false light in which the other was placed would be highly offensive to a reasonable person, and (b) the actor had knowledge of or acted in reckless disregard as to the falsity of the publicized matter and the false light in which the other would be placed.

Toward the end of the twentieth century, various statutes came into existence that limited the ways in which specific organizations may use the information that is provided to them by the individuals with whom they deal. What these statutes protect is often referred to as privacy. Similarly, many organizations have started to assume contractual obligations that limit the ways in which they may use the information that their clients or customers provide; these obligations are also often characterized as protections of privacy. Such statutory and contractual provisions have some affinity with the third of the four ways in which privacy is dealt with by the law of torts, but they go beyond it, in that they are not limited to highly offensive matters. They are also quite similar to what have traditionally been called duties of confidentiality; indeed it appears to be partially a matter of historical accident whether "privacy" or "confidentiality" will be more prominent in characterizing this kind of obligation.

Another area of the law in which the term "privacy" plays a role is the application of the Fourth Amendment of the U.S. Constitution, which protects the people from "unreasonable searches and seizures" by the government. It has thus been said that "[t]he security of one's privacy against arbitrary intrusion by the police . . . is at the core of the Fourth Amendment" (*Wolf v. Colorado*, 27). The term "privacy" became particularly prominent in Fourth Amendment jurisprudence after Justice John Harlan (1899–1971), in 1967, used the phrase "reasonable expectation of privacy" in specifying what triggers the application of the Fourth Amendment (*Katz v. United States*, 360 [concurring opinion]).

The laws involving the term "privacy" that have been referred to so far are not specifically concerned with sexuality. Nevertheless, they have protected a great deal of **sexual activity** from interference. Given that most sexual activity takes place under a "reasonable expectation of privacy," and that much evidence of it is handled with such an expectation, the Fourth Amendment constrains the government's ability to obtain information about people's sexual pursuits. This, in turn, has made difficult government's enforcing laws that criminalize various kinds of sexual acts between consenting partners. The protection of privacy embodied in the Fourth Amendment has thus made it possible for such laws (many of which still remain "on the books" at the beginning of the twenty-first century) to be regularly violated with impunity by millions of people. The provisions regarding privacy that are found in the common law of torts, statutory law, and contracts similarly protect many manifestations of sexuality from scrutiny and interference by private parties.

In contrast to these areas of the law that, even though important to sexuality, are not specifically aimed at it, stands a line of constitutional cases in which the term "privacy" is used in a way that is much more directly concerned with matters related to sexuality. While in the Fourth Amendment jurisprudence privacy functions as a constraint on procedures that police may use in *enforcing* laws, in these other cases privacy functions as a constraint on the *content* of the laws.

This line of cases began in 1965 with *Griswold v. Connecticut*, in which the Supreme Court held that there exists a constitutional right to privacy that makes it unconstitutional for a state to prohibit married couples from using contraceptives. While the majority of the justices agreed that such a right existed, they offered different views on the basis of that right. According to one opinion in the case, authored by Justice William Douglas (1898–1980), the "specific guarantees in the Bill of Rights have penumbras, formed by emanations from those guarantees that help give them life and substance" (484). As several of these "guarantees create zones of privacy," this opinion concludes that there exists a constitutional right to privacy. Another opinion, authored by Justice Arthur Goldberg (1908–1990), adds to these considerations the argument that the right has a basis in the Ninth Amendment ("The enumeration in the Constitution, of certain rights, shall not be construed to deny or disparage others retained by the people"). Justice Harlan, on the other hand, argued that the references to the Bill of Rights in the first two opinions were unnecessary; the Due Process Clause of the Fourteenth Amendment was on its own sufficient to render unconstitutional the prohibition of the use of contraceptives. His argument invoked (but also extended the scope of) the idea, articulated several decades earlier in *Palko v. Connecticut*, that the Due Process Clause prevents states from violating the basic values "implicit in the concept of ordered liberty" (325). Justice Harlan's argument is usually referred to as an argument for a constitutional right to privacy, even though the word "privacy" does not appear in his opinion.

Griswold concerned the use of contraceptives within **marriage**, and it left the impression that the constitutional right to privacy that it invoked is confined to marriage. That impression was dispelled in 1972 when the Court held in *Eisenstadt v. Baird* that distinguishing between married and unmarried persons in access to **contraception** violates the Equal Protection Clause of the Fourteenth Amendment. This holding entailed that the right to privacy is not particularly tied to marriage, notwithstanding the fact that references to the special character of that relationship were prominent in *Griswold*. According to *Eisenstadt*, "the marital couple is not an independent entity with a mind and heart of its own, but an association of two individuals each with a separate intellectual and emotional makeup. If the right of privacy means anything, it is the right of the *individual*, married or single, to be free from unwarranted governmental intrusion into matters so fundamentally affecting a person as the decision whether to bear or beget a child" (453).

Further expansion of what the law treats as constitutionally protected privacy took place in 1973 with *Roe v. Wade*, the decision that grounded the right to **abortion** in the right to privacy. Since then, the precise content and boundaries of the right to abortion have been articulated in a number of other cases. These abortion-related cases refer to the right to privacy recognized in *Griswold* but do not revisit in great detail the fundamental question of precisely how that right is rooted in the Constitution. The most influential post-*Roe* abortion decision, *Planned Parenthood v. Casey* (1992), reaffirmed "the essential holding of *Roe*," yet the concept of privacy was not at all prominent.

The cases about contraception and abortion have served as a stepping stone for extending constitutional protection to other aspects of marital and family life. In *Moore v. City of East Cleveland* (1977), the plurality opinion cited *Griswold* and *Roe* in support of invalidating a housing ordinance that prevented members of an extended family from living together. In *Zablocki v. Redhail* (1978), the right to privacy was held to protect one's decision to marry, as "it would make little sense to recognize a right of privacy with respect to other matters of family life and not with respect to the decision to enter the relationship that is the foundation of the family in our society" (386). The Court thus invalidated a statute that prevented people from marrying if they were not complying with their obligations to support minor children not in their custody, or the children were or were likely to become public charges. An earlier case about the right to enter marriage, *Loving v. Virginia* (1967), which rendered unconstitutional the prohibition of interracial marriages, has an obvious affinity with the cases based on the constitutional right to privacy and is often treated as one of them, even though neither "privacy" nor citations to *Griswold* appears in the Court's opinion.

That the right to privacy might protect a very broad range of interests (much broader than indicated by the cases mentioned above) was suggested by its invocation in *Stanley v. Georgia* (1969), the case in which the Court held that "mere private possession of obscene matter cannot constitutionally be made a crime" (559). The right to privacy, however, plays only a limited role in that decision. On the most straightforward reading of the Court's opinion, it appears to have been invoked merely as an inessential supplement to an argument based on the First Amendment. Later cases have, in any event, greatly limited the impact of *Stanley* on the further development of the law of privacy. *Paris Adult Theatre I v. Slaton* (1973) thus states that the privacy referred to in *Stanley* "is restricted to a place, the home," and is thus different from the kind of privacy that is the subject matter of *Griswold* and *Roe*, which "is not just concerned with a particular place, but with a protected intimate relationship" (66n.13). According to the Court's opinion in *Paris Adult Theatre*, the right to privacy "encompasses and protects the personal intimacies of the home, the family, marriage, motherhood, procreation, and child rearing" (65) and is not relevant to such pursuits as watching obscene movies in a commercial theater.

Another limit to what the Court regards as the right to privacy is visible in *Village of Belle Terre v. Boraas* (1974), which upheld a zoning ordinance preventing more than two unrelated individuals from living together. Whether the intimacy of living in an adulterous relationship is within or outside the protection of the right to privacy is an issue that the Court left unresolved; it declined to hear cases in which individuals who were discharged from public employment for living in such relationships challenged their discharges (*Hollenbaugh v. Carnegie Free Library* [1978]; *City of North Muskegon v. Briggs* [1985]). Lower courts are divided on that issue.

In 2003, however, the Court made a decision that dramatically widened the scope of sexual conduct to which the constitutional doctrine of privacy applies. That was *Lawrence v.*

Texas, in which the Court held that the Constitution protects the right of adults to engage in consensual homosexual conduct. It explicitly overruled the decision to the contrary that it had made only seventeen years earlier in *Bowers v. Hardwick* (1986). The Court in *Lawrence* adopted the position that Justice John Stevens had taken in his dissenting opinion in *Bowers*, according to which "individual decisions by married persons, concerning the intimacies of their physical relationship . . . are a form of 'liberty' that is protected by the Due Process Clause of the Fourteenth Amendment [and] this protection extends to intimate choices by unmarried as well as married persons" (*Lawrence*, 578; quoting *Bowers*, 216). Although the result of *Lawrence* directly concerns only homosexual conduct, the reasoning that led the Court to that result could be adapted to other kinds of sexual conduct, and it is thus possible that *Lawrence* will provide grounds for constitutional challenges to the remaining laws that criminalize private sexual acts between consenting adults, such as **adultery** and fornication.

While the cases that articulate the doctrine of privacy under the federal Constitution get most of the attention in discussions of privacy, it should be noted that individual states may have doctrines of privacy under their own constitutions, which may differ from the federal doctrine.

The laws regarding privacy have been subject to scholarly commentary and discussion in law reviews. Scholars whose background is in philosophy, however, devoted little attention to privacy before the 1970s (as was true for most topics in applied ethics). Two publications that were particularly significant in stimulating the philosophical discussion of privacy were the 1971 volume of the annual *Nomos*, whose topic was privacy (see Pennock and Chapman), and the summer 1975 issue of *Philosophy and Public Affairs*, which contained three articles on the topic. Most of the philosophical literature on privacy that appeared afterward discusses privacy in specific settings (for example, employment, the practice of medicine), but some examine the concept(s) of privacy and the grounds of the right(s) to privacy. Relatively little written by professional philosophers directly focuses on the privacy of sex-related pursuits, but the general philosophical examinations of privacy have implications for the philosophy of sex.

After surveying the different uses of "privacy," one is likely to wonder whether they have anything morally significant in common. One negative answer to that question was defended by Judith Jarvis Thomson, according to whom "the right to privacy is itself a cluster of rights" and "not a distinct cluster of rights" (306) but one that "is everywhere overlapped by other rights" (310). Moreover, "the fact that we have a right to privacy does not explain our having any of the rights in the right to privacy cluster" (312). It is, instead, the other rights that overlap with the cluster that provide the explanation. Consequently, "the right to privacy is 'derivative' in [that] it is possible to explain in the case of each right in the cluster how come we have it without ever once mentioning the right to privacy" (313). The examples Thomson relies on indicate that what she regards as the independent rights within the cluster do not straightforwardly correspond to the different areas of the law that deal with privacy.

Another theory that denies that there is a unified moral ground for what we call the right to privacy is Alexander Rosenberg's. He argues that in the cases in which privacy has moral value it has that value in virtue of its "role in securing other rights" (90). This point, however, applies to only some cases in which the right to privacy is commonly invoked; in other cases it is not a genuine moral right at all. Invoking the right to privacy in these other cases is, for Rosenberg, merely a manifestation of our culture-relative *taste* for privacy.

Unlike Thomson and Rosenberg, most philosophers who have dealt with privacy believe that it is a morally significant concept, and so they present unified accounts of *the* right to privacy. But some philosophers who present such accounts acknowledge that their accounts do not, and are not intended to, accommodate all the ways in which the right to privacy is invoked in the law and everyday discourse. They distinguish between the uses of "privacy" and the "right to privacy" that are illuminating and those that are misleading (even though they may be widespread) and tailor their accounts to the former. Philosophers who make such distinctions differ as to which uses are illuminating and which are misleading. Hyman Gross, for example, analyzed privacy as "the condition under which there is *control* over acquaintance with one's personal affairs by the one enjoying it" (169) and interpreted that in a way that covers most of the legal uses of the term "privacy"—except the one introduced by *Griswold*, which he dismissed because "[t]he [C]ourt's opinion relied heavily on an elaborate *jeu de mots*, in which different senses of the word 'privacy' were punned upon, and the legal concept generally mismanaged" (180).

W. A. Parent criticized those who analyzed privacy in terms of control and argued that it should be understood as "the condition of not having undocumented personal knowledge about one possessed by others" (269), where "undocumented" means not a matter of public record. This results in a narrow concept of privacy: Parent endorses most of the use of that term in connection with the third of the four privacy torts listed above, and some of its use in connection with the first, but criticizes as misguided the remaining ways of using "privacy" in the law of torts, as well as its use in constitutional cases such as *Griswold* and *Roe*. In contrast, for Julie Inness "privacy is the state of the agent having control over a realm of intimacy, which contains her decisions about intimate access to herself (including intimate informational access) and her decisions about her own intimate actions" (56), which entails that the use of "privacy" is perfectly apt in the cases regarding such intimate matters as contraception and abortion. But even though Inness endorses this controversial use of "privacy," she does not endorse all its legal uses: She criticizes its widespread use in various statutes that protect the secrecy of nonintimate information.

There also exist unified accounts of the right to privacy that do not explicitly rule out any of its common uses as misguided but still do so by implication. For example, according to James Rachels (1941–2003), the "ability to control who has access to us and to information about us," which privacy gives us, is valuable because it enables us "to create and maintain different sorts of social relationships with different people" (326). Rachels does not mention the doctrine of privacy introduced by *Griswold* anywhere in his essay, but it seems obvious that his account is not meant to cover that doctrine.

Finally, some philosophers have aimed to encompass all legal uses of "privacy" and show them to be connected in a theoretically significant way. Judith Wagner DeCew argues that we can understand the close relationships among the different legal uses of "privacy" if we think of "the realm of the private" as the realm that is "according to a reasonable person in normal circumstances" (62) "beyond the legitimate concern of others," for such reasons "as freedom from scrutiny, judgment, and pressure to conform or to reveal one's weaknesses and vulnerabilities" (66). DeCew's theoretical integration of the concept of privacy, however, is qualified by her also arguing that it is a "multifaceted cluster concept" (61).

Unlike the philosophers who are interested in privacy in general, and are concerned with sexuality only by implication, Richard Mohr has focused specifically on the relationship between privacy and sexuality. Well before the Supreme Court decided *Lawrence*, Mohr had argued that homosexual conduct should be protected by the constitutional right to privacy. Also of particular interest for the philosophy of sex is Robert Gerstein's thesis that "intimate relationships simply could not exist if we did not continue to insist on privacy for them" (76).

None of the philosophical accounts of privacy has become dominant. It remains an open question whether the different uses of "privacy" are in a state of irreparable disarray or whether sustained philosophical analysis will eventually discern order underneath the apparent chaos.

See also Bestiality; Feminism, Liberal; Fichte, Johann Gottlieb; Harassment, Sexual; Homosexuality, Ethics of; Law, Sex and the; Liberalism; Marriage, Same-Sex; Pornography; Prostitution; Reproductive Technology; Sex Work

REFERENCES

Bowers v. Hardwick. 478 U.S. 186, 106 S.Ct. 2841, 92 L.Ed. 2d 140 (1986); *City of North Muskegon v. Briggs.* 473 U.S. 909, 105 S.Ct. 3535, 87 L.Ed. 2d 659 (1985); DeCew, Judith Wagner. *In Pursuit of Privacy: Law, Ethics, and the Rise of Technology.* Ithaca, N.Y.: Cornell University Press, 1997; *Eisenstadt v. Baird.* 405 U.S. 438, 92 S.Ct. 1029, 31 L.Ed. 2d 349 (1972); Gerstein, Robert S. "Intimacy and Privacy." *Ethics* 89:1 (1978), 76–81; *Griswold v. Connecticut.* 381 U.S. 479, 85 S.Ct. 1678, 14 L.Ed. 2d 510 (1965); Gross, Hyman. "Privacy and Autonomy." In J. Roland Pennock and John W. Chapman, eds., *Nomos XIII: Privacy.* New York: Atherton, 1971, 169–81; *Hollenbaugh v. Carnegie Free Library.* 439 U.S. 1052, 99 S.Ct. 734, 58 L.Ed. 2d 713 (1978); Inness, Julie C. *Privacy, Intimacy, and Isolation.* New York: Oxford University Press, 1992; *Katz v. United States.* 389 U.S. 347, 88 S.Ct. 507, 19 L.Ed. 2d 576 (1967); *Lawrence v. Texas.* 539 U.S. 558, 123 S.Ct. 2472, 156 L.Ed. 2d 508 (2003); *Loving v. Virginia.* 388 U.S. 1, 87 S.Ct. 1817, 18 L.Ed. 2d 1010 (1967); Mohr, Richard D. *Gays/Justice: A Study of Ethics, Society, and Law.* New York: Columbia University Press, 1988; *Moore v. City of East Cleveland.* 431 U.S. 494, 97 S.Ct. 1932, 52 L.Ed. 2d 531 (1977); *Palko v. Connecticut.* 302 U.S. 319, 58 S.Ct. 149, 82 L.Ed. 288 (1937); Parent, W. A. "Privacy, Morality, and the Law." *Philosophy and Public Affairs* 12:4 (1983), 269–88; *Paris Adult Theatre I v. Slaton.* 413 U.S. 49, 93 S.Ct. 2628, 37 L.Ed. 2d 446 (1973); Pennock, J. Roland, and John W. Chapman, eds. *Nomos XIII: Privacy.* New York: Atherton, 1971; *Planned Parenthood v. Casey.* 505 U.S. 833, 112 S.Ct. 2791, 120 L.Ed. 2d 674 (1992); Prosser, William L. "Privacy." *California Law Review* 48:3 (1960), 383–423; Rachels, James. "Why Privacy Is Important." *Philosophy and Public Affairs* 4:4 (1975), 323–33; *Restatement of the Law, Second, Torts 2d,* vol. 3. St. Paul, Minn.: American Law Institute, 1977; *Roe v. Wade.* 410 U.S. 113, 93 S.Ct. 705, 35 L.Ed. 2d 147 (1973); Rosenberg, Alexander. "Privacy as a Matter of Taste and Right." *Social Philosophy and Policy* 17:2 (2000), 68–90; *Stanley v. Georgia.* 394 U.S. 557, 89 S.Ct. 1243, 22 L.Ed. 2d 542 (1969); Thomson, Judith Jarvis. "The Right to Privacy." *Philosophy and Public Affairs* 4:4 (1975), 295–314; *Village of Belle Terre v. Boraas.* 416 U.S. 1, 94 S.Ct. 1536, 39 L.Ed. 2d 797 (1974); Warren, Samuel D., and Louis D. Brandeis. "The Right to Privacy." *Harvard Law Review* 4:5 (1890), 193–220; *Wolf v. Colorado.* 338 U.S. 25, 69 S.Ct. 1359, 93 L.Ed. 1782 (1949); *Zablocki v. Redhail.* 434 U.S. 374, 98 S.Ct. 673, 54 L.Ed. 2d 618 (1978).

Mane Hajdin

ADDITIONAL READING

Allen, Anita L. "Privacy." In Hugh LaFollette, ed., *The Oxford Handbook of Practical Ethics.* Oxford, U.K.: Oxford University Press, 2003, 485–513; Allen, Anita L. *Uneasy Access: Privacy for Women in a Free Society.* Totowa, N.J.: Rowman and Littlefield, 1988; Allen, Anita L. *Why Privacy Isn't Everything: Feminist Reflections on Personal Accountability.* Lanham, Md.: Rowman and Littlefield, 2003; Altman, Andrew. "Liberalism and Campus Hate Speech: A Philosophical Examination." *Ethics* 103 (January 1993), 302–17; Andre, Judith. "Privacy as a Value and as a Right." *Journal of Value Inquiry* 20:4 (1986), 309–17; Baird, Robert, and M. Katherine Baird, eds. *Homosexuality: Debating the Issues.* "Part Three: Homosexuality and the Criminal Law." Amherst, N.Y.:

Prometheus, 1995, 97–147; Ball, Howard. *The Supreme Court in the Intimate Lives of Americans: Birth, Sex, Marriage, Childrearing, and Death*. New York: New York University Press, 2002; Beardsley, Elizabeth L. "Privacy: Autonomy, and Selective Disclosure." In J. Roland Pennock and John W. Chapman, eds., *Nomos XIII: Privacy*. New York: Atherton, 1971, 56–70; Benn, Stanley I. "Privacy, Freedom, and Respect for Persons." In J. Roland Pennock and John W. Chapman, eds., *Nomos XIII: Privacy*. New York: Atherton, 1971, 1–26; Benn, Stanley I. "Privacy and Respect for Persons: A Reply." *Australasian Journal of Philosophy* 58:1 (1980), 54–61; Berlant, Lauren, and Michael Warner. "Sex in Public." *Critical Inquiry* 24:2 (1998), 547–66; Bloustein, Edward J. "Privacy as an Aspect of Human Dignity: An Answer to Dean Prosser." *New York University Law Review* 39:6 (1964), 962–1007. Reprinted in *Individual and Group Privacy*. New Brunswick, N.J.: Transaction, 1978, 1–46; and Ferdinand David Schoeman, ed., *Philosophical Dimensions of Privacy: An Anthology*. Cambridge: Cambridge University Press, 1984, 156–202; Boling, Patricia. *Privacy and the Politics of Intimate Life*. Ithaca, N.Y.: Cornell University Press, 1996; Bork, Robert H. "After Warren: The Burger and Rhenquist Courts." In *The Tempting of America: The Political Seduction of the Law*. New York: Free Press, 1990, 101–28; Califia, Pat. (1994) *Public Sex: The Culture of Radical Sex*, 2nd ed. San Francisco, Calif.: Cleis, 2000; Corlett, Angelo J. "The Nature and Value of the Moral Right to Privacy." *Public Affairs Quarterly* 16:4 (2002), 329–50; Dandekar, Natalie. "Privacy: An Understanding for Embodied Persons." *Philosophical Forum* 24:4 (1993), 331–48; Davenport, Manuel M. "What We Do in Private." *Southwest Philosophy Review* 15:1 (1999), 177–83; Davis, Frederick. "What Do We Mean by 'Right of Privacy'?" *South Dakota Law Review* 4 (1959), 1–24; DeCew, Judith Wagner. "Defending the 'Private' in Constitutional Privacy." *Journal of Value Inquiry* 21:3 (1987), 171–84; DeCew, Judith Wagner. "The Feminist Critique of Privacy." *APA Newsletters* [combined newsletters on *Feminism and Philosophy* and *Philosophy and Law*] 94:2 (1995), 42–45; DeCew, Judith Wagner. "The Scope of Privacy in Law and Ethics." *Law and Philosophy* 5:2 (1986), 145–73; Dickler, Gerald. "The Right to Privacy: A Proposed Redefinition." *United States Law Review* 70:8 (1936), 435–56; Eskridge, William N., Jr., and Nan D. Hunter, eds. *Sexuality, Gender, and the Law*. Westbury, N.Y.: Foundation Press, 1997. 2nd ed., 2004; Feinberg, Joel. *The Moral Limits of the Criminal Law*. Vol. 1: *Harm to Others*. New York: Oxford University Press, 1984. Vol. 2: *Offense to Others*, 1985. Vol. 3: *Harm to Self*, 1986. Vol. 4: *Harmless Wrongdoing*, 1988; Fried, Charles. "Privacy." *Yale Law Journal* 77:3 (1968), 475–93. Reprinted in Ferdinand David Schoeman, ed., *Philosophical Dimensions of Privacy: An Anthology*. Cambridge: Cambridge University Press, 1984, 203–22; Gavison, Ruth. "Privacy and the Limits of the Law." *Yale Law Journal* 89:3 (1980), 421–71. Reprinted in Ferdinand David Schoeman, ed., *Philosophical Dimensions of Privacy: An Anthology*. Cambridge: Cambridge University Press, 1984, 346–402; Gerety, Tom. "Redefining Privacy." *Harvard Civil Rights–Civil Liberties Law Review* 12:2 (1977), 233–96; Gerstein, Robert S. "Intimacy and Privacy." *Ethics* 89:1 (1978), 76–81. Reprinted in Ferdinand David Schoeman, ed., *Philosophical Dimensions of Privacy: An Anthology*. Cambridge: Cambridge University Press, 1984, 265–71; Gould, James. "Abortion: Privacy vs. Liberty." *Journal of Social Philosophy* 21:1 (1990), 98–106; Grcic, Joseph M. "The Right to Privacy: Behavior as Property." *Journal of Value Inquiry* 20:2 (1986), 137–44; Grey, Thomas C. *The Legal Enforcement of Morality*. New York: Knopf, 1983; Gross, Hyman. "Privacy and Autonomy." In J. Roland Pennock and John W. Chapman, eds., *Nomos XIII: Privacy*. New York: Atherton, 1971, 169–81. Reprinted in Joel Feinberg and Hyman Gross, eds., *Philosophy of Law*, 3rd ed. Belmont, Calif.: Wadsworth, 1986, 291–96. 4th ed., 1991, 340–45; Hallborg, Robert B., Jr. "Principles of Liberty and the Right to Privacy." *Law and Philosophy* 5:2 (1986), 175–218; "Has the Supreme Court Gone Too Far? A Symposium." *Commentary* 116:3 (October 2003), 25–48; Hudson, Stephen D., and Douglas N. Husak. "Benn on Privacy and Respect for Persons." *Australasian Journal of Philosophy* 57:4 (1979), 324–29; Inness, Julie. "Information, Access, or Intimate Decisions about One's Actions? The Content of Privacy." *Public Affairs Quarterly* 5:3 (1991), 227–42. Reprinted, revised, in *Privacy, Intimacy, and Isolation*. New York: Oxford University Press, 1992, 56–73; Johnson, Jeffrey L. "Constitutional Privacy." *Law and Philosophy* 13:2 (1994), 161–93; Johnson, Jeffrey L. "Privacy, Liberty, and Integrity." *Public Affairs Quarterly* 3:1 (1989), 15–34; Johnson, Jeffrey L. "Privacy and the Judgment of Others." *Journal of Value*

Inquiry 23:3 (1989), 157–68; Johnson, Jeffery L. "A Theory of the Nature and Value of Privacy." *Public Affairs Quarterly* 6:3 (1992), 271–88; Kalven, Harry, Jr. "Privacy in Tort Law—Were Warren and Brandeis Wrong?" *Law and Contemporary Problems* 31:2 (1966), 326–41; Koppelman, Andrew. "The Right to Privacy?" In *The Gay Rights Question in Contemporary American Law.* Chicago, Ill.: University of Chicago Press, 2002, 35–52; Kupfer, Joseph. "Privacy, Autonomy, and Self-Concept." *American Philosophical Quarterly* 24:1 (1987), 81–89; Mayo, David J., and Martin Gunderson. "Privacy and the Ethics of Outing." In Timothy F. Murphy, ed., *Gay Ethics: Controversies in Outing, Civil Rights, and Sexual Science.* New York: Haworth Press, 1994, 47–65; McCloskey, H. J. "The Political Ideal of Privacy." *Philosophical Quarterly* 21:4 (1971), 303–14; McCloskey, H. J. "Privacy and the Right to Privacy." *Philosophy* 55:211 (1980), 17–38; Mohr, Richard D. "Mr. Justice Douglas at Sodom: Gays and Privacy." In *Gays/Justice: A Study of Ethics, Society, and Law.* New York: Columbia University Press, 1988, 47–133; Mohr, Richard D. "Sexual Privacy." In *A More Perfect Union: Why Straight America Must Stand Up for Gay Rights.* Boston, Mass.: Beacon Press, 1994, 19–30; Mohr, Richard D. "Why Sex Is Private: Gays and the Police." *Public Affairs Quarterly* 1:2 (1987), 57–81; Moore, Adam D. "Privacy: Its Meaning and Value." *American Philosophical Quarterly* 40:3 (2003), 215–27; Nagel, Thomas. "Concealment and Exposure." *Philosophy and Public Affairs* 27:1 (1998), 3–30. Reprinted in *Concealment and Exposure and Other Essays.* Oxford, U.K.: Oxford University Press, 2002, 3–26; Nathan, Daniel O. "Just Looking: Voyeurism and the Grounds of Privacy." *Public Affairs Quarterly* 4:4 (1990), 365–86; Parent, W. A. "A New Definition of Privacy for the Law." *Law and Philosophy* 2:4 (1983), 305–38; Parent, W. A. "Privacy, Morality, and the Law." *Philosophy and Public Affairs* 12:4 (1983), 269–88. Reprinted in Joel Feinberg and Hyman Gross, eds., *Philosophy of Law*, 3rd ed. Belmont, Calif.: Wadsworth, 1986, 297–307; Parent, W. A. "Recent Work on the Concept of Privacy." *American Philosophical Quarterly* 20:4 (1983), 341–55; Parker, Richard. "A Definition of Privacy." *Rutgers Law Review* 27:2 (1974), 275–96; Paul, Ellen Frankel, Fred D. Miller, Jr., and Jeffrey Paul, eds. *The Right to Privacy.* Cambridge: Cambridge University Press, 2000 (*Social Philosophy and Policy* 17:2 [2000]); Pierce, Christine. "AIDS and *Bowers v. Hardwick.*" In Alan Soble, ed., *Sex, Love, and Friendship.* Amsterdam, Holland: Rodopi, 1997, 435–45; Posner, Richard A. "The Sexual Revolution in the Courts." In *Sex and Reason.* Cambridge, Mass.: Harvard University Press, 1992, 324–50; Posner, Richard A., and Katharine B. Silbaugh. "Sodomy." In *A Guide to America's Sex Laws.* Chicago, Ill.: University of Chicago Press, 1996, 65–71; Postow, Betsy C. "Andre on Privacy." *Journal of Value Inquiry* 22:4 (1988), 327–30; Prosser, William L. "Privacy." *California Law Review* 48:3 (1960), 383–423. Reprinted in Ferdinand David Schoeman, ed., *Philosophical Dimensions of Privacy: An Anthology.* Cambridge: Cambridge University Press, 1984, 104–55; Rachels, James. "Why Privacy Is Important." *Philosophy and Public Affairs* 4:4 (1975), 323–33. Reprinted in Ferdinand David Schoeman, ed., *Philosophical Dimensions of Privacy: An Anthology.* Cambridge: Cambridge University Press, 1984, 290–99; Reiman, Jeffrey H. "Privacy, Intimacy, and Personhood." *Philosophy and Public Affairs* 6:1 (1976), 26–44. Reprinted in Ferdinand David Schoeman, ed., *Philosophical Dimensions of Privacy: An Anthology.* Cambridge: Cambridge University Press, 1984, 300–316; Robison, Wade. "The Constitution and the Nature of Law." *Law and Philosophy* 12:1 (1993), 5–23; Rosen, Jeffrey. *The Unwanted Gaze: The Destruction of Privacy in America.* New York: Random House, 2000; Rosenblum, Nancy L. "Democratic Sex: Reynolds v. U.S., Sexual Relations, and Community." In David M. Estlund and Martha C. Nussbaum, eds., *Sex, Preference, and Family: Essays on Law and Nature.* New York: Oxford University Press, 1997, 63–85; Samar, Vincent J. *The Right to Privacy: Gays, Lesbians, and the Constitution.* Philadelphia, Pa.: Temple University Press, 1991; Scanlon, Thomas. "Thomson on Privacy." *Philosophy and Public Affairs* 4:4 (1975), 315–22; Schoeman, Ferdinand D. "Privacy." In Lawrence C. Becker and Charlotte B. Becker, eds., *Encyclopedia of Ethics*, 2nd ed., vol. 3. New York: Routledge, 2001, 1381–84; Schoeman, Ferdinand D. "Privacy and Intimate Information." In Ferdinand David Schoeman, ed., *Philosophical Dimensions of Privacy: An Anthology.* Cambridge: Cambridge University Press, 1984, 403–18; Schoeman, Ferdinand D. *Privacy and Social Freedom.* Cambridge: Cambridge University Press, 1992; Schoeman, Ferdinand D. "Privacy: Philosophical Dimensions." *American Philosophical Quarterly* 21:3 (1984), 199–213. Reprinted, revised, in Ferdinand David

Schoeman, ed., *Philosophical Dimensions of Privacy: An Anthology*. Cambridge: Cambridge University Press, 1984, 1–33; Schoeman, Ferdinand D., ed. *Philosophical Dimensions of Privacy: An Anthology*. Cambridge: Cambridge University Press, 1984; Soifer, Eldon, and Béla Szabados. "Hypocrisy and Privacy." *Journal of Philosophical Research* 27 (2002), 601–18; Stein, Edward. "Bowers v. Hardwick." In Timothy F. Murphy, ed., *Reader's Guide to Lesbian and Gay Studies*. Chicago, Ill.: Fitzroy Dearborn, 2000, 95–96; Steiner, George. "Night Words: High Pornography and Human Privacy." *Encounter* 25:4 (1965), 14–19. Reprinted in *Language and Silence: Essays on Language, Literature, and the Inhuman*. New York: Atheneum, 1967, 68–77; Stramel, James S. "Privacy." In Timothy F. Murphy, ed., *Reader's Guide to Lesbian and Gay Studies*. Chicago, Ill.: Fitzroy Dearborn, 2000, 470–72; Sullivan, Andrew. "Unnatural Law." *The New Republic* (24 March 2003), 18–23; Taylor, James Stacey. "Privacy and Autonomy: A Reappraisal." *Southern Journal of Philosophy* 40:4 (2002), 587–604; Thomson, Judith Jarvis. "The Right to Privacy." *Philosophy and Public Affairs* 4:4 (1975), 295–314. Reprinted in Ferdinand David Schoeman, ed., *Philosophical Dimensions of Privacy: An Anthology*. Cambridge: Cambridge University Press, 1984, 272–89; Tunick, Mark. "Does Privacy Undermine Community?" *Journal of Value Inquiry* 35:4 (2001), 517–34; Warren, Samuel D., and Louis D. Brandeis. "The Right to Privacy." *Harvard Law Review* 4:5 (1890), 193–220. Reprinted in Ferdinand David Schoeman, ed., *Philosophical Dimensions of Privacy: An Anthology*. Cambridge: Cambridge University Press, 1984, 75–103; Wasserstrom, Richard A. "Privacy: Some Arguments and Assumptions." In Richard Bronaugh, ed., *Philosophical Law: Authority, Equality, Adjudication, Privacy*. Westport, Conn.: Greenwood Press, 1978, 148–66. Reprinted in Ferdinand David Schoeman, ed., *Philosophical Dimensions of Privacy: An Anthology*. Cambridge: Cambridge University Press, 1984, 317–32; Weinreb, Lloyd L. "The Right to Privacy." *Social Philosophy and Policy* 17:2 (2000), 25–44; Westin, Alan F. *Privacy and Freedom*. New York: Atheneum, 1967.

PROMISCUITY. *See* Casual Sex

PROSTITUTION. Prostitution is the oldest and most widespread type of mercenary sex. More often than not, it is highly controversial. Opposition to it has traditionally been motivated by religious or moral views of sex but also by considerations of public health and by social and political concerns about the inequality and oppression of women. Arguments in its defense come for the most part from liberal and libertarian thinkers but also from prostitutes' rights activists.

The issue of prostitution has been debated in both moral and legal terms. Accordingly, the main philosophical questions concerning prostitution are two: What is its moral status, and what should its legal standing be? The questions are related, but the legal question is not a mere appendage to the moral. Both the moral rejection of prostitution and its moral toleration, or even acceptance, are compatible with a range of views on how the law should handle it.

The word "prostitution" has two meanings, one primary and narrow, the other derived and wider. In one sense it means, roughly, commercial or mercenary sex, that is, engaging in sex for money or other payment. In a secondary sense it means the use of one's ability or talent in a base or unworthy way. People sometimes speak of artists or politicians prostituting themselves when they allow their artistic creativity or political activity to be motivated by considerations of material gain or (on an extremely purist view of art and politics) by any considerations except artistic value and the common good, respectively. The question about the morality of prostitution could thus be put this way: Is prostitution in the strict sense also prostitution in the derived sense?

Putting the question this way, however, requires some disengagement from the expressive load the word "prostitution" has in everyday usage. For, more often than not, in such usage the word not only refers to a certain kind of sexual transaction but also expresses distaste and, indeed, moral disapproval. Some who do not share this distaste and disapproval are accordingly likely to avoid the word altogether, using **sex work** instead. Replacing "prostitution" with "sex work" has several advantages: One can talk about mercenary sex without appearing to be endorsing the conventional distaste and moral condemnation, and one can talk about it in a gender-neutral way. ("Prostitute" ordinarily restricts the reference to women providing sexual services for payment. A man who does that must be called a "male prostitute." Because men also proffer sexual services for money, it seems helpful to have a term that includes them.) Further, "sex work" suggests that the sale of sex is only another line of work, another way of making a living, and thus may endow mercenary sex with some of the respectability of labor.

While these advantages might justify substituting "sex work" for "prostitution" in certain contexts, they are countervailed by a need for accuracy in other contexts, including the philosophy of sex. For "sex work" is a wider term, covering not only prostitution but also other activities in what is sometimes called the "sex industry," such as providing telephone sex, performing in peep shows, stripping in clubs, and posing for **pornography**. While all these activities cater to the sexual interests of clients and are carried out for payment, they also differ from one another in various ways. Prostitution, in particular, differs from the rest in that it usually involves the client's physical contact with the prostitute's body. That often amounts to coitus, but even when it does not, prostitution (unlike other activities) usually provides sexual satisfaction to the client through physical contact of some sort. Not only does this feature set prostitution apart from other sex work activities, but it also endows the issue of its moral standing with particular gravity.

As in other types of sex work, the provision of sexual service in prostitution is relatively indiscriminate. Within certain limits, a prostitute will accept as a client anybody willing to pay the price. This distinguishes the prostitute from the mistress (kept woman) and the gigolo (kept man) as well as from the spouse in a "**marriage** of convenience." In these cases, the **sexual activity** may be just as mercenary as in prostitution, but it is largely confined to a relationship with a single partner over a period of time. The prostitute differs from them in being promiscuous, and indiscriminately so. Accordingly, prostitution can be defined as the provision of sexual services usually involving physical contact and catering indiscriminately to those willing to pay the price.

The legal status of prostitution differs from one jurisdiction to another. Most Western countries do not legally prohibit prostitution as such. But even when prostitution is not treated as a criminal offense, it is usually restricted or regulated by law. The extent of legal restriction or regulation also varies considerably. In some countries the law prohibits certain activities closely associated with prostitution (in particular, soliciting); this has far-reaching, sometimes crippling, effects on the practice. The question is whether the law should be interfering at all in the liberty of individuals to sell and buy sexual services. The answer depends on the way we answer the more basic question about the proper limits of legal curtailment of individual liberty.

In the philosophical discussion of this fundamental question, four liberty-limiting principles have emerged, principles that specify the considerations that provide *prima facie* justification for legally restricting individual freedom (see Joel Feinberg [1926–2004], 36–54; Wasserstrom). According to the harm principle, individual liberty may be restricted to prevent people from causing harm to others. The offense principle permits laws that restrict liberty by prohibiting acts that are seriously offensive (e.g., noxious, repulsive, repugnant) to others. The principle of paternalism justifies laws that restrict liberty in an attempt to prevent people from harming themselves. And according to the principle of legal moralism, the law may curtail individual liberty by enforcing highly important parts of positive morality, that is, the moral norms widely accepted in society and bound up with strong feelings.

Those who accept only the harm principle are likely to be against the legal prohibition of prostitution as such, as long as only competent and consenting adults are involved. They may support some legal regulation of prostitution for reasons of public health. Some may subscribe to a conception of public harm comprehensive enough to warrant restrictions on soliciting. The offense principle leads to a similar position. In a society where the feelings of the average person tend to be seriously offended by encounters with various aspects of prostitution, the principle will justify restrictions meant to prevent this. One restriction is confining prostitution and its attendant activities to certain venues, so that those likely to be offended are not exposed to it unexpectedly and against their will, while those who choose to engage in it can do so without undue difficulty.

Paternalistic considerations, by contrast, do provide reasons for prohibiting prostitution. These arguments emphasize hazards to which the prostitute exposes herself. One hazard, a threat to her health, is the possibility of contracting venereal and other diseases, including AIDS (acquired immunodeficiency syndrome). Other dangers include the abusive, violent behavior of clients; exploitation by pimps and owners of brothels; and police harassment and extortion. Prostitutes may also experience ostracism by much of society and the ill effects of having low social status. These dangers and harms are real and serious. However, the arguments for legal prohibition of prostitution that focus on them are not sound, for they take for granted the condemnation of prostitution by positive morality—and it is this morality that in large measure informs the law that criminalizes prostitution. The dangers and harms of prostitution are caused or enhanced by criminalization itself. If prostitution were not a crime, those engaging in it could expect to receive the level of health care and police protection from violence, coercion, exploitation, and fraud as everybody else expects; their social status would be higher; and they would not necessarily be treated as outcasts. Any argument from these dangers and harms to the legal prohibition of prostitution is circular.

But one paternalistic argument is not circular, the argument that invokes the damage to the prostitute's personal sexual life or to her personal life in general. The prostitute must perform her job, providing sexual services, with emotional detachment. This detachment is likely to spill over into her personal life, to induce alienation from her sexuality and cause other psychological problems. That harm endured by prostitutes cannot be blamed on social attitudes or the law but seems to be inherent to the nature of the work—to the indiscriminate, promiscuous selling of sex. Yet other types of work (for instance, working as an undercover police agent) are bound up with a high personal cost but are not made illegal on that count. This suggests that a closer examination of the principle of paternalism is required; doing so reveals two versions of the principle. "Weak" paternalism justifies laws protecting individuals from harm caused to themselves by their own choices, when these choices are not (fully) voluntary. Weak paternalism may be seen as a corollary of the harm principle, and those committed to individual liberty need not object to it. But weak paternalism can justify prohibiting only prostitution by minors, incompetent adults, and competent adults compelled or deceived into it. These laws are necessary: Child prostitution is widespread, and some adults enter prostitution without understanding its nature and hazards or as a result of outright fraud or coercion. However, were the law to attempt to prevent a competent, informed adult who chooses freely from engaging in prostitution, that would be "strong" paternalism. This type of paternalism could justify extensive interference with individual liberty in many spheres of life and is therefore rejected by those who hold liberty a paramount moral and political value.

Legal moralism provides a case for criminalizing prostitution in societies where its moral condemnation is widespread, strong, and bound up with intolerance, indignation, and disgust. If one subscribes to this liberty-limiting principle, one will decide for or against prohibiting prostitution on the basis of sociological research into how the positive morality of one's society regards the selling and buying of sex. This principle, too, could justify such extensive restrictions of individual liberty that it is unlikely to be accepted by anyone who places much value on liberty.

The other philosophical question about prostitution concerns its moral standing. This is by no means settled once one opts for or against legal moralism. That principle justifies legal enforcement of a large part of positive morality, the morality accepted by society. Philosophers engage in debate about the morality of prostitution from the standpoint of "critical" morality, a standpoint that exists independently of positive morality and enables us to evaluate the moral views, principles, and values espoused by our society as well as by all others.

In this debate, positive morality provides, at best, a point of departure. Its record on prostitution is deeply flawed. Moral attitudes on prostitution differ from society to society and sometimes change from one period to another in one society's history. That is to be expected, and appeals to positive morality in the course of moral argument have to accommodate this variety. Problems remain even if we disregard the positive moralities of all other societies and historical periods and focus on our own. The sexual morality of contemporary Western societies is still plagued by a sexist double standard, and prostitution is a case in point. This morality condemns prostitution, an occupation populated mostly by women and in which nearly all clients are men. It harshly condemns the prostitute but not so much the client, although both participate in the condemned transaction. Further, our society condemns all prostitutes but not with equal severity. For no good moral reason, the censure varies significantly from the streetwalker to the high-class prostitute: "[T]he higher the fee the less the stigma" (Bullough and Bullough, 313). The question, then, is whether our society's moral condemnation of prostitution can be supported by arguments that withstand critical scrutiny.

One argument for condemning mercenary sex claims that there are things that cannot or must not be bought and sold (see Walzer, 95–103) *and* that sexual activity is one of them. The first part of the argument is unexceptionable: **Friendship** and **love** cannot, for logical reasons, be bought or sold (only their semblance can); political offices and advantages, or votes in elections, can be bought and sold but should not be. As a matter of fact, sex *is* bought and sold; indiscriminate, promiscuous sex motivated by payment is not a logically flawed notion. Nor is there a universally accepted conception of the nature and moral significance of sexuality that would prohibit its being bought and sold. Nevertheless, three different philosophical perspectives on sex support the claim that sex ought not to be bought and sold: the traditional view that the purpose of sex is procreation and that sex is properly confined to marriage (as in Catholicism); the common "romantic" view of sex as something intimately linked with love; and the idea that sex is something that should be enjoyed for its own sake, engaged in only when the people involved experience mutual attraction and desire, not because they have other, ulterior reasons or goals, such as money or social or occupational advancement.

Advocates of the first view condemn prostitution because it involves sexual activity that is both nonmarital and deliberately nonprocreative. Yet it can be argued that they have some reason to mitigate their condemnation of it. Sociological research shows that about three-quarters of the clients are men who are, and mean to remain, married and who go to prostitutes to obtain sexual gratification they do not receive from their spouses (Benjamin and Masters, 201). So prostitution may not be a threat to marriage but complementary to and indeed supportive of it. (Defense of prostitution along these lines antedates sociological research; see, for example, **Bernard Mandeville** [1670–1733], 39–52.) The appropriate attitude toward mercenary sex for those who advocate the procreation-and-marriage view of sex would seem to be tolerance.

Proponents of the romantic view think of sex as properly part of a deeply personal, highly significant, loving relationship. Within such a relationship, sex is a rich, fulfilling, distinctively human experience, while promiscuous, **casual sex** is impersonal, devoid of lasting feeling and significance, and pertains only to our animal nature. On these grounds romantics deprecate and condemn casual sex, including prostitution (see Kristjansson). It is wrong because it "divorce[s] the sexual act from its project of sexual union" (**Roger Scruton**, 156). This condemnation seems too quick. The unfavorable comparison of casual sex, and of mercenary sex in particular, with sex as part of a loving relationship does not establish that casual sex has no value whatsoever, let alone that it is morally wrong. Further, there is something incongruous in a view that ties sex to something so personal and resistant to prescription and proscription as love and proclaims this as a norm, backed up by moral sanction, binding everyone. The romantic view is more plausible as a thesis about human sexuality at its best, offered as an ideal that can be freely adopted and aspired to individually, rather than universally prescribed. When understood in these terms, however, the romantic view cannot justify moral condemnation of those who do not live up to the ideal. It can only advise that those who engage in casual sex, including prostitution, might regret that they are missing out on something much more valuable.

Vulnerable to the same objection is the view that sex ought to be engaged in for its own sake, that is, only out of mutual sexual or personal attraction and not for other, extraneous reasons. This view is advocated from a wide variety of perspectives, by some Marxists (e.g., Friedrich Engels [1820–1895], 94–95), some feminists (see Chamallas), and some liberals (e.g., **Bertrand Russell** [1872–1970], 121). This view may come into its own in some sort of utopia. But where is the convincing argument that it should be adopted as the sexual norm here and now? The norm would prove extremely restrictive of individual liberty. If construed as stating a personal ideal, telling us that we make the most of what sex has to offer when we engage in it out of mutual attraction, the view may be thought plausible. But then it would provide no grounds for condemning prostitution as morally wrong. That which is not ideal is not necessarily worthless or morally suspect.

There are, of course, many other arguments against prostitution. Some argue that it is wrong because it cheapens sex. Elizabeth Anderson, for example, claims that the commodification of sex debases sex proffered as a gift. If mercenary sex were accepted as legitimate, that would make it difficult "to establish insulated social spheres where [sex] can be exclusively and fully valued as a genuinely shared and personal good" and given as a gift (155). Many people do place great value on the opportunity to bestow sexual pleasure—as something that has no price and must be given freely if it is to be given at all—on those they love. If this opportunity were restricted or denied, their freedom would be seriously infringed. But this argument, couched in terms of freedom, is actually one of privilege: X's privilege that Y shall not engage in a certain activity for payment because, if she does, that will make for a social environment in which it is difficult for X to engage in the same activity as a way of bestowing an exclusive gift (see Nussbaum, 290–91).

A widespread objection to prostitution depicts it as a degrading activity (and, therefore, morally wrong). There are four arguments for this claim: that mercenary sex is impersonal; that the client uses the prostitute as a means or treats her as an object; that sex is an intimate activity, yet prostitutes engage in it with strangers and for money; and that the prostitute sells her body or even herself.

The first two arguments are incomplete. Neither the impersonal character of a social transaction or relation, nor the fact that its value for the individuals concerned is instrumental, is enough to make it degrading (and morally wrong). Most social transactions are both impersonal and instrumental (e.g., buying a movie theater ticket, getting the automobile oil changed). That is an inescapable fact of life in any but very small, simple, face-to-face societies. These transactions are impersonal in that we take no interest in the other person as the *particular* person she or he is. Yet it is plausible that they do not offend against the other's personhood, they do not treat the other as a mere object or something other or less than a person, as long as the way we relate to the other is based on or is accompanied by the other's **consent**. These relations are instrumental in that they have no value in themselves and are entered into solely to satisfy a desire or need or promote an interest. Yet we do not thereby reduce the other to a *mere* means, a thing, as long as consent is present, because the giving and receiving of something as both human and complex as consent signals that *persons* (not objects) are involved.

One might reply: "Sex is different." Engaging in sexual activity with another person is not at all the same as those various interactions we have with people in which we do not recognize their particularity but see them only as individuals who can help us attain our goals. But this reply presupposes that sex is not only *at its best* when it is personal but that we *ought* to engage in sex only in that fashion. While the former claim, that such sex is ideal, may be granted, the latter claim, that it is also morally required, is neither obviously true nor clearly sustainable. Besides, it is difficult to maintain that sex *is* (that much) different. This, too, is what is questionable about the argument from intimacy, for it seems to entail that a nurse paid to attend to the intimate hygiene of a disabled patient is doing something degrading and morally wrong, which is implausible (Ericsson, 342).

Some critics of prostitution portray the prostitute as a woman who "sells her body" or "sells herself." Carole Pateman, for example, has argued that sex and sexuality are constitutive of the body and, further, are inseparable from one's understanding of one's gender. One's sexuality, one's body, and one's gender are all linked to one's sense of identity, of who and what one is (562). Therefore, selling sex is tantamount to selling one's body and oneself. One rebuttal to this view is that were it true, we would have to say the same thing about the wet nurse and the surrogate mother, for their bodies and gender, and thus their identity, are just as involved in what they are paid to do. It seems wrong, however, to say that the wet nurse sells her body or herself. Surrogate motherhood is a contested issue, but the standard objections to it do not focus on the connections between body, sexuality, gender, identity, and the self. They claim, rather, that surrogacy undermines the mother-child relationship, or that it is degrading to the child to have been bought for money. (To be sure, there is also the claim that "it is inconsistent with human dignity that a woman should use her uterus for financial profit and treat it as an incubator for someone else's child" [*Report*, 45]. But this claim is neither explained nor backed up by argument.) Another rebuttal of Pateman's position is that it is much too loose to speak of the prostitute as someone who sells her body or herself. That would be an appropriate description if she were selling herself into (sexual) slavery, but she does not do that. What she does sell, strictly speaking, is sexual service (see Schwarzenbach).

The late-twentieth-century feminist critique of prostitution has relied on some of the arguments so far discussed, but it has also frequently emphasized that prostitution epitomizes and reinforces the inequality and oppression of women. Prostitution is claimed to be "an inherently unequal practice defined by the intersection of capitalism and patriarchy" (Overall, 724). It is not merely a commercial transaction but a transaction between a socially inferior seller, the woman, and a socially superior buyer, the man. Indeed, "prostitution occurs within multiple power relations of domination, degradation, and subservience of the pimp and trick [client] over the prostitute: men over women, older over younger, citizen over alien, moneyed over impoverished, violent over victimized, connected over isolated, housed over homeless, tolerated and respected over despised" (**Catharine MacKinnon**, 24–25). Given this inequality, it is untenable to claim that the consent of a prostitute is morally valid and decisive. The elimination of this inequality in our capitalist and patriarchal society is unlikely, but with the demise of this type of society, prostitution will wither away.

This analysis is undermined both by history and a closer look at mercenary sex as it is practiced in capitalist societies. Prostitution existed in precapitalist societies; it did not disappear with the dismantling of capitalism in countries such as the Soviet Union and China. Prostitution within capitalist society displays a complex structure. Much of it does bear out feminist claims of inequality and oppression. But "high-class" prostitution does not. Further, prostitution often occurs between members of the same economic or social class, where inequality between the transacting parties is weak or nonexistent.

Another strand of the feminist critique of prostitution focuses on its complicity in the oppression of women. Prostitution, it has been argued (see Shrage, "Should Feminists Oppose Prostitution?"), both expresses and reinforces certain deeply entrenched assumptions about men, women, and sex that have significant and pernicious repercussions. The most important assumptions are that men are "naturally" dominant and that sex with men pollutes and harms women. This understanding of sex between men and women is said to be implicit in the use of words such as "fuck" and "screw" for sexual intercourse (see Baker). The use of these words implies that the man is the active party in intercourse, while the woman is passive. Further, the same words used in nonsexual contexts describe the taking advantage of someone or harming them. All this indicates an understanding of sexual intercourse as an interaction in which the man is the active party, causing pollution or harm, while the woman is passive, being polluted or harmed. This understanding informs the meaning of sex in general, and of mercenary sex in particular, in modern Western society. It functions as a justification of women's oppression and causes harm both to prostitutes and women in general.

The force of this critique depends on various empirical claims about our society: about the assumptions about sexuality that people generally make and what our linguistic practices reveal about us. But these claims are shaky (see Primoratz, 105–9). The assumption that men are dominant by nature was widespread for a long time but has by now become the preserve of an unenlightened minority, at least in urban environments. Even if it is true that our use of "fuck" or "screw" in sexual contexts frequently implies "hurt," this vocabulary has never been the standard, but rather a substandard, vulgar way of referring to sexual intercourse. Thus it cannot be taken as an indication of general acceptance of the conception of sex said to be implicit in it, let alone that that conception is the only one there is in modern Western society. This line of argument, then, does not provide a critique of prostitution in our society; it is at most a critique of certain instances or types of prostitution in it.

Feminist critics of prostitution invite us to understand and evaluate it in its social context rather than in the abstract. When understood this way, prostitution can be seen to be implicated in the inequality and oppression of women. Now, this is not always the case with many noncapitalist societies nor with all types of mercenary sex in modern capitalist society. However, it may well be true of many if not most varieties of prostitution as it exists in our society. Feminist critics, then, do make an important point—not about prostitution as such but about much of it as it is practiced in our society. When we attend to mercenary sex as it exists in our society, we find that much of it does express and reinforce the inequality and oppression of women. To that extent, it is indeed morally objectionable. At the same time, however, there are ways to improve how prostitution is practiced even in our society, ways that might make it less objectionable or even morally acceptable (see Ericsson, 361–63; Shrage, *Moral Dilemmas*, 158–61).

Thus, it seems that we have not yet disclosed an argument showing that prostitution *as such* is morally wrong. If so, the conclusion is not that we should commend prostitution but only that we should not be so quick to condemn it. For even if prostitution is not wrong, for many people it leaves much to be desired when compared with sex they have just for the fun of it or sex within a personal and loving relationship. It is quite unlike anything that might be put forward as a sexual ideal. It caters to sexual preferences or needs some people have occasionally and others have on a long-term basis. Thus it does serve some socially usefully purposes (see Califia). These facts, as well as the importance of individual liberty (of both the prostitute and the client), are virtually all that can be brought up in prostitution's favor and are typically brought up by its liberal and libertarian defenders (Ericsson; Primoratz, 88–109; Richards, 84–153) and prostitutes' rights activists (see Pheterson). They suggest that prostitution should be viewed like any other service. Such defense is not rebutted, but its application is significantly circumscribed, by feminist arguments referring to the inequality and oppression of women.

See also Addiction, Sexual; Adultery; Bataille, Georges; Casual Sex; Consent; Cybersex; Diseases, Sexually Transmitted; Dworkin, Andrea; Ethics, Sexual; Feminism, Liberal; Feminism, Men's; Fichte, Johann Gottlieb; Kant, Immanuel; Language; Law, Sex and the; Liberalism; MacKinnon, Catharine; Marxism; Objectification, Sexual; Pornography; Rape; Sex Education; Sex Work

REFERENCES

Anderson, Elizabeth. *Value in Ethics and Economics*. Cambridge, Mass.: Harvard University Press, 1993; Baker, Robert B. " 'Pricks' and 'Chicks': A Plea for 'Persons.' " In Robert B. Baker, Kathleen J. Wininger, and Frederick A. Elliston, eds., *Philosophy and Sex*, 3rd ed. Amherst, N.Y.: Prometheus, 1998, 281–305; Benjamin, Harry, and R.E.L. Masters. *Prostitution and Morality*. New York: Julian Press, 1964; Bullough, Vern L., and Bonnie Bullough. *Women and Prostitution: A Social History*. Buffalo, N.Y.: Prometheus, 1987; Califia, Pat. "Whoring in Utopia." In *Public Sex: The Culture of Radical Sex*. Pittsburgh, Pa.: Cleis Press, 1994, 242–48; Chamallas, Martha. "Consent, Equality, and the Legal Control of Sexual Conduct." *Southern California Law Review* 61:4 (1988), 777–862; Engels, Friedrich. (1884) *The Origin of the Family, Private Property, and the State*. New York: International Publishers, 1972; Ericsson, Lars O. "Charges against Prostitution: An Attempt at a Philosophical Assessment." *Ethics* 90:3 (1980), 335–66; Feinberg, Joel. *Social Philosophy*. Englewood Cliffs, N.J.: Prentice-Hall, 1973; Kristjansson, Kristjan. "Casual Sex Revisited." *Journal of Social Philosophy* 29:2 (1998), 97–108; MacKinnon, Catharine A. "Prostitution and Civil Rights." *Michigan Journal of Gender and Law* 1:1 (1993), 13–31; Mandeville,

Bernard. (1724) *A Modest Defence of Publick Stews*. Ed. Richard I. Cook. Los Angeles, Calif.: Augustan Reprint Society, Publication No. 162, 1973; Nussbaum, Martha C. " 'Whether from Reason or Prejudice': Taking Money for Bodily Services." In *Sex and Social Justice*. New York: Oxford University Press, 1999, 276–98; Overall, Christine. "What's Wrong with Prostitution? Evaluating Sex Work." *Signs* 17:4 (1992), 705–24; Pateman, Carole. "Defending Prostitution: Charges against Ericsson." *Ethics* 93:4 (1983), 561–65; Pheterson, Gail, ed. *A Vindication of the Rights of Whores*. Seattle, Wash.: Seal Press, 1989; Primoratz, Igor. *Ethics and Sex*. London: Routledge, 1999; *Report of the Committee of Inquiry into Human Fertilisation and Embryology*. London: HMSO, 1984; Richards, David A. J. *Sex, Drugs, Death, and the Law: An Essay in Human Rights and Overcriminalization*. Totowa, N.J.: Rowman and Littlefield, 1982; Russell, Bertrand. *Marriage and Morals*. London: George Allen and Unwin, 1929; Schwarzenbach, Sibyl. "Contractarians and Feminists Debate Prostitution." *New York University Review of Law and Social Change* 18:1 (1990), 103–30; Scruton, Roger. *Sexual Desire: A Moral Philosophy of the Erotic*. New York: Free Press, 1986; Shrage, Laurie. *Moral Dilemmas of Feminism: Prostitution, Adultery, and Abortion*. New York: Routledge, 1994; Shrage, Laurie. "Should Feminists Oppose Prostitution?" *Ethics* 99:2 (1989), 347–61; Walzer, Michael. *Spheres of Justice: A Defense of Pluralism and Equality*. New York: Basic Books, 1983; Wasserstrom, Richard A., ed. *Morality and the Law*. Belmont, Calif.: Wadsworth, 1971.

Igor Primoratz

ADDITIONAL READING

Alexander, Priscilla. "Prostitution: *Still* a Difficult Issue for Feminists." In Frédérique Delacoste and Priscilla Alexander, eds., *Sex Work: Writings by Women in the Sex Industry*, 2nd ed. San Francisco, Calif.: Cleis Press, 1998, 184–230; Anderson, Clelia Smyth, and Yolanda Estes. "The Myth of the Happy Hooker: Kantian Moral Reflections on a Phenomenology of Prostitution." In Stanley G. French, Wanda Teays, and Laura M. Purdy, eds., *Violence against Women: Philosophical Perspectives*. Ithaca, N.Y.: Cornell University Press, 1998, 152–58; Anderson, Scott A. "Prostitution and Sexual Autonomy: Making Sense of the Prohibition of Prostitution." *Ethics* 112:4 (2002), 748–80; Archard, David. "The Limits of Consensuality I: Incest, Prostitution, and Sadomasochism." In *Sexual Consent*. Boulder, Colo.: Westview, 1998, 98–115; Archard, David. "Sex for Sale: The Morality of Prostitution." *Cogito* 3:1 (1989), 47–51; Baker, Robert B. " 'Pricks' and 'Chicks': A Plea for 'Persons.' " In Robert B. Baker and Frederick A. Elliston, eds., *Philosophy and Sex*, 1st ed. Buffalo, N.Y.: Prometheus, 1975, 45–64. Reprinted in P&S2 (249–67); P&S3 (281–97), with " 'Pricks' and 'Chicks': A Postscript after Twenty-Five Years" (297–305); Bell, Megara. "The Fallen Woman in Fiction and Legislation." *Victoria's Past* (28 September 1999). <www.gober.net/victorian/reports/prostit.html> [accessed 8 September 2004]; Belliotti, Raymond. "Prostitution." In *Good Sex: Perspectives on Sexual Ethics*. Lawrence: University Press of Kansas, 1993, 247–58; Belliotti, Raymond. "The Prostitution in Capitalist Marriage: Marxism." In *Good Sex: Perspectives on Sexual Ethics*. Lawrence: University Press of Kansas, 1993, 111–25; Bloch, Iwan. *Die Prostitution*. Berlin, Ger.: L. Marcus, 1912; Bullough, Bonnie. "Female Prostitution: Current Research and Changing Interpretations." *Annual Review of Sex Research* 7 (1996), 158–80; Bullough, Vern L. *The History of Prostitution*. New Hyde Park, N.Y.: University Books, 1964; Bullough, Vern L., and Bonnie Bullough. *Women and Prostitution: A Social History*. Buffalo, N.Y.: Prometheus, 1987; Califia, Pat. "Whoring in Utopia." In *Public Sex: The Culture of Radical Sex*. Pittsburgh, Pa.: Cleis Press, 1994, 242–48. Reprinted in POS4 (475–81); "Code of Ethics for Prostitutes." *Coyote Howls* 5:1 (1978), 9; Davidson, Julia O'Connell. "Prostitution and the Contours of Control." In Jeffrey Weeks and Janet Holland, eds., *Sexual Cultures: Communities, Values, and Intimacy*. New York: St. Martin's Press, 1996, 180–98; Davidson, Julia O'Connell. "The Rights and Wrongs of Prostitution." *Hypatia* 17:2 (2002), 84–98; Davies, Margaret. "On Prostitution." In M. Daniel Carroll R., David J. A. Clines, and Philip R. Davies, eds., *The Bible in Human Society: Essays in Honour of John Rogerson*. [*Journal for the Study of the Old Testament*, supp. series, no. 200] Sheffield, U.K.: Sheffield Academic Press, 1995, 225–48; Delacoste, Frédérique, and

Priscilla Alexander, eds. *Sex Work: Writings by Women in the Sex Industry*, 1st ed. Pittsburgh, Pa.: Cleis Press, 1987. 2nd ed., San Francisco, Calif.: Cleis Press, 1998; Dworkin, Andrea. "Prostitution and Male Supremacy." *Michigan Journal of Gender and Law* 1:1 (1993), 1–12. Reprinted in Andrea Dworkin, *Life and Death*. New York: Free Press, 1997, 139–51; Elias, James E., Vern L. Bullough, Veronica Elias, and Gwen Brewer, eds. *Prostitution: On Whores, Hustlers, and Johns*. Amherst, N.Y.: Prometheus, 1998; Estes, Yolanda. "Moral Reflections on Prostitution." *Essays in Philosophy* 2:2 (2001). <www.humboldt.edu/~essays/estes.html> [accessed 27 October 2004]; Feinberg, Joel. *The Moral Limits of the Criminal Law*. Vol. 1: *Harm to Others*. New York: Oxford University Press, 1984. Vol. 2: *Offense to Others*, 1985. Vol. 3: *Harm to Self*, 1986. Vol. 4: *Harmless Wrongdoing*, 1988; Freud, Sigmund. (1912) "On the Universal Tendency to Debasement in the Sphere of Love." In *The Standard Edition of the Complete Psychological Works of Sigmund Freud*, vol. 11. Trans. James Strachey. London: Hogarth Press, 1953–1974, 179–90; Garb, Sarah H. "Sex for Money Is Sex for Money: The Illegality of Pornographic Film as Prostitution." *Law and Inequality* 13:2 (1995), 281–301; Goldman, Emma. (1910) "The Traffic in Women." In *Anarchism and Other Essays*. New York: Dover, 1969, 177–94; Green, Karen. "Prostitution, Exploitation and Taboo." *Philosophy* 64:250 (1989): 525–34; Hart, H.L.A. (1962) *Law, Liberty and Morality*. Stanford, Calif.: Stanford University Press, 1963; Hartsock, Nancy C. M. "Gender and Power: Masculinity, Violence, and Domination." In *Money, Sex, and Power: Toward a Feminist Historical Materialism*. New York: Longman, 1983, 155–85; Hughes, Donna M. "Prostitution Online." *Journal of Trauma Practice* 2:3–4 (2003), 115–32. <www.uri.edu/artsci/wms/hughes/prostitution_online.pdf> [accessed 21 September 2004]; Hughes, Donna M. "Sex Tours via the Internet." *Agenda: A Journal about Women and Gender*, no. 28 (1996), 71–76; Jaggar, Alison M. "Prostitution." In Alan Soble, ed., *The Philosophy of Sex: Contemporary Readings*, 1st ed. Totowa, N.J.: Rowman and Littlefield, 1980, 348–68; POS2 (259–80). Reprinted in Marilyn Pearsall, ed., *Women and Values: Readings in Recent Feminist Philosophy*. Belmont, Calif.: Wadsworth, 1999, 132–43; Jeffreys, Sheila. *The Idea of Prostitution*. Melbourne, Australia: Spinifex Press, 1998; Jordan, Bill. *Sex, Money, and Power: The Transformation of Collective Lives*. Malden, Mass.: Polity, 2004; Kulick, Don. (1997) "A Man in the House: The Boyfriends of Brazilian *Travesti* Prostitutes." In Robert J. Corber and Stephen Valocchi, eds., *Queer Studies: An Interdisciplinary Reader*. Malden, Mass.: Blackwell, 2003, 237–54; Kulick, Don. *Travesti: Sex, Gender, and Culture among Brazilian Transgendered Prostitutes*. Chicago, Ill.: University of Chicago Press, 1998; Kupfer, Joseph. "Prostitutes, Musicians, and Self-Respect." *Journal of Social Philosophy* 26:3 (1995), 75–88. Reprinted as "What Is Wrong with Prostitution?" in Thomas Magnell, ed., *Explorations of Value*. Amsterdam, Holland: Rodopi, 1997, 213–20; LeMoncheck, Linda. "I Only Do It for the Money: Pornography, Prostitution, and the Business of Sex." In *Loose Women, Lecherous Men: A Feminist Philosophy of Sex*. New York: Oxford University Press, 1997, 110–54; Lomasky, Loren E. "Gift Relations, Sexual Relations and Freedom." *Philosophical Quarterly* 33:132 (1983), 250–58; MacKinnon, Catharine A. "Prostitution and Civil Rights." *Michigan Journal of Gender and Law* 1:1 (1993), 13–31. Reprinted in *Women's Lives, Men's Laws*. Cambridge, Mass.: Harvard University Press, 2005, 151–61; Madigan, Timothy. "The Discarded Lemon: Kant, Prostitution and Respect for Persons." *Philosophy Now*, no. 21 (Summer–Autumn 1998), 14–16. Reprinted in James E. Elias, Vern L. Bullough, Veronica Elias, and Gwen Brewer, eds., *Prostitution: On Whores, Hustlers, and Johns*. Amherst, N.Y.: Prometheus, 1998, 107–11; Marshall, S. E. "Bodyshopping: The Case of Prostitution." *Journal of Applied Philosophy* 16:2 (1999), 139–50; McGinn, Thomas A. *Prostitution, Sexuality, and the Law in Ancient Rome*. New York: Oxford University Press, 1998; McLeod, Eileen. *Women Working: Prostitution Now*. London: Croom Helm, 1982; Morgan, Seiriol. "Dark Desires." *Ethical Theory and Moral Practice* 6:4 (2003), 377–410; Morgan, Seiriol. "Sex in the Head." *Journal of Applied Philosophy* 20:1 (2003), 1–16; Nagle, Jill, ed. *Whores and Other Feminists*. New York: Routledge, 1997; Olivieri, Achillo. "Eroticism and Social Groups in Sixteenth-Century Venice: The Courtesan." In Philippe Ariès and André Béjin, eds., *Western Sexuality: Practice and Precept in Past and Present Times*. Oxford, U.K.: Blackwell, 1985, 94–102; O'Neill, Maggie. *Prostitution and Feminism: Towards a Politics of Feeling*. Cambridge, U.K.: Polity, 2001; Pateman, Carole. "Sex and Power." *Ethics* 100:2 (1990): 398–407; Pateman,

Carole. "What's Wrong with Prostitution?" In *The Sexual Contract*. Stanford, Calif.: Stanford University Press, 1988, 189–218; Pateman, Carole. "Women and Consent." *Political Theory* 8:2 (1980), 149–68. Reprinted in *The Disorder of Women: Democracy, Feminism, and Political Theory*. Cambridge: Cambridge University Press, 1989, 71–89; Posner, Richard A., and Katharine B. Silbaugh. "Prostitution." In *A Guide to America's Sex Laws*. Chicago, Ill.: University of Chicago Press, 1996, 155–87; Primoratz, Igor. "Prostitution." In Ruth Chadwick, ed., *Encyclopedia of Applied Ethics*, vol. 3. San Diego, Calif.: Academic Press, 1998, 693–702; Primoratz, Igor. "What's Wrong with Prostitution?" *Philosophy* 68:264 (April 1993), 159–82. Reprinted in HS (291–314); POS3 (339–61); POS4 (451–73). Expanded, revised as "Prostitution." In *Ethics and Sex*. London: Routledge, 1999, 88–109; Radin, Margaret-Jane. *Contested Commodities*. Cambridge, Mass.: Harvard University Press, 1996; Reiman, Jeffrey. "Prostitution, Addiction, and the Ideology of Liberalism." *Contemporary Crises* 3 (1979), 53–68; Richards, David A. J. "Commercial Sex and the Rights of the Person." In *Sex, Drugs, Death, and the Law: An Essay in Human Rights and Overcriminalization*. Totowa, N.J.: Rowman and Littlefield, 1982, 84–153; Richards, David A. J. "Commercial Sex in the American Struggle for the Rights of the Person." In James E. Elias, Vern L. Bullough, Veronica Elias, and Gwen Brewer, eds., *Prostitution: On Whores, Hustlers, and Johns*. Amherst, N.Y.: Prometheus, 1998, 501–40; Sappington, Rodney, and Tyler Stallings, eds. *Uncontrollable Bodies: Testimonies of Identity and Culture*. Seattle, Wash.: Bay Press, 1994; Sartorius, Rolf, ed. *Paternalism*. Minneapolis: University of Minnesota Press, 1983, 83–94; Satz, Debra. "Markets in Women's Sexual Labor." *Ethics* 106:1 (1995), 63–85; Schwarzenbach, Sibyl. "Contractarians and Feminists Debate Prostitution." *New York University Review of Law and Social Change* 18:1 (1990), 103–30. Reprinted in HS (315–42); Schwarzenbach, Sibyl. "On Owning the Body." In James E. Elias, Vern L. Bullough, Veronica Elias, and Gwen Brewer, eds., *Prostitution: On Whores, Hustlers, and Johns*. Amherst, N.Y.: Prometheus, 1998, 345–51; Shelby, Tommie. "Parasites, Pimps, and Capitalists: A Naturalistic Conception of Exploitation." *Social Theory and Practice* 28:3 (2002), 381–418; Shrage, Laurie. "Comparing Prostitutions" and "Exotic Erotica and Erotic Exotica: Sex Commerce in Some Contemporary Urban Centers." In *Moral Dilemmas of Feminism: Prostitution, Adultery, and Abortion*. New York: Routledge, 1994, 99–119, 120–61; Shrage, Laurie. "Feminist Perspectives on Sex Markets." In Edward Zalta, ed., *The Stanford Encyclopedia of Philosophy* (18 February 2004). <plato.stanford.edu/entries/feminist-sex-markets/> [accessed 24 August 2004]; Shrage, Laurie. "Is Sexual Desire Raced? The Social Meaning of Interracial Prostitution." *Journal of Social Philosophy* 23:1 (1992), 42–51; Shrage, Laurie. "Prostitution and the Case for Decriminalization." *Dissent* (Spring 1996), 41–45; Shrage, Laurie. "Should Feminists Oppose Prostitution?" *Ethics* 99:2 (1989), 347–61. Reprinted in HS (275–89); POS3 (323–38); POS4 (435–50); STW (71–80); Soble, Alan. "Is Sex Different?" In *Pornography: Marxism, Feminism, and the Future of Sexuality*. New Haven, Conn.: Yale University Press, 1986, 135–41; Soble, Alan. "The Sufficiency of Consent" and "Equality." In *Sexual Investigations*. New York: New York University Press, 1996, 33–37, 204–8; Stewart, Robert M. "Moral Criticism and the Social Meaning of Prostitution." In Robert M. Stewart, ed., *Philosophical Perspectives on Sex and Love*. New York: Oxford University Press, 1995, 81–83; Walkowitz, Judith. *Prostitution and Victorian Society*. Cambridge: Cambridge University Press, 1980; Wartofsky, Marx. "On Doing It for Money." In Thomas A. Mappes and Jane S. Zembaty, eds., *Biomedical Ethics*. New York: McGraw-Hill, 1981, 186–95; Weisberg, D. Kelly, ed. "Prostitution." Section of *Applications of Feminist Legal Theory to Women's Lives: Sex, Violence, Work, and Reproduction*. Philadelphia, Pa.: Temple University Press, 1996, 187–271; Weitzer, Ronald, ed. *Sex for Sale: Prostitution, Pornography, and the Sex Industry*. New York: Routledge, 2000; West, Donald J., with Buz de Villiers. *Male Prostitution*. New York: Haworth, 1993; Wicclair, Mark R. "Is Prostitution Morally Wrong?" *Philosophy Research Archives* 7:3 (1981), 14–29; Winnifrith, Tom. *Fallen Women in the Nineteenth-Century Novel*. New York: St. Martin's Press, 1994; "Wolfenden Report." Report of the Committee on Homosexual Offences and Prostitution (U.K.). Cmd. 247, 1957; Wright, David F. "Homosexuals or Prostitutes? The Meaning of *arsenokoitai* (1 Cor. 6:9, 1 Tim. 1:10)." *Vigiliae Christianae* 38 (June 1984), 125–53.

PROTESTANTISM, HISTORY OF. In the thirteenth century, voices of dissent against the Roman Catholic Church's theological and institutional power surfaced among theologians and members of monastic communities. In the sixteenth century these voices established theological and denominational independence through separation from Rome. "Protestantism" is the generic label that identifies this cluster of reforming and schismatic Christian religious movements and churches, which now constitute about one-third of a worldwide Christian membership of over 2 billion. Protestant attitudes toward **marriage**, family, and sex decisively shaped the **sexual ethics** and practices of the American colonies (most of which were Protestant) and continued to inform attitudes and debates (about **sex education**, premarital sex, **abortion**, **same-sex marriage**) that developed in the United States in the late twentieth century.

Protestants place authority for thinking about the Christian life (including sex) not in the papacy (the Bishop of Rome) or the traditional teachings and offices of the Roman Catholic Church but in the authority of Scripture (the Old and New Testaments) and in the early apostolic teachings and communities of the first century CE. Central to Protestant thought are the biblical doctrines of human sin, alienation, and estrangement from God; the recognition of the need for salvation from such sin; and the belief that salvation is attainable only as a gift from God made possible by the death and resurrection of Jesus Christ, his son. The reception of salvation is not linked to "good works" or to a morally upstanding life on the part of the recipient, although moral rectitude will naturally follow from the reception of the gift of grace. Once salvation is accepted through the recognition of one's sin and a confession of faith in Christ's redemptive power, individuals experience a rebirth into a new life with a reestablished sacred destiny and relationship with God, though persons will still struggle with the realities, limitations, and failings of sin in their lives. New life in Christ establishes a community of faith (the Church) that seeks to live and act in conformity with the spirit and demands of true Christian teaching.

These core theological affirmations shape Protestant thinking about sex. For Protestants, sex is both a gift from God and, because of human sin, a "problem" that challenges individuals and their communities. All Protestants possess an idea of what passes for "good" (that is, morally legitimate) sex. But the complexity and variety of Protestant theological voices and communities, their various, often conflicting, commitments, and the central authority given to individual conscience mean that defining a single Protestant view of sex is not possible.

Protestants reacted to and recast elements of the sexual ethics and practices of early and late medieval Catholicism, which had constructed a sexual ethic in light of the dominant views of **Saint Paul** (5–64?) and **Saint Augustine** (354–430). Paul affirmed celibacy as the preferred sexual ethic and practice of Christians, though he was willing to make tolerable allowances for marriage and marital sex in the face of the problems of controlling human desires (see 1 Cor. 7:1–9). But **sexual desire** and **sexual activity** remained a problem in constant need of management (Brundage, 57–61; Cahill, *Sex, Gender, and Christian Ethics*, 136–39). Although Augustine, too, affirmed celibacy, he embraced a practical middle ground that also celebrated marriage. To the extent that sexual acts reinforced the three desirable qualities of marriage—*fides* (fidelity and sexual obligations to one's spouse), *proles* (offspring), and *sacramentum* (a mystical and indissoluble bond between husband and wife), sex in marriage was affirmed (*On Marriage and Concupiscence*, 1.11.10, 1.19.17, 1.23.21; *On the Good of Marriage*, 3.3, 4.4, 7.7, 15.17). At the same time, however, every act of sexual intercourse was viewed as sinful, a direct result of human rebellion against God and the inability of humans to control their inclinations and genitals (see Clark and Richardson, 69–72).

Building on these tendencies, the late medieval church affirmed virginity and celibacy as the first choice of service to and worship of God (Cahill, *Sex*, 168–83). This commitment was grounded in the notion of "the counsels of perfection" that affirmed a "higher," more morally praiseworthy (and challenging) call to celibacy, poverty, and relinquishing family. Still, marriage, affirmed in the twelfth century as a sacrament (a visible and extraordinary expression of God's grace in human life), was viewed as the natural though compromised state of ordinary persons. **Saint Thomas Aquinas** (1224/25–1274) argued for the goodness of marriage as a legitimate context for the pursuit of a life of faith consistent with the moral norms of God's natural law. Marriage could be considered morally licit if it pursued the natural ends of marriage: first, procreation and the raising of children; and second, the expression of faithfulness, mutual help, and the opportunity to "quiet" or satisfy sexual desire or lust (see *Summa*, vol. 1, 488–91, 516–20: "Treatise on Man," ques. 92, art. 1–4, and ques. 98, art. 1, 2; Cahill, *Sex*, 192–93; Clark and Richardson, 78–85, 95–101 [*Summa*, III Supplement, ques. 39, art. 1; ques. 49, art. 5, 6]). In the context of the rigid interpretation of Natural Law at the foundation of Catholicism's developing penitential and confessional system, sexual intercourse that failed to meet these stipulations (most important, seeking to bring children into the world) was both morally and legally denounced. The standard of Natural Law also prohibited premarital and extramarital liaisons, divorce, concubinage, **incest**, **rape**, **prostitution**, **masturbation**, sexual **fantasy**, homosexual relations, and even remarriage for older widows and widowers (Brundage, 88–108).

In spite of its patriarchal structure, the medieval sex ethic made room for some egalitarian considerations, including the requirement of **consent** by women for marriage. Greater attention was given to the value of marital affection and even sexual intimacy and pleasure (Cahill, *Sex*, 193). Companionship and **friendship**, though not romantic **love** or eroticism, were celebrated within marriage (Brooke, 61–118, 211–27). But rejecting sexual pleasure per se as a worthy end of marriage became a hallmark of official Catholic teaching.

With regard to sexual ethics and practices, the legacy of the Protestant Reformation is essentially one of inverting the hierarchical ranking of marital goods espoused by Roman Catholicism. Martin Luther (1483–1546) and John Calvin (1509–1564) began their pilgrimage of protest as critics of a corrupt church in need of reform. They also rejected church teachings regarding human salvation and the nature of grace; the legitimacy of the counsels of perfection (the special call to celibacy, poverty, and obedience embraced by priests, monks, and nuns); the view of marriage as a sacrament (and therefore indissoluble); and the restrictive and mechanistic interpretation of Natural Law theology as a moral standard for judging particular acts. In its place they introduced a sexual ethic that built on themes found in the Hebrew Bible and modified by the New Testament's spirituality and ethic of love. An understanding of marriage as a legitimate and necessary Christian vocation was central to Reformation theology. The Protestant reformers sought to construct a sexual ethic that could be functional, practical, and sustain the church for many generations. Because all licit sex remained monogamous marital sex, Protestantism rejected all homosexual relationships and activities (with some exceptions in twentieth-century Protestantism) as well as extramarital, unconsented-to, and underage sex. But the Protestant marital sex ethic also led to the denial of nearly all the church's earlier teachings on sexual restrictions *in* marriage (Brundage, 552–57).

Luther's abandoning celibacy as an Augustinian monk and his later marriage informed his gratitude for marriage, sex, and family (Cahill, *Between the Sexes*, 123–37). Luther developed his orientation to sex and marriage in light of his view of the role of moral law and grace in human life. Though all human beings, upon affirmation of faith in Christ, experience the radical freedom that comes from this gift of salvation, the law (in the form of the Ten Commandments as well as other religious and positive laws) serves an essential function in human life. Its primary task (or "first use") is to urge individuals to accept God's grace as the means to salvation, since they are unable to attain salvation through conformity to legal mandates or a "righteous life." For Luther, sin is best appreciated as a state from which to escape, not a series of legal transgressions from which to be absolved of guilt. However, even human beings who are reconciled with God through grace still exist in their "fleshly" state as sinners. They are, in Luther's words, *simul justus et peccatore* (simultaneously justified yet sinners). Thus, in a fallen and sinful yet redeemed world, the law's "second use" is as a tool to constrain and limit sin and rebelliousness through sanctions and coercions (Luther, 585–629).

In light of these understandings of the law, Luther's guidelines for sexual relationships respond to expressions of egoism, rebelliousness, and the persistence of the natural drives that constitute—and consume—our sinful nature. Luther's sexual ethic is fundamentally concerned with the regulation and policing of desire, an orientation for which he is indebted to Paul and Augustine. Still, the normative condition for humans is marriage, God's gift to humanity, which provides a range of blessings to people that transcend, even contradict, the strictly procreative and sacramental benefits asserted by Aquinas (Luther, 630–37; see Clark and Richardson, 143–48 [Luther, *Lecture on Genesis* (1543)]). And because Luther is much more concerned with functional relationships and the long-term maintenance of sex drives, he is less fastidious than earlier Catholic thinkers concerning the rightness or wrongness of individual sexual acts. He focuses, instead, on issues surrounding meeting a spouse's sexual needs, satisfaction and comfort, fidelity, nurture, child rearing, and companionship. Luther downplays concern with premarital and extramarital sex, divorce, remarriage, and deviant sex, although he never really rejects the negative connotations attached to them. Divorce, for example, is discussed by Luther as a practical act permitted in situations not of desire but of **adultery**, the refusal of conjugal duty, coercion into an unchristian way of life, or the (alleged) inability to give children or sexually satisfy one's partner (Brundage, 558–59; Cahill, *Between*, 131).

Luther's reforming movement flourished in central Europe; Calvin's work as a reformer was most decisive in French-speaking western Europe, Holland, and Scotland. His early scholastic and legal training, as well as his identity as a humanist and French Catholic, informed his strong criticisms of the structure and corruptions of the Roman Catholic Church. The loss of his three children in infancy, and his wife of nine years, also illuminates his deemphasizing the procreative dimensions of marriage in favor of companionship, mutuality, and even erotic love (Bouwsma, 23). Calvin's sexual ethic was grounded in his views of the relationship that exists between God's will and His love for humanity, on the one hand, and human desire for meaning, order, and happiness, on the other. For Calvin, sin is best understood not as *rebellion* (as it was with Luther) but as *disorder*, a force that undercuts the integrity and proper functioning of human relationships. Law, including the regulation of sexuality, is appreciated not simply negatively (as with Luther's second use of the law) but, in its "third use," as a positive good, a gift from God, a teacher, and essential for the survival, nurturing, and flourishing of humanity. Calvin is thus more optimistic than Luther about the growth, development, and improvement or progress of the human spirit under the sanctifying grace of God's commands. Biblical and Christian guidelines for sexual intimacy and human relationships are not burdens on freedom but God's means to empower meaningful and "good" sex, both morally and physically. Marriage, attraction and desire, the spiritual and marital equality of men and women, and the joys of marital friendship and companionship are the cornerstones of Calvin's sexual ethic (vol. 20, 406–8; vol. 21, 1248–57; Bouwsma, 136–37; Brundage, 552–60).

A third variety of Protestantism was developed by the Anabaptists and Mennonites in Holland, Switzerland, and central and eastern Europe during the sixteenth century, concurrent with Luther and Calvin. Menno Simons (1496–1561), Thomas Müntzer (1486/89–1525), Michael Sattler (1490–1527), and Huldrych Zwingli (1484–1531) are representatives of the "radical Reformation," best known for its theology of the imitation of Christ, pacifist witness, and rigorous separation from dominant society. Anabaptists and Mennonites embraced communal living, and discussions of marriage and sexuality are prominent in their writings. Celibacy was encouraged by the more austere and spiritualist wings of the movement. But monogamous, lifelong marriage was important for the most successful Mennonite communities in Europe and, later, in North America, not only for communal stability but also because it provided a model of God's covenant and Christ's mystical union with the church (Williams and Mergal, 19–38). Similar to later Calvinists, Mennonite communities emphasized the nurturing of enduring relationships with strong expressions of mutuality and love. A view of the Christian life as one into which a person grows, and the recognition that lust and concerns "of the body" can easily detract from one's spiritual pilgrimage and participation in the experience of communion with Christ, led to a restrained view of sexuality (Brundage, 556).

In spite of their willingness to break new ground both in the theology and morality of marriage and sex, the Protestant cultures of the sixteenth century did not change overnight, and rhetoric and theological reflection often outpaced practice. Restrictive biblical norms remained, their authority now heightened under Reformation theology, and a growing conservatism in the courts gave rise to more restrictive domestic laws and morality (Ozment, 158). Protestant views of sex have always been more conservative than most of the cultures in which the faith took root. Many Protestants asserted that even marital sexual intercourse, because it was accompanied by lust, was a sin—though forgivable, since it allowed other important goods to be realized (Cahill, *Sex*, 124). Even Luther and Calvin remained suspicious of sexual relationships and intimacy. In spite of the often egalitarian **language** of their theological treatises, a significant division of labor and inequality between men and women was maintained, viewed as a regrettable result of Adam and Eve's fall from grace.

Protestantism's most substantive break with the medieval sex ethic occurred in the early seventeenth century. Puritanism, a large and diverse Protestant movement growing out of Calvinist theology and social organization, took root in England and Scotland as a response to Anglican theology and the power of the centralized British monarchy. After 1620 it flourished in New England. John Milton (1608–1674) is perhaps the most well known proponent of a Puritan ethic of marriage and sexual intimacy, though other writers, including Richard Baxter (1615–1691), John Bunyan (1628–1688), and Daniel Defoe (1660–1731), gave significant attention to the theology of sex and marriage. Like Calvin, Puritans asserted the need for the biblical integrity, functionality, and regulation of relationships. A commitment to *moral constancy*—emotional steadiness and self-control as the means to attaining a chaste life in the pursuit of one's personal relationship with God—was Puritanism's defining characteristic (Johnson, 19–49; Leites, 22–33, 51–74). Marriage was affirmed as the fundamental relationship in which persons were destined to discover the true nature and character of a loving and nurturing God. God instituted marriage before the fall of Adam and Eve as humanity's normal and normative state. The Puritans rejected morally assessing sex in terms of its conformity with a natural law of procreation. Marriage's primary purpose was to counter human loneliness and isolation and was not, *pace* Paul and Luther, a "dyke against sin" that channeled and controlled lust. It was viewed as a spiritual rather than a sexual relationship (Clark and Richardson, 149–53; Johnson, 121–53; Milton). In this arrangement, husbands and wives held nearly (but not perfectly) equal status. Marriage is thus not primarily forensic but grounded in mutual assent, compatibility, love, affection, and pleasure (Leites, 76–77). Puritanism, along with Calvinism, largely shaped nineteenth-century and twentieth-century conservative Protestant and Evangelical perspectives on sex and marriage (see Grenz).

Still, given human sin and rebellion against God as well as the symbolic importance and stabilizing force that the marriage bed came to have in early modern society, sex outside marriage was considered profoundly disruptive. However, while divorce was presumptively discouraged, great latitude was given for divorces to which the parties mutually consented, and it could be a moral obligation when a couple felt unfulfilled or unsatisfied in their marriage or irreconcilable differences persisted (Johnson, 177). For Milton and the Puritans, the regulation of premarital and "deviant" sexual activity and the practical subordination of women were essential to guaranteeing purity of soul, good order, and the proper functioning of society (D'Emilio and Freedman, 15–52). The extremes of this conservatism, in the context of a concern with survival and order, surfaced in the exceptional activities surrounding witchcraft in New England beginning in the mid-seventeenth century (Ingebretsen, 23, 34). Later Puritan reflections on sexuality emphasized the language of purity, of separating oneself from the sins and evils of the world and (with regard to premarital sex) of "saving oneself for marriage."

The emerging Protestant denominations of the sixteenth and seventeenth centuries (Lutherans, Calvinist/Presbyterians, Congregationalists, Methodists, Baptists) codified views of sexuality that borrowed largely from earlier Protestant thinkers. Still, Protestantism has never been without its more radical, marginal, and splinter theological and social groups, which often gave rise to more provocative views of celibacy, sex, and marriage. Many such voices arose from the seventeenth to the nineteenth centuries in Europe and North America. Some Protestant groups appropriated more radical interpretations of Scripture, suggesting that the church was called to separate from and act as a witness to "the world" through alternative ethics and social practices. Others, exhibiting a "millennial impulse" and believing in the imminent end of history with the return of Christ (a "second coming"), sought to protect members from the ravages of a fallen world and prepare the faithful community for its final union with the divine. In both cases guidance for a life of purity and dedication to God in a time of trauma, anxiety, and social dislocation was often taken from biblical texts (particularly the Old Testament) and the experiences of early Christian mystics, monastics, and spiritualists (Foster, *Religion and Sexuality*, 3–20; *Women, Family, and Utopia*, 3–13). Utopian thought and the development of utopian communities in America predated the Republic, though they flourished during the Victorian period (1837–1901). When the radical individuality and antiestablishment rhetoric of early Protestantism was coupled with an emphasis on specific, narrow, and literalist readings of Scripture, a range of divergent social arrangements and sexual practices surfaced.

Originating in England in the first part of the eighteenth century, communities of the United Society of Believers in Christ's Second Coming, who came to be known as the Shakers, reached their peak membership in the decades before the Civil War (1861–1865). Under their founder Ann Lee (1736–1784), Shaker theology stressed the task of establishing a community that would usher in the millennial rule of God on earth, a world in which no human authority would be recognized or needed. Their view of God's dual (male/female) nature and the desire to promote deep spirituality resulted in a radical vision of sexual equality (see Whitson). The Shakers introduced total celibacy into their community and thus grew only through conversion and adoption. Radical egalitarianism of male celibates and female virgins was seen as consistent with the spirit of the New Testament Church. They adopted many of the characteristics of monasticism in the religious and ordinary life of their community. Sexual renunciation allowed them to expunge from human activity and God's created order the carnality that brought about the Fall (Lauer and Lauer, 112). As a result, women were freed from the burdens of childbearing, thus reinforcing a commitment to the equality of the sexes (see Humez). But the community seems to have retained hierarchy in many areas, including decision making, work assignments, and appointed community roles (Foster, *Religion*, 21–71; *Women*, 17–71).

Originating in Vermont and New York in the middle of the nineteenth century, John Humphrey Noyes's (1811–1886) Oneida community was a utopian arrangement in which group marriage and free pairings of couples broke decisively with conventional views of sex and marriage. Noyes believed that the required task of his church was to establish Christ's kingdom on earth, to bring earthly existence into conformity with the heavenly kingdom. This required a restructuring of social, economic, marital, and sexual relationships that would overcome the corrosiveness of contemporary society (Foster, *Women*, 81). In the Oneida community, vigorous sexual expression and pleasure were seen as an important part of human life and pleasing to God. Their suspicion of traditional Christian theology, conventional economics, the division of labor in families, Christian institutions of celibacy, and exclusive, monogamous marriage led them to espouse "complex marriage," similar to polygamy and polyandry, though with various regulatory restraints. Sexual relations were theoretically permitted between any man and woman (as young as ten years) in the community, though elders controlled sexual access and discouraged preferential pairing and exclusive relationships (Foster, *Religion*, 72–102). Belief in the imminent end of history and the establishment of the Kingdom of God meant that the community frowned on procreation. (Later, however, regulated births were permitted in the community.) Through the spiritual and physical training of men to avoid ejaculation, sexual intercourse could be enjoyed by community members without incurring the costs, and the "problem" of sex could be largely eliminated (Clark and Richardson, 193–205 [Noyes, *Bible Communism* (1853)]; McClymond, 218–33; Noyes, *Male Continence*). The community, with communal property, flourished for many years, though the corrosive effects of preferential relationships and the demand that all members subsume their personal interests to the good of the community eventually led to its demise.

The Church of Jesus Christ of Latter-day Saints (the Mormon Church) traces its origins to the 1820s and a religious vision experienced by its founder, Joseph Smith (1805–1844). In the 1830s and 1840s the church organized converts into a religious community constructed around Old Testament priestly and prophetic principles. They took on the task of establishing the true Kingdom of God on earth as a means of overcoming the limitations and corruptions of the "old order" that had been taught and practiced by the Christian church and as protection against the rampant social decomposition and erroneous notions of romantic love that were hallmarks of various social and political movements of the time (Foster, *Religion*, 129).

Though Smith died by murder as a result of his promulgating a doctrine of polygamous marriage, his legacy lived on through a remnant of believers who fled Illinois and settled in Utah under the direction of Brigham Young (1801–1877), constructing their New Jerusalem in Salt Lake City. By the early 1850s the church had established itself in its new home. The community adopted models of social and religious organization based on the early Israelite covenant with God, highlighting such biblically informed practices as the priesthood, ritual cleansing and worship, patriarchal division of labor between men and women, missionary work aimed at conversion, and a strict and conservative social ethic with marriage and obedience to the priesthood at its center. The blessings of marriage, and the acceptability, as with the biblical patriarchs, of many wives, and the gifts of progeny, land, and old age were all understood as reflections of righteousness.

Latter-day Saints' doctrines upheld strict gender distinctions and responsibilities in the plan of salvation, asserting that men and women have different roles in a divinely decreed family organization: Women create bodies for spirits and then nurture them, while men, through the priesthood, link mortal existence and the future life (Wallace, 119). Biblical literalism, scriptural images of righteousness, and the priesthood/motherhood division of labor make comprehensible the community's early acceptance of polygamy (Ehat and Cook, 375–77). Though only condoned for sixty years (officially abandoned by the church in 1890), polygamy was seen as a means of overcoming the sexual disorganization and family and social disorientation pervasive during the first half of the nineteenth century. However, ensuing conflicts created by "plural wives," Smith's and Young's establishment of hierarchies among wives, the appointing of "proxy husbands" when a husband might be absent from his wives for months or years, and federal and local pressures against polygamy led to its demise (see Ehat and Cook, 146, 269; Foster, *Religion*, 151–63; Van Wagoner). What survived the official rejection of polygamy in the twentieth century (though polygamy is still faithfully and informally practiced by some Mormons) was the theological vision of a community set apart, a strong commitment to evangelism and conversion, a conventional view of the connection between sexuality and procreation, the maintenance of family life, and a desire to nurture the eternal and celestial bond between a husband and wife (Church Educational System; Foster, *Religion*, 216–20; Wallace, 118–20). Latter-day Saints' attitudes about marital fidelity, gendered role-assignments, child rearing, and **sexual perversion** are widely shared with many other conservative Protestants in the United States (see Olson).

Mainstream Protestant views of sex, at least through the nineteenth century and well into the early twentieth century, can be described as affirming the earlier Christian stance on the legitimacy of sex only in marriage and with a strong predisposition, though not a requirement, toward marriage as the normative state for human beings. Early Protestants sought to nurture marital relationships that permitted personal fulfillment, met the natural sexual needs of married couples, and promoted procreation. Nonmarital sexuality of nearly every stripe was soundly rejected. Various schismatic Protestant sects explored alternative social arrangements and sexual practices, but unless they were able to adapt to the pressures of human needs and adopt practical arrangements that would enhance the integrity of the community, they expired or were abandoned. Many beliefs and practices discussed above remain central to contemporary Protestant thought as we move farther into the twenty-first century, although some Protestant thinking on these matters is more liberal, diverse, and inclusive than the historical record might suggest.

See also African Philosophy; Bible, Sex and the; Catholicism, History of; Marriage; Protestantism, Twentieth- and Twenty-First-Century; Rimmer, Robert; Utopianism

REFERENCES

Augustine. (418?–421) *On Marriage and Concupiscence*. Trans. Peter Holmes and Robert Ernest Wallace. In Philip Schaff, ed., *A Select Library of The Nicene and Post-Nicene Fathers of the Christian Church*. First Series, vol. 5. Reprint of 1887 edition. Grand Rapids, Mich.: Eerdmans, 1971, 258–308; Augustine. (401–402) *On the Good of Marriage*. Trans. C. L. Cornish. In Philip Schaff, ed., *A Select Library of The Nicene and Post-Nicene Fathers of the Christian Church*. First Series, vol 3. Reprint of 1887 ed. Grand Rapids, Mich.: Eerdmans, 1956, 395–413; Bouwsma, William J. *John Calvin: A Sixteenth-Century Portrait*. New York: Oxford University Press, 1988; Brooke, Christopher. *The Medieval Idea of Marriage*. Oxford, U.K.: Oxford University Press, 1989; Brundage, James A. *Law, Sex, and Christian Society in Medieval Europe*. Chicago, Ill.: University of Chicago Press, 1987; Cahill, Lisa Sowle. *Between the Sexes: Foundations for a Christian Ethics of Sexuality*. Philadelphia, Pa.: Fortress Press, 1985; Cahill, Lisa Sowle. *Sex, Gender, and Christian Ethics*. Cambridge: Cambridge University Press, 1996; Calvin, John. (1536–1559) *Institutes of the Christian Religion*. Ed. John T. McNeill. Trans. Ford Lewis Battles. In John Baille, John T. McNeill, and Henry P. Van Dusen, eds., *The Library of Christian Classics*, vols. 20–21. Philadelphia, Pa.: Westminster, 1960; Church Educational System. *Eternal Marriage Student Manual*. Salt Lake City, Utah: Church of Jesus Christ of Latter-Day Saints, 2001; Clark, Elizabeth, and Herbert Richardson, eds. *Women and Religion: A Feminist Sourcebook of Christian Thought*. New York: Harper and Row, 1977; D'Emilio, John, and Estelle B. Freedman. *Intimate Matters: A History of Sexuality in America*. New York: Harper and Row, 1988; Ehat, Andrew F., and Lyndon W. Cook, eds. *The Words of Joseph Smith*. In Ellis T. Rasmussen, dir., *Religious Studies Monograph Series*, vol. 6. Provo, Utah: Religious Studies Center, Brigham Young University, 1980; Foster, Lawrence. *Religion and Sexuality: The Shakers, the Mormons, and the Oneida Community*. New York: Oxford University Press, 1981. Reprinted, Urbana: University of Illinois Press, 1984; Foster, Lawrence. *Women, Family, and Utopia: Communal Experiments of the Shakers, the Oneida Community, and the Mormons*. Syracuse, N.Y.: Syracuse University Press, 1991; Grenz, Stanley. *Sexual Ethics: An Evangelical Perspective*. Louisville, Ky.: Westminster John Knox Press, 1990; Humez, Jean M., ed. *Mother's First-Born Daughters: Early Shaker Writings on Women and Religion*. Bloomington: Indiana University Press, 1993; Ingebretsen, Ed. "Wigglesworth, Mather, Starr: Witch-Hunts and General Wickedness in Public." In Tracy Fessenden, Nicholas F. Radel, and Magdalena J. Zaborowska, eds., *The Puritan Origins of American Sex*. New York: Routledge, 2001, 21–54; Johnson, James Turner. *A Society Ordained by God. English Puritan Marriage Doctrine in the First Half of the Seventeenth Century*. Nashville, Tenn.: Abingdon, 1970; Lauer, Robert K., and Jeanette C. Lauer. *The Spirit and the Flesh: Sex in Utopian Communities*. Metuchen, N.J.: Scarecrow Press, 1983; Leites, Edmund. *The Puritan Conscience and Modern Sexuality*. New Haven, Conn.: Yale University Press, 1986; Luther, Martin. *Martin Luther's Basic Theological Writings*. Trans. Jaroslav Pelikan, Helmut T. Lehman, and others. Ed. Timothy F. Lull. Minneapolis, Minn.: Fortress Press, 1989; McClymond, Michael J. "John Humphrey Noyes, the Oneida Community, and Male Continence." In Colleen McDannell, ed., *Religions of the United States in Practice*, vol. 1. Princeton, N.J.: Princeton University Press, 2001, 218–33; Milton, John. (1643) *The Doctrine and Discipline of Divorce, Restored to the Good of Both Sexes*. In Frank Allen Patterson, gen. ed., *The Works of John Milton*, vol. 3, pt. 2. New York: Columbia University Press, 1931, 366–512; Noyes, John Humphrey. (1872) *Male Continence*. New York: AMS Press, 1976; Olson, Terrance D. "Sexuality." In Daniel H. Ludlow, ed., *Encyclopedia of Mormonism*, vol. 3. New York: Macmillan, 1992, 1306–8; Ozment, Stephen. *Protestants: The Birth of a Revolution*. New York: Doubleday, 1992; Thomas Aquinas. (1265–1273) *Summa theologica*, 2 vols. Trans. Fr. Laurence Sharpcote and Fathers of the English Dominican Province. Rev. Daniel J. Sullivan. In Robert Maynard Hutchins, ed., *Chief Great Books of the Western World*, vols. 19–20. Chicago, Ill.: Encyclopaedia Britannica, 1952; Van Wagoner, Richard S. *Mormon Polygamy: A History*, 2nd. ed. Salt Lake City, Utah: Signature Books, 1989; Wallace, Caroline. "The Priesthood and Motherhood in the Church of Jesus Christ of Latter-Day Saints." In Caroline Walter Bynum, Stevan Harrell, and Paula Richman, eds., *Gender and Religion: On the Complexity of Symbols*. Boston,

Mass.: Beacon Press, 1986, 117–40; Whitson, Robley Edward, ed. *The Shakers: Two Centuries of Spiritual Reflection*. Mahwah, N.J.: Paulist Press, 1984; Williams, George Hunston, and Angel M. Mergal, eds. *Spiritual and Anabaptist Writers*. Philadelphia, Pa.: Westminster, 1957.

Joel Zimbelman

ADDITIONAL READING

Brown, Peter. *The Body and Society: Men, Women, and Sexual Renunciation in Early Christianity*. New York: Columbia University Press, 1988; Bullough, Vern L. "Christianity and Sexuality." In Ronald M. Green, ed., *Religion and Sexual Health: Ethical, Theological, and Clinical Perspectives*. Boston, Mass.: Kluwer, 1992, 3–16; Childress, James F., and John Macquarrie, eds. *The Westminster Dictionary of Christian Ethics*. Philadelphia, Pa.: Westminster, 1986; Corcoran, Brent. *Multiply and Replenish: Mormon Essays on Sex and Family*. Salt Lake City, Utah: Signature Books, 1994; Crompton, Louis. "Calvinism and Repression" and "Puritanism and the Restoration." In *Homosexuality and Civilization*. Cambridge, Mass.: Harvard University Press, 2003, 324–28, 391–97; De Rougemont, Denis. (1939) *Love in the Western World*. Trans. Montgomery Belgion. Rev. ed. New York: Pantheon, 1956; Doriani, Daniel. "The Puritans, Sex, and Pleasure." In Elizabeth Stuart and Adrian Thatcher, eds., *Christian Perspectives on Sexuality and Gender*. Grand Rapids, Mich.: Eerdmans, 1996, 33–51; Duby, Georges. *Medieval Marriage: Two Models from Twelfth-Century France*. Trans. Elborg Forester. Baltimore, Md.: Johns Hopkins University Press, 1978; Edwards, Robert R., and Stephen Spector, eds. *The Olde Daunce: Love, Friendship, Sex, and Marriage in the Medieval World*. Albany: State University of New York Press, 1991; Ellison, Marvin M. "Homosexuality and Protestantism." In Arlene Swidler, ed., *Homosexuality and World Religions*. Valley Forge, Pa.: Trinity Press, 1993, 149–79; Ellison, Marvin M. "A Protestant Christian Perspective." In John C. Raines and Daniel C. Maguire, eds., *What Men Owe to Women: Men's Voices from World Religions*. Albany: State University of New York Press, 2001, 41–67; Fessenden, Tracy, Nicholas F. Radel, and Magdalena J. Zaborowska, eds. *The Puritan Origins of American Sex*. New York: Routledge, 2001; Fuchs, Eric. (1979) *Sexual Desire and Love: Origins and History of the Christian Ethic of Sexuality and Marriage*. Trans. Marsha Daigle. Cambridge, U.K.: James Clarke, 1983; Gies, Frances, and Joseph Gies. *Marriage and Family in the Middle Ages*. New York: Harper and Row, 1987; Gudorf, Christine. *Body, Sex, and Pleasure: Reconstructing Christian Sexual Ethics*. Cleveland, Ohio: Pilgrim Press, 1994; Karlsen, Carol F. *The Devil in the Shape of a Woman: Witchcraft in Colonial New England*. New York: Norton, 1987; Kern, Louis J. *An Ordered Love: Sex Roles and Sexuality in Victorian Utopias. The Shakers, the Mormons, and the Oneida Community*. Chapel Hill: University of North Carolina Press, 1981; Klaw, Spencer. *Without Sin: The Life and Death of the Oneida Community*. New York: Penguin, 1993; Kooper, Erik. "Loving the Unequal Equal: Medieval Theologians and Marital Affection." In Robert R. Edwards and Stephen Spector, eds., *The Olde Daunce: Love, Friendship, Sex, and Marriage in the Medieval World*. Albany: State University of New York Press, 1991, 44–56; Lindberg, Carter. *The European Reformations*. Cambridge, Mass.: Blackwell, 1996; Mace, David, and Vera Mace. *The Sacred Fire: Christian Marriage through the Ages*. Nashville, Tenn.: Abingdon Press, 1978; Mahoney, John. *The Making of Moral Theology: A Study of the Roman Catholic Tradition*. Oxford, U.K.: Clarendon Press, 1989; Morgan, Edmund S. *The Puritan Family*. Boston, Mass.: Public Library, 1944; Oberman, Heiko A. (1982) *Luther: Man between God and the Devil*. Trans. Eileen Walliser-Schwarzbart. New York: Doubleday/Image Books, 1992; Percy, William A. "Protestantism." In Wayne R. Dynes, ed., *The Encyclopedia of Homosexuality*, vol. 1. New York: Garland, 1990, 1058–69; Rogers, Eugene, ed. *Theology and Sexuality: Classic and Contemporary Readings*. Oxford, U.K.: Blackwell, 2002; Singer, Irving. "Luther versus Caritas." In *The Nature of Love*, vol. 1: *Plato to Luther*, 2nd ed. Chicago, Ill.: University of Chicago Press, 1984, 312–63; Witte, John, Jr. *From Sacrament to Contract: Marriage, Religion, and Law in the Western Tradition*. Louisville, Ky.: Westminster John Knox Press, 1997; Witte, John, Jr., and Robert M. Kingdon. *Sex, Marriage, and Family in John Calvin's Geneva*, 3 vols. Grand Rapids, Mich.: Eerdmans, 2004– .

PROTESTANTISM, TWENTIETH- AND TWENTY-FIRST-CENTURY.
Conflict about human sexuality within the Christian tradition is hardly new. Even so, Protestant Christians in the late twentieth and early twenty-first centuries have been noticeably embroiled in fierce controversies about sexuality, spirituality, and the moral life. Across the spectrum of Protestant denominations, both leaders and the general membership have engaged in contentious debate. They have risked denominational schism to promote or resist change on such issues as the ordination of women, adolescent **sex education**, clerical sexual misconduct, divorce, remarriage, **abortion**, **homosexuality**, and **same-sex marriage**.

Given this religious ferment, by the mid-1990s two Protestant theologians plausibly claimed that "the past twenty-five years [have been] without parallel in the long history of the church in terms of the amount of critical focus on sexuality issues" (Nelson and Longfellow, xvi). Among the evidence cited was the sheer number of books, articles, and denominational task force reports on religion and sexuality produced in recent years. Reaching a similar conclusion, an educator at the World Council of Churches put the matter theologically: "The fact that the churches are so exercised on the subject suggests that God is calling us to rethink it" (Smith, 167).

Identifying a singular Protestant voice or perspective on sexuality (or any other subject) is difficult, because of denominational diversity and because of the absence of a centralized teaching authority. Hence, speaking of Protestantisms instead of a unified Protestantism is more accurate. However, some commonalities exist across denominations. United Methodist theologian John Cobb points out that in a post-Freudian era "most Christians acknowledge that humans are sexual beings and that the desire for sexual contact with others is natural and inevitable" (94). At the same time, debate among Protestants continues over whether sexual expression should be limited to heterosexual (and procreative) **marriage** and how the church should respond to sexually active single persons, including gays, lesbians, and bisexuals, as well as transgender persons. Dealing with these questions has been complicated by the fact that the dominant Christian tradition has long reflected a fear of and negativity toward sexuality. This negativity has been reinforced over the centuries by two interlocking dualisms: body-spirit and male-female. The first elevates the superior spirit over the inferior body, which must be disciplined and kept under control. Gender dualism reflects a patriarchal hierarchy of value, status, and power in which good order requires male control of women's lives, bodies, and labor, including their procreative power (Harrison, 135–51; Nelson, *Embodiment*, 37–69).

Under the influence of these dualisms, Christianity, including its Protestant streams, has long given credence to the notion that sex is unclean and should be avoided or perhaps tolerated but restricted as a necessary evil. As historian and sexologist **Vern L. Bullough** has concluded, "[T]he Christian Church brought an overlay of sinfulness to almost every aspect of human sexuality. Masturbation, fornication outside marriage, homosexuality, transvestism, adultery, and in fact almost any aspect of sexual behavior was sinful and ultimately against church law." Even though church authorities may not have been particularly effective in curtailing this activity, Protestants and other Christians have helped "breed a deep feeling of guilt about sexual activity which remains one of the more troubling aspects of the Christian heritage. Though there were modifications of the basic teachings by various Protestant writers, and a general weakening of religious influence in the nineteenth and twentieth centuries, the guilt feelings remain" (15). In popular culture the very notion of morality is typically equated with sexual behavior, and sex is frequently associated with sin. For this reason, cultural anthropologist Gayle Rubin suggests that it is not surprising that in a culture so strongly influenced by Protestant Christian sensibilities sex is "presumed guilty until proven innocent," cast perennially as a "problem," treated with suspicion, and "burdened with an excess of significance" (278–79).

While Roman Catholicism has regarded virginity and celibacy as superior to the married life, Protestantism early on rejected the celibate life for its clergy and developed a more positive view of marriage as a companionate relationship. Not only was the celibacy/marriage dichotomy upended, but Protestant culture consistently encouraged marriage for all believers as a matter of Christian duty. Men and women alike have been pressured to assume their proper marital roles and obligations as husband/father and wife/mother, a pressure that some feminist theorists (e.g., Rich) have critiqued as "compulsory heterosexuality" and monogamy. It is also worth noting that the elevation of marriage occurred not because marriage was regarded as spiritually or morally preferable but because the Reformers were alert to the power of sinful lust and strongly doubted that a consistent lifestyle of **abstinence** was attainable. Within the Protestant tradition, sexuality continues to be viewed as a dangerous force requiring regulatory controls and ongoing supervision.

Early Protestant theologians regarded marriage as a hedge against immorality in keeping with **Saint Paul**'s (5–64?) admonitions (1 Cor. 7:2–5). Even among the married, sinful lust was viewed as a serious problem. At the same time, they insisted that marital sex was permissible because it served the good ends of procreation and companionship. Moreover, although husband and wife were spiritually equal, the conventional assumption has been that the husband should be in charge of the family (Jordan, 107–30). Accordingly, Martin Luther (1483–1546) and other Protestant Reformers failed to critique, much less transform, the sex-negative and patriarchal biases of the Christian tradition. "All *should* marry," the Reformers argued, "because God's intention from the beginning had been to unite men and women in marital union and bid them to procreate. Almost all *must* marry because the lustful urges that had arisen from the Fall could be contained without sin only in marriage" (Ruether, 74). Thus, the only sex the Protestant tradition has officially sanctioned has been marital sex under male direction; even then, human sexuality is understood as necessarily marred by human sinfulness. Only more recently have Protestants questioned this marriage paradigm and sought to develop a more comprehensive, sex-positive, women-friendly ethic of sexuality. However, even during the modern period, Protestants have, by and large, promulgated not so much a *sexual* ethic but a more limited and often highly restrictive *marriage* ethic. The Protestant focus has been on control of the body, on containing passion and strong feeling, and on the rightness of men's power and authority in exercising "headship" over women in family and society. (See the Blankenhorn et al. volume.)

From the 1960s, efforts to reevaluate the meaning and place of sexuality in family and public life have intensified within liberal Protestantism in a context of accelerated economic and cultural change, social crisis, and heightened conflict. Historians trace significant shifts in the United States from an early republican and family-centered procreative sexual morality to a nineteenth-century Victorian morality that emphasized emotional intimacy between marriage partners, then to a twentieth-century "public sexuality" sparked by both the idealization of sexuality as central to human fulfillment and the commercialization of sexuality (see D'Emilio and Freedman). Further, population migration from rural to urban centers, the widening split between workplace and home, the rising affluence of the middle class, increased health and longevity, and the disruptions caused by major wars together created the conditions that enabled increasing numbers of people to shape independent lives outside the confines of the biological family—including single women, divorced women, gay men, and lesbian women (D'Emilio, 187–200). Medical developments (for example, effective, inexpensive **contraception**; safe, legalized abortion; assisted **reproductive technology**) have also greatly affected sexual practices. So, too, concerns about the incidence of **sexually transmitted diseases**, about the rise in nonmarital births among Euro-American and other women, and about pervasive patterns of domestic and child sexual abuse have affected sexual practices. Moreover, by the mid-1960s, the family model of two adults with dependent children, the post–World War II cultural icon, was no longer the statistical norm. While the loss of familial hegemony distressed many, the U.S. situation only replicates a pattern common to other advanced industrialized nations.

At its best the Protestant tradition has encouraged openness to new empirical knowledge and nondefensive engagement with changing cultural patterns. The adaptability of this religious tradition to new conditions has been its major strength, along with its emphasis on human freedom, creativity, and responsibility for promoting personal and communal well-being. One set of challenges has come from revisionist understandings of the human person and, in particular, fresh insights about psychosexual development from the social and natural sciences. Another set of challenges has come from the encounter of Protestants with the feminist and gay liberation movements. The social and moral struggle to reorder power relations between men and women has precipitated a reexamination of social and family roles, a critique of patriarchal religious teachings about sexuality, gender, family, and community, and heightened awareness of the deficits of gendered religious **language** and symbol systems (see Harrison; Kimmel). As a 1991 Presbyterian study acknowledges, "The crisis of sexuality we are experiencing is . . . a massive cultural earthquake, a loosening of the hold of an unjust, patriarchal structure built on dehumanizing assumptions, roles, and relationships." In responding to this crisis, Protestant Christians face a decisive choice: People of faith "can retreat into silence or, worse yet, participate in a reactionary effort to buttress traditional patterns of oppression and sexual exclusion," or "the church can work diligently to dismantle this dehumanizing edifice" and "extend to people struggling with questions of sexuality the church's longstanding commitment to human liberation and justice" (*Presbyterians and Human Sexuality*, 3–4).

In responding to cultural change and the crisis in sexuality and family, Protestants have had to decide whether to join the forces of change or of resistance. Sexually conservative evangelicals and fundamentalists interpret the crisis of sexuality as a decline in fidelity to traditional values and as a lack of respect for and adherence to established authority. In their view sexual decency requires confining **sexual activity** exclusively to heterosexual marriage. Politically active proponents of traditional values, committed to restoring sexuality to a reproductive marital context, expend considerable energy and financial resources to oppose abortion, the widespread availability of contraception, sex education in public schools, no-fault divorce, and the extension of civil rights to sexual minorities (see Grenz; Pharr). It can be argued that in appealing to absolute biblical norms, traditionalists fail to see how they endorse historically relative, class-bound, sex-bound, and race-bound norms as divinely sanctioned.

In reaction to the most vocal, politically active traditionalists, sexual libertarians have argued for unrestricted sexual freedom and the loosening of sex from institutional regulation (see Warner). Although liberal Protestants share libertarian discontent with conventional Christian approaches, agreeing that fear, guilt, and shame should be removed from sex, they seek to affirm the goodness of a healthy eroticism without questioning either normative heterosexuality or the framework of long-term, heterosexual, monogamous relationships (see Fletcher). Good sex remains heterosexual and marital even as some latitude is given to sexually active, unmarried heterosexual couples—if they do not publicly reject the institution of marriage or deviate far from conventional gender roles.

In contrast, liberation theologians and progressive Christians push liberal Protestants toward a more radical rethinking of sexuality. Feminist theologian Beverly Harrison notes, "Traditional Christianity has . . . confused sexual mores with genuine morals, assuming that earlier patterns of practice continue to have value for their own sake, quite apart from our need as rational beings . . . to justify past norms and practices in light of new conditions" (146). These new conditions include a world in which women no longer accept inferiority, in which overpopulation threatens, and in which there is growing insistence that human sexual intimacy avoid exploitation and communicate respect. Thus, an overhaul of Christian teaching is called for, precisely because the Protestant tradition has constructed its theological and ethical framework on the basis of devaluing the body, women, and nonheterosexual persons. A progressive church report states the case:

> A gap now exists between official church teaching and the sexual practices of most people, including many church members. This gap is occurring, not because people are suddenly less moral or conscientious in their ethical deliberations, but because the conventional moral code is inadequate for large numbers of people today—young and old, male and female, gay and straight, married and unmarried. . . . No ethic can be adequate if it is constructed upon—or continued to perpetuate—sexual injustice and the oppression of women and gay and lesbian persons. (*Presbyterians*, 5)

Throughout the twentieth century, whenever Protestants have departed from the inherited Christian tradition, they have justified their efforts to reframe sexuality, marriage, and family by arguing that a dynamic, evolving tradition calls each generation to discern anew how best to embody the values and commitments of Christian faithfulness. At the close of the nineteenth century and into the first decades of the twentieth, Protestant leaders opposed family planning, in keeping with their vision of a Protestant America and concerns not to be outnumbered by Catholic immigrants. However, in response to a reproductive freedom movement associated with Margaret Sanger (1879–1966) and because of the Protestant Christian emphasis on faithful love rather than procreation as the primary purpose of marriage, by the 1930s mainstream Protestants, led by the Episcopalians at their 1930 Lambeth Conference, accepted contraceptive practices that they had come to recognize as strengthening rather than endangering marriage bonds. Such developments had echoes in Roman Catholicism, as well, even as Pope Pius XI's (1876–1958) encyclical *Casti connubii* (1930) permitted use of the "rhythm method" as a natural means of pregnancy regulation, while it also reaffirmed official teaching against "unnatural" contraceptive practices.

In light of long-standing Christian sex-negativity, contemporary Protestants have had to struggle with the place of desire and eroticism in intimate relationships. Anders Nygren's (1890–1978) *Agape and Eros* influenced a generation of preachers and scholars by characterizing Christian love as disinterested and selfless, something much different from a "carnal love" that seeks self-interested gratification at the expense of others. Christian love, said this theologian, has nothing to do with passion, desire, or sexual fulfillment. In contrast, Paul Tillich (1886–1965) spoke appreciatively of *eros* as the moving power of life, as that which drives everything now separated toward unity (see Tillich; Irwin). More recently, a United Methodist theologian has observed, "Most Christians today, thanks to the sexual revolution, have rediscovered the biblical affirmation of sexuality in general, and of the physical pleasure of sexual intercourse in particular, as gifts of God" (Cobb, 95).

If Protestants early on celebrated, as the ideal model, the lifelong, heterosexual union of two adults who refrain from sexual activity outside marriage, at least mainstream Protestants were realistic enough to accept divorce and remarriage. The Protestant emphasis on the unitive rather than the procreative purpose of marriage made possible giving considerable weight to the personal and sexual fulfillment of both parties. Divorce has come to be regarded as the unfortunate but necessary cessation of a loveless or even destructive union. Consistently with the importance of the quality of personal intimacy, by the middle of the twentieth century Protestant theologians were promoting a shift from a rule-based, act-focused legalism toward more flexible decision making that gave greater attention to relationships, motivations, and specific contexts (Nelson, *Embodiment*, 104–29). This shift also instigated a rethinking of premarital sexual relations, for many young heterosexual adults were reaching physical and sexual maturity long before achieving economic independence and were postponing marriage to complete their education and establish themselves in the workforce. Some contemporary theologians argue that the church should offer rituals of commitment for young adults who are sexually active, not ready to marry, and yet seek their religious community's support for and encouragement of their committed, though not (yet) permanent relationships (Spong, 177–87; Thatcher, 103–31).

In the late 1980s a leading American religious journal, *The Christian Century*, published a series of essays, "After the Revolution," on rethinking Christian **sexual ethics** (that is, after the sexual revolution). James B. Nelson, speaking in favor of a "continuing revolution," challenged Protestant churches to "deal more forthrightly and creatively" with sexuality and spirituality, in large part because "organized religion has been, and in some ways still is, the major institution of ideological legitimation for sexual oppression in Western culture" (Nelson, *Body Theology*, 16). What Nelson took as bad news he offset with positive news: "There are more voices speaking and sometimes heard," he noted, and "more indications of movement on sexual issues, than we might have imagined not many years ago" (18). In particular, the feminist and gay liberation movements have had favorable impact on both church and society, even though "the surface of sexual oppression is just being scratched" (16). Progressive Protestants share a characteristic commitment to a comprehensive justice vision, including sexual justice: honoring the goodness of sexuality as the capacity for intimate communication; promoting sexual diversity (**sexual orientation** and family patterns) as an enrichment of community life; advocating for the sexually abused, exploited, and oppressed; and demonstrating accountability both for personal behavior and for the well-being of the community (Ellison, *Erotic Justice*, 24–29).

Among contemporary Protestants, a theological and ideological split is widening between conservative and fundamentalist groups, on one side, and progressive groups, on the other. These internal divisions are reflected in their disparate responses to nonheterosexuality, ranging from rejection and exclusion of gay persons from the church to full and unqualified acceptance of gay, lesbian, bisexual, and transgender (GLBT) persons as members and leaders. Conservative evangelicals and biblical fundamentalists find no reason to debate the morality of homosexuality, much less to reconsider church teaching. In their view, biblical sources condemning homosexual practices are unambiguous and provide definitive guidance. Homosexuality is properly handled by prohibition. Southern Baptists, at their 1976 convention, passed a resolution affirming their "commitment to the biblical truth regarding the practice of homosexuality as sin" and urged churches "not to afford the practice of homosexuality any degree of approval" (Percy, 1062). In 1988 the Southern Baptist

Convention passed, after ten minutes of debate, a similar resolution condemning "homosexuality as an abomination in the eyes of God, a perversion of divine standards and a violation of nature" (Nugent and Gramick, 25).

Protestants more moderate than Southern Baptists may also view homosexuality with suspicion and disapproval but tend to call for greater tolerance and forbearance. Evangelical Protestant theologian Stanley Grenz encourages churches to adopt a stance of "welcoming but not affirming" gay persons. All persons, regardless of sexual orientation, should be invited into the life of the church, but at the same time everyone should be held to the standard that only sexual activity within heterosexual marriage is permissible. If the church is to be the church, it must not condone immorality, including sexual immorality. For Grenz, joining the discipleship community must be done "on God's terms, not [our] own," and this entails "being willing to leave behind old sinful practices—including unchaste sexual behaviors—so that together we might become a holy people" (157). From this perspective, a holy people should welcome gay people but not affirm gay sex or gay unions.

Even progressive Protestants have engaged in considerable debate about the inclusion of GLBT persons in the church. In most denominations there are gay-affirming caucuses, such as Integrity (Episcopal), Lutherans Concerned, More Light Presbyterians, Affirmation (United Methodist), Brethren/Mennonite Council on Gay Concerns, and the Seventh Day Adventist Kinship. These groups provide support for gay church members and their families and friends, as well as resources for education and advocacy. Some congregations challenge exclusionary denominational policies by declaring themselves "More Light" congregations, "Open and Affirming" congregations, or "Welcoming" and "Reconciling" congregations, thereby signaling their commitment to the full participation of GLBT persons in the life and ministry of the church. In 1988 the United Church of Canada, following the lead of the United Church of Christ, the Unitarian Universalist Association, and the Universal Fellowship of Metropolitan Community Churches, approved the ordination of qualified homosexuals as clergy. The decision generated much controversy, and there were threats of congregational secession across the denomination.

Despite these developments, most analysts of the Protestant debates conclude that "the tensions in the churches between homosexuality and traditional Christian beliefs and values will not . . . be resolved quickly or effortlessly" (Nugent and Gramick, 43). One factor is the cultural, institutionalized stigmatizing of homosexuality. Other factors include a "middle-class therapeutic mentality ill at ease with moral argument"; a fear of conflict and divisiveness, especially disruption that might be costly in terms of church membership or financial contributions; a tendency to be reactive rather than proactive regarding sexual issues; and finally, "the very complexity of sexuality itself" (Nelson, "Needed," 65). For these reasons, many denominations have followed the lead of the United Church of Christ in its 1977 *Human Sexuality: A Preliminary Study*; it incorporated gay and lesbian issues within a comprehensive framework dealing with a broad range of sexuality issues. As a 1992 United Methodist report acknowledges, "Homosexuality is best considered in the context of a more general Christian understanding of human sexuality" (Yamasaki, 5).

Same-sex relations clearly deviate from the patriarchal cultural pattern of male-dominant and female-subordinate sexual and social relations. Beverly Harrison notes that homoeroticism "represents a break with the strongest and most familiar control on sexuality—compulsory heterosexuality" and the ideology of male control of women (146–47). In Western culture, gay men in particular have been stereotyped as highly sexualized. As a result, they are envied but also despised as "carriers" of repressed sexuality and as visible nonconformists to male-dominant heterosexual marriage.

For Protestants, four factors have precipitated a reexamination of homosexuality. First, homosexuality, according to reputable medical judgment, has been recognized as non-pathological, a benign variation among human sexualities. This judgment is in keeping with the 1973 decision by the Board of Trustees of the American Psychiatric Association to eliminate homosexuality *per se* from its list of mental disorders (Conrad and Schneider, 207–8). Second, fear of same-sex eroticism and hostility toward gay men and lesbians are commonplace in Western societies. Third, Christianity, including Protestantism, has played its own large role in the oppression of sexual minorities. Fourth, and most important, gay people have insisted on being subjects of their own lives, including their religious lives, and not mere objects for the scrutiny and judgment of others (Gomes, 144–72).

Progressive Protestants argue that the "homosexuality problem" is more accurately a problem of sexual oppression, namely, the intertwined dynamics of homophobia and **heterosexism**. Protestant Christianity is now being challenged to break with its legacy of sexual exclusivism, which limits acceptable sexual expression to heterosexual marriage. On this score, GLBT people, the consummate outsiders, are the ones (along with their allies) who are calling the church to repentance and moral transformation, this time to dismantle sexually oppressive norms and practices within religious traditions (and elsewhere). Even progressive Protestants resist this call for renewal. In 1983, the liberal National Council of Churches of Christ voted "not to vote," thereby refusing to accept into membership the Universal Fellowship of Metropolitan Community Churches (UFMCC), even though this small, young denomination, founded in 1968, met all the formal requirements for membership in the ecumenical organization. At issue was UFMCC's predominantly gay membership and its policy as a church not to discriminate on the basis of sexual orientation. Admitting the UFMCC to the Council would have contributed to Christian unity by healing the brokenness of the faith community brought about by the majority's sexual exclusionism. Further, because "a principle of exclusion necessarily suggests what is most important theologically, ethically, and politically," rejecting the UFMCC acutely demonstrated how "sexuality remains Christianity's 'dirty little secret,' for those who occupy the liberal middle ground no less than for those on the reactionary right" (Ellison, "NCC on the Hook," 982; see Gorsline).

Among the most pressing tasks for Protestants is developing a "new ecumenism" that would align progressive wings of various denominations and allow them to pursue egalitarian policies within and beyond their own specific traditions (Ruether, 223–24). Progressive Roman Catholics, Jews, and Protestants often discover that they have more in common theologically, ethically, and politically about such contested matters as sexuality than they do with more conservative colleagues in their own traditions. While Southern Baptists have, by and large, condemned homosexuality as incompatible with a Christian lifestyle, not all Southern Baptists toe the line. In 1992 the Southern Baptist Convention ousted two "renegade" congregations from membership on the grounds that one had ordained a gay man and the other had solemnized a same-sex union (Siler). Progressive Southern Baptists have more affinity with progressive Presbyterians, Episcopalians, and Lutherans than they do with most of their Baptist kin.

If the past is a reliable indicator, Protestants will likely continue to endure significant conflict over sexuality. The challenge for progressive religionists will be to insist on placing sexuality within a comprehensive social justice framework (Ellison and Thorson-Smith) while exploring the particularities, as well as the intersections, of sexuality and racism (Douglas), sexuality and economic justice (Hobgood), sexuality and violence (Fortune), and sexuality and ecology (Spencer).

See also Abstinence; Bible, Sex and the; Catholicism, History of; Catholicism, Twentieth- and Twenty-First-Century; Heterosexism; Homosexuality, Ethics of; Judaism, History of; Judaism, Twentieth- and Twenty-First-Century; Paul (Saint); Protestantism, History of; Violence, Sexual

REFERENCES

Blankenhorn, David, Don Browning, and Mary Stewart Van Leeuwen, eds. *Does Christianity Teach Male Headship? The Equal-Regard Marriage and Its Critics.* Grand Rapids, Mich.: Eerdmans, 2004; Bullough, Vern L. "Christianity and Sexuality." In Ronald M. Green, ed., *Religion and Sexual Health: Ethical, Theological, and Clinical Perspectives.* Boston, Mass.: Kluwer, 1992, 3–16; Cobb, John B., Jr. *Matters of Life and Death.* Louisville, Ky.: Westminster John Knox, 1991; Conrad, Peter, and Joseph W. Schneider. "Homosexuality: From Sin to Sickness to Life-Style." In *Deviance and Medicalization: From Badness to Sickness.* St. Louis, Mo.: 1980, 172–214; D'Emilio, John. "Capitalism and Gay Identity." In Karen Lebacqz and David Sinacore-Guinn, eds., *Sexuality: A Reader.* Cleveland, Ohio: Pilgrim Press, 1999, 187–200; D'Emilio, John, and Estelle B. Freedman. *Intimate Matters: A History of Sexuality in America.* New York: Harper and Row, 1988; Douglas, Kelly Brown. *Sexuality and the Black Church: A Womanist Perspective.* Maryknoll, N.Y.: Orbis Books, 1999; Ellison, Marvin M. *Erotic Justice: A Liberating Ethic of Sexuality.* Louisville, Ky.: Westminster John Knox, 1996; Ellison, Marvin M. "The NCC on the Hook." *The Christian Century* 100 (2 November 1983), 981–82; Ellison, Marvin M., and Sylvia Thorson-Smith, eds. *Body and Soul: Rethinking Sexuality as Justice-Love.* Cleveland, Ohio: Pilgrim Press, 2003; Fletcher, Joseph F. *Situation Ethics: The New Morality.* Philadelphia, Pa.: Westminster, 1966; Fortune, Marie M. *Sexual Violence: The Unmentionable Sin.* New York: Pilgrim, 1983; Gomes, Peter J. *The Good Book: Reading the Bible with Mind and Heart.* New York: Morrow, 1996; Gorsline, Robin Hawley. "A Queer Church, Open to All." *Union Seminary Quarterly Review* 57:1–2 (2003), 46–66; Grenz, Stanley J. *Welcoming But Not Affirming: An Evangelical Response to Homosexuality.* Louisville, Ky.: Westminster John Knox, 1998; Harrison, Beverly Wildung. *Making the Connections: Essays in Feminist Social Ethics.* Ed. Carol S. Robb. Boston, Mass.: Beacon Press, 1985; Hobgood, Mary E. *Dismantling Privilege: An Ethic of Accountability.* Cleveland, Ohio: Pilgrim, 2000; Irwin, Alexander C. *Eros toward the World: Paul Tillich and the Theology of the Erotic.* Minneapolis, Minn.: Fortress, 1991; Jordan, Mark D. *The Ethics of Sex.* Malden, Mass.: Blackwell, 2002; Kimmel, Michael S. *The Gendered Society.* New York: Oxford University Press, 2000; Nelson, James B. *Body Theology.* Louisville, Ky.: Westminster John Knox, 1992; Nelson, James B. *Embodiment: An Approach to Sexuality and Christian Theology.* Minneapolis, Minn.: Augsburg, 1978; Nelson, James B. "Needed: A Continuing Sexual Revolution." In *Sexual Ethics and the Church: After the Revolution; A Christian Century Symposium.* Chicago, Ill.: The Christian Century, 1989, 63–70; Nelson, James B., and Sandra P. Longfellow. "Introduction." In James B. Nelson and Sandra P. Longfellow, eds., *Sexuality and the Sacred: Sources for Theological Reflection.* Louisville, Ky.: Westminster John Knox, 1994, xiii–xviii; Nugent, Robert, and Jeannine Gramick. "Homosexuality: Protestant, Catholic, and Jewish Issues: A Fishbone Tale." In Richard Hasbany, ed., *Homosexuality and Religion.* New York: Harrington Park Press, 1989, 4–76; Nygren, Anders. (1930, 1936) *Agape and Eros.* Trans. Philip S. Watson. Chicago, Ill.: University of Chicago Press, 1982; Percy, William A. "Protestantism." In Wayne R. Dynes, ed., *The Encyclopedia of Homosexuality*, vol. 1. New York: Garland, 1990, 1058–69; Pharr, Suzanne. *In the Time of the Right: Reflections on Liberation.* Berkeley, Calif.: Chardon Press, 1996; Pius XI (Pope). "On Christian Marriage." [*Casti connubii*] *Catholic Mind* 29:2 (1931), 21–64; *Presbyterians and Human Sexuality 1991.* Louisville, Ky.: Office of the General Assembly Presbyterian Church (U.S.A.), 1991; Rich, Adrienne. "Compulsory Heterosexuality and Lesbian Existence." *Signs* 5:4 (1980), 631–60; Rubin, Gayle S. "Thinking Sex: Notes for a Radical Theory of the Politics of Sexuality." In Carole S. Vance, ed., *Pleasure and Danger: Exploring Female Sexuality.* Boston, Mass.: Routledge and Kegan Paul, 1984, 267–319; Ruether, Rosemary Radford. *Christianity and the Making of the Modern Family.* Boston, Mass.: Beacon Press, 2000; Siler, Mahan. "The Blessing of a Gay Union: Reflections of a Pastoral Journey." *Baptists Today* (19 March 1992), 11; Smith, Robin. *Living in Covenant with God and One Another.* Geneva, Switz.: World Council of Churches Family

Education Office, 1990; Spencer, Daniel T. *Gay and Gaia: Ethics, Ecology, and the Erotic*. Cleveland, Ohio: Pilgrim Press, 1996; Spong, John Shelby. *Living in Sin? A Bishop Rethinks Human Sexuality*. San Francisco, Calif.: Harper and Row, 1988; Thatcher, Adrian. *Marriage after Modernity: Christian Marriage in Postmodern Times*. Sheffield, U.K.: Sheffield Academic Press, 1999; Tillich, Paul. *Love, Power, and Justice: Ontological Analyses and Ethical Applications*. New York: Oxford University Press, 1954; United Church of Christ. *Human Sexuality: A Preliminary Study*. New York: United Church Press, 1977; Warner, Michael. *The Trouble with Normal: Sex, Politics, and the Ethics of Queer Life*. New York: Free Press, 1999; Yamasaki, Nancy C. "The Committee to Study Homosexuality Offer the Church . . . Its Report, Its Conclusions, Its Recommendations!" *Circuit Rider* 15:10 (1992), 4–7.

Marvin M. Ellison

ADDITIONAL READING

Abelove, Henry, Michèle Aina Barale, and David M. Halperin, eds. *The Lesbian and Gay Studies Reader*. New York: Routledge, 1993; Cahill, Lisa Sowle. *Between the Sexes: Foundations for a Christian Ethics of Sexuality*. Philadelphia, Pa.: Fortress Press, 1985; Cahill, Lisa Sowle. *Sex, Gender, and Christian Ethics*. Cambridge: Cambridge University Press, 1996; Douglas, Kelly Brown. "The Black Church and Homosexuality: The Black and White of It." *Union Seminary Quarterly Review* 57:1–2 (2003), 32–45; Ellison, Marvin M. "Homosexuality and Protestantism." In Arlene Swidler, ed., *Homosexuality and World Religions*. Valley Forge, Pa.: Trinity Press, 1993, 149–79; Ellison, Marvin M. "A Protestant Christian Perspective." In John C. Raines and Daniel C. Maguire, eds., *What Men Owe to Women: Men's Voices from World Religions*. Albany: State University of New York Press, 2001, 41–67; Ellison, Marvin M. *Same-Sex Marriage? A Christian Ethical Analysis*. Cleveland, Ohio: Pilgrim Press, 2004; Gudorf, Christine E. *Body, Sex and Pleasure: Reconstructing Christian Sexual Ethics*. Cleveland, Ohio: Pilgrim Press, 1994; Haffner, Debra W. *A Time to Speak: Faith Communities and Sexuality Education*. New York: Sexuality Information and Education Council of the United States (SIECUS), 1998; Harrison, Beverly Wildung. *Our Right to Choose: Toward a New Ethic of Abortion*. Boston, Mass.: Beacon Press, 1983; Johansson, Warren. "Judeo-Christian Tradition." In Wayne R. Dynes, ed., *The Encyclopedia of Homosexuality*, vol. 1. New York: Garland, 1990, 648–49; Lebacqz, Karen, and David Sinacore-Guinn, eds. *Sexuality: A Reader*. Cleveland, Ohio: Pilgrim Press, 1999; Nelson, James B. "Sources for Body Theology: Homosexuality as a Test Case." In Patricia Beattie Jung and Shannon Jung, eds., *Moral Issues and Christian Responses*, 7th ed. Belmont, Calif.: Wadsworth, 2003, 276–84; Nelson, James B., and Sandra P. Longfellow, eds. *Sexuality and the Sacred: Sources for Theological Reflection*. Louisville, Ky.: Westminster John Knox, 1994; Nygren, Anders. *Den kristna kärlekstanken genom tiderna* (Part I, 1930; Part II, 1936). *Agape and Eros*. London: S.P.C.K. House, 1932, 1938. Philadelphia, Pa.: Westminster Press, 1953. Trans. Philip S. Watson. Chicago, Ill.: University of Chicago Press, 1982; Rauch, Jonathan. *Gay Marriage: Why It Is Good for Gays, Good for Straights, and Good for America*. New York: Times Books, 2004; Rich, Adrienne. "Compulsory Heterosexuality and Lesbian Existence." *Signs* 5:4 (1980), 631–60. Reprinted in *Blood, Bread, and Poetry: Selected Prose 1979–1985*. New York: Norton, 1986, 23–75; and Henry Abelove, Michèle Aina Barale, and David M. Halperin, eds., *The Lesbian and Gay Studies Reader*. New York: Routledge, 1993, 227–54; Rogers, Eugene, ed. *Theology and Sexuality: Classic and Contemporary Readings*. Oxford, U.K.: Blackwell, 2002; Rubin, Gayle S. "Thinking Sex: Notes for a Radical Theory of the Politics of Sexuality." In Carole S. Vance, ed., *Pleasure and Danger: Exploring Female Sexuality*. Boston, Mass.: Routledge and Kegan Paul, 1984, 267–319. Reprinted in Henry Abelove, Michèle Aina Barale, and David M. Halperin, eds., *The Lesbian and Gay Studies Reader*. New York: Routledge, 1993, 3–44; Rudy, Kathy. *Sex and the Church: Gender, Homosexuality, and the Transformation of Christian Ethics*. Boston, Mass.: Beacon Press, 1997; Sands, Kathleen M., ed. *God Forbid: Religion and Sex in American Public Life*. New York: Oxford University Press, 2000; Seidman, Steven. *Beyond the Closet: The Transformation of Gay and Lesbian Life*. New York: Routledge, 2002; Siker, Jeffrey S., ed. *Homosexuality in the Church: Both Sides of the Debate*. Louisville, Ky.: Westminster John Knox, 1994; Soble, Alan. Review of

Christian Perspectives on Sexuality and Gender, ed. Adrian Thatcher and Elizabeth Stuart. *Ethics* 108:3 (1998), 654; Stuart, Elizabeth. *Religion Is a Queer Thing: A Guide to the Christian Faith for Lesbian, Gay, Bisexual, and Transgendered Persons*. Cleveland, Ohio: Pilgrim Press, 1997; Thatcher, Adrian, and Elizabeth Stuart, eds. *Christian Perspectives on Sexuality and Gender*. Grand Rapids, Mich.: Eerdmans, 1996; Tillich, Paul. *Love, Power, and Justice: Ontological Analyses and Ethical Applications*. New York: Oxford University Press, 1954; Williams, Rowan D. "The Body's Grace." In Eugene F. Rogers, Jr., ed., *Theology and Sexuality: Classic and Contemporary Readings*. Oxford, U.K.: Blackwell, 2002, 309–21.

PSYCHOLOGY, EVOLUTIONARY. Simone de Beauvoir (1908–1986) captures the complexity of romantic **love** when she writes that its "supreme goal" is "identification with the loved one. . . . [I]t is not enough to serve him. The woman in love tries to see with his eyes; she reads the books he reads, prefers the pictures and the music he prefers; she is interested only in . . . ideas that come from him" (*The Second Sex*, 613–14). There seems little possibility of science's explaining such a baffling emotion. Yet from other philosophical perspectives, the attempt to ground a comprehensive understanding of human sexuality in evolutionary biology would be cheered. Consider Donald Symons's aspirations:

> If selection has always been potent at the level of the individual, individuals must have "innate" mechanisms, probably best conceived as emotional/motivational mechanisms, to recognize and look after their own reproductive "interests." . . . [T]he complexity of sexual opportunity and constraint in natural human environments . . . made adaptive a human psyche uniquely informed by sexuality. That individual reproductive "interests" must in some degree conflict with one another may account for the intensity of human sexual emotions, the pervasive interest in other people's sex lives, the frequency with which sex is a subject of gossip, the universal seeking of privacy for sexual intercourse, [and] the secrecy and deception that surround sexual activities. (308)

If so, Beauvoir's woman who sees everything through her beloved's eyes is ultimately, although not proximately, simply managing her reproductive interests.

This is why the evolutionary project is often accused of reducing the psychological complexities of love to a mating ritual of sexually charged agents. It is also accused of genetic determinism, of neglecting developmental and environmental influences on a trait's expression in favor of its genotypic basis (see Rose). But despite the fact that its initial rejection by the social sciences arguably endures, E. O. Wilson's sociobiology has been the source of many vibrant research studies. And though evolutionary accounts of human behavior and cultural phenomena are controversial, the development of the application of **evolution** to human behavior has become a growth industry, attracting the attention of scholars in many fields. Whether the accusations of reductionism and determinism, which had been powerfully leveled by Philip Kitcher against "pop sociobiology," continue to be legitimate is unclear. Evolutionary theory is now interdisciplinary, drawing from, among other areas, cognitive psychology and ethology. From this convergence, approaches more subtle than Wilson's have emerged, producing surprising new findings about cognition and behavior. According to Kevin Laland and Gillian Brown, whose survey includes human behavioral ecology, memetics, and gene-culture evolution, evolutionary psychology has proven to be "enormously creative" (195).

Evolutionary psychology's guiding assumption is that many behaviors are adaptations to the ecological settings of an organism's lineage or exist in virtue of broader psychological mechanisms and anatomical features that are themselves adaptive. It attempts to *explain* the adaptive function of observed traits: **Jealousy** might be an adaptive solution to the problem of avoiding cuckoldry (Daly et al.). Or it attempts to *predict* psychological traits from known evolutionary forces: Humans today possess information-processing algorithms for recognizing degrees of kinship or detecting "cheaters" in swapping benefits for payments (Cosmides and Tooby, "Cognitive Adaptations"). The explanatory project generally gets a more favorable assessment (Davies; Grantham and Nichols). Evolutionary psychology's findings range over many areas. For example, logical reasoning improves dramatically when problems are stated in terms of social norms rather than in terms of truth or falsity. Evolutionary psychology explains this by positing a preference, an adaptation in our cognitive architecture, that emerged in response to repeated pressure to reason about social dominance hierarchies (Cosmides and Tooby, "Cognitive Adaptations") and to "check . . . up on our neighbors" (Morton, 104). Politically sensitive claims often raise eyebrows: that **rape** is an adaptation to sexual exclusion (Thornhill and Palmer; Thornhill and Thornhill; see Smuts); that **sexual harassment** and the phenomenon of "trophy wives" (Kenrick et al.; Studd) have an evolutionary basis; that the universality of Cinderella stories involving an evil stepparent results from the decreased rewards felt, and hence decreased investment made, by substitute parents in caring for the young (Daly and Wilson, 83 ff.).

There are weak and strong versions of evolutionary psychology's guiding assumption. In the weak version, human behavioral traits are rooted in general cognitive mechanisms and learning rules that are adaptations explainable in evolutionary terms. The strong version claims that the specific forms our behaviors take are explainable by natural selection. The weak thesis, in postulating general cognitive mechanisms, extrapolates from the existence of one such mechanism, the culturally complex skill of **language** (Plotkin, chap. 4). Each human is genotypically programmed with a universal grammar, which manifests itself phenotypically in the ability to speak a language. The mind comprises other general mechanisms designed to solve problems that arose in our evolutionary past.

The strong version of evolutionary psychology involves the application of sociobiology to psychology. The idea is that humans are "inclusive fitness maximizers" in the sense that "the major goals toward which humans direct action" are resolutions of "problems that historically had to be solved to enable reproductive success" (Buss, "Evolutionary Personality," 484). The weak version, by contrast, limits itself to providing evolutionary explanations of cognitive mechanisms, learning rules, or so-called Darwinian algorithms, as opposed to explaining specific behaviors (like rape). Leda Cosmides and John Tooby have sociobiology in mind when they write, "In the rush to apply evolutionary insights to a science of human behavior, many researchers have made a conceptual 'wrong turn.' . . . This wrong turn [is] . . . attempting to apply evolutionary theory directly to . . . manifest behavior, rather than using it as a heuristic guide for the discovery of innate psychological mechanisms" ("From Evolution," 278 ff.). Observed behaviors are better understood as enhancing fitness, not necessarily maximizing it (as sociobiology has it), and perhaps only in the particular settings within which human brains evolved. For weak evolutionary psychology (I omit "weak" henceforth, considering the strong version equivalent to sociobiology), **homosexuality**, homicide, and **violence** might enhance fitness in less direct ways than permitted by Wilsonian sociobiology. Nonetheless, evolutionary psychology and sociobiology share commitments to five principles: (1) the ancient provenance of current traits, (2) some degree of adaptationism (natural selection is the only important factor in a trait's evolution), (3) a close fit between an organism's design and the environmental problems pressuring that design, (4) the plausibility of speculations about the Pleistocene environment, and (5) the existence of universals across diverse contemporary cultural settings. The best illustration of a universal cognitive capacity is language. Theorists such as Steven Pinker (*Language*) point to Noam Chomsky's *Language and Mind* and its universal grammar as a paradigmatic finding of evolutionary psychology. There are, of course, sexual examples. David Schmitt employed evolutionary psychology, in particular parental investment theory, to predict that he would find universal sexual differences: Human males desire partner variety more than females, and males are less discriminating in sexual partner selection. He found this to be true in "52 Nations, 6 Continents, and 13 Islands" (85).

If there is, as David Buss ("Mate Preference") claims, an innate device, "a mate preference mechanism," that governs human sexual strategy, it developed over long periods of history. Since the approximately 500 generations that have lived since the end of the Paleolithic age (and the agricultural revolution) represent less than half of 1 percent of all generations of *Homo sapiens*, principle (1) says that we are essentially now what we were long ago. (Rose and Rose dispute this [2].) Principle (2) claims that Buss's sexual selection mechanism is, like other complex psychological traits, the result of an inherited modification of our ancestral gene pool, is therefore built by genes, and is not an accident of random evolutionary forces such as genetic drift. Adaptationism is a much debated view (see Ferguson's typology), and to avoid "Panglossian" extremism (i.e., every trait is perfectly suited to its environment), evolutionary psychology must supply criteria for a property to be considered an actual trait. It argues, for example, that the mechanisms involved in mate selection are adaptive traits because strong selection pressures operate on choice, and choosing a mate is psychologically complex. Principle (3) claims that we are able to individuate adaptations and traits because there is a close fit between design problems (e.g., to have humans "hook up" for a reasonably long portion of their mature lives) and the observed design solutions (in this case, romantic love). The existence of dating rituals and other strategies males and females adopt (coyness, chastity) illustrate this principle.

It is perhaps the Pleistocenic cast of these psychological speculations (see principle [4]) that draws most of the informed criticism of evolutionary psychology. Its *modus operandi* is a sort of bootstrapping operation, in which anthropological theorizing about human origins helps identify problems humans faced *then*, and psychological studies done *now* are meant to show the ways humans have solved them. This procedure is fraught with difficulty. The very idea of an "environment of evolutionary adaptedness" has changed from a historical time and place (the Pleistocene's African savannah) to a "statistical composite" of ancient niches faced (and of course partly constructed!) by our ancestors (see Laland and Brown, 179). Of course, the mere existence of culture and industrial civilization presents obstacles to drawing analogies between ancient and contemporary behaviors. For instance, Randy Thornhill and Craig Palmer's ascription of a reproductive function to rape involves not only massive speculations about the psychology of Pleistocene man but also problematic "zoomorphic" comparisons of animal and human sexual acts (Tobach and Reed, 112; see also Sanday).

These similarities between evolutionary psychology and sociobiology led Kim Sterelny and Paul Griffiths to call evolutionary psychology the "second-wave sociobiology of the 1990s" (14). The charge of reductionism attendant with this association does not, however, obviously stick to evolutionary psychology. Its unique problems and advantages are best seen regarding culturally complex and psychologically anomalous phenomena. Consider how Pinker, following Robert Frank, explains the behavior of "fools for love" (*How the Mind*, 417–19). He wants to explain "why . . . romantic love leave[s] us bewitched, bothered, and bewildered" (a version of Beauvoir's woman in love). He proceeds to "reverse engineer" this "mad love" by connecting it to the choice and promise to "spend your life and raise children with someone." Given that this promise is most credible when the "promiser" cannot back out, our brains have evolved an emotion that is involuntarily "triggered" not by you and your loved one's respective "mate-values" but by "a glance, a laugh, a manner that steals the heart." As far back as **Plato**'s (427–347 BCE) *Phaedrus*, the folk-psychological account of love's madness has turned on the strength of its appetitive desire; love's passion overcomes reason's restraint (245c). Pinker's account is consistent with this but goes farther. Evolutionary psychology trades in "ultimate explanations" and in turn explains the adaptive function of this cognitive-affective phenomenon. The emotions, being nonvoluntary, serve as subpersonal, noncognitive, motivational states, executing Darwinian algorithms within us unbeknownst to us. In addition, being so closely tied to physiology, emotions are harder to fake than the result of a hedonic or pragmatic calculation.

Evolutionary psychology's response, then, to the accusation of reductionism is that it is merely bridging the gap between emergent features of human cognition and their biological substrates. Evolutionary psychology recognizes, indeed emphasizes, the importance of individual development and historical contingencies in the behavioral expression of innate mechanisms. If evolutionary psychology reduces anything, it reduces a range of behavior to a (narrower) range of mental modules, thus leaving open their eventual reduction to biology. But evolutionary psychology does not necessarily diminish the cultural or historical vectors in language, love, and other psychological phenomena (see the rejection of the biology-is-destiny model by Cosmides and Tooby ["Cognitive Adaptations"]). A case can be made that **Sigmund Freud**'s (1856–1939) theory of the instincts (1933) is no more or less reductionistic than Pinker's theory of the language instinct. (See Glymour for parallels between Freud and cognitive psychology.)

In his "fools for love" example, Pinker can be seen as starting either with a behavioral observation—the apparent irrationality involved in choosing a mate on romantic grounds—or, alternatively, with a design problem of Mother Nature: How can humans be designed to mate for as long as it takes to raise a child? The first strategy is "reverse engineering," the second "adaptive thinking." Both make strong assumptions about the selective history and current function of the trait in question.

Evolutionary psychology must assume that the current utility of a trait in a modern setting is at least a useful guide to its selective history in a Pleistocene environment. But given the differences between these and modern environments and the fact that traits are a function of genetic expression within specific ecological and social settings, the assumption is dubious. Further, the interaction of genetic and environmental factors in a trait's expression and fitness might make it impossible to decide whether a particular behavior is an inherited adaptation or learned. The research programs of memetics (Aunger), human behavioral ecology (Hrdy), and developmental systems theory (Oyama et al.) are predicated in large part on this problem. Outside the biological sciences, in Marxist and feminist theory in particular, much is made of the influence of culture and the inextricable interaction of the social and the biological (see Lewontin et al.).

Pinker's account of romantic love also emphasizes one dimension of the phenomenon to the exclusion of others. Romantic love is more than falling head over heels over someone (e.g., crazily seeing everything through their eyes), even if this was its adaptive function. He recognizes that the irrationalities of romantic love have to be tempered by "the other component of courtship, smart shopping," and claims that "the contradiction of courtship—flaunt your desire while playing hard to get—comes from the two parts of romantic love:

setting a minimal standard for candidates in the mate market and capriciously committing body and soul to one of them" (419). This yields a situation full of tension. One Darwinian algorithm tells me I should not accept a partner who wants me for rational reasons, while another instructs me to employ those same rational reasons. Should I mate with someone who has nonvoluntarily fallen for me or with one who has calculated that I am the best thing going?

The problem is not that Pinker's account cannot make some sense of the stuff of soaps and sonnets. Rather, problems internal to evolutionary theory and cognitive psychology weaken the inference to the best explanation that his conclusions rest on. There is, first, the problem of identifying adaptive traits. Without cross-species comparisons—close relatives of *Homo sapiens* are extinct—evolutionary psychology might not be able to separate genuine adaptationist explanations from "just so stories" (Sterelny and Griffiths, 214). Theorists do have, however, other means to isolate adaptive problems and the complex mechanisms that are their solutions. For instance, Pinker establishes the "language module" in part through its capacity to be selectively damaged. That is, one can lose the ability to perform certain linguistic tasks without losing general cognitive function, and modularity is indicative of an adaptation (*Language Instinct*, 45–46). Yet as Stephen Jay Gould (1941–2002) emphasizes, natural selection is given too much explanatory work to do; it is best thought of as the first-among-equal forces at work in evolution. "Fundamentalists" such as Daniel Dennett distort the pluralist approach of most working biologists and of Charles Darwin (1809–1882) himself, by claiming exclusive explanatory efficacy for natural selection (see *Darwin's Dangerous Idea*, 229 ff.). As Gould reminds us, not every contingent property or cluster is an adaptation: "Reading and writing are now highly adaptive for humans, but the mental machinery for these . . . capacities must have originated as" *by-products*. They were "coopted later, for the brain reached its current size and conformation tens of thousands of years before any human invented reading or writing" (113–14).

Thus, that romantic love has the function for which Frank and Pinker claim it has been adapted is questionable; who may have sex with whom and who may have children is regulated by the social group to such a degree that romantic attachment might not be, and might never have been, linked that closely with **marriage** and sexuality and their resulting parentage. (See Geoffrey Gorer [1905–1985] on the rareness of romantic love.) Melvin Konner speculates that the function of romantic love may have been to get people out of arranged relationships (315–16), and others in the field (Buss, "Mate Preference," 261) put more emphasis on male competition for females, and hence on jealousy, in their understanding of the ties that bind. Similarly, consider speculation about the function of concealed ovulation in human females: It fosters cooperation among (male-led) groups by keeping their minds off the fertile females; it fosters a long-term parental pair bond by minimizing a female's attractiveness to other males based on her procreative power; it conceals paternity, which is adaptive among (primate) species that regularly kill the offspring of others; and because ovulation is concealed from the females themselves, it increases the likelihood of their engaging in the costly affair of motherhood. Still other functions have been proposed (Diamond, 79 ff.). Now, if it is hard to find expert consensus on this physiological trait ("there is an excess of speculation over fact"; Jones, 41), which is as closely linked to procreation as any, then why expect more than well-grounded hunches about the function of romantic love?

Further, there is the conundrum of individuating traits. Is romantic love one trait or many? If our descriptions are too coarse-grained, if love is taken to be whatever draws us toward an object, we will not be able to trace a selective history for what might be in fact multifaceted.

But if we analyze love too narrowly, as the emotion responsible for procreative mating-for-life, we will not see that it is part of a larger emotional/cognitive nexus, that pair bonds might have variable utility in different environments, or that nonprocreative (e.g., homosexual) relationships based on love are perhaps equally adaptive. (Michael Ruse has tried to explain homosexuality on the basis of inclusive fitness theory or kin selection: Benefits to extended kin can outweigh the individual's costs of not breeding ["Are There Gay Genes?"; *Homosexuality*, 203–35]. But see Rice and Barbone, who in part complain that Ruse homogenizes homosexuality.) Sterelny and Griffiths's criticism of Wilson's sociobiology has some purchase here: "Our behavior is produced by mental mechanisms that play a role in many different behaviors. Some of the mental mechanisms used in hunting are also used in storytelling. So speculations about the adaptive significance of rape, xenophobia, child abuse, or homosexuality seem to be at the wrong grain of analysis" (321). In part this is a problem of the constraints and constants we propose about early humans. Are we essentially social, bonding, even (which is rare) parenting mammals, or do these represent problems the solutions to which are still operative within our unconscious minds?

Mention of the unconscious raises another possible confusion, this one concerning levels of description. It is responsible for some of the confusion over reductionism in evolutionary psychology. For example, according to Terry Burnham and Jay Phelan,

> Men throughout the world show a preference for younger women and for traits associated with youth—full lips, big eyes, and radiant hair. There's nothing specifically desirable about youth per se: it's simply that fertility tends to decrease with age. (163)

That the sociological status, economic benefits, psychological appeal, and sensuous pleasures a young woman offers a man can be explained in terms of increased fertility strikes many as facile. Antireductionists argue that one-dimensionalizing motives by viewing humans as "fitness maximizers" is to commit the "socio-biological fallacy," in which "a theory of the origins of mechanisms (inclusive-fitness theory)" is conflated with "a theory of the nature of those mechanisms" (Buller, 106, citing Buss). The standard view is that evolutionary psychology avoids this by considering humans not as "fitness maximizers" but as "adaptation executers," so that while fertility does not "motivate" male preference in women, men have evolved in a manner that leads them to prefer features historically linked to fertility. The difference is subtle but important in distinguishing the reductionist aspects of sociobiology from evolutionary psychology's naturalistic agenda.

Motives are not functions. But the neurochemistry underlying our emotions and feelings does have a functional, adaptive history. Instead of fearing for the loss of the self at the hands of evolutionary psychology, we (properly forewarned) can look forward to a deeper understanding of the origins both of our personal goals and of the subpersonal, neurobiological nature of our motivational states.

See also Animal Sexuality; Beauty; Evolution; Homosexuality and Science; Jealousy; Love; Psychology, Twentieth- and Twenty-First-Century; Sexology; Spencer, Herbert; Westermarck, Edward

REFERENCES

Aunger, Robert, ed. *Darwinizing Culture: The Status of Memetics as a Science.* Oxford, U.K.: Oxford University Press, 2000; Beauvoir, Simone de. (1949) *The Second Sex.* Trans. Howard M. Parshley. New York: Bantam, 1961; Buller, David J. "DeFreuding Evolutionary Psychology." In V. Gray Hardcastle, ed., *Where Biology Meets Psychology: Philosophical Essays.* Cambridge, Mass.: MIT Press, 1999, 99–114; Burnham, Terry, and Jay Phelan. *Mean Genes: From Sex to Money to Food,*

Taming Our Primal Instincts. Cambridge, Mass.: Perseus, 2000; Buss, David M. "Evolutionary Personality Psychology." *Annual Review of Psychology* 42 (1991), 459–91; Buss, David M. "Mate Preference Mechanisms: Consequences for Partner Choice and Intrasexual Competition." In Jerome Barkow, Leda Cosmides, and John Tooby, eds., *The Adapted Mind: Evolutionary Psychology and the Generation of Culture*. New York: Oxford University Press, 1992, 250–66; Chomsky, Noam. *Language and Mind*. New York: Harcourt Brace Jovanovich, 1968; Cosmides, Leda, and John Tooby. "Cognitive Adaptations for Social Exchange." In Jerome Barkow, Leda Cosmides, and John Tooby, eds., *The Adapted Mind: Evolutionary Psychology and the Generation of Culture*. New York: Oxford University Press, 1992, 163–228; Cosmides, Leda, and John Tooby. "From Evolution to Behavior: Evolutionary Psychology as the Missing Link." In Jared Dupre, ed., *The Latest on the Best: Essays on Evolution and Optimality*. Cambridge, Mass.: MIT Press, 1987, 277–306; Daly, Martin, and Margo Wilson. *Homicide*. New York: Aldine, 1988; Daly, Martin, Margo Wilson, and Suzanne Weghorst. "Male Sexual Jealousy." *Ethology and Sociobiology* 3:1 (1982), 11–27; Davies, Paul. "The Conflict of Evolutionary Psychology." In V. Gray Hardcastle, ed., *Where Biology Meets Psychology: Philosophical Essays*. Cambridge, Mass.: MIT Press, 1999, 67–82; Dennett, Daniel. *Darwin's Dangerous Idea*. New York: Simon and Schuster, 1995; Diamond, Jared M. *The Third Chimpanzee: The Evolution and Future of the Human Animal*. New York: HarperCollins, 1992; Ferguson, Sally. "Methodology in Evolutionary Psychology." *Biology and Philosophy* 17:5 (2002), 635–50; Frank, Robert. *Passion within Reason: The Strategic Role of the Emotions*. New York: Norton, 1988; Freud, Sigmund. (1933) *New Introductory Lectures on Psycho-analysis*. In *The Standard Edition of the Complete Psychological Works of Sigmund Freud*, vol. 22. Trans. James Strachey. London: Hogarth Press, 1953–1974, 1–182; Glymour, Clark. "Freud's Androids." In Jerome Neu, ed., *The Cambridge Companion to Freud*. Cambridge: Cambridge University Press, 1991, 44–85; Gorer, Geoffrey. "On Falling in Love." In *The Danger of Equality*. New York: Weybright and Talley, 1966, 126–32; Gould, Stephen J. "More Things in Heaven and Earth." In Hillary Rose and Steven Rose, eds., *Alas Poor Darwin: Arguments against Evolutionary Psychology*. New York: Harmony Books, 2000, 101–25; Grantham, Tod, and Shaun Nichols. "Evolutionary Psychology: Ultimate Explanations and Panglossian Predictions." In V. Gray Hardcastle, ed., *Where Biology Meets Psychology: Philosophical Essays*. Cambridge, Mass.: MIT Press, 1999, 47–66; Hrdy, Sarah B. "The Past, Present, and Future of the Human Family." In Grethe Peterson, ed., *The Tanner Lectures on Human Values*, vol. 23. Salt Lake City: University of Utah Press, 2002, 57–110; Jones, Steve. "Go Milk a Fruit Bat!" [Review of *Why Is Sex Fun? The Evolution of Human Sexuality*, by Jared Diamond] *New York Review of Books* (17 July 1997), 39–41; Kenrick, Douglas T., Melanie R. Trost, and Virgil L. Sheets. "Power, Harassment, and Trophy Mates: The Feminist Advantages of an Evolutionary Perspective." In David M. Buss and Neil M. Malamuth, eds., *Sex, Power, Conflict: Evolutionary and Feminist Perspectives*. New York: Oxford University Press, 1996, 29–53; Kitcher, Philip. *Vaulting Ambition: Sociobiology and the Quest for Human Nature*. Cambridge, Mass.: MIT Press, 1985; Konner, Melvin. *The Tangled Wing: Biological Constraints on the Human Spirit*. New York: Harper and Row, 1983; Laland, Kevin N., and Gillian R. Brown. *Sense and Nonsense: Evolutionary Perspectives on Human Behavior*. Oxford, U.K.: Oxford University Press, 2002; Lewontin, Richard C., Steven Rose, and Leon J. Kamin. *Not in Our Genes: Biology, Ideology, and Human Nature*. New York: Pantheon, 1984; Morton, Oliver. "Doing What Comes Naturally." *The New Yorker* (3 November 1997), 102–7; Oyama, Susan, Paul E. Griffiths, and Russell D. Gray, eds. *Cycles of Contingency: Developmental Systems and Evolution*. Harvard, Mass.: MIT Press, 2001; Pinker, Steven. *How the Mind Works*. New York: Norton, 1997; Pinker, Steven. *The Language Instinct*. New York: Morrow, 1994; Plato. (ca. 365 BCE) *Phaedrus*. In Edith Hamilton and Huntington Cairns, eds., *The Collected Dialogues of Plato*. Trans. R. Hackforth. New York: Pantheon, 1961, 475–525; Plotkin, Henry. *Evolution in Mind: An Introduction to Evolutionary Psychology*. Cambridge, Mass.: Harvard University Press, 1998; Rice, Lee, and Steven Barbone. "Hatching Your Genes Before They're Counted." In Alan Soble, ed., *Sex, Love, and Friendship*. Amsterdam, Holland: Rodopi, 1997, 89–98; Rose, Hillary, and Steven Rose, eds. *Alas Poor Darwin: Arguments against Evolutionary Psychology*. New York: Harmony Books, 2000; Rose, Steven. "Escaping Evolutionary Psychology." In Hillary Rose and Steven Rose, eds., *Alas Poor*

Darwin: Arguments against Evolutionary Psychology. New York: Harmony Books, 2000, 299–320; Ruse, Michael. "Are There Gay Genes? Sociobiology Looks at Homosexuality." *Journal of Homosexuality* 4:1 (1981), 5–34; Ruse, Michael. *Homosexuality: A Philosophical Inquiry.* New York: Blackwell, 1988; Sanday, Peggy Reeves. "The Socio-Cultural Context of Rape: A Cross-Cultural Study." *Journal of Social Issues* 37:4 (1981), 5–27; Schmitt, David P., and 118 members of the International Sexuality Description Project. "Universal Sex Differences in the Desire for Sexual Variety: Tests from 52 Nations, 6 Continents, and 13 Islands." *Journal of Personality and Social Psychology* 85:1 (2003), 85–104; Smuts, Barbara. "Male Aggression against Women: An Evolutionary Perspective." In David M. Buss and Neil M. Malamuth, eds., *Sex, Power, Conflict: Evolutionary and Feminist Perspectives.* New York: Oxford University Press, 1996, 231–68; Sterelny, Kim, and Paul E. Griffiths. *Sex and Death: An Introduction to Philosophy of Biology.* Chicago, Ill.: University of Chicago Press, 1999; Studd, Michael V. "Sexual Harassment." In David M. Buss and Neil M. Malamuth, eds., *Sex, Power, Conflict: Evolutionary and Feminist Perspectives.* New York: Oxford University Press, 1996, 54–89; Symons, Donald. *The Evolution of Human Sexuality.* Oxford, U.K.: Oxford University Press, 1979; Thornhill, Randy, and Craig Palmer. *A Natural History of Rape: Biological Bases of Sexual Coercion.* Cambridge, Mass.: MIT Press, 2000; Thornhill, Randy, and Nancy Thornhill. "The Evolutionary Psychology of Men's Coercive Sexuality." *Brain and Behavioral Sciences* 15:3 (1992), 363–421; Tobach, Ethel, and Rachel Reed. "Understanding Rape." In Cheryl Travis, ed., *Evolution, Gender, and Rape.* Cambridge, Mass.: MIT Press, 2003, 105–38; Wilson, Edward O. *Sociobiology: The New Synthesis.* Cambridge, Mass.: Harvard University Press, 1975.

Nicholas P. Power

ADDITIONAL READING

Barkow, Jerome, Leda Cosmides, and John Tooby, eds. *The Adapted Mind: Evolutionary Psychology and the Generation of Culture.* New York: Oxford University Press, 1992; Barnett, Rosalind, and Caryl Rivers. "The Mating Game." In *Same Difference: How Gender Myths Are Hurting Our Relationships, Our Children, Our Jobs.* New York: Basic Books, 2004, 71–97; Birkhead, Tim. *Promiscuity: An Evolutionary History of Sperm Competition and Sexual Conflict.* London: Faber and Faber, 2000; Blackburn, Simon. "Evolution and Desire." In *Lust.* New York: New York Public Library/Oxford University Press, 2004, 111–25; Buss, David M. *The Evolution of Desire: Strategies of Human Mating.* New York: Basic Books, 1994; Buss, David M. "Evolutionary Psychology: A New Paradigm for Psychological Science." *Psychological Inquiry* 6:1 (1995), 1–30; Buss, David M. *Evolutionary Psychology: The New Science of the Mind.* Boston, Mass.: Allyn and Bacon, 1999; Buss, David M. "Sex Differences in Human Mate Preferences: Evolutionary Hypotheses Tested in Thirty-Seven Cultures." *Behavioral and Brain Sciences* 12:1 (1989), 1–49; Buss, David M., and Neil M. Malamuth, eds. *Sex, Power, Conflict: Evolutionary and Feminist Perspectives.* New York: Oxford University Press, 1996; Buss, David M., and David P. Schmitt. "Sexual Strategies Theory: An Evolutionary Perspective on Human Mating." *Psychological Review* 100:2 (1993), 204–32; Byrne, Robert. *The Thinking Ape.* Oxford, U.K.: Oxford University Press, 1995; Caulfield, Mina Davis. "Sexuality in Human Evolution: What Is 'Natural' in Sex?" *Feminist Studies* 11:2 (1985), 343–63; Cosmides, Leda, and John Tooby. *Evolutionary Psychology: A Primer.* <www.psych.ucsb.edu/research/cep/primer.html> [accessed 2 February 2005]; Daly, Martin, and Margo Wilson. *Sex, Evolution, and Behavior,* 2nd ed. Belmont, Calif.: Wadsworth, 1983; Diamond, Jared M. *Why Is Sex Fun? The Evolution of Human Sexuality.* New York: Basic Books, 1997; Geertz, Clifford. "Sociosexology." [Review of *The Evolution of Human Sexuality,* by Donald Symons] *New York Review of Books* (24 January 1980), 3–4; Gould, Stephen J. "Male Nipples and Clitoral Ripples." In *Bully for Brontosaurus: Reflections in Natural History.* New York: Norton, 1991, 124–38; Gould, Stephen J. *Ontogeny and Phylogeny.* Cambridge, Mass.: Harvard University Press, 1977; Griffiths, Paul. *What Emotions Really Are.* Chicago, Ill.: University of Chicago Press, 1997; Horgan, John. "Darwin on His Mind." *Lingua Franca* (November 1997), 40–48; Hrdy, Sarah Blaffer. "The Evolution of Human Sexuality: The Latest Word and the Last." *Quarterly Review of Biology* 54:3 (1979), 309–14; Hrdy, Sarah Blaffer. *The Language of Abu: Female and Male*

Reproductive Strategies. Cambridge, Mass.: Harvard University Press, 1977; Hrdy, Sarah Blaffer. *Mother Nature: Natural Selection and the Female of the Species.* London: Chatto and Windus, 1999; Hrdy, Sarah Blaffer. *The Woman That Never Evolved.* Cambridge, Mass.: Harvard University Press, 1981; Jones, Owen D. "Sex, Culture, and the Biology of Rape: Toward Explanation and Prevention." *California Law Review* 87:4 (1999), 827–941; Lehrman, Sally. "The Virtues of Promiscuity." *AlterNet* (22 July 2002). <www.alternet.org/story.html?StoryID=13648> [accessed 16 February 2005]; Lewontin, Richard C. *Biology as Ideology: The Doctrine of DNA.* New York: Harper, 1991; Lieberman, Debra, John Tooby, and Leda Cosmides. "Does Morality Have a Biological Basis? An Empirical Test of the Factors Governing Moral Sentiments Relating to Incest." *Proceedings of the Royal Society (Biological Sciences)* 270:1517 (2003), 819–26; Menand, Louis. "What Comes Naturally: Does Evolution Explain Who We Are?" *The New Yorker* (25 November 2002), 96–101; Murphy, Dominic. "Darwinian Models of Psychopathology." In Jennifer Radden, ed., *The Philosophy of Psychiatry: A Companion.* New York: Oxford University Press, 2004, 329–37; Pinker, Steven. "Boys Will Be Boys." *The New Yorker* (9 February 1998), 30–31; Posner, Richard A. "The Biology of Sex." In *Sex and Reason.* Cambridge, Mass.: Harvard University Press, 1992, 85–110; Radcliffe Richards, Janet. "The Evolutionary Psychology of Sex." In *Human Nature after Darwin: A Philosophical Introduction.* London: Routledge, 2000, 67–82; Regan, Pamela C. "Functional Features: An Evolutionary Perspective on Inappropriate Relationships." In Robin Goodwin and Duncan Cramer, eds., *Inappropriate Relationships: The Unconventional, the Disapproved, and the Forbidden.* Mahwah, N.J.: Lawrence Erlbaum, 2002, 25–42; Ridley, Matt. *The Red Queen: Sex and the Evolution of Human Nature.* New York: Macmillan, 1993; Ruse, Michael. "Are There Gay Genes? Sociobiology Looks at Homosexuality." *Journal of Homosexuality* 4:1 (1981), 5–34. Reprinted, "Are There Gay Genes? Sociobiology and Homosexuality," in SLF (61–86); Ruse, Michael. *Darwin and Design: Does Evolution Have a Purpose?* Cambridge, Mass.: Harvard University Press, 2003; Ruse, Michael. *Taking Darwin Seriously.* Oxford, U.K.: Blackwell, 1986; Small, Meredith. *What's Love Got to Do with It? The Evolution of Human Mating.* New York: Anchor, 1995; Symons, Donald. "Another Woman That Never Existed." *Quarterly Review of Biology* 57:3 (1982), 297–300; Symons, Donald. "Beauty Is in the Adaptations of the Beholder: The Evolutionary Psychology of Human Female Sexual Attractiveness." In Paul R. Abramson and Steven D. Pinkerton, eds., *Sexual Nature Sexual Culture.* Chicago, Ill.: University of Chicago Press, 1995, 80–118; Symons, Donald. "A Critique of Darwinian Anthropology." *Ethology and Sociobiology* 10:1–3 (1989), 427–44; Symons, Donald. "On the Use and Misuse of Darwinism in the Study of Human Behavior." In Jerome Barkow, Leda Cosmides, and John Tooby, eds., *The Adapted Mind: Evolutionary Psychology and the Generation of Culture.* New York: Oxford University Press, 1992, 137–59; Travis, Cheryl, ed. *Evolution, Gender, and Rape.* Cambridge, Mass.: MIT Press, 2003; Wertheimer, Alan. "The Psychology of Sex." In *Consent to Sexual Relations.* Cambridge: Cambridge University Press, 2003, 37–69; Wiederman, Michael W., and Elizabeth Rice Allgeier. "Mate Selection." In Vern L. Bullough and Bonnie Bullough, eds., *Human Sexuality: An Encyclopedia.* New York: Garland, 1994, 386–90; Wilson, Edward O. *On Human Nature.* Cambridge, Mass.: Harvard University Press, 1978; Wright, Robert. (1994) *The Moral Animal: Evolutionary Psychology and Everyday Life.* New York: Vintage, 1995.

PSYCHOLOGY, TWENTIETH- AND TWENTY-FIRST-CENTURY. The philosophy underlying psychological perspectives on human sexuality is largely unexplored. One primary source for social scientific approaches to sexuality, *Theories of Human Sexuality* (Geer and O'Donohue), is typical: Key frameworks for understanding sexuality are discussed (for example, evolutionary, developmental, learning, cognitive, scripting, psychoanalytic), but their philosophical bases are insufficiently identified, examined, or compared. Moreover, it often seems that the theories that dominate the psychology of sex have been developed outside psychology. The epistemological positivism that has been prevalent in contemporary psychology has, perhaps, relegated theory to a secondary role. Yet if the philosophy of the psychology of sex has often been ignored or is still rudimentary, divining the philosophical foundations of this psychology should be a simple yet creative task. In the most general sense, psychological investigations began the twentieth century with questions about sexual taxonomies, grounded in theories linking anatomical sex with psychological sexuality. Later, a positivistic, scientific approach became the primary focus. Near the end of the twentieth century, postmodernist trends radically contested much of the earlier groundwork, and this has led to an increase in philosophical debate.

Several features of the late 1800s set the stage for twentieth-century developments. Sexuality, in this late Victorian period, was widely viewed as an impulse requiring control and expressible only within intimate relationships (see Robinson). John D'Emilio and Estelle Freedman, for example, observe that it has been common to characterize Victorian sexuality as repressed and that this period was followed in the early twentieth century by a gradual increase in sexual freedom. This is certainly one possible story about Victorian and post-Victorian sexuality. Historians have noted, however, that sexual repression and control (as in the Victorian period) are often responses to an underlying reality of sexual freedom (see, for example, Gay). People during this period were talking about sex a great deal, indeed sex discourse exploded, with repression working as an "incitement to discourse" (see **Michel Foucault** [1926–1984]). Early sexual health practitioners were sought out by the state to intervene in the expanding sexual liberation, for sex, which had been primarily associated with reproduction and the family, was becoming increasingly connected, instead, with romantic **love**, happiness, and emotional or psychological intimacy.

One of the first significant efforts in psychological **sexology** was ontological: The earliest psychological studies on sexuality sought to determine the "kinds" of sexuality that exist. These late-nineteenth-century studies—by Karl Ulrichs (1825–1895), Richard von Krafft-Ebing (1840–1902), Magnus Hirschfeld (1868–1935), and **Havelock Ellis** (1859–1939)—were principally concerned with crafting sexual taxonomies based on sexual behaviors and desires. For instance, Ulrichs, in a series of pamphlets published in the 1860s and beyond, sought to identify people based on the "sex" of their minds and the "sex" of their bodies. His typology identified all the permutations; for example, most homosexuals had the brain of one sex and the body of another. Krafft-Ebing put a different spin on the search for sexual kinds, trying to classify the various kinds of perverts. He thought that **masturbation**, or giving in to sexual self-gratification more generally, would lead to a wide range of pathologies, which was an idea prevalent among physicians of the day. Magnus Hirschfeld was liberal (even, in a sense, anarchistic) in his nomenclature. He argued that sexual taxonomies were pointless: If one considers all the various indicators of sexuality (genetic, anatomical, psychological, and so forth), there were literally millions of kinds of sexual persons. Like Krafft-Ebing, Ellis also sought to chart diversity in **sexual desire** and behavior, but unlike Krafft-Ebing he believed most sexual expression was fundamentally natural and healthy.

Creating medical categories for sexual behaviors and desires had a profound effect. Jeffrey Weeks suggests that the mapping of sexual behavior onto distinct psychological entities worked to construct sexual identities. That is, these early taxonomic efforts transformed how people thought about others and themselves. Part of the sense of self, in particular sexual identity, was now something one *was* (e.g., a homosexual, a masturbator) instead of something one *did* (e.g., a person who engages in homosexual acts or who masturbates). This led, further, to the notion that sexual disorders are primarily disorders of identity, of personhood itself, an idea developed later in Freudian theory.

Sigmund Freud (1856–1939) extended the medical approach to sexuality. Beginning with his studies on hysteria carried out with Josef Breuer (1842–1925), he linked sexual functioning with mental health, proposing that disorders or distortions in psychosexual development produced broader psychopathology. By 1905, soon after the turn of the century, Freud was arguing that childhood sexual development laid the groundwork for adult psychosexual maturity (*Three Essays on the Theory of Sexuality*). In retrospect, Freud's "anatomy is destiny" thesis turns out to have been one of his most provocative and controversial claims. He argues that bodily sexual differences have psychological consequences. Having a penis leads to castration anxiety, contempt for womanly characteristics, and identification with the same-sex parent; having a clitoris/vagina leads to penis envy, feelings of inferiority, and a longing to forgo clitoral pleasure for the vaginal pleasure related to childbirth ("Some Psychical Consequences"). Disruptions in this process (say, if a female fails to abandon clitoral sexuality) causes immaturity and ultimately (in some cases) the same-sex desires of phallic women. The reduction of psychology to the biological in Freudian theory implies a connection between gender (masculinity, femininity) and sexuality, a notion pervasive in contemporary lay accounts of **sexual orientation**, such that femininely stereotyped males and masculinely stereotyped females are assumed *prima facie* to be homosexual. (For one place in Freud's writings in which the expression "anatomy is destiny" appears but does not imply psychological consequences of differing male and female sexual anatomy, see "On the Universal Tendency," 189.)

Freud's contemporaries responded with compelling philosophical challenges. For Karen Horney (1885–1952), Freud's error, in focusing on only one Gestalt, was getting everything backwards. It is not that women are inferior because they lack a phallus; rather, they are superior by virtue of their capacity for motherhood. Moreover, in Horney's gynocentric critique, women's actual sense of inferiority does not result from their missing a phallus but from the patriarchal nature of culture. Horney thus located the origin of psychological sex differences in society and not anatomy. Joan Rivière's (1883–1962) challenge to Freud was even more radical, asserting that women use their womanliness as a mask to hide their inherent masculinity. The masquerade of femininity allows them secretly to dominate men sexually. Horney rebuts Freud's notion of biology as destiny by arguing that culture has a role in shaping psychosexual development. Rivière, by contrast, is a kind of biological determinist.

Psychological approaches to sexuality underwent a transformation during the 1930s, near the beginning of the modern period. Psychologists who tired of Freudian speculation and clinical case studies shifted from issues of ontology to epistemology. "Physics envy," we might say, dominated psychological sex studies in the early modern period. Psychological positivism relegated theoretical issues to secondary importance in favor of (ideally) logically generated predictions (from hypotheses) that could be either confirmed or falsified by empirical observations. This sense of rationalism governed views about sexuality as well. Researchers assumed that sexuality, and human action in general, was a thoughtful and deliberate process. One early example of this was the work of Lewis Terman (1877–1956) and his colleagues, who surveyed Americans about their attitudes toward premarital sex and the prevalence of multiple orgasm.

Perhaps the best known psychologist in this early scientific tradition was Alfred Kinsey (1894–1956), who believed that the diversity of human sexual experience could be catalogued by using objectively scientific surveys. Kinsey's studies established the extreme breadth of human sexual experience, a fact that (in the late 1940s and early 1950s) was unsettling for those who preferred to think of human sexuality in narrower terms. Moreover, one of Kinsey's key conceptual contributions, which provided a contrast to earlier static ontological models, was the idea that sexual behavior fell on a continuum ranging from exclusive **homosexuality** to exclusive heterosexuality. The abundant number of people who were neither exclusively heterosexual nor homosexual, who fell somewhere between the two extremes, disrupted the notion of sexual identity. Hence sexual types, if there are any such things, are fluid and flexible. As a result, sexual identity was not explicitly part of Kinsey's model: There is no, say, homosexual person, but just people who engage with various frequencies in a wide variety of sexual acts. Kinsey's survey technique to investigate orgasmic experience (when it first occurred, how many times, under what conditions, etc.) only weakly elucidated the subjectivity of human sexual pleasure. The physician William Masters (1915–2001) and Virginia Johnson, also in the modern scientific tradition, literally mapped bodily responses to sexual arousal. Masters and Johnson's studies were remarkable for their efforts to document, with fastidious detail, the physiological processes that occurred during the experience of sexual pleasure. By connecting human subjects to recording devices, they were able to measure many physiological parameters during all phases of a person's sexual experience, whether alone during masturbation or with a partner.

If the modern period was a quest for the "truth" of sex, Masters and Johnson delineated it. Or had they? Some psychologists were opposed to this cold scientific exploration—the "wires and gauges" approach to sexuality—believing that sexuality was more than blood flow and muscle tension. Perhaps the strongest antithesis to these early modern explorations of sexuality during the first half of the twentieth century was the humanistic approach. Reacting to mechanistic medical models of sexuality, humanists sought to invigorate the study of sexuality with deeper meaning. The German sexologist Wilhelm Reich (1897–1957), for instance, proposed profound connections between the body, emotions, and sexuality, such that developing orgastic potency could lead to healing. Moreover, healing life energies, such as that released through **sexual activity**, were often blocked by repression. The focus here is quite different. At least for some psychologists, sexuality was more than biological processes and population variability. The pleasures of the body as connected with expressions of emotional intimacy were suggesting a more romantic view of sexuality.

Up to this point in twentieth-century psychology, explorations of sexuality were moderately unsophisticated, at least philosophically. Most historians agree, however, that by the 1960s there had been a dramatic shift in the approach to sexuality. In the period of late modernity or, as some call it, postmodernity, the sexual revolution and a widespread, incisive questioning of dominant ideologies and institutions in the Western world cleared the way for more complex conceptions of sexuality. However, in a typically postmodern turn, as much as things changed, they also stayed the same. For instance, while the active pursuit of sexual pleasure was deemed more acceptable, biologically reductionistic theories and physiological empiricism were still relied on to chart the border between normal and abnormal sexuality. Further, the sexually liberationist impulses of the 1960s were often met with attempts at control and containment. Critics of early modernism agree that we can use logic and observations to develop and test theories of sexuality, but in the postmodern view there is no one, universal, true reality. Truth, then, is highly dependent on perspective, on one's social, economic, ethnic, gender (and so forth) location. There is no "view from nowhere." And humans beings ultimately fail to be perfectly rational, often acting on impulse, passion, or vested interest. This late modern period offers interesting answers to questions asked by early moderns; it also prompts innovative concerns about the relations between gender, sexuality, power, love, and desire.

One of the most significant disruptions in modern thinking occurred when **John Money** severed the long-held association between biological sex and gendered behavior or psychology. Money had found, especially in his research with the ambiguously sexed, that "sex" referred (equivocally) to both biological maleness and femaleness and to psychological masculinity and femininity. In 1955, he borrowed "gender" from philology and linguistics to describe more accurately people with a psychological sense of masculinity or femininity incongruent with their biological sex. This distinction would have radical impact on future conceptualizations of crossdressing, transsexualism, and **intersexuality**. It also anticipated the later distinction feminists made between one's sex and gender, an important aspect of most Second Wave feminist thought. Money also represented a loosening of Freud's "anatomy is destiny" legacy, asserting that gender, not sex, shaped a person's "gendermaps" or "lovemaps," that is, patterns of sexual relations during critical periods of development.

The latter half of the twentieth century also witnesses widespread revisions of psychoanalysis. Many thinkers were involved in developing postmodern psychoanalysis, including Julia Kristeva, Hélène Cixous, Dorothy Dinnerstein, and Jane Flax. French psychoanalyst **Jacques Lacan** (1901–1981) importantly thought that Freud had been interpreted too literally and not symbolically: Penis envy is not literally a desire to possess an organ but a desire for the symbolic power of the phallus. Lacan also reinterprets female sexuality, in which he deconstructs Freud's characterization of women's sexuality as frigid and passive. Rather than seeing the vagina as passive (waiting for and receiving the active, penetrating penis), it can be construed as "castrating, devouring" (92). Lacan also argues that "feminine" lesbians are impossible (a contradiction) in Freudian thought, yet "nonphallic" love of this sort is abundant.

Like Freud, Lacan has had his feminist critics. Luce Irigaray finds Lacan masculine and patriarchal in presupposing that women are defined by what they lack (a phallus). Irigaray is most famous for her 1974 book *Speculum of the Other Woman*, in which she rewrites the relationship between mother and daughter in terms of female experience. Her work on female sexuality is remarkably unique. She reconceptualizes feminine sexuality without any reference to masculinity; and she constructs women's experience of sexuality as essentially different from men's, but plural in its essence due to the multiple sites of pleasure on a woman's body. Nancy Chodorow, another feminist critic of psychoanalysis, crafts a "post-Oedipal" model of sexuality, in which female-dominated parenting produces different emotional and sexual needs in men and women. Because girls establish a close bond with their mother, which is rarely severed, they develop a nurturing emotionality. Boys, however, have to detach themselves from their mother, so they come to deny and denigrate interpersonal connection and emotional closeness, defining themselves as "not woman." Adults then seek out sexual relationships that satisfy these early relational styles, a notion common in object relations and attachment theory.

Underlying these debates are deep concerns and wonderment about the nature of sexual desire. Historically, much psychological discourse on sexual desire has been unsatisfying; only recently have psychologists begun to reflect more acutely on this matter. One failure in modern approaches to desire was to focus on a specific desire, usually homosexuality, and then attempt to articulate the basic motivations of this desire. But this tactic seems fruitless, for each desire "type" would require a different conceptualization. Further, the search for a "grand theory" of sexual desire *tout court* has given way to looking for theories for specific desires in particular contexts. Reflecting on two decades of thought on sexual desire, Steven Levine, at the beginning of the twenty-first century, described elements common to most views about sexual desire. In Levine's analysis, desire (as in **Plato**'s [427–347 BCE] *Symposium*, 200a–e) reflects what we lack and need but more specifically is a manifestation of our private sense of our wants, relative to our social context. Desire is conceived as a broad motivator that varies in strength across needs, persons, and life circumstances (health and gender, for example).

We may know little about sexual desire, but there has a good deal of work on love. Robert Sternberg has developed perhaps the most comprehensive psychological theory. His "triangular theory of love" implies that love has three components: intimacy (feelings of closeness), passion (intense longing), and commitment. Intimacy usually builds up gradually during a relationship; passion might at the beginning be strong and later drop off; and commitment takes some time to develop. Passion, then, is the least stable and controllable dimension. Sternberg's model is the basis of a taxonomy of various kinds of love. For instance, if all three elements are balanced and high, this is what is called "consummate" love.

New questions about sexual desire and love challenged models of sexual orientation. Kinsey's continuum model of sexual orientation came under broad criticism in the latter half of the twentieth century. His model, for example, fails to consider that sexual feelings (desires and so forth) and sexual behavior may not always be concordant. Further, by presuming a continuum from pure heterosexuality to pure homosexuality, Kinsey made it difficult to appraise oneself (or others) as asexual, bisexual, polysexual, or at one time homosexual and at another time heterosexual. Newer models have done much to resolve these problems. Michael Storms suggests that a person can be high or low on both the heteroeroticism dimension and the homoeroticism dimension. Bisexuals are high on both, asexuals low on both, heterosexuals high on heteroeroticism, and homosexuals high on homoeroticism. But others criticized this model as still being too simple. Physical and emotional preferences may or may not coincide, and other important dimensions of sexuality must be considered. Fritz Klein and his colleagues attempted to address the weakness in earlier models by postulating multiple dimensions in sexual orientation: sexual attraction, sexual behavior, sexual fantasies, emotional preferences, social preferences, self-identification, and lifestyle. A person's dimensions need not remain constant but may vary across time. Some people may now identify their sexual orientation as heterosexual but may have or have had sexual experiences or desires inconsistent with that identification. Pursuing a model of sexual orientation and desire has led psychologists to challenge and upset previously cherished notions: the strong connection between desire and behavior; consistency in sexual desire; and links between self-identification and desire. From a philosophical perspective, these developments in psychological models of desire reflect a growing awareness that the classification of human sexual desire is far more complex than assumed by earlier scientific studies.

In the context of late modern or postmodern studies, the taxonomical issue arises again, but now the debate is more philosophical. John DeLamater and Janet Hyde have contributed substantially to this discourse. After comparing classical (say, Platonic) and modern essentialist (whether evolutionary, biological, or cultural) views of human sexuality with social constructionist views (according to which sexuality is shaped by cultural symbols and scripts), they explore the possibilities of theories that integrate essentialist and constructionist perspectives. Daryl Bem's "exotic becomes erotic" theory is one such attempt, albeit controversial. Bem grounds sexual orientation initially in biologically antecedent conditions (genes, prenatal hormones, neurology), which influence a child's preference for sex-stereotypical activities and peers. On his view, a predilection for peers and activities that are atypical leads to a sense of "exotic-ness," a difference from same-sex peers. Interacting with someone who is "exotic," according to Bem, increases physiological arousal that is, importantly, interpreted as sexual arousal. In some ways, this model repeats features common to much psychological theory in the twentieth century: Even though sexuality is strongly grounded in physiological processes, gender nonconformity is associated with homosexual behavior. Critics contend that Bem's model is not supported by the evidence (see Peplau et al.). Many people who are gender nonconformists are nevertheless heterosexual, and many gender conformists are gay or lesbian.

Perhaps the most salient case of the postmodern turn in the philosophy of the psychology of sex is **queer theory**. Although queer theory has strongly influenced other disciplines in the social sciences and the philosophy of sex, it has yet to establish a wide influence in psychology. Queer theorists, drawing on poststructural social theorists like Foucault, argue that psychiatric taxonomies are nothing more than regimes of social control that attempt to regulate behavior and acceptable sexual identities. Moreover, queer theory questions theories that are based on fixed categories of sexual identity and the pathologization of dynamic or fluid identities. This has led psychologists to begin disputing whether psychiatric diagnoses of gender identity disorders, such as transsexualism and transvestism, are valid mental disorders at all (see Gert's critique). Much of this debate is reminiscent of the early 1970s debate about the depathologization of homosexuality. Taking the queer theory argument to its logical conclusion, psychology has been asking whether any necessary connection between gender and sexuality exists, thereby undoing Freudian gender inversion theories of homosexuality, and whether the notion of a sexual mental disorder makes any sense to begin with. (On this, see the early "late modern" work of Szasz.)

The central philosophical questions in the psychology of sex in the twentieth century have, of course, spilled over into the twenty-first. Approaches to sexuality early in the twentieth century were (with hindsight) simplistic and have given way to much more complex assumptions and investigations in the latter half of the century. The older questions about taxonomy yielded to intriguing inquiries about the correspondence between biological sex, gender, and sexual orientation. Early modern studies were dominated by medical and psychoanalytic views and then the ascendance of largely atheoretical scientific positivism. The postmodern period has been contesting much of what went before and is finally focusing more explicitly on the philosophical assumptions underlying the study of sexuality. Moreover, queer and feminist challenges to modern models of sexuality have raised significant questions about the contextual nature and categories of desire. The philosophy of the psychology of sex is currently fertile ground awaiting continued exploration in the twenty-first century.

See also Bisexuality; Ellis, Albert; Feminism, French; Firestone, Shulamith; Freud, Sigmund; Freudian Left, The; Intersexuality; Lacan, Jacques; Love; Money, John; Orientation, Sexual; Poststructuralism; Psychology, Evolutionary; Queer Theory; Rimmer, Robert; Sexology; Sherfey, Mary Jane; Social Constructionism

REFERENCES

Bem, Daryl. "Exotic Becomes Erotic: A Developmental Theory of Sexual Orientation." *Psychological Review* 103:2 (1996), 320–35; Breuer, Josef, and Sigmund Freud. (1895) *Studies in Hysteria*. Trans. James Strachey. Oxford, U.K.: Basic Books, 1957; Chodorow, Nancy. *The Reproduction of Mothering: Psychoanalysis and the Sociology of Gender*. Berkeley: University of California Press, 1978; Cixous, Hélène, and Catherine Clément. *The Newly Born Woman*. Trans. Betsy Wing. Minneapolis: University of Minnesota Press, 1975; DeLamater, John, and Janet Hyde. "Essentialism vs. Social Constructionism in the Study of Human Sexuality." *Journal of Sex Research* 35:1 (1998), 10–18; D'Emilio, John, and Estelle Freedman. *Intimate Matters: A History of Sexuality in America*. New

York: Harper and Row, 1997; Dinnerstein, Dorothy. *The Mermaid and the Minotaur: Sexual Arrangements and Human Malaise*. New York: Harper and Row, 1976; Ellis, Havelock. (1905) *Studies in the Psychology of Sex*. New York: Random House, 1936; Flax, Jane. *Disputed Subjects: Essays on Psychoanalysis, Politics, and Philosophy*. New York: Routledge, 1993; Foucault, Michel. (1976) *The History of Sexuality*, vol. 1: *An Introduction*. Trans. Robert Hurley. New York: Vintage, 1978; Freud, Sigmund. (1912) "On the Universal Tendency to Debasement in the Sphere of Love." In *The Standard Edition of the Complete Psychological Works of Sigmund Freud*, vol. 11. Trans. James Strachey. London: Hogarth Press, 1953–1974, 179–90; Freud, Sigmund. (1925) "Some Psychical Consequences of the Anatomical Distinction between the Sexes." In *The Standard Edition of the Complete Psychological Works of Sigmund Freud*, vol. 19. Trans. James Strachey. London: Hogarth Press, 1953–1974, 248–60; Freud, Sigmund. (1905) *Three Essays on the Theory of Sexuality*. In *The Standard Edition of the Complete Psychological Works of Sigmund Freud*, vol. 7. Trans. James Strachey. London: Hogarth Press, 1953–1974, 125–245; Gay, Peter. *The Bourgeois Experience*. Vol. 1: *Education of the Senses*. Oxford, U.K.: Oxford University Press, 1984. Vol. 2: *The Tender Passion*, 1986; Geer, James, and William O'Donohue, eds. *Theories of Human Sexuality*. New York: Plenum, 1987; Gert, Bernard. "A Sex Caused Inconsistency in DSM-III-R: The Definition of Mental Disorder and the Definition of Paraphilias." *Journal of Medicine and Philosophy* 17 (1992), 155–71; Hirschfeld, Magnus. (1910) *Transvestites: The Erotic Drive to Cross-Dress*. Trans. Michael A. Lombardi-Nash. Buffalo, N.Y.: Prometheus, 1991; Horney, Karen. "Flight from Womanhood: The Masculinity Complex in Women, as Viewed by Men and by Women." *International Journal of Psychoanalysis* 7 (1926), 324–29; Irigaray, Luce. (1974) *Speculum of the Other Woman*. Trans. Gillian C. Gill. Ithaca, N.Y.: Cornell University Press, 1985; Kinsey, Alfred C., Wardell B. Pomeroy, and Clyde E. Martin. *Sexual Behavior in the Human Male*. Philadelphia, Pa.: W. B. Saunders, 1948; Kinsey, Alfred C., Wardell B. Pomeroy, Clyde E. Martin, and Paul H. Gebhard. *Sexual Behavior in the Human Female*. Philadelphia, Pa.: W. B. Saunders, 1953; Klein, Fritz, Barry Sepekoff, and Timothy Wolf. "Sexual Orientation: A Multi-Variable Dynamic Process." *Journal of Homosexuality* 11:1–2 (1985), 35–49; Krafft-Ebing, Richard von. (1868) *Psychopathia Sexualis*. New York: Physicians and Surgeons Book Company, 1924; Kristeva, Julia. (1983) *Tales of Love*. Trans. Leon S. Roudiez. New York: Columbia University Press, 1987; Lacan, Jacques. (1966) "Guiding Remarks for a Congress on Feminine Sexuality." Trans. Jacqueline Rose. In Juliet Mitchell and Jacqueline Rose, eds., *Feminine Sexuality: Jacques Lacan and the École Freudienne*. New York: Norton, 1985, 86–98; Levine, Steven. "Re-exploring the Concept of Sexual Desire." *Journal of Sex and Marital Therapy* 28:1 (2002), 39–51; Masters, William H., and Virginia E. Johnson. *Human Sexual Response*. Boston, Mass.: Little, Brown, 1966; Money, John. *Clinical Concepts of Sexual/Erotic Health and Pathology, Paraphilia, and Gender Transposition in Childhood, Adolescence, and Maturity*. New York: Irvington, 1986; Money, John. *Gendermaps: Social Constructionism, Feminism, and Sexosophical History*. New York: Continuum, 1995; Money, John. "Linguistic Resources and Psychodynamic Theory." *British Journal of Medical Psychology* 28:4 (1955), 264–66; Peplau, Letitia, Linda Garnets, Leah Spalding, Terri Conley, and Rosemary Veniegas. "A Critique of Bem's 'Exotic Becomes Erotic' Theory of Sexual Orientation." *Psychological Review* 105:2 (1998), 387–94; Plato. (ca. 380 BCE) *Symposium of Plato*. Trans. Tom Griffith. (1986) Berkeley: University of California Press, 1989; Reich, Wilhelm. (1942) *The Discovery of the Orgone*, vol. 1: *The Function of the Orgasm. The Sex-Economic Problems of Biological Energy*. Trans. Vincent R. Carfagno. Oxford, U.K.: Touchstone, 1973; Rivière, Joan. "Womanliness as Masquerade." *International Journal of Psychoanalysis* 10 (1929), 303–13; Robinson, Paul. *The Modernization of Sex: Alfred Kinsey, William Masters, and Virginia Johnson*. New York: Harper and Row, 1976; Sternberg, Robert. *The Triangular Theory of Love: Intimacy, Passion, and Commitment*. New York: Basic Books, 1988; Storms, Michael. "Theories of Sexual Orientation." *Journal of Personality and Social Psychology* 38:5 (1980), 783–92; Szasz, Thomas S. *The Manufacture of Madness: A Comparative Study of the Inquisition and the Mental Health Movement*. New York: Harper and Row, 1970; Terman, Lewis, P. Buttenwieser, Leonard Ferguson, Winifred Johnson, and Donald Wilson. *Psychological Factors in Marital Happiness*. New York: McGraw-Hill, 1938; Ulrichs, Karl Heinrich. (1864–1880) *The Riddle of "Man-Manly" Love:*

The Pioneering Work on Male Homosexuality, 2 vols. Trans. Michael A. Lombardi-Nash. Buffalo, N.Y.: Prometheus, 1994; Weeks, Jeffrey. *Coming Out: Homosexual Politics in Britain, from the Nineteenth Century to the Present*. New York: Quartet, 1977.

Darryl B. Hill

ADDITIONAL READING

American Psychiatric Association. *Diagnostic and Statistical Manual of Mental Disorders*, 4th ed. Washington, D.C.: Author, 1994. Text revision, 2000; Bancroft, John, ed. *The Role of Theory in Sex Research*. Bloomington: Indiana University Press, 2000; Bergo, Bettina. "Freud's Debt to Philosophy and His Copernican Revolution." In Jennifer Radden, ed., *The Philosophy of Psychiatry: A Companion*. New York: Oxford University Press, 2004, 338–50; Bohan, Janice. *Psychology and Sexual Orientation: Coming to Terms*. New York: Routledge, 1996; Deutsch, Helene. "On Female Homosexuality." *Psychoanalytic Quarterly* 1 (1932), 484–510; Deutsch, Helene. *The Psychology of Women*. Oxford, U.K.: Grune and Stratton, 1945; Deutsch, Helene. "The Significance of Masochism in the Mental Life of Women." *International Journal of Psychoanalysis* 11 (1930), 48–60; Devereux, George. "The Irrational in Sexual Research." In *From Anxiety to Method in the Behavioral Sciences*. The Hague: Mouton, 1967, 103–17; Ellis, Albert. *Reason and Emotion in Psychotherapy*. New York: Lyle Stuart, 1962. Revised ed., New York: Birch Lane Press, 1994; Ellis, Albert. *Sex without Guilt in the 21st Century*. Fort Lee, N.J.: Barricade Books, 2003; Erikson, Erik. *Childhood and Society*. New York: Norton, 1964; Foucault, Michel. (1976/1984/1984) *The History of Sexuality*. Vol. 1: *An Introduction*. Trans. Robert Hurley. New York: Vintage, 1978. Vol. 2: *The Use of Pleasure*. Trans. Robert Hurley. New York: Pantheon, 1985. Vol. 3: *The Care of the Self*. Trans. Robert Hurley. New York: Vintage, 1986; Freedman, Estelle B. (1987) " 'Uncontrolled Desires': The Response to the Sexual Psychopath, 1920–1960." In Kathy Peiss and Christina Simmons, eds., *Passion and Power: Sexuality in History*. Philadelphia, Pa.: Temple University Press, 1989, 199–225; Freud, Sigmund. (1895) *Studies on Hysteria*. In *The Standard Edition of the Complete Psychological Works of Sigmund Freud*, vol. 2. Trans. James Strachey. London: Hogarth Press, 1953–1974, 1–335; Frosh, Steven. (1987) *The Politics of Psychoanalysis: An Introduction to Freudian and Post-Freudian Theory*, 2nd ed. New York: New York University Press, 1999; Giles, James. "A Theory of Love and Sexual Desire." *Journal for the Theory of Social Behavior* 24:4 (1994), 339–57; Gilligan, Carol. *In a Different Voice: Psychological Theory and Women's Development*. Cambridge, Mass.: Harvard University Press, 1982; Gilligan, Carol. "Moral Orientation and Moral Development." In Eva Feder Kittay and Diana T. Meyers, eds., *Women and Moral Theory*. Totowa, N.J.: Rowman and Littlefield, 1987, 19–33; Hall, Marny. "Not Tonight, Dear, I'm Deconstructing a Headache: Confessions of a Lesbian Sex Therapist." In Karla Jay, ed., *Lesbian Erotics*. New York: New York University Press, 1995, 15–27; Hill, Darryl B. "Transvestism." In Timothy F. Murphy, ed., *Reader's Guide to Lesbian and Gay Studies*. Chicago, Ill.: Fitzroy Dearborn, 2000, 592–94; Hill, Darryl B., and Michael Kral, eds. *About Psychology: Essays at the Crossroads of History, Theory, and Philosophy*. Albany: State University of New York Press, 2003; Horney, Karen. *Feminine Psychology*. New York: Norton, 1937; Horney, Karen. "Flight from Womanhood: The Masculinity Complex in Women, as Viewed by Men and by Women." *International Journal of Psycho-analysis* 7 (1926), 324–29. Reprinted in *Feminine Psychology*. Ed. Harold Kelman. New York: Norton, 1967, 54–70; Irigaray, Luce. (1977) *This Sex Which Is Not One*. Trans. Catherine Porter, with Carolyn Burke. Ithaca, N.Y.: Cornell University Press, 1985. Reprinted in Claudia Zanardi, ed., *Essential Papers on the Psychology of Women*. New York: New York University Press, 1990, 344–51; Irvine, Janice. *Disorders of Desire: Sex and Gender in Modern American Sexology*. Philadelphia, Pa.: Temple University Press, 1990; Jacoby, Russell. *Social Amnesia: A Critique of Conformist Psychology from Adler to Laing*. Boston, Mass.: Beacon Press, 1975. With a new introduction, New Brunswick, N.J.: Transaction, 1996; Kaplan, Louise J. "Women Masquerading as Women." In Gerald I. Fogel and Wayne A. Myers, eds., *Perversions and Near-Perversions in Clinical Practice: New Psychoanalytic Perspectives*. New Haven, Conn.: Yale University Press, 1991, 127–52; Keller, Evelyn Fox. *Reflections on Gender and Science*. New Haven,

Conn.: Yale University Press, 1985; Keller, Evelyn Fox. *Secrets of Life, Secrets of Death: Essays on Language, Gender and Science*. New York: Routledge, 1992; Keller, Evelyn Fox, and Jane Flax. "Missing Relations in Psychoanalysis: A Feminist Critique of Traditional and Contemporary Accounts of Analytic Theory and Practice." In Stanley B. Messer, Louis A. Sass, and Robert L. Woolfolk, eds., *Hermeneutics and Psychological Theory: Interpretive Perspectives on Personality, Psychotherapy, and Psychopathology*. New Brunswick, N.J.: Rutgers University Press, 1988, 334–66; Lorber, Judith, Rose Laub Coser, Alice S. Rossi, and Nancy Chodorow. "On *The Reproduction of Mothering*: A Methodological Debate." *Signs* 6:3 (1981), 482–514; Masson, Jeffrey Moussaieff. *A Dark Science: Women, Sexuality, and Psychiatry in the Nineteenth Century*. New York: Farrar, Straus and Giroux, 1986; Miller, Jean Baker, ed. *Psychoanalysis and Women*. Baltimore, Md.: Penguin, 1973; Minton, Henry L. "American Psychology and the Study of Human Sexuality." *Journal of Psychology and Human Sexuality* 1:1 (1988), 17–34; Minton, Henry L. "Queer Theory: Historical Roots and Implications for Psychology." *Theory and Psychology* 7:3 (1997), 337–53; Mitchell, Juliet. "On Freud and the Distinction between the Sexes." In Jean Strouse, ed., *Women and Analysis: Dialogues on Psychoanalytic Views of Femininity*. New York: Grossman, 1974, 27–36; Mitchell, Juliet. *Psychoanalysis and Feminism: Freud, Reich, Laing, and Women*. New York: Vintage, 1975; Mitchell, Juliet, and Jacqueline Rose, eds. *Feminine Sexuality: Jacques Lacan and the École Freudienne*. New York: Norton, 1985; Money, John. *Lovemaps: Clinical Concepts of Sexual/Erotic Health and Pathology, Paraphilia, and Gender Transposition in Childhood, Adolescence, and Maturity*. New York: Irvington, 1986. Paperback reprint, Buffalo, N.Y.: Prometheus, 1988; Money, John, and Anke Ehrhardt. *Man and Woman, Boy and Girl: The Differentiation and Dimorphism of Gender Identity from Conception to Maturity*. Baltimore, Md.: Johns Hopkins University Press, 1972; Parlee, Mary B. "Situated Knowledges of Personal Embodiment: Transgender Activists' and Psychological Theorists' Perspectives on 'Sex' and 'Gender.'" *Theory and Psychology* 6:4 (1996), 625–45; "Psychology and Sex." Appendix B in Robert Trevas, Arthur Zucker, and Donald Borchert, eds., *Philosophy of Sex and Love: A Reader*. Upper Saddle River, N.J.: Prentice-Hall, 1997, 429–50; Reik, Theodor. *A Psychologist Looks at Love*. Oxford, U.K.: Farrar and Rinehart, 1944; Reik, Theodor. *The Psychology of Sex Relations*. Oxford, U.K.: Farrar and Rinehart, 1945; Rubin, Lillian B. *Erotic Wars: What Happened to the Sexual Revolution?* New York: Farrar, Straus and Giroux, 1990; Rubin, Lillian B. *Intimate Strangers: Men and Women Together*. New York: Harper and Row, 1983; Ryan, Joanna. "Psychoanalysis and Women Loving Women." In Sue Cartledge and Joanna Ryan, eds., *Sex and Love: New Thoughts on Old Contradictions*. London: Women's Press, 1983, 196–209; Skinner, B. F. *Beyond Freedom and Dignity*. New York: Knopf, 1971; Stein, Edward. *The Mismeasure of Desire: The Science, Theory, and Ethics of Sexual Orientation*. New York: Oxford University Press, 1999; Stein, Edward, ed. *Forms of Desire: Sexual Orientation and the Social Constructionist Controversy*, 1st pnt. New York: Garland, 1990. 2nd pnt., New York: Routledge, 1992; Sternberg, Robert, and Michael Barnes, eds. *The Psychology of Love*. New Haven, Conn.: Yale University Press, 1988; Strouse, Jean, ed. *Women and Analysis: Dialogues on Psychoanalytic Views of Femininity*. New York: Grossman, 1974; Thurber, James, and E. B. White. (1929) *Is Sex Necessary? Or Why You Feel the Way You Do*. New York: Harper and Row, 1975; Updike, John. "Libido Lite." [Review of *Is Sex Necessary?* by James Thurber and E. B. White] *New York Review of Books* (18 November 2004), 30–31; Weeks, Jeffrey. "Necessary Fictions: Sexual Identities and the Politics of Diversity." In *Invented Moralities: Sexual Values in an Age of Uncertainty*. New York: Columbia University Press, 1995, 82–123; Weis, David. "The Need to Integrate Sexual Theory and Research." In Michael W. Wiederman and Bernard E. Whitley, Jr., eds., *Handbook for Conducting Research on Human Sexuality*. Mahwah, N.J.: Erlbaum, 2002, 2–24; Weis, David. "The Use of Theory in Sexuality Research." *Journal of Sex Research* 35:1 (1998), 1–9; Zanardi, Claudia, ed. *Essential Papers on the Psychology of Women*. New York: New York University Press, 1990.

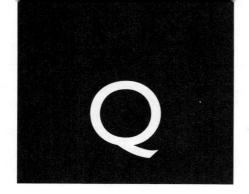

QUEER THEORY. Even though the interdisciplinary area called "queer theory" developed alongside lesbian and gay studies in the 1990s, "queer theory" is not another name for lesbian and gay studies. It has been importantly influenced by **poststructuralism**'s criticism of "identity" as something fixed, unified, natural, and essential. In particular, queer theory challenges the claim that relations between sex, gender, and desire are stable, a claim that underpins the belief that heterosexuality is normal and natural. Not only does queer theory explore the contingency of these relations; it also questions the coherence of the very categories "man," "woman," "male," "female," "lesbian," "gay," "bisexual," and "heterosexual." For queer theorists, categories of sex and gender are "constantly subject to negotiation and renegotiation" (Duggan, "Making It," 167).

Despite the popular use of "queer" as an umbrella term covering lesbian, gay, bisexual, transgendered, and transsexual people, queer theorists use "queer" otherwise than merely to refer to sexual minorities. "Queer" implies a confrontation with mainstream society's pathologization of "perverse" sexual desires, embodiments, practices, and identities. It also implies criticism of the **liberalism** and quest for legitimacy that has shaped the majority voice of the lesbian and gay rights movement (see Duggan, *Twilight*; Goldstein; Warner). Queer theorists do not seek a place at the heteronormative, capitalist, white supremacist, able-bodied table. Instead, they try to imagine new worlds, "new ways of thinking and acting politically" (Duggan, "Making It," 155; Warner, 139). The word "queer," historically, has been disparaging. Queer theorists and activists have reclaimed it to encompass practices and embodiments that undermine heteronormativity.

In *Epistemology of the Closet*, a groundbreaking book, Eve Sedgwick proposed that queer theory was central for understanding modern Western culture, since the homo/heterosexual divide is foundational for that culture. Building on **Michel Foucault**'s (1926–1984) studies, Sedgwick emphasized the significance of the fact that the term "homosexual" appeared only in the last third of the nineteenth century. That term marked some individuals as "homosexual" and inaugurated the idea that sexuality is deeply involved in and explains much human personality and experience. Western culture thereby embraced the idea that sexuality makes an individual a certain kind of person, precisely the sort of reification of identity rejected by queer theory.

David Halperin also argues that Foucault's *History of Sexuality* is significant for queer politics: It articulates a theory of power that enables queer activists to understand how liberalism operates to normalize and discipline, as opposed to overtly coerce, people who (perhaps wrongly) see themselves as free (*Saint Foucault*, 18, 26). Foucault famously contends that the history of the relationship between sex and power is not primarily a history of the repression and silencing of sex by power (*History*, 8–13, 17–18). Instead, power operates, in various historical and cultural contexts, to construct "truths" about sexuality and sexual subjects. Foucault examined how scientific discourse in the late nineteenth century produced visible sexual subjects (for example, "the" homosexual). Far from being a time of silence about sexuality, it exhibited a proliferation of sexual discourses. While these discourses contributed to the oppression of "homosexuals," they also created the conditions for "the formation of a 'reverse' discourse: homosexuality began to speak in its own behalf, to demand that its legitimacy or 'naturality' be acknowledged, often in the same vocabulary, using the same categories by which it was medically disqualified" (101). Thus, for Foucault, the power of discourse brings the subject into existence, subjugates the subject, but also provides the subject with mechanisms of resistance.

This theory of power underlies queer criticisms of identity-based liberation movements. When gay, lesbian, or feminist movements seek to liberate common, oppressed identities, they accommodate norms that privilege white, dominant-class, Western members of their respective groups (Butler, *Gender Trouble*, 3–4; Duggan, "Making It," 162). For queer theory, focusing on liberating repressed identities is the wrong tactic, since identity is unstable and itself an effect of discourse. For example, queer analyses of acquired immunodeficiency syndrome (AIDS) explored how biomedical, racist, classist, nationalist, sexist, and homophobic discourses worked together to produce the meanings of AIDS and "public health" that shaped public responses (see Crimp; Treichler). In confronting these dominant meanings, AIDS activists, to generate safer sex campaigns, moved from matters of identity (which groups are at risk?) to questions about which practices likely facilitate human immunodeficiency virus (HIV) transmission. Consistently with the queer critique of the relationship between sexuality and identity, a shift was effected from understanding AIDS as a problem only for specific groups (gay men, intravenous drug users, hemophiliacs, etc.) to understanding it as a problem for everyone.

Identities must always be regarded with suspicion because they tend to be instruments of regulation; claiming identity is risky. And establishing identity is fraught with both theoretical and political difficulties: "What, if anything, can lesbians be said to share? And who will decide this question, and in the name of whom?" (Butler, "Imitation," 15). "Lesbian" and other identities are permanently troubled. But this situation is, for queer theorists, also full of potential and not just a cause for despair. Taking identity as always provisional calls into question, for example, the judgment that coming out of the closet is liberatory for lesbians and gays. Instead of being simply the liberation of a repressed identity, coming out is a demand for visibility, an aspect of normalizing power.

Queer theory's "provisionality of identity" departs from how identity was mobilized in the various homophile movements from the late nineteenth century to the 1970s. This is not to say that the movements were not crucial in the quest for justice for lesbians, gays, bisexuals, transsexuals, and transgendered people. Queers of the late twentieth and early twenty-first centuries owe a great debt to these movements. The earlier homophile movements must be appreciated and judged in their historical context rather than dismissed as assimilationist (D'Emilio, *Making Trouble*, 239; *Sexual Politics*, 2–3). Further, gay liberation's desire to transform society is consistent with queer theory's effort to denaturalize heterosexual norms and create a world, relationships, and ways of being that cannot be known in advance and are always open to transformation (Butler, "Imitation," 19; Duggan, "Making It," 155, 167; Halperin, 62, 76–79; Warner, 71, 139, 166).

The Mattachine Society (1951) and the Daughters of Bilitis (1955) were homophile organizations in the United States that educated heterosexuals about lesbians and gays, increased social tolerance of **homosexuality**, and pushed for the decriminalization and depathologization of homosexuality (D'Emilio, *Making Trouble*, 238–39; Duggan, *Twilight*, 52). The Mattachine Society was composed mostly of men; it focused on issues that affected gays and ignored issues of concern to lesbians. The Daughters of Bilitis was formed to offer lesbians an alternative to the 1950s bar scene. They have been criticized as anti-butch/femme, classist, and assimilationist, to the extent that they favored feminine styles of dress and behavior that they believed would facilitate the acceptance of lesbians by mainstream society (Jagose, 27). While these homophile groups seem conservative and counterproductive from a twenty-first-century queer perspective, they were radical in the 1950s. They made themselves visible and argued for their rights even though there were no antidiscrimination laws to protect them from losing their jobs, homes, and lives. One might point out that some states still lack such laws in the early twenty-first century. But lesbians and gay men are able to come out into a visible community in which there are far more sources of support than existed in the 1950s. Homophile organizations were also effective in working against, even if they did not eradicate, police violence against gays and lesbians. Their efforts, assimilationist by twenty-first-century queer standards, nevertheless created a context hospitable to more radical politics (D'Emilio, *Making Trouble*, 239–40; *Sexual Politics*, 2–3).

When police raided the Stonewall Inn in New York City (27 June 1969), the patrons resisted, and afterward rioting went on for several days. While criticism of liberalism had existed earlier in the homophile movement, Stonewall can be seen as the moment of the radicalization of the lesbian and gay movement, taking it beyond mere assimilationist politics (D'Emilio, *Making Trouble*, 242; *Sexual Politics*, 231–33). The activism of the New Left, feminist, Black Power, Chicano, and American Indian movements also contributed to the context in which gays and lesbians began to critique a politics of conformity to dominant norms. Gay liberation demanded the transformation of heteronormative society, proclaiming that gays and lesbians should mobilize an unapologetic, proud, "in-your-face" politics and move "out of the closets [and] into the streets" (Young, 6).

Gay liberation's critique of psychiatry, militarism, imperialism, capitalism, sexism, racism, and religion continues to influence the split between assimilationist and queer politics (see Goldstein). Queer theorists have criticized the liberalism of the mainstream gay and lesbian rights movement, whose goal is for lesbians and gays to be accepted as "normal" and for which achieving **same-sex marriage** is the culmination of the struggle (Goldstein, 106; Warner, 81–147). By contrast, queer theorists question the appropriateness of government's granting legitimacy to any relationships. Further, what is needed is not marriage but full citizenship rights for everyone, regardless of whether they conform to gender or relationship norms (Duggan, "Holy"; *Twilight*, 64–65; Warner, 117–19). This does not mean that lesbians and gays should be denied a right to marry. It does mean rejecting a strategy of securing state benefits for people who conform to the norm of the monogamous couple while denying benefits to those who do not conform.

Queer theory has also influenced an emerging area, queer **disability** studies, which builds both on queer theory's critique of heteronormativity and on disability studies' critique of cultural norms of bodily appearance and function (see Hall; McRuer and Wilkerson). In queer disability studies, able-bodiment is compulsory and not "natural," just as heterosexuality is compulsory and not "natural" (see McRuer; Rich). Probing the cultural norms that enable some bodies and dis-able others connects queer disability studies to queer theory's impeachment of normalization.

Queer theory, ethics, and politics incorporate the values created in the project of queer world-making, in parks, public restrooms, **pornography** theaters, sex parties, and bars; in the relationships between leatherdyke boys and their daddies; by drag queens, drag kings, butches, femmes, tops, bottoms, transsexuals, and transgendered people (see Delany;

Halberstam; Hale; Warner). Queer theory, ethics, and politics are generated in the places where people are "at odds with [and resist] the norms of straight culture" (Warner, 38), in the places where queer sex, desires, and bodies are recognized as sites of creativity and transformation rather than considered shameful secrets.

See also Beauty; Bisexuality; Boswell, John; Disability; Diseases, Sexually Transmitted; Dysfunction, Sexual; Feminism, French; Foucault, Michel; Heterosexism; Judaism, Twentieth- and Twenty-First-Century; Orientation, Sexual; Perversion, Sexual; Psychology, Twentieth- and Twenty-First-Century; Sexology; Social Constructionism

REFERENCES

Butler, Judith. *Gender Trouble: Feminism and the Subversion of Identity*. New York: Routledge, 1990; Butler, Judith. "Imitation and Gender Insubordination." In Diana Fuss, ed., *Inside/Out: Lesbian Theories, Gay Theories*. New York: Routledge, 1991, 13–31; Crimp, Douglas, ed. *AIDS: Cultural Analysis, Cultural Activism*. Cambridge, Mass.: MIT Press, 1987; Delany, Samuel R. *Times Square Red, Times Square Blue*. New York: New York University Press, 1999; D'Emilio, John. *Making Trouble: Essays on Gay History, Politics, and the University*. New York: Routledge, 1992; D'Emilio, John. *Sexual Politics, Sexual Communities: The Making of a Homosexual Minority in the United States 1940–1970*. Chicago, Ill.: University of Chicago Press, 1983; Duggan, Lisa. "Holy Matrimony!" *The Nation* (15 March 2004), 14–16, 18–19; Duggan, Lisa. "Making It Perfectly Queer." In Lisa Duggan and Nan D. Hunter, *Sex Wars: Sexual Dissent and Political Culture*. New York: Routledge, 1995, 155–72; Duggan, Lisa. *The Twilight of Equality? Neoliberalism, Cultural Politics, and the Attack on Democracy*. Boston, Mass.: Beacon Press, 2003; Foucault, Michel. (1976) *The History of Sexuality*, vol. 1: *An Introduction*. Trans. Robert Hurley. New York: Vintage, 1978; Goldstein, Richard. *The Attack Queers: Liberal Society and the Gay Right*. London: Verso, 2002; Halberstam, Judith. *Female Masculinity*. Durham, N.C.: Duke University Press, 1998; Hale, C. Jacob. "Leatherdyke Boys and Their Daddies: How to Have Sex without Women or Men." *Social Text* 15:3–4 (1997), 222–36; Hall, Kim Q. "Queerness, Disability, and the Vagina Monologues." *Hypatia* 20:1 (2005), 99–119; Halperin, David M. *Saint Foucault: Towards a Gay Hagiography*. New York: Oxford University Press, 1995; Jagose, Annamarie. *Queer Theory: An Introduction*. New York: New York University Press, 1996; McRuer, Robert. "Compulsory Able-Bodiedness and Queer/Disabled Existence." In Sharon L. Snyder, Brenda Jo Brueggemann, and Rosemarie Garland-Thomson, eds., *Disability Studies: Enabling the Humanities*. New York: Modern Language Association, 2002, 88–99; McRuer, Robert, and Abby Wilkerson, eds. *Desiring Disability: Queer Theory Meets Disability Studies*. Special double issue of *GLQ: A Journal of Lesbian and Gay Studies* 9:1–2 (2003); Rich, Adrienne. "Compulsory Heterosexuality and Lesbian Existence." *Signs* 5:4 (1980), 631–60; Sedgwick, Eve Kosofsky. *Epistemology of the Closet*. Berkeley: University of California Press, 1990; Treichler, Paula A. "AIDS, Homophobia, and Biomedical Discourse: An Epidemic of Signification." *Cultural Studies* 1:3 (1987), 263–305; Warner, Michael. *The Trouble with Normal: Sex, Politics, and the Ethics of Queer Life*. Cambridge, Mass.: Harvard University Press, 1999; Young, Allen. "Out of the Closets, into the Streets." In Karla Jay and Allen Young, eds., *Out of the Closets: Voices of Gay Liberation*. New York: Douglas, 1972, 6–31.

Kim Q. Hall

ADDITIONAL READING

Abelove, Henry, Michèle Aina Barale, and David Halperin, eds. *The Lesbian and Gay Studies Reader*. New York: Routledge, 1993; Bawer, Bruce. "Notes on Stonewall." In Robert Baird and M. Katherine Baird, eds., *Homosexuality: Debating the Issues*. Amherst, N.Y.: Prometheus, 1995, 23–30; Beemyn, Brett, and Mickey Eliason, eds. *Queer Studies: A Lesbian, Gay, Bisexual, and Transgender Anthology*. New York: New York University Press, 1996; Brett, Philip, Elizabeth Wood, and Gary C. Thomas, eds. *Queering the Pitch: The New Gay and Lesbian Musicology*. New York:

Routledge, 1994; Bruhm, Steven, and Natasha Hurley, eds. *Curiouser: On the Queerness of Children*. Minneapolis: University of Minnesota Press, 2004; Burgess, Susan R. Review of *Sex Wars: Sexual Dissent and Political Culture*, by Lisa Duggan and Nan D. Hunter. *Law and Politics Book Review* 6:1 (1996), 16–19. <www.bsos.umd.edu/gvpt/lpbr/subpages/reviews/duggan.htm> [accessed 5 April 2004]; Butler, Judith. *Bodies That Matter: On the Discursive Limits of "Sex."* New York: Routledge, 1993; Califia, Pat. "Feminism and Sadomasochism." *Heresies* #12 ["Sex Issue"] 3:4 (1981), 30–34. Reprinted in Stevi Jackson and Sue Scott, eds., *Feminism and Sexuality: A Reader*. New York: Columbia University Press, 1996, 230–37; Califia, Pat. *Public Sex: The Culture of Radical Sex*. Pittsburgh, Pa.: Cleis Press, 1994; Califia, Pat. *Sex Changes: The Politics of Transgenderism*. San Francisco, Calif.: Cleis, 1997; Califia, Pat [Califia-Rice, Patrick]. *Speaking Sex to Power: The Politics of Queer Sex*. San Francisco, Calif.: Cleis, 2002; Clare, Eli. *Exile and Pride: Disability, Queerness, and Liberation*. Cambridge, Mass.: South End Press, 1999; Comstock, Gary David, and Susan E. Henking, eds. *Que(e)rying Religion: A Critical Anthology*. New York: Continuum, 1997; Corber, Robert J., and Stephen Valocchi, eds. *Queer Studies: An Interdisciplinary Reader*. Malden, Mass.: Blackwell, 2003; Cuomo, Chris J., and Kim Q. Hall, eds. *Whiteness: Feminist Philosophical Reflections*. Totowa, N.J.: Rowman and Littlefield, 1999; Daumer, Elizabeth. "Queer Ethics, or the Challenge of Bisexuality to Lesbian Ethics." *Hypatia* 7:4 (1992), 91–106; Dever, Carolyn. "Either/And: Lesbian Theories, Queer Theories." *GLQ: A Journal of Lesbian and Gay Studies* 5:3 (1999), 413–24. <muse.jhu.edu/demo/journal_of_lesbian_and_gay_studies/v005/5.3dever.html> [accessed 4 January 2005]; Doty, Alexander. *Making Things Perfectly Queer: Interpreting Mass Culture*. Minneapolis: University of Minnesota Press, 1993; Duggan, Lisa. "The Discipline Problem: Queer Theory Meets Lesbian and Gay History." In Lisa Duggan and Nan D. Hunter, *Sex Wars: Sexual Dissent and Political Culture*. New York: Routledge, 1995, 194–206; Duggan, Lisa, and Nan D. Hunter. *Sex Wars: Sexual Dissent and Political Culture*. New York: Routledge, 1995; Epstein, Julia, and Kristin Straub, eds. *Body Guards: The Cultural Politics of Gender Ambiguity*. New York: Routledge, 1991; Ferguson, Roderick A. *Aberrations in Black: Toward a Queer of Color Critique*. Minneapolis: University of Minnesota Press, 2004; Garber, Linda. *Tilting the Tower: Lesbians, Teaching, Queer Subjects*. New York: Routledge, 1994; Golden, Carla. "Diversity and Variability in Women's Sexual Identities." In Boston Women's Psychologies Collective, ed., *Lesbian Psychologies: Explorations and Challenges*. Urbana: University of Illinois Press, 1987, 18–34. Reprinted in John Corvino, ed., *Same Sex: Debating the Ethics, Science, and Culture of Homosexuality*. Lanham, Md.: Rowman and Littlefield, 1997, 149–66; Grant, Catherine. (1994–1995) "Queer Theorrhea (and What It Might Mean for Feminists)." In Stevi Jackson and Sue Scott, eds., *Feminism and Sexuality: A Reader*. New York: Columbia University Press, 1996, 166–71; Hall, Kim Q. "Learning to Touch Honestly: A White Lesbian's Struggle with Racism." In Jeffner Allen, ed., *Lesbian Philosophies and Cultures*. Albany: State University of New York Press, 1990, 317–26; Halperin, David M. *One Hundred Years of Homosexuality: And Other Essays on Greek Love*. New York: Routledge, 1990; Halperin, David M. *Saint Foucault: Towards a Gay Hagiography*. New York: Oxford University Press, 1995; Hammill, Graham. "The Epistemology of Expurgation: Bacon and *The Masculine Birth of Time*." In Jonathan Goldberg, ed., *Queering the Renaissance*. Durham, N.C.: Duke University Press, 1994, 236–52; Heyes, Cressida. "Feminist Solidarity after Queer Theory: The Case of Transgender." *Signs* 28:4 (2003), 1093–1120; Jeffreys, Sheila. *Unpacking Queer Politics: A Lesbian Feminist Perspective*. Malden, Mass.: Blackwell, 2003; Kumashiro, Kevin K., ed. *Troubling Intersections of Race and Sexuality: Queer Students of Color and Anti-Oppressive Education*. Lanham, Md.: Rowman and Littlefield, 2001; Levinson, Nan. "Stalemate in the Sex Wars." [Review of *Sex Wars: Sexual Dissent and Political Culture*, by Lisa Duggan and Nan D. Hunter] *Women's Review of Books* 13:4 (1996), 14; Martin, Biddy. "Sexualities without Genders and Other Queer Utopias." In Mandy Merck, Naomi Segal, and Elizabeth Wright, eds., *Coming Out of Feminism?* Oxford, U.K.: Blackwell, 1998, 11–35; Meyerowitz, Joanne. *How Sex Changed: A History of Transsexuality in the United States*. Cambridge, Mass.: Harvard University Press, 2002; Minton, Henry L. "Queer Theory: Historical Roots and Implications for Psychology." *Theory and Psychology* 7:3 (1997), 337–53; Morrison, James. "Queer Theory." In Timothy F. Murphy, ed., *Reader's Guide to Lesbian and Gay Studies*. Chicago, Ill.: Fitzroy Dearborn, 2000,

491–93; Pendleton, Eva. "Love for Sale: Queering Heterosexuality." In Jill Nagle, ed., *Whores and Other Feminists*. New York: Routledge, 1997, 73–82; Penn, Donna, and Janice Irvine. "Gay/Lesbian/Queer Studies." *Contemporary Sociology* 24:3 (1995), 328–30; Phelan, Shane, ed. *Playing with Fire: Queer Politics, Queer Theories*. New York: Routledge, 1997; Poulsen, Rachel E. "Queer Studies." In Timothy F. Murphy, ed., *Reader's Guide to Lesbian and Gay Studies*. Chicago, Ill.: Fitzroy Dearborn, 2000, 488–91; Queen, Carol. "Strangers at Home: Bisexuals in the Queer Movement." *Out/Look*, no. 16 (Spring 1992), 23, 29–33. Reprinted, revised, in John Corvino, ed., *Same Sex: Debating the Ethics, Science, and Culture of Homosexuality*. Lanham, Md.: Rowman and Littlefield, 1997, 258–63; Queen, Carol, and Laurence Schimel, eds. *PoMoSexuals: Challenging Assumptions about Gender and Sexuality*. San Francisco, Calif.: Cleis Press, 1997; Rich, Adrienne. "Compulsory Heterosexuality and Lesbian Existence." *Signs* 5:4 (1980), 631–60. Reprinted in *Blood, Bread, and Poetry: Selected Prose 1979–1985*. New York: Norton, 1986, 23–75; in Ann Snitow, Christine Stansell, and Sharon Thompson, eds., *Powers of Desire: The Politics of Sexuality*. New York: Monthly Review Press, 1983, 177–205; and Henry Abelove, Michèle Aina Barale, and David M. Halperin, eds., *The Lesbian and Gay Studies Reader*. New York: Routledge, 1993, 227–54; Rubin, Gayle S. "Thinking Sex: Notes for a Radical Theory of the Politics of Sexuality." In Carole S. Vance, ed., *Pleasure and Danger: Exploring Female Sexuality*. London: Routledge and Kegan Paul, 1984, 267–319. Reprinted in Henry Abelove, Michèle Aina Barale, and David Halperin, eds., *The Lesbian and Gay Studies Reader*. New York: Routledge, 1993, 3–44; and Peter M. Nardi and Beth E. Schneider, eds., *Social Perspectives in Lesbian and Gay Studies*. New York: Routledge, 1998, 100–133; Somerville, Siobhan B. *Queering the Color Line: Race and the Invention of Homosexuality in American Culture*. Durham, N.C.: Duke University Press, 2000; Stone, Sandy [Allucquère Rosanne Stone]. "The Empire Strikes Back: A Posttranssexual Manifesto." In Julia Epstein and Kristin Straub, eds., *Body Guards: The Cultural Politics of Gender Ambiguity*. New York: Routledge, 1991, 280–304; Stone, Sandy. *The War of Desire and Technology at the Close of the Mechanical Age*. Cambridge, Mass.: MIT Press, 1995; Stuart, Elizabeth. *Religion Is a Queer Thing: A Guide to the Christian Faith for Lesbian, Gay, Bisexual, and Transgendered Persons*. Cleveland, Ohio: Pilgrim Press, 1997; Tierney, William G. *Academic Outlaws: Queer Theory and Cultural Studies in the Academy*. Thousand Oaks, Calif.: Sage, 1997; Warner, Michael, ed. *Fear of a Queer Planet: Queer Politics and Social Theory*. Minneapolis: University of Minnesota Press, 1993; Weeks, Jeffrey. "Necessary Fictions: Sexual Identities and the Politics of Diversity." In *Invented Moralities: Sexual Values in an Age of Uncertainty*. New York: Columbia University Press, 1995, 82–123.

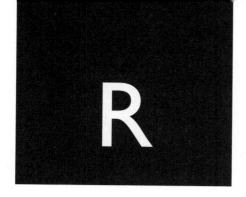

RAPE. Almost everyone agrees that rape is a very serious moral wrong and that it should be counted as one of the most serious crimes. In popular estimation, rape ranks second only to murder. Some, however, while not disputing that rape is wrong, argue that it is not *very* wrong or not as wrong as ordinarily alleged. At the same time, even though everyone "agrees that rape is a terrible thing, . . . we don't agree on what rape is" (Roiphe, 54). What exactly should be counted as rape is deeply contested (see Reitan). For example, feminists point to the unacceptable narrowness of traditional legal definitions of rape, yet they in turn are charged with improperly extending its scope. So there are a number of important disputes about rape: How should it be defined? In what does the wrongness of rape consist? And how much of a wrong is it? (In what follows, rape is discussed as something done by men to women. Of course men rape men, for example, in prison, and some women have been found guilty of raping or being accomplices to the rape of men. Still, rape is principally perpetrated by men against women.)

A widely shared view is that rape is a distinctive, special kind of wrong. It does not follow that all rapes share a single common feature, although on one prominent view they do: Every instance of nonconsensual sex is rape. This definition might seem to expand unduly the scope of "rape." One paradigm of rape is using force or threatening violence to obtain sex. Yet some cases of nonconsensual sex do not result from force or fear: sex that results from fraud or the administration of drugs. Hence either this paradigm of rape yields an inadequate definition (because it is too narrow) or defining "rape" as nonconsensual sex is wrong (because it is too inclusive). However, there need be nothing amiss in extending the definition of rape beyond this paradigm, as long as all rapes falling within the extended definition have the property (see below) that makes rape a special and serious wrong. Those defending an extended definition of rape (e.g., Burgess-Jackson, chap. 1) do insist that *all* rapes, of any type, are very wrong. On this view, considered as rapes, forcible and nonconsensual rapes are equally wrong.

One worry that arises about extended definitions is that the effective administration of law requires that criminal categories correspond at least roughly to popular discriminations. A legal system that sets itself to punish a class of actions, some of which are not generally believed to be as serious as others (nonconsensual versus forced sex), might not be efficiently administered. Law officers might be reluctant to pursue alleged criminals or be unenthusiastic in prosecuting the crime; juries might hesitate to convict. This worry, however, underestimates the extent to which popular perceptions change over time and sells short the role of the law in encouraging such changes. Bear in mind that we have moved a long way from the view that wives cannot be raped by their husbands. Hence this worry is not a decisive objection to an expanded definition of rape. It can be acknowledged that some sex obtained by force can be worse than some nonconsensual sex. We could still define rape as nonconsensual sex while allowing that particular instances of rape might have, as other crimes do, aggravating features. After all, robbery occurs with varying degrees of violence.

Rape seems to be a *sexual* crime, but this has been disputed by some feminists and for understandable reasons. It implies, because sex is generally pleasurable, that *some* part of rape must be enjoyable. Further, it misunderstands the rapist's motivation as the pursuit of pleasure rather than the exercise of domination. We can, however, represent rape as sexual without asserting that its victim must feel pleasure. To assert that is to make the mistake of seeing rape simply as sex with **consent** subtracted, instead of the indivisible wrong of nonconsensual sex. Rapists *do* exercise domination, but this is compatible with the act's being sexual, if rapists exercise domination by assaulting the sexual integrity of victims. Not to conceive of rape as sexual thus runs the risk of missing or understating its wrongfulness (see below).

In what respect is rape sexual? The basic idea is that the genitalia are somehow involved. (This might be what distinguishes rape from battery.) Legal terms such as "unlawful intercourse" might seem to imply that emission is necessary, but it is not. If rape is considered to involve at least "penetration," there are still disagreements about what is penetrated and what penetrates. Some jurisdictions define penetration as vaginal or anal. But oral penetration can be as great a violation of a person's sexual integrity (maybe sometimes greater). Some laws distinguish between penetration by the penis (rape proper) and penetration by a finger or object, which is categorized as the lesser offense of sexual assault (Home Office, vol. 1, sec. 2.8, 2.9, 15–17; see **Richard Posner** and Silbaugh, 5–34). Yet it might be that penetration in itself, a physical invasion of a person's body, makes the act seriously wrongful. Empirical studies of rape victims suggest that the trauma does not depend on how or in what orifice penetration occurs (Burgess and Holmstrom, 1974, 1985).

What makes a sex act rape is the absence of the victim's agreement. But "absence of agreement," as we have seen, can be taken narrowly or broadly. Historically, rape was seen as forced sex. Not only must a woman have been forcibly overcome, but she must have resisted her attacker to the "utmost," which showed the necessity of his using force and her unwillingness to have sex with him (her "absence of agreement"). Further, a woman is raped if she submits as the result of a man's credible threat to use force. Thus coerced sex is rape. But rape can encompass sex that is nonconsensual, even if not coerced. A woman who has sex with a man she mistakes for another, or a woman who undergoes what she does not realize is sex, or a woman who has sex when rendered by another incapable of consenting (e.g., by drugs) is raped. In all these cases, there is "absence of agreement."

Of course, "consent" must be clarified. There are ontological questions about whether consent is an act, a mental state, or some combination. Whatever consent is, it is vital that consent as giving permission, as *agreeing* to something, be distinguished from approving of, agreeing with, *that thing*. A woman who has sex she would prefer not to have or a kind she finds distasteful does not approve of *that thing*, but she still might have consented, agreed to it. She is raped, however, if she has not consented at all. It is therefore irrelevant whether a rape victim might have welcomed a man's sexual advances (approving of *that thing*), as juries have been misleadingly invited to consider. All that matters is whether the man had sex with her without her agreement.

Consent to sex need not be given explicitly, although some writers (e.g., Pineau; Remick; Schulhofer) defend the view that consent is given only if "yes" or its unambiguous equivalent is uttered. This view is different from the view that the *evidence* of consent (say, in a courtroom) is verbal affirmation. This view is stringent enough, and the view that consent itself requires "yes" strikes many as far too demanding. To insist that men have an obligation to ensure that women do consent is legitimate. But this obligation can sometimes be met by men's acting *reasonably* on a presumption that some behaviors by women betoken their willingness. Moreover, many sexual interactions, especially between long-standing partners, are conducted on the basis of reciprocal, unstated understandings.

Still, there are dangers in tacit consent, which is consent given by the performance (or the intentional nonperformance) of some action. It is different from "indirect" consent: consent to what must follow from or is indissolubly connected to that which *is* explicitly consented to. My consenting to your using my car is also consent to your consuming my fuel. But consenting to a certain level of sexual intimacy is not consenting to coitus, since the "indissoluble" link is missing. Tacit consent relies crucially on shared conventions whereby an action (or inaction) may be taken as having a specific meaning. In sexual contexts, there must be some assurance that both parties are aware of and subscribe to the relevant conventions. Some have argued that it is reasonable for men to rely on social conventions whereby women express agreement to sex (e.g., Husak and Thomas). There are problems, however, with relying solely on such conventions (see Archard, "Nod"). First, men must be able to distinguish behaviors that indicate that consent might be forthcoming from behaviors that directly signify consent. (Note the difference between indicating that one might later agree to have sex and indicating one's agreement, now, to have sex later.) Second, it is doubtful that men and women share a set of conventions whereby behaviors can reasonably be interpreted by both sexes as giving consent. What a hopeful man takes as a woman's signifying definite interest she may never have intended to be taken that way. Third, men have means, should they be in doubt, of ascertaining whether a woman is consenting: direct, explicit questions.

It is also crucial to specify the conditions under which consent is absent or invalidated. It is defeated by a person's incapacity, the nonvoluntariness of agreement, or ignorance. Puzzles about coercion that are much discussed by philosophers have application to rape. A woman who has sex with a man who threatens to kill her child is raped; her agreement is not voluntary. But is she raped if a man offers to provide the surgery she cannot afford to save the life of her ill child? Which threats or offers coerce such that sex resulting from them are rapes? The law has defined them as threats that would overcome resistance by an ordinary woman. But there are problem cases: Contrast, for example, a man's threat to harm a woman's child and a threat to expose her criminal past.

Deception also raises problems. In the law, a distinction is made between fraud in the *factum* and fraud in the inducement. The first is deception about the act performed (it is not a medical procedure, after all, but sex) or about identity of the person performing the act (he is not her husband but someone in disguise). The second involves misrepresenting facts that motivate a woman to have sex she otherwise would not have (a married man says he is single). Fraud in the *factum* is often seen as rape, while fraud in inducement is not, as amounting at most to a lesser offense. Why, if rape is nonconsensual sex and consent in both cases is vitiated by deception?

One answer is that in fraud in the inducement a woman *does* consent to the act of sex and is deceived only about "collateral matters." By contrast, a woman does *not* consent to the act of sex when she is deceived about what the act is or with whom it is done. Yet, arguably, what one consents to must be specified *de dicto*, not *de re*. Consider a classic example of fraud in the inducement: A woman is told falsely that she will be paid for sex. Did she consent *to sex* (specified *de re*) and simply not get the money? Or did she consent to *sex-for-money* (specified *de dicto*) and thus did not consent to the sex that actually occurred? At any rate, the range of "collateral matters" must be limited. It seems implausible that a woman is raped if she has sex with a man because he falsely promises **marriage**.

A woman who is incapable, permanently or temporarily, of giving consent is raped by someone who has sex with her. Incapacity can be cognitive or volitional. A woman must know enough about sex and its reasonably foreseeable consequences to have the capacity to consent to it. She must also be able to will that something happen or not happen and to express her will. Temporary incapacitation results frequently from intoxication. In some legal contexts voluntary self-intoxication excuses the commission of an offense. I get myself drunk but when drunk do not know what I am doing and thus avoid liability. But the fact that a woman gets herself drunk to the point of incapacity does not excuse a *nonintoxicated* man from the charge of rape if he knowingly has sex with her. Intoxication to the point of insensibility vitiates consent. However, no bright line exists between being drunk (and relaxed) but still able to consent and being so drunk that consent is impossible. This problem influences our treatment of **acquaintance and date rape**.

Some feminists claim that all sexual relations between men and women are nonconsensual and thus amount to rape. This claim is associated with **Catharine MacKinnon** (1982; 1983; 1989a; 1989b, chap. 9), **Andrea Dworkin** (1946–2005), and Carole Pateman. There are three distinct grounds for the claim. One is the fact that men have more social, economic, and political power than do women. It follows, on their view, that no woman truly consents to sex with a man. The argument succeeds only if inequalities *as such* render agreements null and void. Of course, a man might use his power to issue threats against a woman. But if so, the woman is coerced into sex. In this case, the exercise of power, not the fact that it is possessed, vitiates consent. A second ground is that heterosexual sex *is* the subordination of women by men. Dworkin, for instance, writes that coitus makes "a woman inferior: communicating to her cell by cell her own inferior status, impressing it on her, burning it into her by shoving it into her, over and over, pushing and thrusting until she gives in" (138). And MacKinnon defines heterosexuality as the "eroticization of dominance and submission" (1983, 635). But descriptions of heterosexual coitus as "possession" or "invasion" are pejorative and question-begging. It need not be described in these terms (Susan Brownmiller says that she has "no basic quarrel with the procedure" itself; 14) and could easily be described alternatively as the subordination of men (Dworkin notices this; *Intercourse*, 64–65). The third argument is that women have no alternative but to be heterosexual (Overall; Rich). "Compulsory heterosexuality" is accomplished by a range of social, economic, political, and cultural measures, including the systematic derogation of alternatives such as lesbianism and sexual abstention. Of course I may knowingly and willingly (i.e., consensually) do what I have no alternative but to do. Anyway, it is not obvious that women, if provided with alternatives and not subject to the alleged pressures, would choose to foreswear sex with men. After all, powerful women continue to have sex with weak men.

Suppose, then, that rape is the subset of the class of penetrative sexual acts to which no consent is given. Why is it seriously wrong? What is wrongful is "sex-without-consent." The hyphens are important; they dissuade us from thinking of rape as consisting of sex, which is normally pleasurable, without consent, the subtraction of which detracts from an otherwise enjoyable experience. Many discussions of rape maintain that the only difference between rape and ordinary sex is the absence of consent (Davis, 89; Harrison, 52; Posner, 388). This may be misleading. Nonconsensual sex can be seen as an indivisible whole whose wrongfulness is best appreciated by seeing it that way. It also helps avoid the line of thought, notoriously displayed in the courtroom questioning of rape victims, that a woman who has in the past greatly enjoyed sex must not have found entirely unwelcome the sex she endured, in which only her agreement to it was missing. Research on rape trauma syndrome does not identify prior sexual experience as a salient factor in the severity of that trauma (Burgess and Holmstrom; Koss and Harvey, chap. 2; Mazur, chaps. 4, 14).

Some insist that the wrongfulness of rape is not captured by its nonconsensuality, because rape is more than just sex without agreement. On one version of this view, a man expresses hatred of women by rape. The evidence suggests, however, that even though some men rape out of anger against women or wanting to dominate them, men rape from a variety of other motives. Another version of the view says that rape serves the social function of terrorizing and oppressing women (Brownmiller, 15, 209; Card). This claim might be true even if individual rapists do not seek by their actions to dominate women. However, the claim being made is stronger than the claim that a set of actions just happens to have a particular outcome. On functional accounts, the outcome *explains* the actions. Functional explanations are controversial. They are rendered less so by some story about how the outcomes, beneficial for but not intended by the agents, causally influence the commission of the actions. But it is unclear what the causal influence is in the case of rape. Men in general may benefit from the occurrence of rape. (This does not mean that men as a group are responsible for rape, as argued by May and Strikwerda.) Women are, generally, harmed by rape, even those (as Brownmiller claims) who are not victims. The incidence of rape exposes all women to anxiety and insecurity, and it encourages them to depend on men for protection and security. But it does not follow that every rape is directed at women as a group. Brownmiller discusses the systematic rape of women by soldiers during war (31–113). In situations like this, victorious armies might seek the "social death" of the women in a defeated populace (MacKinnon, 1993a, 1993b). This is plausible about the rapes of Muslim women by Serbs in the Balkan wars of the 1990s. Yet the awful efficacy of these rapes in socially "killing" the women is explained as much by their ethnic and religious identity as by gender. It was part of the ethnic cleansing carried out by the Serbs, not the organized domination of women *qua* women (for discussion, see Stiglmayer).

Rape may be viewed as causing various, different harms that can be listed (see Bogart; Wertheimer, 97). Or it may be viewed as having an essential wrongfulness (Henderson thinks of rape as "a form of soul murder"; 225). Rape can be seriously harmful even if, in exceptional cases, it is not experienced as a harm. Further, the degree of felt harmfulness varies with contingent social and psychological factors. Insisting that rapes that are especially traumatic merit higher penalties does not mean that rapes causing little or no distress deserve no penalty. Rape is wrong as the violation of bodily integrity, an overruling of another's corporeal sovereignty. It is a sexual violation in virtue of involving the penetration of genital orifices or of bodily orifices by genitalia. Some see the wrongfulness of rape in Kantian terms as objectification, the "sheer use of a person" (Gardner and Shute, 205). In violation of **Immanuel Kant**'s (1724–1804) Categorical Imperative, the rapist treats his victim as an object, as merely a means to his own ends. However, prostitutes consent to being used as mere instruments of satisfaction by their clients. Such consensual **sexual objectification** might be undesirable and morally suboptimal. Yet, arguably, it is not wrong. This suggests that rape is wrong primarily as nonconsensual instead of objectifying. To subject another to sex to which she does not consent is already to treat her merely as a means.

Any rape can include aggravating harms, such as accompanying physical violence, and contingent harms due to social and psychological factors. A woman might deem a particular sex act disgusting or her culture might accord a special value to chastity. Then what is the core harm of rape, and how serious is it? On one account, harmfulness is measured by the extent to which a person's other interests are interfered with or damaged. Rape, then, is not particularly harmful: It is episodic and the interests set back are local (see Baber). On another account, rape damages something central to a person's sense of personhood and identity: her sexual bodily integrity (Hampton; Shafer and Frye). This account requires that we recognize humans as sexed beings, not that we think that everyone is sexually active or values sex.

Men commit rapes for which they can be held responsible. What are the conditions for holding them responsible? Most jurisdictions hold men liable for rape if they intentionally, knowingly, or *recklessly* have sex with a woman who has not consented. A man is reckless if he continues to pursue a course of action he knows has serious risks of harm. By contrast, few jurisdictions hold men liable for *negligence*. A man is negligent when he has sex with a woman that he does not know at the time is not consenting, but whom he ought, if he is reasonable, to know is not consenting. In a notorious British legal case, *Director of Public Prosecutions v. Morgan* (1975), it was held that an honest but unreasonable mistake about a woman's consent constituted a defense to the charge of rape. The reasoning in this and similar cases has received much critical attention (see Berliner; Bienen; Curley; Pickard; Thornton).

Some argue that it is not possible for a man to be mistaken about a woman's nonconsent (Duff; Telling). True, reasonable sexual actors *ought* to know whether a woman is consenting and would, if in doubt, seek assurances. The most obvious way to avoid reasonable *or* unreasonable mistakes, both of which cause great harm, is by asking the woman if she consents. But not all men are reasonable; further, even honest, reasonable mistakes are possible. The difficult question is how to decide which mistakes are unreasonable and whether (or how much) we should punish those who act on them. It is arguable, though, that a man who relies on variable and sometimes misleading social conventions in assessing whether a woman is consenting, instead of the woman's authoritative voice, acts culpably insofar as he is ignoring, and thereby defying, the only legitimate source of consent and permission to proceed (Archard, "*Mens Rea*").

See also Abortion; Activity, Sexual; Coercion (by Sexually Aggressive Women); Consent; Contraception; Dworkin, Andrea; Ethics, Sexual; Flirting; Harassment, Sexual; Kant, Immanuel; MacKinnon, Catharine; Military, Sex and the; Rape, Acquaintance and Date; Seduction; Violence, Sexual

REFERENCES

Archard, David. "The *Mens Rea* of Rape: Reasonableness and Culpable Mistakes." In Keith Burgess-Jackson, ed., *A Most Detestable Crime: New Philosophical Essays on Rape*. New York: Oxford University Press, 1999, 213–29; Archard, David. " 'A Nod's as Good as a Wink': Consent, Convention, and Reasonable Belief." *Legal Theory* 3:3 (1997), 273–90; Baber, H. E. "How Bad Is Rape?" *Hypatia* 2:2 (1987), 125–38; Berliner, Dana. "Rethinking the Reasonable Belief Defense to Rape." *Yale Law Journal* 100 (1991), 2687–2706; Bienen, Leigh. "Mistakes." *Philosophy and Public Affairs* 7 (Spring 1978), 224–45; Bogart, John H. "On the Nature of Rape." *Public Affairs Quarterly* 5:2 (1991), 117–36; Brownmiller, Susan. *Against Our Will: Men, Women, and Rape*. New York: Simon and Schuster, 1975; Burgess, Ann Wolbert, and Lynda Lytle Holmstrom. "Rape Trauma Syndrome." *American Journal of Psychiatry* 131:9 (1974), 981–86; Burgess, Ann Wolbert, and Lynda Lytle Holmstrom. "Rape Trauma Syndrome and Post-Traumatic Stress Response." In Ann Wolbert Burgess, ed., *Rape and Sexual Assault: A Research Handbook*. New York: Garland, 1985, 46–69;

Burgess-Jackson, Keith. *Rape: A Philosophical Investigation*. Aldershot, U.K.: Dartmouth, 1996; Card, Claudia. "Rape as a Weapon of War." *Hypatia* 11:4 (1996), 5–18; Curley, E. M. "Excusing Rape." *Philosophy and Public Affairs* 5:4 (1996), 325–60; Davis, Michael. "Setting Penalties: What Does Rape Deserve?" *Law and Philosophy* 3:1 (1984), 61–110; *Director of Public Prosecutions v. Morgan*. 2 All. E.R. 347, 1976 App. Cas. 182 (H.L. 1975); Duff, Antony. "Recklessness and Rape." *Liverpool Law Review* 3:2 (1981), 49–64; Dworkin, Andrea. *Intercourse*. New York: Free Press, 1987; Estrich, Susan. *Real Rape: How the Legal System Victimizes Women Who Say No*. Cambridge, Mass.: Harvard University Press, 1987; Gardner, John, and Stephen Shute. "The Wrongness of Rape." In Jeremy Horder, ed., *Oxford Essays in Jurisprudence*, 4th series. Oxford, U.K.: Oxford University Press, 2000, 193–217; Hampton, Jean. "Defining Wrong and Defining Rape." In Keith Burgess-Jackson, ed., *A Most Detestable Crime: New Philosophical Essays on Rape*. New York: Oxford University Press, 1999, 118–56; Harrison, Ross. "Rape: A Case Study in Political Philosophy." In Sylvana Tomaselli and Roy Porter, eds., *Rape: An Historical and Cultural Inquiry*. Oxford, U.K.: Blackwell, 1986, 41–56; Henderson, Lynne N. "What Makes Rape a Crime?" [Review of *Real Rape*, by Susan Estrich] *Berkeley Women's Law Journal* 3 (1988), 193–229; Home Office (United Kingdom). *Setting the Boundaries: Reforming the Law on Sex Offences*, vol. 1. Vol. 2: *Supporting Evidence*. London: Home Office Communication Directorate, 2000; Husak, Douglas N., and George C. Thomas III. "Date Rape, Social Convention, and Reasonable Mistakes." *Law and Philosophy* 11:1–2 (1992), 95–126; Koss, Mary P., and Mary R. Harvey. (1987) *The Rape Victim: Clinical and Community Interventions*, 2nd ed. London: Sage, 1991; MacKinnon, Catharine A. "Crimes of War, Crimes of Peace." In Stephen Shute and Susan Hurley, eds., *On Human Rights: The Oxford Amnesty Lectures 1993*. New York: Basic Books, 1993a, 83–109; MacKinnon, Catharine A. "Feminism, Marxism, Method, and the State: An Agenda for Theory." *Signs* 7:3 (1982), 515–44; MacKinnon, Catharine A. "Feminism, Marxism, Method, and the State: Toward Feminist Jurisprudence." *Signs* 8:4 (1983), 635–58; MacKinnon, Catharine A. "Rape: On Coercion and Consent." In *Toward a Feminist Theory of the State*. Cambridge, Mass.: Harvard University Press, 1989b, 171–83; MacKinnon, Catharine A. "Sexuality, Pornography, and Method: 'Pleasure under Patriarchy.' " *Ethics* 99:2 (1989a), 314–46; MacKinnon, Catharine A. "Turning Rape into Pornography: Postmodern Genocide." *Ms.* (July–August 1993b), 24–30; May, Larry, and Robert Strikwerda. "Men in Groups: Collective Responsibility for Rape." *Hypatia* 9:2 (1994), 134–51; Mazur, Mary Ann. *Understanding the Rape Victim: A Synthesis of Research Findings*. New York: John Wiley, 1979; Overall, Christine. "Heterosexuality and Feminist Theory." *Canadian Journal of Philosophy* 20:1 (1990), 1–17; Pateman, Carol. "Women and Consent." *Political Theory* 8:2 (1980), 149–68; Pickard, Toni. "Culpable Mistakes and Rape: Relating *Mens Rea* to the Crime." *University of Toronto Law Review* 30 (1980), 5–98; Pineau, Lois. "Date Rape: A Feminist Analysis." *Law and Philosophy* 8:2 (1989), 217–43; Posner, Richard A. "Coercive Sex." In *Sex and Reason*. Cambridge, Mass.: Harvard University Press, 1992, 383–404; Posner, Richard A., and Katharine B. Silbaugh. "Rape and Sexual Assault." In *A Guide to America's Sex Laws*. Chicago, Ill.: University of Chicago Press, 1996, 5–34; Reitan, Eric. "Rape as an Essentially Contested Concept." *Hypatia* 16:2 (2001), 43–66; Remick, Lani Anne. "Read Her Lips: An Argument for a Verbal Consent Standard in Rape." *University of Pennsylvania Law Review* 141:3 (1993), 1103–51; Rich, Adrienne. "Compulsory Heterosexuality and Lesbian Existence." *Signs* 5:4 (1980), 631–60; Roiphe, Katie. *The Morning After: Sex, Fear, and Feminism on Campus*. New York: Little, Brown, 1993; Schulhofer, Stephen J. "The Gender Question in Criminal Law." *Social Philosophy and Policy* 7 (Spring 1990), 105–37; Shafer, Carolyn M., and Marilyn Frye. "Rape and Respect." In Mary Vetterling-Braggin, Frederick Elliston, and Jane English, eds., *Feminism and Philosophy*. Totowa, N.J.: Littlefield, Adams, 1977, 333–46; Stiglmayer, Alexandra, ed. *Mass Rape: The War against Women in Bosnia-Herzegovina*. Lincoln: University of Nebraska Press, 1994; Telling, David. "Rape—Consent and Belief." *Journal of Criminal Law* 47:3 (1983), 129–39; Thornton, Mark T. "Rape and *Mens Rea*." *Canadian Journal of Philosophy*, supp. vol. 8 (1982), 119–46; Wertheimer, Alan. "Consent and Sexual Relations." *Legal Theory* 2:2 (1996), 89–112.

David Archard

ADDITIONAL READING

Abbey, Antonia. "Sex Differences in Attributions for Friendly Behavior: Do Males Misperceive Females' Friendliness?" *Journal of Personality and Social Psychology* 42:5 (1982), 830–38; Alexander, Larry. "The Moral Magic of Consent (II)." *Legal Theory* 2:3 (1996), 165–74; Allen, Beverly. *Rape Warfare: The Hidden Genocide in Bosnia-Herzegovina and Croatia*. Minneapolis: University of Minnesota Press, 1996; American Law Institute. *Model Penal Code and Commentaries* (Official Draft and Revised Commentaries). Philadelphia, Pa.: Author, 1980; Archard, David. "Negligent Rape." *Australian Journal of Professional and Applied Ethics* 1:2 (1999), 40–48; Archard, David. *Sexual Consent*. Oxford, U.K.: Westview, 1998; Askin, Kelly Dawn. *War Crimes against Women: Prosecution in International War Crimes Tribunal*. The Hague: Martinus Nijhoff, 1997; Baber, H. E. "How Bad Is Rape?" *Hypatia* 2:2 (1987), 125–38. Reprinted in POS2 (243–58); POS3 (249–62); POS4 (303–16); Baker, Brenda M. "Consent, Assault and Sexual Assault." In Anne Bayefsky, ed., *Legal Theory Meets Legal Practice*. Edmonton, Can.: Academic Press, 1988, 223–38; Baker, Brenda M. "*Mens Rea*, Negligence, and Criminal Law Reform." *Law and Philosophy* 6:1 (1987), 53–88; Baker, Brenda M. "Understanding Consent in Sexual Assault." In Keith Burgess-Jackson, ed., *A Most Detestable Crime: New Philosophical Essays on Rape*. New York: Oxford University Press, 1999, 49–70; Benatar, David. "Two Views of Sexual Ethics: Promiscuity, Pedophilia, and Rape." *Public Affairs Quarterly* 16:3 (2002), 191–201; "Beyond Prosecution: Sexual Assault Victim's Rights in Theory and Practice." [Symposium] *Suffolk University Law Review* 38:2 (2005); Bogart, John H. "Commodification and Phenomenology: Evading Consent in Theory Regarding Rape." *Legal Theory* 2:3 (1996), 253–64; Bogart, John H. "On the Nature of Rape." *Public Affairs Quarterly* 5:2 (1991), 117–36. Reprinted in STW (168–80); Bogart, John H. "Reconsidering Rape: Rethinking the Conceptual Foundations of Rape Law." *Canadian Journal of Law and Jurisprudence* 8:1 (1995), 159–82; Bonilla, Margaret D. "What Feminists Are Doing to Rape Ought to Be a Crime." *Policy Review* 66 (1993), 22–29; Bostwick, Tracy D., and Janice L. Deluica. "Effects of Gender and Specific Dating Behaviors on Perceptions of Sex Willingness and Date Rape." *Journal of Social and Clinical Psychology* 11:1 (1992), 14–25; Brett, Nathan. "Sexual Offences and Consent." *Canadian Journal of Law and Jurisprudence* 11:1 (1998), 69–88; Brundage, James A. "Implied Consent to Intercourse." In Angeliki E. Laiou, ed., *Consent and Coercion to Sex and Marriage in Ancient and Medieval Societies*. Washington, D.C.: Dumbarton Oaks, 1993, 245–56; Burgess-Jackson, Keith. "A History of Rape Law." In Keith Burgess-Jackson, ed., *A Most Detestable Crime: New Philosophical Essays on Rape*. New York: Oxford University Press, 1999, 15–31; Burgess-Jackson, Keith. "Rape and Persuasive Definition." *Canadian Journal of Philosophy* 25 (September 1995), 415–54; Burgess-Jackson, Keith. "Statutory Rape: A Philosophical Analysis." *Canadian Journal of Law and Jurisprudence* 8:1 (1995), 139–58. Reprinted in HS (463–82); Burgess-Jackson, Keith. "A Theory of Rape." In Keith Burgess-Jackson, ed., *A Most Detestable Crime: New Philosophical Essays on Rape*. New York: Oxford University Press, 1999, 92–117; Burgess-Jackson, Keith, ed. *A Most Detestable Crime: New Philosophical Essays on Rape*. New York: Oxford University Press, 1999; Chamallas, Martha. "Consent, Equality, and the Legal Control of Sexual Conduct." *Southern California Law Review* 61:4 (1988), 777–862; Clark, Lorenne M. G., and Debra J. Lewis. *Rape: The Price of Coercive Sexuality*. Toronto, Can.: Women's Press, 1977; Cowling, Mark. "Rape, and Other Sexual Assaults: Towards a Philosophical Analysis." *Essays in Philosophy* 2:2 (2001). <www.humboldt.edu/~essays/cowling.html> [accessed 3 June 2005]; Davion, Victoria. "Rape, Group Responsibility, and Trust." *Hypatia* 10:2 (1995), 153–56; Denno, Deborah W. "Why the Model Penal Code's Sexual Offense Provisions Should Be Pulled and Replaced." *Ohio State Journal of Criminal Law* 1 (2003), 207–18; Dibbell, Julian. "A Rape in Cyberspace; or How an Evil Clown, a Haitian Trickster Spirit, Two Wizards, and a Cast of Dozens Turned a Database into a Society." In Peter Ludlow, ed., *High Noon on the Electronic Frontier: Conceptual Issues in Cyberspace*. Cambridge, Mass.: MIT Press, 1996, 375–95; Dripps, Donald D. "Beyond Rape: An Essay on the Difference between the Presence of Force and the Absence of Consent." *Columbia Law Review* 92:8 (1992), 1780–1809; Dworkin, Andrea. *Pornography: Men Possessing Women*. New York: Perigee, 1981; Estrich, Susan. "Rape." *Yale Law Journal* 95 (May

1986), 1087–1184; Foa, Pamela. "What's Wrong with Rape." In Mary Vetterling-Braggin, Frederick A. Elliston, and Jane English, eds., *Feminism and Philosophy*. Totowa, N.J.: Littlefield, Adams, 1977, 347–59. Reprinted in Hugh LaFollette, ed., *Ethics in Practice: An Anthology*, 2nd ed. Malden, Mass.: Blackwell, 2002, 212–19; P&S3 (583–93); Francis, Leslie P. "Rape." In Ruth Chadwick, ed., *Encyclopedia of Applied Ethics*, vol. 3. San Diego, Calif.: Academic Press, 1998, 791–98; Friedman, Marilyn, and Larry May. "Harming Women as a Group." *Social Theory and Practice* 11:2 (1985), 207–34; Gauthier, Jeffrey A. "Consent, Coercion, and Sexual Autonomy." In Keith Burgess-Jackson, ed., *A Most Detestable Crime: New Philosophical Essays on Rape*. New York: Oxford University Press, 1999, 71–91; Gilbert, Neil. "Realities and Mythologies of Rape." *Society* 29 (May–June 1992), 4–10; Girshick, Lori B. *Woman-to-Woman Sexual Violence: Does She Call It Rape?* Boston, Mass.: Northeastern University Press, 2002; Groth, A. Nicholas. (1979) *Men Who Rape: The Psychology of the Offender*. New York: Plenum, 1979; Helliwell, Christine. "It's Only a Penis: Rape, Feminism, and Difference." *Signs* 25:3 (2000), 789–816; Hubin, Don C., and Karen Haely. "Rape and the Reasonable Man." *Law and Philosophy* 18:2 (1999), 113–31; Husak, Douglas N., and George C. Thomas III. "Date Rape, Social Convention, and Reasonable Mistakes." *Law and Philosophy* 11:1–2 (1992), 95–126. Reprinted, abridged, in Lori Gruen and George Panichas, eds., *Sex, Morality, and the Law*. New York: Routledge, 1997, 444–54; Husak, Douglas N., and George C. Thomas III. "Rapes without Rapists: Consent and Reasonable Mistake." *Noûs*, supp. 11 (2001), 86–117; Jones, Owen D. "Sex, Culture, and the Biology of Rape: Toward Explanation and Prevention." *California Law Review* 87:4 (1999), 827–941; Katz, Bonnie. "The Psychological Impact of Stranger versus Nonstranger Rape on Victims' Recovery." In Andrea Parrot and Laurie Bechhofer, eds., *Acquaintance Rape: The Hidden Crime*. New York: John Wiley, 1991, 251–69; Krahé, Barbara. "Police Officers' Definition of Rape: A Prototype Study." *Journal of Community and Applied Social Psychology* 1:3 (1991), 223–44; Lacey, Nicola. "Unspeakable Subjects, Impossible Rights: Sexuality, Integrity and Criminal Law." In *Unspeakable Subjects: Feminist Essays in Legal and Social Theory*. Oxford, U.K.: Hart, 1998, 98–124; Lees, Sue. *Carnal Knowledge: Rape on Trial*. London: Hamish Hamilton, 1996; MacKinnon, Catharine A. *Toward a Feminist Theory of the State*. Cambridge, Mass.: Harvard University Press, 1989; MacKinnon, Catharine A. "Turning Rape into Pornography: Postmodern Genocide." *Ms*. (July–August 1993), 24–30. Reprinted in Alexandra Stiglmayer, ed., *Mass Rape: The War against Women in Bosnia-Herzegovina*. Lincoln: University of Nebraska Press, 1994, 73–81; Malm, H. M. "The Ontological Status of Consent and Its Implications for the Law on Rape." *Legal Theory* 2:2 (1996), 147–64; May, Larry. *Masculinity and Morality*. Ithaca, N.Y.: Cornell University Press, 1998; May, Larry. *The Morality of Groups: Collective Responsibility, Group-Based Harm, and Corporate Rights*. Notre Dame: University of Notre Dame Press, 1987; May, Larry, and Robert Strikwerda. "Men in Groups: Collective Responsibility for Rape." *Hypatia* 9:2 (1994), 134–51. Reprinted in P&S3 (594–610). Reprinted as "Rape and Collective Responsibility," in Larry May, *Masculinity and Morality*. Ithaca, N.Y.: Cornell University Press, 1998, 79–97. Revised version in Hugh LaFollette, ed., *Ethics in Practice: An Anthology*, 1st ed. Cambridge, Mass.: Blackwell, 1997, 418–28. 2nd ed., 2002, 418–27; May, Larry, and Robert Strikwerda. "Reply to Victoria Davion's Comments on May and Strikwerda." *Hypatia* 10 (Spring 1995), 157–58; McGregor, Joan. "Force, Consent, and the Reasonable Woman." In Jules Coleman and Allen Buchanan, eds., *In Harm's Way: Essays in Honor of Joel Feinberg*. Cambridge: Cambridge University Press, 1994, 231–54; McGregor, Joan. "Why When She Says No She Doesn't Mean Maybe and Doesn't Mean Yes: A Critical Reconstruction of Consent, Sex, and the Law." *Legal Theory* 2:3 (1996), 175–208; Muehlenhard, Charlene L. "Misinterpreted Dating Behaviors and the Risk of Date Rape." *Journal of Social and Clinical Psychology* 6:1 (1988), 20–37; Muehlenhard, Charlene L., Irene G. Powich, Joi L. Phelps, and Laura M. Givsi. "Definitions of Rape: Scientific and Political Implications." *Journal of Social Issues* 48:1 (1992), 23–44; Muehlenhard, Charlene L., and Jennifer L. Schrag. "Nonviolent Sexual Coercion." In Andrea Parrot and Laurie Bechhofer, eds., *Acquaintance Rape: The Hidden Crime*. New York: John Wiley, 1991, 115–28; Murphy, Jeffrie G. "Some Ruminations on Women, Violence, and the Criminal Law." In Jules Coleman and Allen Buchanan, eds., *In Harm's Way: Essays in Honor of Joel Feinberg*. Cambridge: Cambridge University Press, 1994,

209–30; Norris, Jeanette, and Shirley Feldman-Summers. "Factors Related to the Psychological Impact of Rape on the Victim." *Journal of Abnormal Psychology* 90:6 (1981), 562–67; Ng, Vivien W. "Ideology and Sexuality: Rape Laws in Qing China." *Journal of Asian Studies* 46:1 (1987), 57–70; Oberman, Michelle. "Turning Girls into Women: Re-evaluating Modern Statutory Rape Law." *Journal of Criminal Law and Criminology* 85:1 (1994), 15–79; Palmer, Craig T. "Twelve Reasons Why Rape Is Not Sexually Motivated: A Skeptical Examination." *Journal of Sex Research* 25:4 (1988), 521–30. Reprinted in Roy Baumeister, ed., *Social Psychology and Human Sexuality: Essential Readings*. Philadelphia, Pa.: Psychology Press, 2001, 225–35; Patel, Krishna R. "Recognizing the Rape of Bosnian Women as Gender-Based Persecution." *Brooklyn Law Review* 60 (Fall 1994), 929–58; Pateman, Carole. " 'The Disorder of Women': Women, Love, and the Sense of Justice." *Ethics* 91:1 (1980), 20–34; Pateman, Carole. *The Sexual Contract*. Cambridge, U.K.: Polity Press, 1988; Pateman, Carole. "Women and Consent." *Political Theory* 8:2 (1980), 149–68. Reprinted in *The Disorder of Women: Democracy, Feminism, and Political Theory*. Cambridge: Cambridge University Press, 1989, 71–89; Peterson, Susan Rae. "Coercion and Rape: The State as a Male Protection Racket." In Mary Vetterling-Braggin, Frederick A. Elliston, and Jane English, eds., *Feminism and Philosophy*. Totowa, N.J.: Littlefield, Adams, 1977, 360–71; Pineau, Lois. "Date Rape: A Feminist Analysis." *Law and Philosophy* 8:2 (1989), 217–43. Reprinted in Hugh LaFollette, ed., *Ethics in Practice: An Anthology*, 1st ed. Cambridge, Mass.: Blackwell, 1997, 418–28; 2nd ed., 2002, 410–17; Leslie P. Francis, ed., *Date Rape: Feminism, Philosophy, and the Law*. State College: Pennsylvania State University Press, 1996, 1–26; HS (483–509); Posner, Richard A., and Katharine B. Silbaugh. "Marital Exemptions from Rape and Sexual Assault." In *A Guide to America's Sex Laws*. Chicago, Ill.: University of Chicago Press, 1996, 35–43; Rich, Adrienne. "Compulsory Heterosexuality and Lesbian Existence." *Signs* 5:4 (1980), 631–60. Reprinted in *Blood, Bread, and Poetry: Selected Prose 1979–1985*. New York: Norton, 1986, 23–75; and Henry Abelove, Michèle Aina Barale, and David M. Halperin, eds., *The Lesbian and Gay Studies Reader*. New York: Routledge, 1993, 227–54; Sanday, Peggy Reeves. "The Socio-Cultural Context of Rape: A Cross-Cultural Study." *Journal of Social Issues* 37:4 (1981), 5–27; Schulhofer, Stephen J. "The Gender Question in Criminal Law." *Social Philosophy and Policy* 7 (Spring 1990), 105–37. Reprinted in Ellen Frankel Paul, Fred Miller, and Jeffrey Paul, eds., *Crime, Culpability, and Remedy*. Oxford, U.K.: Blackwell, 1990, 105–37; Schulhofer, Stephen J. "Taking Sexual Autonomy Seriously: Rape Law and Beyond." *Law and Philosophy* 11:1–2 (1992), 35–94; Schulhofer, Stephen J. *Unwanted Sex: The Culture of Intimidation and the Failure of the Law*. Cambridge, Mass.: Harvard University Press, 1998; Scully, Diana. *Understanding Sexual Violence: A Study of Convicted Rapists*. Boston, Mass.: Unwin Hyman, 1990; Seifert, Ruth. "War and Rape: A Preliminary Analysis." In Alexandra Stiglmayer, ed., *Mass Rape: The War against Women in Bosnia-Herzegovina*. Lincoln: University of Nebraska Press, 1994, 54–72; Sherwin, Emily. "Infelicitous Sex." *Legal Theory* 2:3 (1996), 209–31; Stock, Wendy. "Women's Sexual Coercion of Men: A Feminist Analysis." In Peter B. Anderson and Cindy Struckman-Johnson, eds., *Sexually Aggressive Women: Current Perspectives and Controversies*. New York: Guilford, 1998, 169–84; Sweet, Ellen. "Date Rape: The Story of an Epidemic and of Those Who Deny It." *Ms.* (October 1985), 56–85; Syrota, George. "Rape: When Does Fraud Vitiate Consent?" *Western Australian Law Review* 25 (December 1995), 334–45; Tadros, Victor. "No Consent: A Historical Critique of the *Actus Reus* of Rape." *Edinburgh Law Review* 3:1 (1999), 318–40; Temkin, Jennifer. *Rape and the Legal Process*. London: Sweet and Maxwell, 1987; Thornhill, Randy, and Craig Palmer. *A Natural History of Rape: Biological Bases of Sexual Coercion*. Cambridge, Mass.: MIT Press, 2000; Thornton, Mark T. "Rape and *Mens Rea*." *Canadian Journal of Philosophy*, supp. vol. 8 (1982), 119–46. Also published in Kai Nielsen and Steven C. Patten, eds., *New Essays in Ethics and Public Policy*. Guelph, Can.: Canadian Association for Publishing in Philosophy, 1982, 119–46. Reprinted in HS (435–62); Tomaselli, Sylvana, and Roy Porter, eds. *Rape: An Historical and Social Enquiry*. Oxford, U.K.: Blackwell, 1986; Tur, Richard H. S. "Rape: Reasonableness and Time." *Oxford Journal of Legal Studies* 1 (Winter 1981), 432–41; Weisberg, D. Kelly, ed. "Rape." In *Applications of Feminist Legal Theory to Women's Lives: Sex, Violence, Work, and Reproduction*. Philadelphia, Pa.: Temple University Press, 1996, 405–527; Wertheimer, Alan. "Consent and Sexual

Relations." *Legal Theory* 2:2 (1996), 89–112. Reprinted in POS4 (341–66); Wertheimer, Alan. *Consent to Sexual Relations*. Cambridge: Cambridge University Press, 2003; Wertheimer, Alan. "What Is Consent? And Is It Important?" *Buffalo Criminal Law Review* 3:2 (2001), 557–83; West, Robin. "A Comment on Consent, Sex, and Rape." *Legal Theory* 2:3 (1996), 233–51; Wing, Adrien Kallentine, and Sylke Merchán. "Rape, Ethnicity, and Culture: Spirit Injury from Bosnia to Black America." *Columbia Human Rights Law Review* 25:1 (1993), 25–72; Wyre, Ray, and Anthony Swift. *Women, Men and Rape*. London: Hodder and Stoughton, 1990.

RAPE, ACQUAINTANCE AND DATE. **Rape**, defined most broadly, is sex with a person who is not consenting. Narrower definitions limit rape to penetration, by a male against a female, accompanied by force or threatened force. The mental element required for the offense of rape may be that the perpetrator intended or knew that the female was not consenting. Or, more expansively, it may be reckless indifference or negligence about **consent** (see Baron). Acquaintance rape is rape by someone the victim knows, including family members, friends, neighbors, colleagues, or casual associates. Date rape is rape between individuals who are currently in a dating relationship (Wiehe and Richards, 4). It does not include rapes that occur after a romantic affair has ended or rapes that are planned to occur during a date (Cowling, 34).

In the United States, 77 percent of completed rapes involved offenders who were known to the victim (1997 data, from the National Center for Victims of Crime). Estimates are that between 18 percent (Johnson and Sigler, 43) and 25 percent (Bohmer and Parrot, 26) of women at universities in the United States have been victims of date rape, although there are methodological problems with studies that rely on self-reports (Johnson and Sigler, 36–37; Sommers, 209–26). Rates at **military** academies or in the military may be even higher (Cowling, 42), as may rates among athletes (Benedict, 89). Reports to authorities notoriously underestimate actual prevalence (Campbell-Ruggaard and Van Ryswyk, 288; Russell and Bolen, 26). Estimates are that about 10 percent of rape victims are male (Scarce, 9), although some characterizations exclude male victims from the definition of the offense.

In *Real Rape* (1987), Susan Estrich famously distinguished between "real rape," a violent attack by a stranger, and nonviolent "simple" rape, in which the victim knows the rapist. Estrich argued that simple rapes are real rapes, too: Forced intercourse is rape, even if violence is not involved and the victim knows the rapist. Society, the law, and even victims failed to recognize simple rape as rape, Estrich contended, because they identified rape with force and the resistance of the victim. Legal and philosophical controversies attend whether acquaintance rape is "really" rape, on a par with stranger rape. At the heart of these controversies is how the wrongfulness of rape should be understood. Is rape fundamentally a crime of violence or an offense against sexual autonomy? Radical feminists view rape in the context of power relationships between men and women (e.g., **Catharine MacKinnon**), while liberals focus on the failure of consent (e.g., Schulhofer). Or should forced sex and nonconsensual sex be understood as two different wrongs, one against bodily integrity and the other against autonomy (McGregor, 181; West, 243)? Other central questions in understanding acquaintance rape concern the differences and similarities between stranger, acquaintance, date, and spousal rape; the meaning and role of consent (and of coercion); and the significance of problems of proof.

In defining rape, Anglo-American courts have (historically) insisted on resistance "to the utmost." Even if women screamed, scratched, and punched, if they eventually succumbed, courts concluded that they consented (Estrich, 31; Schulhofer, 3). This utmost resistance requirement was modified by problematic evaluations of the relationship between rapist and victim: Courts demanded less resistance for white victims assailed by blacks, more when victim and assailant were acquainted (Estrich, 37). The contemporary standard is "reasonable resistance," with courts more inclined to find the standard satisfied for stranger rapes than for acquaintance rapes. Many jurisdictions now require proof of force rather than resistance, yet legal decisions in some jurisdictions continue to measure force by resistance (Schulhofer, 31).

According to Estrich, gendered attitudes continue to inform judgments about whether women demonstrate sufficient resistance. Some think women's resistance is ambivalent and equivocal and hence that "no" may mean "yes" (see "Comment"; Muehlenhard and Hollabaugh). Moreover, surveys indicate that with a prior relationship between accuser and accused, attitudes diverge by gender about whether the woman consented, whether the man was blameworthy, whether the woman contributed to the result, and whether the sex seriously harmed her (Estrich, 24–25; Wiehe and Richards, 17). Traditional attitudes toward gender roles also correlate with these differences (Wiehe and Richards, 77–79). These gendered attitudes commonly downplay the seriousness of acquaintance rape. The Model Penal Code (American Law Institute) designates rape generally as a second-degree felony (sec. 213.1 [1]). Moreover, for rape to count as a first-degree felony, there must have been serious bodily harm to someone *or* it must be the case that the victim was both not acquainted with the perpetrator and had not previously permitted him sexual liberties. Thus acquaintance rape is merely a second-degree felony.

The distinction between "real" and "simple" rape persists in the narratives of rape survivors such as Estrich herself (see also Brison; Francisco; Raine). Survivors of "real" rape report that they feel "lucky" (Sebold) because they suffered actual injury and thus are believed. Public validation of their having been wronged is important (Francisco, 43), but difficult to obtain in a "simple" rape committed by an acquaintance, due to social attitudes that acquaintance rape does not victimize the way stranger rape does (Warshaw and Parrot, 75–77). But acquaintance rape, some claim, can be as traumatic a violation of a woman's embodiment and agency as stranger rape (Cahill, 197). Indeed, some contend that the violation of trust involved in acquaintance rape may be worse than a stranger's coercion (Byers and O'Sullivan, 2). "People are more afraid of stranger crime because they assume, often wrongly, that no one they know would victimize them. But . . . betrayal by someone you know may be every bit as terrifying, or more so, than random violence" (Estrich, 25).

Does the wrongfulness of rape depend on whether the actor was an acquaintance or a stranger? Arguably, someone whose life has been threatened and who has been sexually assaulted has been violated more seriously than someone who, not fearing for her life, has had unwanted sex. Threats, however, are not restricted to stranger rapes; acquaintances, too, may threaten, even lethally. Ultimately, the relevant differences are not whether the perpetrator was an acquaintance or a stranger but the extent and type of sexual imposition and sexual violation (see below).

Traditionally, the definition of rape excluded forced sex between spouses: "[T]he husband cannot be guilty of a rape committed by himself upon his lawful wife, for by their mutual matrimonial consent and contract the wife hath given up herself in this kind unto her husband, which she cannot retract" (Matthew Hale [1609–1676], vol. 1, chap. 58, 629). Although this rule is no longer generally accepted, many jurisdictions in the United States still exclude spousal rape (see Hasday, 1375; **Richard Posner** and Silbaugh). The Model Penal Code also excludes nonmarried but cohabiting couples (213.6 [2]). Yet spousal sex can have all the features of rape: It can be against her most vigorous protests, threatening, violent, even deadly.

One explanation for the spousal exclusion is the conception of rape as a property crime, like **adultery** and **seduction**, and hence a trespass on the property of a woman's father or husband (see **Thomas Aquinas** [1224/25–1274], *Summa theologiae* IIaIIae, ques. 154, art. 6–7). Because trespassing on one's own property is impossible, it followed that a husband could not rape his wife (Burgess-Jackson, 44). Another explanation is the idea that a woman's getting married includes her consent, in advance, to sex whenever her husband wants it. (This is the "conjugal debt" or "**marriage** debt"; see Schroeder, 1195–99. Note, however, that the debt, as originally articulated by **Saint Paul** [5–64?] in 1 Cor. 7:4–5, was egalitarian: Each spouse owed sex to the other.) Even now, the Model Penal Code explains the exclusion by contending that marriage gives "a blanket [*sic*] consent to sexual intimacy" (213.1 [comment]). Yet nonconsensual sex within marriage can be just as harmful as nonconsensual sex outside marriage (Burgess-Jackson, 116). Nonetheless, legal-institutional reasons may count against criminalizing spousal rape. The state may choose not to interfere with intimate family matters. Difficulties surrounding evidence and proof may seem especially acute, particularly if rape is defined as nonconsensual (rather than forceful) sex. Despite these institutional concerns, the decision against criminalizing spousal rape is a failure to protect women from **sexual violence** in intimate relationships.

That two people are acquainted or even dating does not in itself imply their willingness to have a sexual relationship. But especially within a dating relationship, the meanings of consent and coercion may be complex. The Model Penal Code grades the offense of rape differently, depending on whether the victim was a voluntary social companion of the rapist and they had previously had sexual contact. If she was not a voluntary social companion and they had never had sexual contact, rape is a first-degree felony, but if she was a voluntary social companion or they had had prior sexual contact, it is second-degree (213.1[1]). This gradation points out the difficult questions about consent and coercion that lie at the heart of distinguishing acquaintance and especially date rape from merely bad sex.

In understanding consent, a crucial task is to distinguish unwanted but voluntary sex from sex that is "chosen" but only in response to undue coercion (see Baker, 53–55). On one liberal view of rape, consent is the critical dividing line between date rape and a "bad sex" experience. But what is consent? If rape is an offense against sexual autonomy (see Pineau; Schulhofer) or a nonconsensual invasion of the body (Burgess-Jackson, 49), consent here should be understood on the model of consent in other circumstances in which autonomy or bodily integrity is at issue. The models most often suggested are drawn from political philosophy (consent to political authority) and bioethics (informed consent to medical treatment). In these circumstances, consent is an *act* that changes relationships among people, not merely a report about the mental state of the consenting person (Baker, 52). The consenting individual must have the capacity to consent, be informed about what is at stake, and have a range of reasonable alternatives. She must also be free of coercion. Rejected here is a model of tacit or implicit consent, according to which consenting to go on a date might, in some situations, encompass or imply consenting to other things that might happen on the date, including sex (Schulhofer, 271).

The most complete account of rape as a violation of sexual autonomy and of informed consent as that which divides sexual offense from bad sex has been developed by Stephen Schulhofer. On his view, "rape" should be reserved for cases of violence, while a new category, "sexual assault," should be used for nonconsensual sex. This includes coercive offers, impermissible threats, decisional incapacity, abuse of trust or authority (e.g., on the part of teachers, physicians, lawyers), and negligent failure to ascertain consent in the face of either protests or silence from the victim. Along the lines of the medical model of informed consent, this model requires that persons have adequate information about the proposed social encounter and the alternatives (see Mappes). Is he planning to ply her with alcohol and get her into bed? Is he seeking a long-range relationship or a one-night stand? Does he have a **sexually transmitted disease**? Is he romantically involved with someone else? What might happen if she does not consent to sex—will he end the relationship? By contrast, a far more limited informed consent requirement is found in statutes that define intercourse induced by a false promise of marriage as a lesser sexual offense. (It is a misdemeanor in the Model Penal Code; see 213.3 [1][d], 213.3 [2].)

The medical model also requires decision-making capacity. Rape statutes typically categorize rape as more serious if the victim is very young or unconscious, the obvious cases of incapacity (Schulhofer, 101). Statutes also typically categorize it as more serious if the victim, without her knowledge, was given a substance by the rapist intended to impair her judgment. Most difficult are cases in which the parties voluntarily ingest a substance that impairs judgment or diminishes inhibitions (see Richardson and Hammock; Wertheimer, *Consent*, 232–57). In the Model Penal Code, the offense in these cases could be at most "sexual assault," the misdemeanor offense of sexual contact known to be offensive to the victim (213.4 [1]). On the medical model of consent, taking advantage of a victim's impaired state is a serious violation of her autonomy. Critics of this broader understanding of rape argue that it is unfair to the male who, in the context of mutual drinking, may have reasonably believed she consented. It might also be unjustifiably paternalistic to the woman: She is seen as someone who needs protection from her own mistaken choices, such as getting into unpleasant or risky situations (see Roiphe). These cases illustrate the more general problem of determining when background conditions render consent not fully voluntary. What if a woman begins by saying "no," but he keeps insisting and she eventually acquiesces, engaging in sex she does not want? Lois Pineau's idea of "communicative sexuality" speaks to this problem by requiring step-by-step, active consent to sexual escalation in a dating context. Antioch University's sexual offense policy (in Francis, 135–54; Leone and Koster, 10–22) implements this approach. It has been praised for its efforts to promote and protect autonomy and criticized as paternalistic and for misunderstanding the nature and function of consent (see Kittay; Soble).

If date rape is wrong because it violates a woman's sexual autonomy, the absence of consent should define the offense. But defining rape this way instead of by the use of force poses difficulties for prosecutor and victim. If rape is defined by the absence of consent, the prosecution has to prove beyond a reasonable doubt that the woman did not consent. This sets a high barrier, since it means proving a negative. Furthermore, it puts evidence about the victim at the center of the case, opening her to examination about her sexuality and prior relations with the rapist. (By contrast, evidence about victim consent is not required for proof of crimes against property; there is no need to show that the victim did not consent to the transfer of goods.) For these reasons the consent requirement has been a target of legal reformers. "Reformed" statutes define rape by the use of force; the Model Penal Code, for example, requires proof of force for conviction of rape and relegates proof that the victim was consenting to the status of a defense (213.1, 213.6 [comment]). However, the effect of this approach is that nonviolent, nonconsensual sex—much date rape—is removed from the category of rape and is relegated to a lesser offense category (if it even remains an offense). The insistence on violence ignores much culpable interference with sexual autonomy (Schulhofer, 115).

Another question in determining consent is the relevance of threats and offers, either of which can be coercive and undermine consent. Threats may range from acts of mild violence that seem harbingers of worse to come (the "light choking" of *State v. Rusk*), to refusals of what is legitimately expected (a ride home), to warnings about the status of the relationship (it will end unless she "goes all the way"). Determining the legitimacy of these threats—which, if enacted, make someone worse off—requires an account of the morality of coercion. The issues are complex. Still, getting sex through threatened violence is wrongful, as are threats to renege on agreements or legitimate expectations (the ride home). By contrast, autonomous agents generally have a right to bring relationships to an end if they are not receiving the satisfactions they were hoping for (see Murphy; Wertheimer, "Consent"). Absent special circumstances, "If you don't have sex with me, I won't marry you" is a coercive threat that may be no more or no less blameworthy than "If you don't marry me soon, I won't have sex with you any longer." But perhaps we accept these judgments too quickly, especially when victims are in vulnerable circumstances. And there is the complication of gender differences in attitudes about what is permissible coercion or pressure (Johnson and Sigler, 77).

Coercive offers, affirmations that someone will be made better off, are similarly morally problematic. Indeed, the distinction between a threat ("Have sex with me or I'll beat you") and an offer ("Have sex with me and I won't beat you *today*") is itself problematic (Malm, 151–52). "If you promise to marry me, I will have sex with you" and "If you have sex with me, I promise to marry you" are coercive offers—they imply making the recipient better off, but at a cost—yet they might not be morally objectionable. A morally suspicious coercive offer in a date rape context might be an offer by a professor (dating a student) to write an especially glowing letter of recommendation, or an offer by a wealthy gentleman to pay a woman's college tuition in exchange for sex. As with threats, the morality of offers depends on the background legitimacy of what is promised in the offer.

In addition to the physical element of nonconsensual sex, rape as a crime has a mental element. Otherwise, rape would be a "strict liability" offense, one that consists of a physical act alone without any mental culpability on the part of the offender. Defining the mental element of rape, its *mens rea*, is a controversial undertaking. In perhaps the most notorious example, a woman's husband told his male companions that his wife liked sex with multiple partners but would nevertheless pretend to be protesting (*Director of Public Prosecutions v. Morgan*). The British House of Lords held that an honest or sincere, even if unreasonable, belief that a woman consented provided a defense to an allegation of rape. *Morgan* unleashed a stream of critical reactions (see Archard; Bienen; Curley).

For some scholars, the most serious offense category should be reserved for rapes in which a man knew or should have known that the woman was not consenting. Negligent failure to ascertain whether a woman is consenting should suffice for the mental element of a lesser sexual assault offense (Schulhofer, 258). Other commentators argue that negligence in ascertaining consent is an appropriate *mens rea* for rape: Marcia Baron writes, in much the spirit of Pineau, "It is reasonable to require everyone to attend to whether or not their (supposed) partner is consenting to sexual intimacy, and, if there is reason to suspect that he or she is not consenting, to ask" (9).

Douglas Husak and George Thomas (1992, 2001) argue that a man's reasonable belief that sex was consensual should be a defense to a charge of rape and, moreover, that "reasonableness" should be understood expansively. On their view, whether beliefs about consent are reasonable should be assessed in terms of generalizations about how consent is commonly given, which they think is typically nonverbally (see Hickman and Muehlenhard). They contend that law that intervenes to alter these social conventions is unacceptably moralistic. They cite an empirical study that found that over a third of female subjects express nonconsent indirectly and another study that showed that over half of those refusing overtures did so nonverbally. For Husak and Thomas, men are more likely to construe behavior as signaling consent than are women, and this must figure into the assessment of the reasonableness of their beliefs. (This is why MacKinnon insists that relying on "reasonable belief as a standard without asking . . . to whom the belief is reasonable and why—meaning, what conditions make it reasonable—is one-sided: male-sided"; 183.) Some studies do point to gender differences in beliefs about consent. Charlene Muehlenhard and her colleagues ("Is Date Rape Justifiable?") found that "traditional" and "nontraditional" males vary in their estimates of what women want. Further, beliefs about reasonable expectations differ and depend on the circumstances: whether, for example, the date is attending a religious event or watching television in the man's apartment. Susan Ehrlich, in analyzing the transcript of a sexual assault proceeding at the University of York, found that gendered ideology influences whether responses to sexual advances are understood as consenting or nonconsenting. Schulhofer (59–68) details the difficulty of legal reforms that cut against such folkways. But along with other commentators (e.g., McGregor), he argues that the law must take seriously that "no" means no, at least to the point that it affirms that men are criminally negligent if they proceed to intercourse, ignoring the possibility that the "no" might very well be genuine.

Rape is also beset with problems of proof. Gendered attitudes color rape allegations with the suspicion that "women lie" (Estrich, 43). Rules of evidence in rape cases have included the requirements of corroboration and of a "fresh" complaint. The Model Penal Code, for example, requires that sexual offenses be reported within three months (213.6 [4]). A rationale for this requirement is that a consenting partner could become a vindictive accuser in response to later regrets or events. Satisfying the freshness requirement, however, might be more difficult in cases involving acquaintances than in cases involving strangers, if women are more ambivalent about reporting events involving acquaintances. Further, because acquaintance and date rapes often take place in private settings, corroborating evidence is difficult to provide. The woman's sexual history has been examined for evidence concerning several factors: her propensity to fabricate, the likelihood that she actually did consent, the reasonableness of the man's belief that she consented, and whether the sexual act really did cause her harm. Although in many jurisdictions these evidentiary rules are no longer formally imposed, in practice they still affect rape trials (Schulhofer, 25–27). Like the definitions of rape as an offense, the evidentiary rules of rape tend to favor conviction in stranger rape and to make conviction more difficult in acquaintance rape. They have also been the basis for suggestions that acquaintance rape should be regarded as a lesser criminal offense or even that it should be moved from the criminal law altogether to civil damage remedies (see Bohmer and Parrot, 140–66).

Although these epistemological difficulties are real, they are insufficient for concluding that only stranger rapes are "real" rapes. Rape accompanied by violence might be more traumatic and more easily identified. Nevertheless, sex imposed by an acquaintance or by a dating partner, without consent, is a violation of autonomy in an intimate matter. Problems in proving that it has occurred should be recognized in maintaining due process protections for offenders, but they are not grounds for devaluing the seriousness of either acquaintance or date rape.

See also Abortion; Coercion (by Sexually Aggressive Women); Consent; Contraception; Ethics, Professional Codes of; Ethics, Sexual; Flirting; Incest; Law, Sex and the; Paglia, Camille; Rape; Seduction; Violence, Sexual

REFERENCES

American Law Institute. *Model Penal Code*. Philadelphia, Pa.: Author, 1962; Archard, David. "The *Mens Rea* of Rape: Reasonableness and Culpable Mistakes." In Keith Burgess-Jackson, ed., *A Most Detestable Crime: New Philosophical Essays on Rape*. New York: Oxford University Press, 1999, 213–29; Baker, Brenda M. "Understanding Consent in Sexual Assault." In Keith Burgess-Jackson, ed., *A Most Detestable Crime: New Philosophical Essays on Rape*. New York: Oxford University Press, 1999, 49–70; Baron, Marcia. "I Thought She Consented." *Noûs*, supp. 11 (2001), 1–32; Benedict, Jeffrey R. *Athletes and Acquaintance Rape*. Thousand Oaks, Calif.: Sage, 1998; Bienen, Leigh. "Mistakes." *Philosophy and Public Affairs* 7 (Spring 1978), 224–45; Bohmer, Carol, and Andrea Parrot. *Sexual Assault on Campus: The Problem and the Solution*. New York: Lexington Books, 1993; Brison, Susan J. *Aftermath: Violence and the Remaking of a Self*. Princeton, N.J.: Princeton University Press, 2000; Burgess-Jackson, Keith. *Rape: A Philosophical Investigation*. Aldershot, U.K.: Dartmouth, 1996; Byers, E. Sandra, and Lucia F. O'Sullivan, eds. *Sexual Coercion in Dating Relationships*. New York: Haworth Press, 1996; Cahill, Ann J. *Rethinking Rape*. Ithaca, N.Y.: Cornell University Press, 2001; Campbell-Ruggaard, Julie, and Jami Van Ryswyk. "Rape on Campus: Numbers Tell Less Than Half the Story." In Merril D. Smith, ed., *Sex without Consent: Rape and Sexual Coercion in America*. New York: New York University Press, 2001, 283–99; "Comment: Forcible and Statutory Rape: An Exploration of the Operation and Objectives of the Consent Standard." *Yale Law Journal* 52:1 (1952), 55–83; Cowling, Mark. *Date Rape and Consent*. Aldershot, U.K.: Ashgate, 1998; Curley, E. M. "Excusing Rape." *Philosophy and Public Affairs* 5:4 (1976), 325–60; *Director of Public Prosecutions v. Morgan*. 2 All. E. R. 347, 1976 App. Cas. 182 (H.L. 1975); Ehrlich, Susan. "The Discursive Reconstruction of Sexual Consent." *Discourse and Society* 9:2 (1998), 149–71; Estrich, Susan. *Real Rape: How the Legal System Victimizes Women Who Say No*. Cambridge, Mass.: Harvard University Press, 1987; Francis, Leslie P., ed. *Date Rape: Feminism, Philosophy, and the Law*. State College: Pennsylvania State University Press, 1996; Francisco, Patricia Weaver. *Telling: A Memoir of Rape and Recovery*. New York: HarperCollins, 1999; Hale, Matthew (Sir). (1736) *The History of the Pleas of the Crown*, 2 vols. London: Professional Books Limited, 1971; Hasday, Jill. "Contest and Consent: A Legal History of Marital Rape." *California Law Review* 88 (October 2000), 1373–1505; Hickman, Susan, and Charlene L. Muehlenhard. "By the Semi-Mystical Appearance of a Condom: How Young Women and Men Communicate Sexual Consent in Heterosexual Situations." *Journal of Sex Research* 36:3 (1999), 258–72; Husak, Douglas N., and George C. Thomas III. "Date Rape, Social Convention, and Reasonable Mistakes." *Law and Philosophy* 11:1–2 (1992), 95–126; Husak, Douglas N., and George C. Thomas III. "Rapes without Rapists: Consent and Reasonable Mistake." *Noûs*, supp. 11 (2001), 86–117; Johnson, Ida M., and Robert T. Sigler. *Forced Sexual Intercourse in Intimate Relationships*. Aldershot, U.K.: Ashgate, 1997; Kittay, Eva Feder. "AH! My Foolish Heart: A Reply to Alan Soble's 'Antioch's "Sexual Offense Policy": A Philosophical Exploration.'" *Journal of Social Philosophy* 28:2 (1997), 153–59; Leone, Bruno, and Katie de Koster, eds. *Rape on Campus*. San Diego, Calif.: Greenhaven, 1995; MacKinnon, Catharine. *Toward a Feminist Theory of the State*. Cambridge, Mass.: Harvard University Press, 1989; Malm, H. M. "The Ontological Status of Consent and Its Implications for the Law on Rape." *Legal Theory* 2:2 (1996), 147–64; Mappes, Thomas A. "Sexual Morality and the Concept of Using Another Person." In Thomas A. Mappes and Jane S. Zembaty, eds., *Social Ethics: Morality and Social Policy*, 6th ed. Boston, Mass.: McGraw-Hill, 2002, 170–83; McGregor, Joan. "Why When She Says No She Doesn't Mean Maybe and Doesn't Mean Yes: A Critical Reconstruction of Consent, Sex, and the Law." *Legal Theory* 2:3 (1996), 175–208; Muehlenhard, Charlene L., Debra E. Friedman, and Celeste M. Thomas. "Is Date Rape Justifiable? The Effects of Dating Activity, Who Initiated, Who Paid, and Men's Attitudes toward Women." *Psychology of Women Quarterly* 9:3 (1985), 297–310; Muehlenhard, Charlene L., and Lisa C. Hollabaugh. "Do Women Sometimes Say No When They Mean Yes?

The Prevalence and Correlates of Women's Token Resistance to Sex." *Journal of Personality and Social Psychology* 54:5 (1988), 872–79; Murphy, Jeffrie G. "Some Ruminations on Women, Violence, and the Criminal Law." In Jules Coleman and Allen Buchanan, eds., *In Harm's Way: Essays in Honor of Joel Feinberg*. Cambridge: Cambridge University Press, 1994, 209–30; National Center for Victims of Crime. (2004) "Victim Assistance." <www.ncvc.org/gethelp/acquaintancerape> [accessed 19 May 2004]; Pineau, Lois. "Date Rape: A Feminist Analysis." *Law and Philosophy* 8:2 (1989), 217–43; Posner, Richard A., and Katharine B. Silbaugh. "Marital Exemptions from Rape and Sexual Assault." In *A Guide to America's Sex Laws*. Chicago, Ill.: University of Chicago Press, 1996, 35–43; Raine, Nancy Venable. *After Silence: Rape and My Journey Back*. New York: Crown, 1998; Richardson, Deborah R., and Georgina S. Hammock. "Alcohol and Acquaintance Rape." In Andrea Parrot and Laurie Bechhofer, eds., *Acquaintance Rape: The Hidden Crime*. New York: Wiley, 1991, 83–95; Roiphe, Katie. *The Morning After: Sex, Fear, and Feminism on Campus*. New York: Little, Brown, 1993; Russell, Diana E. H., and Rebecca M. Bolen. *The Epidemic of Rape and Child Sexual Abuse in the United States*. Thousand Oaks, Calif.: Sage, 2000; Scarce, Michael. *Male on Male Rape: The Hidden Toll of Stigma and Shame*. New York: Plenum Press, 1997; Schroeder, Jeanne L. "Feminism Historicized: Medieval Misogynist Stereotypes in Contemporary Feminist Jurisprudence." *Iowa Law Review* 75 (July 1990), 1135–1217; Schulhofer, Stephen. *Unwanted Sex: The Culture of Intimidation and the Failure of Law*. Cambridge, Mass.: Harvard University Press, 1998; Sebold, Alice. *Lucky*. Boston, Mass.: Back Bay Books, 2002; Soble, Alan. "Antioch's 'Sexual Offense Policy': A Philosophical Exploration." *Journal of Social Philosophy* 28:1 (1997): 22–36; Sommers, Christina Hoff. *Who Stole Feminism? How Women Have Betrayed Women*. New York: Simon and Schuster, 1994; *State v. Rusk*. 289 Md. 230, 424 A.2d 720 (1981); Thomas Aquinas. (1265–1273) *Summa theologiae*, 60 vols. Trans. Blackfriars. Cambridge, U.K.: Blackfriars, 1964–1976; Warshaw, Robin, and Andrea Parrot. "The Contribution of Sex-Role Socialization to Acquaintance Rape." In Andrea Parrot and Laurie Bechhofer, eds., *Acquaintance Rape: The Hidden Crime*. New York: Wiley, 1991, 73–82; Wertheimer, Alan. "Consent and Sexual Relations." *Legal Theory* 2:2 (1996), 89–112; Wertheimer, Alan. *Consent to Sexual Relations*. Cambridge: Cambridge University Press, 2003; West, Robin. "A Comment on Consent, Sex, and Rape." *Legal Theory* 2:3 (1996), 233–51; Wiehe, Vernon R., and Ann L. Richards. *Intimate Betrayal: Understanding and Responding to the Trauma of Acquaintance Rape*. Thousand Oaks, Calif.: Sage, 1995.

Leslie P. Francis

ADDITIONAL READING

Abbey, Antonio. "Sex Differences in Attributions for Friendly Behavior: Do Males Misperceive Females' Friendliness?" *Journal of Personality and Social Psychology* 42:5 (1982), 830–38; Anderson, Peter B., and Cindy Struckman-Johnson, eds. *Sexually Aggressive Women: Current Perspectives and Controversies*. New York: Guilford, 1998; Antioch College. "The Antioch College Sexual Offense Prevention Policy." In P&S3 (640–60). Reprinted, abridged, in Robert Trevas, Arthur Zucker, and Donald Borchert, eds., *Philosophy of Sex and Love: A Reader*. Upper Saddle River, N.J.: Prentice-Hall, 1997, 384–93; and Jodi Gold and Susan Villari, eds., *Just Sex: Students Rewrite the Rules on Sex, Violence, Activism, and Equality*. Lanham, Md.: Rowman and Littlefield, 2000, 292–93; Archard, David. " 'A Nod's as Good as a Wink': Consent, Convention, and Reasonable Belief." *Legal Theory* 3:3 (1997), 273–90; Archard, David. *Sexual Consent*. Boulder, Colo.: Westview, 1998; Baker, Katharine K. "Sex, Rape, and Shame." *Boston University Law Review* 79:3 (1999), 663–716; Balos, Beverly, and Mary Louise Fellows. "Guilty of the Crime of Trust: Nonstranger Rape." *Minnesota Law Review* 75 (February 1991), 599–618; Belliotti, Raymond. "A Philosophical Analysis of Sexual Ethics." *Journal of Social Philosophy* 10:3 (1979), 8–11; Bogart, John H. "On the Nature of Rape." *Public Affairs Quarterly* 5:2 (1991), 117–36. Reprinted in STW (168–80); Bogart, John H. "Reconsidering Rape: Rethinking the Conceptual Foundations of Rape Law." *Canadian Journal of Law and Jurisprudence* 8:1 (1995), 159–82; Burchard, Melissa. "Feminist Jurisprudence." In James Fieser, ed., *The Internet Encyclopedia of Philosophy*. <www.iep.utm.edu/j/jurisfem.htm> [accessed 8 September 2004]; Burgess, Ann Wolbert, ed. *Rape and Sexual Assault: A Research Handbook*. New York: Garland, 1985; Burgess, Ann Wolbert, ed. *Rape and Sexual Assault II*. New York: Garland, 1988; Burgess, Ann Wolbert, ed. *Rape and Sexual Assault III: A Research Handbook*. New York: Garland, 1991; Burgess-Jackson, Keith. "Rape and Persuasive Definition." *Canadian Journal of Philosophy* 25 (September 1995), 415–54; Burgess-Jackson, Keith. "Wife Rape." *Public Affairs Quarterly* 12 (January 1998), 1–22; Burgess-Jackson, Keith, ed. *A Most Detestable Crime: New Philosophical Essays on Rape*. New York: Oxford University Press, 1999; Cowling, Mark, and Paul Reynolds, eds. *Making Sense of Sexual Consent*. Aldershot, U.K.: Ashgate, 2004; Crowley, Ray. " 'Consent Condoms'? No Thanks." *Spiked* (4 July 2001). <www.spiked-online.com/Articles/00000002D16E.htm> [accessed 31 August 2004]; Doniger, Wendy. "Sex, Lies, and Tall Tales." *Social Research* 63:3 (1996), 663–99; Estrich, Susan. "Rape." In Patricia Smith, ed., *Feminist Jurisprudence*. New York: Oxford University Press, 1993, 158–87; Francis, Leslie P. "Rape." In Ruth Chadwick, ed., *Encyclopedia of Applied Ethics*, vol. 3. San Diego, Calif.: Academic Press, 1998, 791–98; Frederick, Sharon, and the Award Committee on Rape. *Rape: Weapon of Terror*. River Edge, N.J.: Global, 2001; Gilbert, Neil. "Realities and Mythologies of Rape." *Society* 29 (May–June 1992), 4–10; Gold, Jodi, and Susan Villari, eds. *Just Sex: Students Rewrite the Rules on Sex, Violence, Activism, and Equality*. Lanham, Md.: Rowman and Littlefield, 2000; Hampton, Jean. "Defining Wrong and Defining Rape." In Keith Burgess-Jackson, ed., *A Most Detestable Crime: New Philosophical Essays on Rape*. New York: Oxford University Press, 1999, 118–56; Henley, Nancy M., and Cheris Kramarae. "Gender, Power, and Miscommunication." In Nikolas Coupland, Howard Giles, and John M. Wiemann, eds., *"Miscommunication" and Problematic Talk*. Newbury Park, Calif.: Sage, 1991, 18–43; Hershfield, Jeffrey. "The Threat of Acquaintance Rape: A Reply to Reitan." *Southwest Philosophy Review* 20:2 (2004), 171–73; Hickman, Susan E., and Charlene L. Muehlenhard. "College Women's Fears and Precautionary Behaviors Related to Acquaintance Rape and Stranger Rape." *Psychology of Women Quarterly* 21:4 (1997), 527–47; Hurd, Heidi M. "The Moral Magic of Consent." *Legal Theory* 2:2 (1996), 121–46; Husak, Douglas N., and George C. Thomas III. "Date Rape, Social Convention, and Reasonable Mistakes." *Law and Philosophy* 11:1–2 (1992), 95–126. Reprinted, abridged, in Lori Gruen and George Panichas, eds., *Sex, Morality, and the Law*. New York: Routledge, 1997, 444–54; Iannone, Carol. "Sex and the Feminists." *Commentary* 96:3 (September 1993), 51–54; Kamen, Paula. "Acquaintance Rape: Revolution and Reaction." In Nan Bauer Maglin and Donna Perry, eds., *"Bad Girls"/"Good Girls": Women, Sex, and Power in the Nineties*. New Brunswick, N.J.: Rutgers University Press, 1996, 137–49; Kittay, Eva Feder. "AH! My Foolish Heart: A Reply to Alan Soble's 'Antioch's "Sexual Offense Policy": A Philosophical Exploration.' " *Journal of Social Philosophy* 28:2 (1997), 153–59. Reprinted in Ellen K. Feder, Karmen MacKendrick, and Sybol S. Cook, eds., *A Passion for Wisdom: Readings in Western Philosophy on Love and Desire*. Upper Saddle River, N.J.: Prentice Hall, 2004, 755–60; Kramer, Karen M. "Rule by Myth: The Social and Legal Dynamics Governing Alcohol-Related Acquaintance Rapes." *Stanford Law Review* 47 (November 1994), 115–60; Lim, Grace, and Michael Roloff. "Attributing Sexual Consent." *Journal of Applied Communication Research* 27:1 (1999), 1–24; M., Jack. "Confessions of a Date Rapist." In Michael S. Kimmel and Michael A. Messner, eds., *Men's Lives*, 3rd ed. Needham Heights, Mass.: Allyn and Bacon, 1995, 318–21; Mappes, Thomas A. "Sexual Morality and the Concept of Using Another Person." In Thomas A. Mappes and Jane S. Zembaty, eds., *Social Ethics: Morality and Social Policy*, 5th ed. Boston, Mass.: McGraw-Hill, 1997, 163–76. 6th ed., Boston, Mass.: McGraw-Hill, 2002, 170–83. Reprinted in POS4 (207–23); McGregor, Joan. *Is It Rape? On Acquaintance Rape and Taking Women's Consent Seriously*. Aldershot, U.K.: Ashgate, 2005; Muehlenhard, Charlene L., and Jennifer L. Schrag. "Nonviolent Sexual Coercion." In Andrea Parrot and Laurie Bechhofer, eds., *Acquaintance Rape: The Hidden Crime*. New York: John Wiley, 1991, 115–28; Newman, Graeme. *Global Report on Crime and Justice*. New York: Oxford University Press, 1999; Paglia, Camille. *Sex, Art, and American Culture: Essays*. New York: Vintage Books, 1992; Parrot, Andrea, and Laurie Bechhofer, eds. *Acquaintance Rape: The Hidden Crime*. New York: John Wiley, 1991; Phillips, Lynn M. *Flirting with Danger: Young Women's Reflections on Sexuality and Domination*. New York: New York University Press, 2000; Pineau, Lois. "Date Rape: A Feminist Analysis." *Law and Philosophy* 8:2 (1989), 217–43. Reprinted in Hugh LaFollette, ed., *Ethics in Practice: An Anthology*, 1st ed. Cambridge, Mass.: Blackwell, 1997, 418–28; 2nd ed., 2002, 410–17; in Leslie P. Francis, ed., *Date Rape: Feminism, Philosophy, and the Law*. State College: Pennsylvania State University Press, 1996, 1–26; HS (483–509); Pirog-Good, Maureen, and Jan E. Stets, eds. *Violence in Dating Relationships: Emerging Social Issues*. New York: Praeger, 1989; Pollitt, Katha. "Not Just Bad Sex." *The New Yorker* (4 October 1993), 220–24. Reprinted in *Reasonable Creatures: Essays on Women and Feminism*. New York: Knopf, 1994, 157–68; and Adele M. Stan, ed., *Debating Sexual Correctness: Pornography, Sexual Harassment, Date Rape, and the Politics of Sexual Equality*. New York: Delta, 1995, 161–71; Primoratz, Igor. "Sexual Morality: Is Consent Enough?" *Ethical Theory and Moral Practice* 4:3 (2001), 201–18; Reitan, Eric. "Date Rape and Seduction: Towards a Defense of Pineau's Definition of 'Date Rape.'" *Southwest Philosophy Review* 20:1 (2004), 99–106; Reitan, Eric. "Rape as an Essentially Contested Concept." *Hypatia* 16:2 (2001), 43–66; Russell, Diana E. H. (1982) *Rape in Marriage*, rev. ed. Bloomington: Indiana University Press, 1990; Russell, Gordon W., ed. *Violence in Intimate Relationships*. New York: PMA Publishing, 1988; Sanday, Peggy Reeves. *Fraternity Gang Rape: Sex, Brotherhood, and Privilege on Campus*. New York: New York University Press, 1990; Sanday, Peggy Reeves. *A Woman Scorned: Acquaintance Rape on Trial*. New York: Doubleday, 1996; Schulhofer, Stephen J. "The Gender Question in Criminal Law." *Social Philosophy and Policy* 7 (Spring 1990), 105–37. Reprinted in Ellen Frankel Paul, Fred Miller, and Jeffrey Paul, eds., *Crime, Culpability, and Remedy*. Oxford, U.K.: Blackwell, 1990, 105–37; Schulhofer, Stephen J. "Rape in the Twilight Zone: When Sex Is Unwanted but Not Illegal." *Suffolk University Law Review* 38:2 (2005), 415–25; Shalit, Wendy. "The Fallout." In *A Return to Modesty: Discovering the Lost Virtue*. New York: Free Press, 1999, 39–57; Soble, Alan. "Antioch's 'Sexual Offense Policy': A Philosophical Exploration." *Journal of Social Philosophy* 28:1 (1997), 22–36. Reprinted in Ellen K. Feder, Karmen MacKendrick, and Sybol S. Cook, eds., *A Passion for Wisdom: Readings in Western Philosophy on Love and Desire*. Upper Saddle River, N.J.: Prentice Hall, 2004, 742–54; in David Boonin and Graham Oddie, eds., *What's Wrong? Applied Ethicists and Their Critics*. New York: Oxford University Press, 2005, 241–49; POS4 (323–40); Sommers, Christina Hoff. *Who Stole Feminism? How Women Have Betrayed Women*. New York: Simon and Schuster, 1994. Expanded paperback edition, 1995; Stan, Adele M., ed. *Debating Sexual Correctness: Pornography, Sexual Harassment, Date Rape, and the Politics of Sexual Equality*. New York: Delta, 1995; Stock, Wendy. "Women's Sexual Coercion of Men: A Feminist Analysis." In Peter B. Anderson and Cindy Struckman-Johnson, eds., *Sexually Aggressive Women: Current Perspectives and Controversies*. New York: Guilford, 1998, 169–84; Struckman-Johnson, Cindy. "Forced Sex on Dates: It Happens to Men, Too." *Journal of Sex Research* 24:1–4 (1988), 234–41; Struckman-Johnson, Cindy. "Male Victims of Acquaintance Rape." In Andrea Parrot and Laurie Bechhofer, eds., *Acquaintance Rape: The Hidden Crime*. New York: John Wiley, 1991, 192–214; Thornton, Mark T. "Rape and *Mens Rea.*" *Canadian Journal of Philosophy*, supp. vol. 8 (1982), 119–46. Also published in Kai Nielsen and Steven C. Patten, eds., *New Essays in Ethics and Public Policy*. Guelph, Can.: Canadian Association for Publishing in Philosophy, 1982, 119–46. Reprinted in HS (435–62); Tong, Rosemarie. *Women, Sex, and the Law*. Totowa, N.J.: Rowman and Littlefield, 1984; Tuana, Nancy. "Sexual Harassment in Academe: Issues of Power and Coercion." *College Teaching* 33:2 (1985), 53–63. Reprinted, abridged, in Edmund Wall, ed., *Sexual Harassment: Confrontations and Decisions*. Buffalo, N.Y.: Prometheus, 1992, 49–60; Ward, Sally K., Jennifer Dziuba-Leatherman, Jane Gerard Stapleton, and Carrie L. Yodanis, eds. *Acquaintance and Date Rape: An Annotated Bibliography*. Westport, Conn.: Greenwood Press, 1994; Warshaw, Robin. *I Never Called It Rape: The Ms. Report on Recognizing, Fighting, and Surviving Date and Acquaintance Rape*. New York: Harper and Row, 1988; Weisberg, D. Kelly, ed. "Rape." In *Applications of Feminist Legal Theory to Women's Lives: Sex, Violence, Work, and Reproduction*. Philadelphia, Pa.: Temple University Press, 1996, 405–527; Wertheimer, Alan. "Consent and Sexual Relations." *Legal Theory* 2:2 (1996), 89–112. Reprinted in POS4 (341–66).

REICH, WILHELM. *See* Freudian Left, The

REPRODUCTIVE TECHNOLOGY. Technological prevention and facilitation of reproduction constitute schemes for human control of the natural consequences of human **sexual activity**. One set of questions, to be explored here, has to do with the ethical and ontological dimensions of the technologies of assisted reproduction.

It is worth remembering that need for assisted reproduction comes in part as an indirect consequence of the sexual liberation made possible by pharmacological suppression of female fertility. Liberation led to increased sexual activity with multiple partners whose sexual histories were not known; that increase brought increased exposure to **sexually transmitted diseases**; and these (chlamydia, gonorrhea) are common causes of infertility. Reduced fertility, however, has other causes. Some are environmental (heavy use of marijuana); others involve physical injury, endocrine, and other disorders (endometriosis); and genetic or developmental conditions also play a role (cryptorchidism, undescended testis).

Humans have sought sterilization through chemical or surgical means as a way of putting off generation of children while permitting the enjoyment of sexual intercourse. Pharmacological substances that prevent ovulation offer temporary, reversible sterilization to women. Comparable drugs that suppress production of sperm have not been developed and accepted by men, perhaps because the consequences of conception are not so immediate and unavoidable for them. Surgical sterilization for both men and women has long been available but generally restricted in voluntary contexts to those couples whose reproductive goals have been realized. Even in those cases (for example, vasectomy), reversal is sometimes sought when reproductive aims change on remarriage or the death of children. Unsuccessful reversal in someone strongly motivated to reproduce constitutes a powerful motive for seeking reproduction assistance.

Involuntary sterilization has been imposed on persons under multiple felony convictions or on those judged incapable of following contraceptive regimens or of being responsible parents (*Buck v. Bell*). However, the right to reproduce has been found to be so fundamental (*Skinner v. Oklahoma*; *Stanley v. Illinois*) that involuntary measures are constitutionally controversial and applied justly only to protect individuals from the medical harm to themselves of unintended pregnancy. The practice remains highly controversial either as a eugenic measure (since mental retardation is generally not genetic in etiology) or as a convenient way for guardians to avoid unwanted minor charges, chiefly due to the lack of competent understanding on the part of those sterilized (see Lapon).

Estimates run as high as 14 percent of couples of childbearing age that experience involuntary infertility (Fox). In most cases, the causes are correctable with minimal medical or surgical interventions. But chronic infertility can be a devastating condition that provides enormous stress and strong motivation to achieve child rearing in other ways. Prior to the emergence of earlier assisted reproductive technologies, couples suffering from infertility—defined as an inability to conceive over the course of twelve months of unprotected intercourse—typically resorted to adoption to satisfy their desire for children. With the development of technologically assisted reproduction, adoption rates have dropped. But the number of domestic children available for adoption has also dropped as a result of the technologies of **contraception** and **abortion**. Couples seeking adoption must turn, increasingly, to adoptable children of other races and nationalities, which raises questions about transcultural adoption (Montalvo).

Discussion of the ethics of reproductive technology was forestalled by its unavailability. What discussion there was centered on the question of the licitness of low-tech measures, such as artificial insemination, and on worries about the prospects of more sophisticated technologies under experimental development. The announcement of the birth of Louise Brown by British doctors Patrick Steptoe and Robert Edwards (25 July 1978) marked a major turning point in the ethical discussion of the new technologies. Louise was the first baby to result from *in vitro* fertilization (IVF), in which ova surgically removed from a woman's ovaries are mixed with sperm in a Petri dish and a selection of one or more fertilized ova are placed in the fallopian tubes or the uterus. Louise was promptly dubbed the "test-tube" baby. Steptoe and Edwards had implanted sixty fertilized ova over the previous ten years, but any resulting pregnancy always failed in its earliest weeks. The high previous mortality rate, combined with worries about whether exteriorization of the egg for two days had harmed it, stimulated some ethicists to criticize the attempt as too risky and premature. Because informed **consent** cannot be obtained from an embryo, and because the prospective parents had a conflict of interest and thus could not properly represent the embryo's interests, some even suggested appointing guardians *ad litem* to represent the prospective embryo in deciding whether to try the procedure.

Such safety concerns have abated as IVF has become widely used. Although success rates of IVF vary widely with the experience of each assisted reproduction clinic, in the most successful clinics the rates approximate normal pregnancy success rates; viewed from the perspective of an ethics of **consequentialism**, comparable success rates imply no moral difference. But viewed from the perspective of nonconsequentialist (or deontological) moral systems, artificial reproductive techniques remain inherently problematic due to the foreseeable exposure of potential offspring to the risks inherent in the technologies. The fact that natural fertilization through coitus is also risky is discounted by nonconsequentialist critics, who distinguish morally between natural harms, which might be permissible, and harms, not permitted, that attach to deliberate acts undertaken as means to admittedly laudable ends.

To concerns about medical risk to the conceptus, other concerns were added: those of religious views, chiefly those voiced by Roman Catholicism. Its criticisms arise from its position on the optimal nature of human reproduction, which partly but not completely depends on its view of the ontological status of the conceptus as a person throughout all stages of development. The Catholic view of the ontological status of the fetus as a person from the point of completion of the ovum's fertilization—often confusingly called the point of conception—imposes duties of respect for the life of the fetus over the interests of the parent; it also influences Catholic moral judgments about reproductive technologies. Criticism of this ontological position has persisted. For example, zygotes and their successor morulas and blastocysts, prior to gastrulation or the emergence of the first cells predestined to give rise to different cell types, lack "nondivisibility," a chief property necessary to all organisms (see Smith and Brogaard). Any one cell of the zygote through blastocyst sequence, if separated from the cluster of identical cells, can give rise to a complete human being, a twin. So prior to the point after which twinning is no longer possible, the product of fertilization and subsequent cell division bears no necessary numerical identity with any future person. The phase in which the specialized cells that give rise to the nervous system, neuralization, begins at day sixteen after fertilization, and it is this point that marks the emergence of the entity that satisfies the full set of criteria for being a distinct human substance. On this view, duties owed to humans are not occurrent until day sixteen after fertilization.

But the Church also holds that reproduction must be through normal conjugal relations that preserve the connection between the "unitive and procreative functions" of intercourse (Congregation for the Doctrine of the Faith; Paul VI). For individuals with fertility problems, correction through surgical or hormonal means restores a natural ability and is therefore licit; the Church did not condemn these restorative reproductive technologies. But technologies that introduce third parties into the actual process of fertilization (with one exception; see below) were condemned because they separated the unitive (spousal support and bonding) and procreative aspects of reproduction. Adoption was seen as not only licit but an (imperfect) duty, because it involved the rescue of an already existing child from a desperate situation.

Various techniques of assisted *in vivo* fertilization have been developed to circumvent specific fertility problems. Artificial insemination (AI) is the simplest of these, used to give the male's sperm access to the female's ovum when erectile disorders, low sperm count, or sperm motility problems have reduced the male's ability to deliver his genetic material. The Catholic condemnation included (with one exception) all forms of artificial insemination: AI with the husband's sperm was illicit because the means of introducing sperm into the vagina was unnatural; AI with a mix of husband's and a donor's sperm, or with a donor's sperm alone (AID), was illicit not only for the unnaturalness of the method but also because offspring were possible whose biological father was not the women's husband. Similarly condemned were means that involved donor ova or embryo transfer to a host mother (biological surrogacy). Contracts with women to provide ova for AI with a husband's sperm, and afterwards gestational services, followed by the surrender of the newborn to the biological father and his wife, were condemned. In all these cases, two principles operated: No substitute for coitus between husband and wife was allowable, and the child had an absolute natural right to be born to and raised by its married biological parents.

The one pragmatic exception made by Catholicism was a technique developed to assist in overcoming infertility due either to low concentrations of sperm in a given ejaculate or to sperm with low motility. It was judged licit for sperm to be collected during coitus between husband and wife in a condom and subsequently introduced through artificial insemination, provided that the condom was constructed with a small opening, such that sperm could have passed through it into the vagina during intercourse. This exception appears to be based on the assumption that sperm from the same source are fungible, so that a pregnancy resulting from this technique could be regarded as resulting from a natural act of coitus, thus preserving the act's unitive and procreative functions (Congregation, n.36).

The Ethics Committee of the American Fertility Society responded to the Congregation's *Instruction* in a 1988 article ("Ethical Considerations") that reconsidered the conclusions of two earlier Ethics Committee articles ("Constitutional Aspects," "Moral Right to Reproduce") in light of the Congregation's differing conclusions. The Committee observed that the legal right to reproduce is virtually unlimited in the United States and is recognized even for unmarried individuals ("Moral Right"). The Committee argued that the right should be extended to assisted means of reproduction, but only as a negative liberty right (government may not interfere), not as a positive legal claim or welfare right to financial assistance in obtaining access to reproductive technology ("Constitutional Aspects"). These arguments illustrate the difference in approach to the issue of AI's moral permissibility between the Vatican's "thick" moral-doctrine-guided position and the "thin" moral-doctrine stance of the American Fertility Society, which argues from a secular standpoint—in particular, one that recognizes the importance of avoiding laws respecting the establishment of any religion. The Vatican's arguments conclude with a call for legislators to institute the *Instruction*'s prohibitions of AI; much of the American Fertility Society's response was to this call, arguing that a zone of **privacy** recognized by the U.S. Supreme Court would preclude legislation restricting reproductive decisions made by patients and their physicians. Thus the Vatican and the American Fertility Society did not usefully engage at the level of "thick" morality. (Another illustration is the difference between the Vatican's approach to abortion and that taken by the U.S. Supreme Court in *Roe v. Wade*.)

The legal status of AID children as illegitimate was another powerful issue that societies wrestled with as the issue of paternity came to the fore in legislative bodies (see Smart). Further, because identities of sperm donors are usually withheld from their offspring, as a requirement of donation, a subtle evolutionary issue arises. Does the assurance and requirement of anonymity select for males who have no interest in their offspring? A bold experiment in Sweden, undertaken under pressure from AID-sired children, eliminated anonymity. Initially, sperm donation dropped precipitously as potential and regular donors were faced with disclosure to their offspring. But a different group of donors emerged, men who wanted contact with their offspring (Hull, *Ethical Issues in the New Reproductive Technologies*, 97). This phenomenon lends support to the evolutionary concern that anonymity may select for parental irresponsibility.

In response to each new advance in technology, similar objections were raised (see Tiefel). The most common objection to advancing reproductive technology invokes the risk that unproven technology holds for prospective children. Management of risk has dictated careful development of the methods employed in nonhuman animal models, followed by application of those methods to ova not intended to be brought through gestation (Zaner). Developing technology gradually recognizes, if only implicitly, the substantially different status of human cell clusters before and after neuralization (Caplan; Cohnitz and Smith; Smith and Brogaard): Clusters before neuralization are not individual human beings with interests that need protection and may be treated as material for research so long as development past neuralization is not involved. The criterion of reliable normal progress through the stages prior to neuralization stands as the threshold of permissible introduction of a new technique into human trials, for this threshold marks the point at which risks to the future child may be assumed to be no greater than those of natural, unassisted conception (Zaner).

Various techniques for circumventing female fertility problems have been devised. Among these are removal of ova from the ovaries of a woman whose fallopian tubes are blocked and reinsertion of the ova below the point of blockage ("gamete intrafallopian transfer," or "GIFT"; see Hull, "Gamete Intrafallopian Transfer"). This is often combined with artificial insemination. More complex, expensive techniques involve IVF (Gore-Langton and Daniel; Mullen et al.). To minimize the risks that come with multiple surgeries, fertility drugs are often administered to guarantee ripening of multiple follicles and removal of numerous ova. Because multiple zygotes are likely to result during IVF, healthy specimens not selected for immediate implantation are cryo-preserved in liquid nitrogen for use in the future, if pregnancy does not occur in the first attempt or more children are desired. Typically, several zygotes are implanted in each attempt to increase the chance of a successful pregnancy.

The practices of multiple implantation and the use of fertility drugs to stimulate ovulation prior to normal, unassisted fertilization through coitus frequently result in multiple pregnancies. The dilemma that arises in these cases is the choice between allowing all fetuses to proceed to delivery (but who will almost assuredly be premature with a high likelihood of severe developmental problems) and selectively reducing the number of fetuses through "therapeutic" abortion. Because confirmation that multiple pregnancy has occurred is generally not possible before neuralization, a choice must be made between impaired lives for all the progeny versus quality of life for some offspring and early death for the others. Few dilemmas for would-be parents are more troublesome.

In this situation, consequentialism would focus on outcomes and would contend that the best (or maximal) consequences are attained by the abortion of all but two of the conceptuses. (Perinatal mortality rates for triplets are nearly twenty times higher than for singleton pregnancies; Henifin.) The decision as to which fetuses would survive would be made either arbitrarily or on medically identifiable grounds of likely healthy survival. (Abortion for sex selection is, as a general policy, problematic for consequentialists.) Deontological approaches, which focus on the nature of the act and not its consequences, commonly condemn the deliberate taking of innocent life, in which case selective abortion in multiple pregnancies is not permitted. Women who utilize the multiple implantation technique therefore bear moral responsibility for potentially imperiling their future children, a consideration that prompts deontologists to oppose the practice itself.

The term "surrogate motherhood" is applied to two distinct strategies. In the correct use of the term, a woman outside a marriage agrees to serve as a gestational host for a fetus resulting from the union of the gametes of a husband and wife. The usual reason for this procedure is the inability of the wife to carry a pregnancy to term, as when a hysterectomy has previously been performed. The gestational surrogate provides the fetus with all the biological support that the genetic mother would provide, were she able to, but surrenders the child to the couple at birth (Purdy and Holmes; Robertson).

The other form occurred in the "Baby M" case, which made "surrogacy" a household word (albeit, used incorrectly). Mary Beth Whitehead, a married woman, contracted in early 1985 with William and Elizabeth Stern to have a child by the husband through artificial insemination. The child, the product of Whitehead's ovum and his sperm, was to be surrendered to the Sterns after its birth. Elizabeth Stern's medical condition, multiple sclerosis, would likely be exacerbated by pregnancy, and she agreed to the arrangement, intending to adopt the issue of her husband's sperm and Mary Beth Whitehead's ovum. But during the pregnancy Mrs. Whitehead bonded with the developing child and as a result refused to turn the child (born on March 27, 1986) over to the Sterns, thereby violating the contract. The Sterns went to court to have the contract enforced. The New Jersey Supreme Court voided the contract on the grounds that such a contract was prohibited by New Jersey's statutes against baby selling. Nevertheless, the court (on February 3, 1988) awarded the child to the Sterns in accordance with the court's determination of the best interests of the child (Whitehead and Schwartz-Nobel; Wilentz). Visitation rights were granted to Mrs. Whitehead.

Reproductive technologies, initially developed to treat medical problems of infertility, have lent themselves to nonmedical uses. Medicine as a profession has not been successful in restricting the use of reproductive technologies to married, childless, heterosexual couples. AI employing the husband's sperm was quickly followed by the employment of donor gametes, and GIFT employing a woman's own ova was soon followed by the fallopian transfer of donor ova. The implantation of fertilized ova from a Petri dish was modified to permit selection of abnormality-free zygotes, a step that required their spending longer time in the artificial environment. Thus further analysis for other, nonlethal characteristics, such as sex and eye color, became possible. The production of multiple zygotes, done to minimize the risk of repetitive surgery, led first to cryopreservation, then to unwanted, "spare" embryos that were sometimes made available for "adoption," and then to fetal stem cell research. It seems that we should expect advances in reproductive technology to be applied eventually beyond the range of medical conditions that provided their initial warrant. Such extensions often fuel slippery-slope moral objections to reproductive technology (Tiefel).

Groups of people who are "infertile" as a result of lifestyle choices, namely, single men, single women, gay men, and lesbian women, have sought to avail themselves of reproductive technology to make raising their own biological children possible. For Roman Catholicism, a child has a right to heterosexual parents, and some preference is expressed for the traditional family unit. Still, single parents or those in same-sex relationships may very well prove to raise children adequately. Women who by circumstance or choice are not married can, with the assistance of reproductive technology as simple as artificial insemination, satisfy their desire to exercise their reproductive capacity and their desire for children. With the support of courts' interpretations of the Fourteenth Amendment (*Eisenstadt v. Baird*; *Meyer v. Nebraska*), it was easy for physicians to progress from providing reproductive assistance to economically secure single women to providing it to women in stable lesbian relationships. Single men and gay men have sought gestational surrogacy using donor ova.

Advances in plant and animal husbandry have created the possibility of the cloning of genetically similar younger "twins" of existing humans. Part of what drives research into cloning is the challenge of understanding reproductive biology well enough to master the process of unlocking and sequencing any given cell's genetic code. Cloning is also attractive to a small number of infertile couples who wish to reproduce using only their own rather than donor genetic material, to keep reproduction "in the family" (see Nelson, 133–50). It is also appealing to the occasional individual who wishes to achieve a kind of immortality. Perhaps most important is cloning's offering the possibility of repairing the tissues and organs of diseased people by using fully genetically compatible organs grown from totipotent fetal stem cells, thereby avoiding the need for and dangers of immunosuppressive drugs chronically employed in organ transplant cases.

Now existing only in the realm of science fiction, but to be viewed as a live possibility, is ectogenesis—gestating a human fetus to term wholly outside a woman's womb. A remarkable amount of research effort has gone into developing this technique (Corea, 250–59). Speculation has run high that this technology would permit, and perhaps lead to, a modification of abortion procedures so as to restrict them to the safe transfer of an embryo or fetus from the womb of a woman who wants to exercise her right to be free of a pregnancy (see James; Singer and Wells). More far-reaching and to many minds sinister possibilities were envisioned by Aldous Huxley in his 1932 novel *Brave New World*.

One of the truths we struggle repeatedly to recognize in our social and medical ethics is that no action, development, or piece of technology has a sole consequence. To put it briefly: You cannot do just one thing. Nowhere is that lesson learned more profoundly than from the burgeoning field of reproductive technology. Every new piece of technology, made for the specific purpose of addressing some clearly compelling medical need, has led to controversial applications and moral and social issues only dimly apprehended, if at all, by its inventors. They take us, as it were, by surprise, which is one reason reproductive ethics is among the most active areas of philosophical reflection and debate.

See also Abortion; Anscombe, G.E.M.; Contraception; Disability; Diseases, Sexually Transmitted; Firestone, Shulamith; Homosexuality and Science; Intersexuality; Natural Law (New); Privacy; Utopianism

REFERENCES

Buck v. Bell. 274 U.S. 200 (1927); Caplan, Arthur L. "The Ethics of *In Vitro* Fertilization." *Primary Care* 13:2 (1986), 241–53; Cohnitz, Daniel, and Barry Smith. "Assessing Ontologies: The Question of Its Ethical Significance." In E. Runggaldier and C. Kanzian, eds., *Persons: An Interdisciplinary Approach.* Vienna, Austria: Hoelder-Pichler-Tempsky und Österreichischer Bundesverlag, 2003, 243–59; Congregation for the Doctrine of the Faith. *Instruction on Respect for Human Life in Its Origin and on the Dignity of Procreation.* Vatican City: Vatican Polyglot Press, 1987; Corea, Gena. *The Mother Machine: Reproductive Technologies from Artificial Insemination to Artificial Wombs.* New York: Harper and Row, 1986; *Eisenstadt v. Baird.* 405 U.S. 438, 92 S.Ct. 1029, 31 L.Ed. 2d 349 (1972); Ethics Committee of the American Fertility Society. "The Constitutional Aspects of Procreative Liberty." *Fertility and Sterility* 46, supp. 1 (1986), 2S–6S; Ethics Committee of the American Fertility Society. "Ethical Considerations of the New Reproductive Technologies." *Fertility and Sterility* 49, supp. 2 (1988), 2S–10S; Ethics Committee of the American Fertility Society. "The Moral Right to Reproduce and Its Limitations." *Fertility and Sterility* 46, supp. 1 (1986), 21S–23S; Fox, Michael. "Age and Infertility: The Biological Clock: Fact or Fiction?" *Jacksonville Medicine* (May 2000). <www.dcmsonline.org/jax-medicine/2000journals/may2000/ageinf.htm> [accessed 9 December 2004]; Gore-Langton, Robert, and Susan Daniel. "*In Vitro* Fertilization—Overview and Historical Development." In Annette Burfoot, ed., *Encyclopedia of Reproductive Technologies.* Boulder, Colo.: Westview, 1999, 211–17; Henifin, Mary Sue. "Commentary: Selective Termination of Pregnancy." *Hastings Center Report* 18:1 (1988), 22; Hull, Richard T. "Gamete Intrafallopian Transfer (GIFT)." In Annette Burfoot, ed., *Encyclopedia of Reproductive Technologies.* Boulder, Colo.: Westview, 1999, 251–54; Hull, Richard T., ed. (1990) *Ethical Issues in the New Reproductive Technologies.* Amherst, N.Y.: Prometheus, 2005; Huxley, Aldous. *Brave New World.* New York: Harper and Row, 1932; James, David N. "Ectogenesis." In Annette Burfoot, ed., *Encyclopedia of Reproductive Technologies.* Boulder, Colo.: Westview, 1999, 370–72; Lapon, Lenny. "Mass Murderers in White Coats (From Harvard to Buchenwald: A Chronology of Psychiatry and Eugenics)." <www.mindfreedom.org/mindfreedom/news/mass.shtml> [accessed 9 December 2004]; *Meyer v. Nebraska.* 414 U.S. 632, 639–40 (1974); Montalvo, Elba. "Identity Development in Children Adopted Transracially." Paper delivered at a Conference of the North American Council on Adoptable Children: "Winds of Change: New Directions for Families and Children" (3 August 2002), Chicago, Ill. <www.chcfinc.org/speeches/Transracial%20adoption.pdf> [accessed 9 December 2004]; Mullen, Michelle A., Judith Lorber, and Linda S. Williams. "*In Vitro* Fertilization—Risks." In Annette Burfoot, ed., *Encyclopedia of Reproductive Technologies.* Boulder, Colo.: Westview, 1999, 255–60; Nelson, James Lindemann. *Hippocrates' Maze: Ethical Explorations of the Medical Labyrinth.* Lanham, Md.: Rowman and Littlefield, 2003; Paul VI (Pope). *"Humanae vitae." Acta Apostolicae Sedis* 60:9 (1968), 481–503; Purdy, Laura, and Helen B. Holmes. "Surrogacy." In Annette Burfoot, ed., *Encyclopedia of Reproductive Technologies.* Boulder, Colo.: Westview, 1999, 272–79; Robertson, John A. "Surrogate Mothers: Not So Novel After All." *Hastings Center Report* 13:5 (1983), 28–34; *Roe v. Wade.* 410 U.S. 113, 93 S.Ct. 705, 35 L.Ed. 2d 147 (1973); Singer, Peter, and Deane Wells. *Making Babies: The New Science and Ethics of Conception.* New York: Charles Scribner's Sons, 1985; *Skinner v. Oklahoma.* 316 U.S. 535 (1942); Smart, Carol. " 'There Is of Course the Distinction Dictated by Nature': Law and the Problem of Paternity." In Michelle Stanworth, ed., *Reproductive Technologies: Gender, Motherhood, and Medicine.* Minneapolis: University of Minnesota Press, 1987, 98–117; Smith, Barry, and Berit Brogaard. "Sixteen Days." *Journal of Medicine and Philosophy* 28:1 (2003), 45–78; *Stanley v. Illinois.* 405 U.S. 645, 651 (1972); Tiefel, Hans O. "Human *In Vitro* Fertilization: A Conservative View." *Journal of the American Medical Association* 247:23 (1982), 3235–42; Whitehead, Mary Beth, and Loretta Schwartz-Nobel. *A Mother's Story: The Truth about the Baby M Case.* New York: St. Martin's Press, 1989; Wilentz, Hon. Robert

N., Chief Justice, New Jersey Supreme Court. "In the Matter of Baby M, a Pseudonym for an Actual Person." 109 N.J. 396 (1988), 421–74; Zaner, Richard M. "A Criticism of Moral Conservatism's View of *In Vitro* Fertilization and Embryo Transfer." *Perspectives in Biology and Medicine* 27:2 (1984), 201–12.

Richard T. Hull

ADDITIONAL READING

American Society for Reproductive Medicine. "Fact Sheet: *In Vitro* Fertilization (IVF)" (2002). <www.asrm.org/Patients/FactSheets/invitro.html> [accessed 9 December 2004]; Andrews, Lori B. "The Aftermath of Baby M: Proposed State Laws on Surrogate Motherhood." *Hastings Center Report* 17:5 (1987), 31–40. Reprinted in Richard T. Hull, ed., *Ethical Issues*, 2005 (q.v.), 186–201; Andrews, Lori B. *New Conceptions: A Consumer's Guide to the Newest Infertility Treatments, Including In Vitro Fertilization, Artificial Insemination, and Surrogate Motherhood*. New York: St. Martin's Press, 1984; Annas, George J., and Sherman Elias. "*In Vitro* Fertilization and Embryo Transfer: Medicolegal Aspects of a New Technique to Create a Family." *Family Law Quarterly* 17:2 (1983), 199–223; Atwood, Margaret. *The Handmaid's Tale*. New York: Houghton Mifflin, 1986; Baron, C. H. " 'If You Prick Us, Do We Not Bleed?' Of Shylock, Fetuses, and the Concept of Person in the Law." *Law, Medicine, and Health Care* 11:2 (1983), 52–63; Bayles, Michael D. "Harm to the Unconceived." *Philosophy and Public Affairs* 5:3 (1976), 292–304; Bayles, Michael D. "Limits to a Right to Procreate." In Onora O'Neill and William Ruddick, eds., *Having Children: Philosophical and Legal Reflections on Parenthood*. New York: Oxford University Press, 1979, 13–24; Bayles, Michael D., ed. *Reproductive Ethics*. Englewood Cliffs, N.J.: Prentice-Hall, 1984; Belliotti, Raymond A. "Morality and *In Vitro* Fertilization." *Bioethics Quarterly* 2:1 (1980), 6–19; Blank, R. H. "Making Babies: The State of the Art." *The Futurist* 19:1 (1985), 1–17; Boss, Judith A., ed. "Genetic Engineering and Cloning." In *Analyzing Moral Issues*, 3rd ed. New York: McGraw Hill, 2005, 132–80; Brannigan, Michael C., ed. *Ethical Issues in Human Cloning: Cross-Disciplinary Perspectives*. New York: Seven Bridges Press, 2001; Burfoot, Annette, ed. *Encyclopedia of Reproductive Technologies*. Boulder, Colo.: Westview, 1999; Caplan, Arthur L. "The Ethics of *In Vitro* Fertilization." *Primary Care* 13:2 (1986), 241–53. Reprinted in Richard T. Hull, ed., *Ethical Issues*, 2005 (q.v.), 96–108; "Case Conference. Lesbian Couples: Should Help Extend to AID?" *Journal of Medical Ethics* 4:2 (1978), 91–95; Congregation for the Doctrine of the Faith. *"Donum vitae." Acta Apostolicae Sedis* 80 (1988), 70–162; Corea, Gena. "The Subversive Sperm: 'A False Strain of Blood.' " In *The Mother Machine: Reproductive Technologies from Artificial Insemination to Artificial Wombs*. New York: Harper and Row, 1986, 34–48. Reprinted in Richard T. Hull, ed., *Ethical Issues*, 2005 (q.v.), 56–68; Dorff, Elliot N. *Matters of Life and Death: A Jewish Approach to Modern Medical Ethics*. Philadelphia, Pa.: Jewish Publication Society, 1998; Edwards, R. G. "Fertilization of Human Eggs *In Vitro*: Morals, Ethics and the Law." *Quarterly Review of Biology* 40:1 (1974), 3–26; Ethics Advisory Board. "Protection of Human Subjects; U.S. Department of Health, Education, and Welfare Support of Human *In Vitro* Fertilization and Embryo Transfer." *Federal Register* 44 (1979), 35033–58; Flannery, D. M., C. D. Weisman, and C. R. Limpest. "Test Tube Babies: Legal Issues Raised by *In Vitro* Fertilization." *Georgetown Law Journal* 67:6 (1979), 1295–1345; Fletcher, Joseph. *The Ethics of Genetic Control: Ending Reproductive Roulette*. Garden City, N.Y.: Anchor/Doubleday, 1974; Francoeur, Robert T. *Utopian Motherhood: New Trends in Human Reproduction*. Garden City, N.Y.: Doubleday, 1970; Freitas, Robert A., Jr. "Fetal Adoption: A Technological Solution to the Problem of Abortion Ethics." *The Humanist* 40 (May–June 1980), 22–23; Friedman, S. "Artificial Donor Insemination with Frozen Human Semen." *Fertility and Sterility* 28:11 (1977), 1230–33; Genetic Science Learning Center at the Eccles Institute of Human Genetics, University of Utah. "What is Cloning?" <gslc.genetics.utah.edu/units/cloning/whatiscloning/> [accessed 30 August 2004]; *Griswold v. Connecticut*. 381 U.S. 479, 85 S.Ct. 1678, 14 L.Ed. 2d 510 (1965); Hodgen, G. D. "*In Vitro* Fertilization and Alternatives." *Journal of the American Medical Association* 246:6 (7 August 1981), 590–97; Holland, Suzanne, Karen Leblaqz, and Laurie Zoloth, eds. *The Human Embryonic Stem Cell*

Debate: Science, Ethics, and Public Policy. Cambridge, Mass.: MIT Press, 2001; Holmes, Helen B., Betty Hoskins, and Michael Gross, eds. *The Custom-Made Child? Women-Centered Perspectives*. Clifton, N.J.: Humana Press, 1981; Hubbard, Ruth. "Test Tube Babies: Solution or Problem?" *Technology Review* 5 (March–April 1980), 10–12; Hull, Richard T., ed. *Ethical Issues in the New Reproductive Technologies*. Belmont, Calif.: Wadsworth, 1990. 2nd ed., *Ethical Issues in the New Reproductive Technologies*. Amherst, N.Y.: Prometheus, 2005; Jonas, Hans. *Philosophical Essays: From Current Creed to Technological Man*. Chicago, Ill.: University of Chicago Press, 1980; Kass, Leon R. "Making Babies Revisited." *Public Interest* 54 (Winter 1979), 32–60; Knight, James W. "Birth-Control Technology." In Ruth Chadwick, ed., *Encyclopedia of Applied Ethics*, vol. 1. San Diego, Calif.: Academic Press, 1998, 353–68; Kritchevsky, Barbara. "The Unmarried Woman's Right to Artificial Insemination: A Call for an Expanded Definition of Family." *Harvard Women's Law Journal* 4:1 (1981), 1–42; McGee, Glenn, ed. *The Human Cloning Debate*. Berkeley, Calif.: Berkeley Hill Books, 2002; Menning, Barbara. "In Defense of *In Vitro* Fertilization." In Helen B. Holmes, Betty Hoskins, and Michael Gross, eds., *The Custom-Made Child? Women-Centered Perspectives*. Clifton, N.J.: Humana Press, 1981, 263–67; Nelson, Hilde Lindemann, and James Lindemann Nelson. "Cutting Motherhood in Two: Some Suspicions Concerning Surrogacy." *Hypatia* 4:3 (1989), 85–94; Nussbaum, Martha C., and Cass R. Sunstein, eds. *Clones and Clones: Facts and Fantasies about Human Cloning*. New York: Norton, 1998; Okin, Susan M. "A Critique of Pregnancy Contracts." *Politics and the Life Sciences* 8:2 (1990), 205–10; O'Neill, Onora, and William Ruddick, eds. *Having Children: Philosophical and Legal Reflections on Parenthood*. New York: Oxford University Press, 1979; Paul VI (Pope). *"Humanae vitae." Acta Apostolicae Sedis* 60:9 (1968), 481–503. Also *Catholic Mind* 66 (September 1968), 35–48. Reprinted in Claudia Carlen, ed., *The Papal Encyclicals 1958–1981*. Raleigh, N.C.: Pierian Press, 1990, 223–36; P&S1 (131–49); P&S2 (167–84); P&S3 (96–105); Ramsey, Paul. *Fabricated Man: The Ethics of Genetic Control*. New Haven, Conn.: Yale University Press, 1970; Robertson, John A. "Surrogate Mothers: Not So Novel After All." *Hastings Center Report* 13:5 (1983), 28–34. Reprinted in Richard T. Hull, ed., *Ethical Issues*, 2005 (q.v.), 156–66; Ryan, Michael. "Countdown to a Baby." *The New Yorker* (1 July 2002), 68–77; Schoeman, Ferdinand. "Rights of Children, Rights of Parents, and the Moral Basis of the Family." *Ethics* 91:1 (1980), 6–19; Smart, Carol. "'There Is of Course the Distinction Dictated by Nature': Law and the Problem of Paternity." In Michelle Stanworth, ed., *Reproductive Technologies: Gender, Motherhood, and Medicine*. Minneapolis: University of Minnesota Press, 1987, 98–117. Reprinted in Richard T. Hull, ed., *Ethical Issues*, 2005 (q.v.), 69–86; Solomon, Lewis D. *The Jewish Tradition, Sexuality, and Procreation*. Lanham, Md.: University Press of America, 2002; Tiefel, Hans O. "Human *In Vitro* Fertilization: A Conservative View." *Journal of the American Medical Association* 247:23 (1982), 3235–42. Reprinted in Richard T. Hull, ed., *Ethical Issues*, 2005 (q.v.), 120–36; Tong, Rosemarie. "Reproductive Technologies: Surrogacy." In Warren T. Reich, ed., *Encyclopedia of Bioethics*, 2nd ed., vol. 4. New York: Simon Schuster Macmillan, 1995, 2225–29; Veatch, Robert M. "Artificial Insemination from a Father-in-Law." In Robert M. Veatch, ed., *Case Studies in Medical Ethics*. Cambridge, Mass.: Harvard University Press, 1976, 214–21. Reprinted, abridged, in Richard T. Hull, ed., *Ethical Issues*, 2005 (q.v.), 50; Weisberg, D. Kelly, ed. "Reproductive Technology and Adoption." Section of *Applications of Feminist Legal Theory to Women's Lives: Sex, Violence, Work, and Reproduction*. Philadelphia, Pa.: Temple University Press, 1996, 1041–1166; Wilentz, Hon. Robert N., Chief Justice, New Jersey Supreme Court. "In the Matter of Baby M, a Pseudonym for an Actual Person." 109 N.J. 396 (1988), 421–74. Reprinted in Richard T. Hull, ed., *Ethical Issues*, 2005 (q.v.), 167–81; Zaner, Richard M. "A Criticism of Moral Conservatism's View of *In Vitro* Fertilization and Embryo Transfer." *Perspectives in Biology and Medicine* 27:2 (1984), 201–12. Reprinted in Richard T. Hull, ed., *Ethical Issues*, 2005 (q.v.), 137–47.

RIMMER, ROBERT (1917–2001).

In a number of popular novels, sometimes erotic, Robert Henry Rimmer wrote about what he described as "achievable utopias." He believed that "the novel can be a vehicle to show people how they can recreate their environment and live more self-fulfilling lives" ("Robert H. Rimmer," 281). Born in Quincy, Massachusetts, Rimmer discovered writing early in life and in his teens helped publish a mimeographed boy's magazine. He earned a B.A. in English (Bates College, 1939) and an M.B.A. (Harvard, 1941). In World War II, he served in the China-Burma-Indian theater. After the war, Rimmer entered the family business, Relief Printing Corporation, becoming its president at forty. Meanwhile, he developed a **love** of ideas and spent his "other life" reading and absorbing knowledge in the arts, sciences, and humanities, especially about sexuality and love.

Rimmer and his wife Erma (1918–   ), who married in 1941, became involved in an intimate sexual relationship with another couple that began in 1955 (*Harrad Experiment* [1990], 291) and lasted for over twenty years. The two-couple **marriage** dissolved with the death of the other couple's wife in 1976 ("Robert H. Rimmer," 301). Inspired by this experience and his intensive reading, Rimmer began to write novels about alternatives to monogamous marriage. From age forty-five to his death, he wrote eighteen novels and wrote or edited seven works of nonfiction. Rimmer's first book (although published second) was *The Rebellion of Yale Marratt*. Thinking his wife has been killed, Yale marries again, to an old flame. When his original wife reappears, alive, Yale realizes that he loves both women. After the three resolve their chaotic emotions, Yale attempts to persuade their state to repeal its antibigamy statute.

Rimmer's best-known book, *The Harrad Experiment* ("Harrad" is a contraction of "Harvard" and "Radcliffe"), consists of the diaries of six students who enter an experimental college program offering intense intellectual and sensitivity training for intimacy, coupled with co-ed rooming. After graduation, these students form a group marriage. David Allyn described the novel, many years later, as "both an erotic tale and a serious-minded plea for more scientific sexual attitudes. . . . If individuals took a rational view of sex, there would be no more jealousy, no more monogamy, no more shame. . . . In fact, by eliminating shame and self-loathing, sexual rationalism would solve virtually all of society's remaining problems" (72).

In appealing to scientific attitudes and rationalism, Rimmer's philosophy was similar to that of **Albert Ellis** (1913–   ), one of his contemporaries. But Ellis had little expectation about making extensive progress (in his sense), while Rimmer was utopian. About Ellis, Rimmer wrote, "Albert's approaches, based on his theories of rational-emotive therapy, appeal to me. While he has written some freaky books in the last few years, this one [*Civilized Couple's Guide to Extramarital Adventure*] is up to his past standards and is interesting reading" (*Adventures in Loving*, 371). Rimmer's applauding this book was consistent both with his personal life and the substance of his writings. In *Civilized*, Ellis wrote that although he was pessimistic, many authors, including Rimmer, were optimistic about communal marriage (39).

Harrad sold millions of copies and attracted wide attention among the inquisitive intelligentsia of the 1960s. College students eagerly passed it around, faculty assigned it in courses, and people of all ages considered it permission to enjoy sex before and outside marriage (Allyn, 71–84). Its bibliography added to the book's depth and charm, challenging readers to obtain the intellectual education offered at Harrad. Letters from readers poured in (*The Harrad Letters*; *You and I*), including their accounts of alternative marital arrangements (collected in Rimmer, *Adventures in Loving*). Rimmer later expanded *Harrad*'s thesis to embrace social, racial, and income diversity (*The Premar Experiments*) and applied it to secondary schools (*The Lov-Ed Solution*). In 1990, *Harrad* was reissued with supplementary material.

As a result of *Harrad*, Rimmer was hailed as a guru of alternative lifestyles (Allyn, chap. 6; Rubin). Its success fired his utopian imagination. *Proposition 31* ends with a resolution put before California voters to legalize group marriage. *Thursday, My Love* describes "synergamous" marriage, in which a married couple maintains a legal, committed sexual relationship with a third person. In *The Trade Off—My Husband/Your Wife*, two long-term married couples agree to enjoy each other's spouses for brief periods in a "succedenam" marriage. A similar idea is proposed as "LovXchange" in *Come Live My Life*. Other themes emerged in subsequent novels: sex as sacrament, sex as play in the corporate subculture, and time travel.

Rimmer's later novels never did as well as *Harrad*, and publishers came to spurn his utopian fiction. Financially secure in his mid-60s but looking to continue writing, Rimmer, always appreciative of nudity and erotic depictions, undertook to prepare an intelligent directory of pornographic videos (*The Adult X-Rated Videotape Guide*). His thought that open-minded intellectuals would enjoy the "best" of what he called "sexvids" came during liberal opposition to the antipornography agendas of the conservative Meese Commission (1986) and the feminists **Catharine MacKinnon** and **Andrea Dworkin** (1946–2005). Rimmer's guide, which annotated thousands of videos, went through several editions between 1983 and 1995. It broke new ground; nothing had been available to separate "good" from "bad" **pornography**, however these might be defined. Rimmer's guide was even reviewed as a serious reference work (but sometimes sneeringly; contrast Solomon and Palmer) and opened the door for later guides (Blue; Winks).

Rimmer was a humanist. He counted Paul Kurtz (1926–) among his mentors and in 1980 signed the Humanist Manifesto (Briggs). He felt that sexual rationalism could solve many of society's problems. But although he crusaded for the joy of learning and the joy of sex, his recommendations for widespread **sex education** (see *Let's Really Make Love*), which run counter to **abstinence**-only sex education, never made progress. Rimmer expressed his philosophy as the "Five Ls—Living, Loving, Laughter, Learning, and Ludamus [play]" (*Let's Really Make Love*, 195). He is remembered mostly for "polyfidelity," being faithful to more than one person at the same time. He favored stable, expanded marital structures in contrast to recreational "swinging," serial monogamy, casual affairs, or transient relationships (Hall and Poteete). Academic and nonacademic intellectuals and aficionados interested in alternative marriage arrangements have been encouraged by his work (Anapol; Constantine and Constantine; Francoeur; Francoeur et al.; Nearing; Smith and Smith).

Rimmer was part of the American sexual utopian tradition, going back to the polygynous Mormons and the collective marital practices of the Oneida community (1848–1879) of John Noyes ([1811–1886]; see Foster). Both groups ran into legal problems. Rimmer's novelistic characters crusade for legal changes in marriage, but no such changes occurred in his lifetime. Stanley Kurtz, however, wrote in 2003 that the acceptance of **same-sex marriage** could lead to "legalized polygamy." Kurtz also described how the trial of Mormon polygamist Tom Green (2001) evoked "a surprising number of mainstream defenses of polygamy" (27; see Rubin).

Rimmer's endorsement of alternative marital structures earned him puzzlement and some animosity among more radical sexual liberals, who thought that two- or three-couple marriages were still "monogamous" and too restrictive in requiring intramarriage fidelity (Rimmer, *Adventures*, 295–96). He was also criticized for writing badly and for being naive about human relationships. He was once described as a "businessman-writer of philosophical tracts poorly disguised as novels" and "the true swami" of the alternative lifestyle subculture with "colossal" influence, despite "dreadful" writing (Seligson, 108). In one study, over 50 percent of group marriages failed within a year, and only 7 percent remained intact after five (Constantine and Constantine, 69, 249). Despite these bleak figures, Rimmer's cheerful, friendly optimism combined with intellectual and personal passion carried his point with many people.

Rimmer's goal was not to found a real Harrad College or to fight a Proposition 31 through a legislature but to create "[m]illions of me[s] who can't walk into a bookstore or library without feeling a tingle of excitement at all the things there are to know in this world. . . . [B]ooks are one of the few intimate ways *to become* another human being" (*You and I*, 420). His prescription for sex as a key to intimacy has probably been more often filled than his prescription for learning.

See also Adultery; Bisexuality; Casual Sex; Dworkin, Andrea; Ellis, Albert; MacKinnon, Catharine; Marriage; Pornography; Protestantism, History of; Sex Education; Utopianism

REFERENCES

Allyn, David. *Make Love Not War: The Sexual Revolution. An Unfettered History*. New York: Little, Brown, 2000; Anapol, Deborah M. *Love without Limits: The Quest for Sustainable Intimate Relationships*. San Rafael, Calif.: IntiNet Resource Center, 1992; Blue, Violet. *The Ultimate Guide to Adult Videos: How to Watch Adult Videos and Make Your Sex Life Sizzle*. San Francisco, Calif.: Cleis, 2003; Briggs, Kenneth A. "Secular Humanists Attack a Rise in Fundamentalism." *New York Times* (15 October 1980), A18; Constantine, Larry L., and Joan M. Constantine. *Group Marriage: A Study of Contemporary Multilateral Marriage*. New York: Collier/Macmillan, 1973; Ellis, Albert. *The Civilized Couple's Guide to Extramarital Adventure*. New York: Wyden, 1972; Foster, Lawrence. "That All May Be One: John Humphrey Noyes and the Origins of Oneida Community Complex Marriage." In *Religion and Sexuality: The Shakers, the Mormons, and the Oneida Community*. Urbana: University of Illinois Press, 1984, 72–122; Francoeur, Robert T. *Eve's New Rib: Twenty Faces of Sex, Marriage, and Family*. New York: Delta/Dell, 1972; Francoeur, Robert T., Martha Cornog, and Timothy Perper. *Sex, Love, and Marriage in the 21st Century: The Next Sexual Revolution*. San Jose, Calif.: toExcel, 1999; Hall, Elizabeth, and Robert A. Poteete. "Do You, Mary, and Anne, and Beverly, and Ruth, Take These Men . . . A Conversation with Robert H. Rimmer about Harrad, Group Marriage, and Other Loving Arrangements." *Psychology Today* (January 1972), 57–64, 78–82; Kurtz, Stanley. "Beyond Gay Marriage." *The Weekly Standard* (4–11 August 2003), 26–33; Nearing, Ryam. *Loving More: The Polyfidelity Primer*. Captain Cook, Hawaii: PEP Publishing, 1992; Palmer, Joseph W. "799. Rimmer, Robert H., *The X-Rated Videotape Guide. Revised and Updated*." [Review] In Bohdan S. Wynar, ed., *American Reference Books Annual*, vol. 16. Littleton, Colo.: Libraries Unlimited, 1985, 294; Rimmer, Robert H. *The Adult X-Rated Videotape Guide*. New York: Arlington House, 1983; Rimmer, Robert H. *Come Live My Life*. New York: New American Library, 1977; Rimmer, Robert H. *The Harrad Experiment*. Los Angeles, Calif.: Sherbourne Press, 1966; Rimmer, Robert H. *The Harrad Experiment*. 25th Anniversary Edition. Buffalo, N.Y.: Prometheus, 1990; Rimmer, Robert H. *Let's Really Make Love: Sex, the Family, and Education in the Twenty-First Century*. Amherst, N.Y.: Prometheus, 1995; Rimmer, Robert H. *The Lov-Ed Solution*. San Jose, Calif.: Writers Club Press, 2000; Rimmer, Robert H. *The Premar Experiments*. New York: Crown, 1975; Rimmer, Robert H. *Proposition 31*. New York: New American Library, 1968; Rimmer, Robert H. *The Rebellion of Yale Marratt*. Boston, Mass.: Challenge Press, 1964; Rimmer, Robert H. "Robert H. Rimmer, 1917–   ." In Mark Zadrozny, ed., *Contemporary Authors Autobiography Series*, vol. 10. Detroit, Mich.: Gale Research, 1989, 281–306; Rimmer, Robert H. *Thursday, My Love*. New York: New American Library, 1972; Rimmer, Robert H. *The Trade Off—My Husband/Your Wife*. San Jose, Calif.: Writers Club Press, 2000; Rimmer, Robert H., ed. *Adventures in Loving*. New York: New American Library, 1973; Rimmer, Robert H., ed. *The Harrad Letters to Robert H. Rimmer*. New York: New American Library, 1969; Rimmer, Robert H., ed. *You and I . . . Searching for Tomorrow:*

The Second Book of Letters to Robert Rimmer. New York: New American Library, 1971; Rubin, Roger H. "Alternative Lifestyles Revisited, or Whatever Happened to Swingers, Group Marriages, and Communes?" *Journal of Family Issues* 22:6 (2001), 711–16; Seligson, Marcia. *Options: A Personal Expedition through the Sexual Frontier*. New York: Charter Books/Grosset and Dunlap, 1978; Smith, James R., and Lynn G. Smith, eds. *Beyond Monogamy: Recent Studies of Sexual Alternatives in Marriage*. Baltimore, Md.: Johns Hopkins University Press, 1974; Solomon, Charles. "The X-Rated Videotape Guide II." [Review] *Los Angeles Times Book Review* (16 February 1992), 10; Winks, Cathy. *The Good Vibrations Guide: Adult Videos*. San Francisco: Down There Press, 1998.

Martha Cornog

ADDITIONAL READING

Anapol, Deborah M. *Polyamory: The New Love within Limits: Secrets of Sustainable Intimate Relationships*. San Rafael, Calif.: IntiNet Resource Center, 1997; Clark, Stephen R. L. "Sexual Ontology and the Group Marriage." *Philosophy* 58 (1983), 215–27. Reprinted in P&S3, 165–76; Ertman, Martha M. "Marriage as a Trade: Bridging the Private/Private Distinction." *Harvard Civil Rights—Civil Liberties Law Review* 36:1 (2001), 79–132; Gay, William T. "The Prophet of Group Marriage." *The Futurist* 4:2 (1970), 46–47; Gould, Terry. *The Lifestyle: A Look at the Erotic Rites of Swingers*. New York: Firefly, 2000; Heinlein, Robert. *Stranger in a Strange Land*. New York: Putnam, 1961; Kirkendall, Lester A. "Adventures in Loving." [Review] *Journal of Marriage and the Family* 36:4 (1974), 829; Levin, Martin. "The Harrad Experiment." [Review] *New York Times Book Review* (12 June 1966), 33; Levin, Martin. "The Premar Experiments." [Review] *New York Times Book Review* (28 September 1975), 37; Levin, Martin. "Proposition Thirty-one." [Review] *New York Times Book Review* (8 December 1968), 78; Martin, Douglas. "Robert H. Rimmer, 84, Author of 'The Harrad Experiment.'" *New York Times* (11 August 2001), A14; O'Neill, Nena, and George O'Neill. *Open Marriage: A New Life Style for Couples*. New York: M. Evans, 1972; Rimmer, Robert H. "Playing Pygmalion." In Robert T. Francoeur, Martha Cornog, and Timothy Perper, eds., *Sex, Love, and Marriage in the 21st Century: The Next Sexual Revolution*. San Jose, Calif.: toExcel, 1999, 137–50; Webb, Randall, and Doug Raynor. "The Connubial Utopias of Robert Rimmer." *The Futurist* 2:5 (1968), 99–100.

ROMAN SEXUALITY AND PHILOSOPHY, ANCIENT. For many years Latin was a requirement for acceptance to American universities, and Roman values had a distinctive influence on American ideals, from the Founding Fathers onward. Not so for Roman sexuality: The Latin texts that were read by students were heavily censored for sexual content, and even when books on Roman sexuality were published, there was little understanding of the radically different system of sexual categories in ancient Rome. Only when contemporary **feminism** (Pomeroy; Richlin) and the growing interest in same-sex relationships reached into classical scholarship did a better understanding evolve. A comparison of (for example) Jean Marcadé with Craig Williams reveals the difference between the traditional approach, in which similarities between the ancients and the moderns are stressed, and contemporary scholarship, which analyzes the ancient evidence on the basis of recent hermeneutical and anthropological theories. **Michel Foucault**'s (1926–1984) *History of Sexuality* (vol. 2 deals with ancient Rome) has been a major inspiration.

There were two opposing attitudes toward sex in the ancient Roman world. One was that sex was something strictly within the life of a married couple and not to be talked about in public. An example of this attitude is found in the story told about the foundation of the Roman Republic. The young Etruscan Prince Tarquinius decided to seduce Lucretia, another man's wife, and after he raped her, she took her own life because she could not bear the shame. Her husband and his friends became so enraged that they overthrew the monarchic government and established the Roman Republic (Livy [59 BCE–17 CE], *History of Rome*, 1.58). (For opposing philosophical views about the propriety of Lucretia's suicide, see **Saint Augustine** [354–430], *City of God*, bk. 1, chaps. 15–19, esp. pp. 20–21, 23, and **Immanuel Kant** [1724–1804], 145–46.) Another example of this particular attitude is illustrated by Caesar's divorce from his wife Pompeia in 61 BCE after the rumor circulated that she had been involved with the infamous Clodius. Caesar, however, defended Clodius at a subsequent trial, declaring that he was of the opinion that his wife ought not even to be suspected of sexual impropriety (Plutarch, 10).

In stark contrast to this Roman outlook on **sexual activity**, many modern sources portray Rome from the first century BCE as a society with fairly relaxed and liberal attitudes toward sex and **love** outside **marriage**. This impression is to a large extent derived from accounts of numerous scandals reported in our historical and literary sources and in particular from several popular works of Roman love poetry. They include passionate lyrical poems by Catullus (ca. 85–55 BCE) and love elegies by the later Augustan writers Propertius (born ca. 50 BCE), Tibullus (ca. 50–19 BCE), and Ovid (43 BCE–17 CE), among them the latter's (in)famous mock-didactic poem *Ars Amatoria*, or *Art of Love*. Ovid's *Art of Love* is more a manual for successful **seduction** than a handbook of sexual behavior generally, but it does contribute to the impression of a relatively tolerant climate for sexual self-fulfillment in the Rome of Ovid's days. According to these poems, the male lover can be compared with a soldier whose one and only goal is to meet with his beloved and have sex with her. According to Ovid, there were circumstances in Rome in which it was fairly easy to seduce women and to launch amorous relationships (for example, when watching games in the Circus Maximus or attending a private dinner party), and Ovid offered to teach both men and women the skills and effort required to keep an affair going. Women were often described by the Augustan poets as being unfaithful, not only to their husbands but also to their lovers; the male lovers were by no means faithful themselves, having other female or male lovers, but this situation seems not to have bothered anybody, at least according to the male authors who are our sources.

Reality was probably more complicated than, and attitudes toward extramarital sexual activity not as lax as, this world of poetry suggests. The best piece of evidence that this sexual permissiveness was more than a poetic **fantasy** is provided by the laws proposed by the Emperor Augustus (63 BCE–14 CE) in 18 BCE that attempted to prohibit **adultery** and extramarital sexuality—not that these laws seem to have had much effect. More, Augustus's own behavior as a young man did not accord with them. But this was the first time in Roman history that sexual conduct as such became a matter of concern for the state. Previously, inappropriate sexual behavior was a private affair and subject only to the authority of the male head of the family, the *paterfamilias*. Despite Augustus's laws, the Roman attitude toward sexual activity seems to have been more or less the same from about 200 BCE to late in the Roman Empire, when Christianity began to make a difference (ca. 200).

As was the case in classical Greece, social attitudes focused largely on male sexual conduct. The Romans were concerned with the distinction between active and passive roles, that is, penetrative and penetrated behavior, not whether the activity was heterosexual or homosexual. Indeed, the terms "heterosexual" and "homosexual," despite their obvious Greco-Latin elements, were coined in modern times and make no sense in the ancient Roman world (Williams, chap. 5). A slave in Plautus's (born ca. 254 BCE) comedy *Curculio* says to his young master:

Nobody prevents you or forbids you to buy what is openly for sale, if you have the money. Nobody prevents anyone from walking on a public road. As long as you do not walk across a fenced-off farm, as long as you keep away from married or widowed women, from virgins, from young men and freeborn boys, make love to whatever you like! (lines 33–38)

As long as a man did not transgress against the property or family of another Roman male citizen, any sexual act was acceptable, provided that the man performed in the active role, that is, he penetrated another human being. The main difference from the ancient Greek world was that sexual relationships between free men in the Roman world were not considered acceptable under any circumstances. In a society in which marriage, at least among the upper classes, was often a matter of political or economical convenience, it is not remarkable that sexual relations between free men and slaves, male or female, flourished, and that **prostitution** was readily available to any man willing to pay for sex. Not only do literary sources attest to this attitude, but it is also clear from the archaeological remains in a small but fashionable provincial town like Pompeii, where both inscriptions and wall paintings illustrate that sex was a commodity to be bought along with wine and food (see Clarke). Erotic paintings and other objects were also found in the living quarters of ordinary people (see Grant). One striking feature of these erotic representations is the frequent depiction of large male sexual organs; it seems as if the Greek god Priapus was more often portrayed in Italy than in Greece. Statues of this god with his erect penis were in fact used as scarecrows in urban gardens and rural fields.

The phallocentric attitude of Roman men is also reflected in the rich Latin vocabulary denoting sexual acts. The verbs for "to penetrate vaginally" (*futuere*), "to penetrate anally" (*pedicare*), and "to penetrate orally" (*irrumare*) are all active and can be used without any negative connotations: A man is allowed to do all three with another man or woman. In fact, a "real" man *will* do them, provided that he does not violate the principles described above or allow himself to be penetrated. In the passive voice, however, these verbs describe the behavior of the other (passive) partner in such activities, usually with negative connotations. The same goes for the expressions that describe nonpenetrative activities: *Fellare* ("to suck man's penis") and in particular the noun *cunnilingus* are very negative terms. While women were considered passive by nature, men who preferred to be penetrated anally or orally were not considered "real" men (*viri*). The fact that they were referred to by terms derived from the Greek rather than the Latin (*pathici, cinaedi, catamiti*—the last was derived from the name of Zeus's young mortal beloved, Ganymedes) need not mean that their activities were considered Greek. These terms often emphasized not what such men did but how they acted excessively. Some of the same men who were accused of womanizing were also accused of being not merely "homosexual" but the passive partner in a same-sex relationship. When Julius Caesar conducted his triumph after the Gallic Wars, the soldier sang that he conquered Gaul, while the King of Bithynia conquered (= penetrated) him (Suetonius, *Life of Julius Caesar*, 49). Even if the accusations were untrue, as they very well might have been, they clearly indicate how the passive role was scorned. Conversely, women who engaged in same-sex sexual activities were sometimes described as acting like men and were called by the Greek term *tribas* ("one who rubs"). But we know little about female sexuality in Rome (or in Greece).

Roman literature seems to be more willing to describe sexual practices in detail than Greek literature. In addition to the works of poetry mentioned above, we find much useful and titillating information in both Petronius's (first century CE) novel *Satyrica* and in Suetonius's (b. ca. 70–d. after 122) biographies of the Roman emperors. In contrast, such information about sexual mores is absent from the biographies of famous Greek and Roman men by Suetonius's Greek predecessor Plutarch (ca. 50–120). The sexual details prominent in the collection of *Priapea*, erotic poems about male sexuality (see Hooper), and in Martial's (ca. 40–104) satirical epigrams are also absent from Greek erotic poetry.

While Roman philosophers discuss feelings and passions often enough, it is rare for them to mention sexual matters specifically in their treatises. This phenomenon is in part explained by the fact that most of the Roman philosophers were either Stoics or Epicureans and thus more concerned with controlling and eliminating passions than with evaluating them. As the philosopher Seneca (ca. 4 BCE–65 CE) says: "The wise man ought to love his wife deliberately, not passionately. He controls the impulse to pleasure and is not led headlong to intercourse" (from "On Marriage," translated by Nussbaum, in *Therapy of Desire*, 473).

We are fortunate, however, to have two discussions of sexuality by Roman philosophers, one from each of the two major philosophical schools. Lucretius (ca. 99/95–55 BCE) wrote his *De rerum natura* in the 50s BCE about the Epicurean explanation of the world as consisting of atoms and the void, a view that freed human beings from religious superstition and fear of death. In Book Four of *De rerum* (lines 1036–1287), Lucretius discusses love and sex. Love, he claims, is the result of a natural desire but is often burdened with false perceptions and sense impressions. Thus, love may be complicated, while sex is relatively simple and the same for both animals and human beings. He maintains, too, that an upsurge in bodily fluids, as children mature, causes them to seek physical relief in the form of sexual intercourse. Since all humans have the same urges, and all humans have a reason for finding pleasure, he concludes that sexual activity is the best way to achieve physical satisfaction and that both man and woman have the right to experience this pleasure. Even though this recognition of equal sexual rights is not often expressed in other ancient Roman sources (see, however, Ovid's *Art of Love* 2.757–58), Lucretius's discussion of sexuality is perhaps an indication that women in Roman society were more independent than women in the Greek world, even though females who were actively engaged in sex outside marriage were not looked on with approving eyes, at least outside Augustan poetry.

A century after Lucretius we find the Roman knight Gaius Musonius Rufus (ca. 25–95 CE) advocating a Stoic view of life. He lectured in Greek, and though he published nothing, his lectures were later published, as was the case with his pupil Epictetus (ca. 55–135 CE). Musonius's main philosophy was concerned with ethical matters (see texts translated by Nussbaum in "Incomplete Feminism," 314–20). Since he accepted the Stoic idea that men and women by birth possess identical qualifications, he argued fervently in favor of sexual equality and contended that marriage should be a partnership. In fact, he says that men have no good reason to have sexual relations with women other than their wives (contrary to Roman practice) and maintained that men lost their claim to moral superiority if they admitted to being overwhelmed by physical desire. Musonius even opposed sexual intercourse for the sake of pure pleasure, although he was convinced that the wish to have children was not sufficient reason to get married. While hardly a feminist, he was able, as a result of his Stoic background, to formulate a more consistent view of the relationship between the sexes than most other Stoic philosophers. His view of sexuality, however, is far from the antisexual attitude of the Christians.

See also Catholicism, History of; Chinese Philosophy; Foucault, Michel; Greek Sexuality and Philosophy, Ancient; Language; Orientation, Sexual; Social Constructionism

REFERENCES

Adams, James N. *The Latin Sexual Vocabulary*. Baltimore, Md.: Johns Hopkins University Press, 1982; Augustine. (413–427) *The City of God*. Trans. John Healey. Ed. R.V.G. Tasker. London: J. M. Dent and Sons, 1945; Clarke, John R. *Looking at Lovemaking: Constructions of Sexuality in Roman Art, 100 B.C.–250 A.D.* Berkeley: University of California Press, 1998; Foucault, Michel. (1984) *The History of Sexuality*, vol. 2: *The Use of Pleasure*. Trans. Robert Hurley. New York: Pantheon, 1985; Grant, Michael. *Eros in Pompei: The Secret Rooms of the National Museum of Naples*. New York: Morrow, 1975; Hooper, Richard W., trans. *The Priapus Poems: Erotic Epigrams from Ancient Rome*. Urbana: University of Illinois Press, 1999; Kant, Immanuel. (ca. 1762–1794) *Lectures on Ethics*. Trans. Peter Heath. Cambridge: Cambridge University Press, 1997; Livy. (26 BCE–17 CE) *The Early History of Rome. Books I-V*, rev. ed. Trans. Aubrey de Selincourt and Robert Oglevie. Harmondsworth, U.K.: Penguin, 2002. <mcadams.posc.mu.edu/txt/ah/Livy/> [accessed 1 October 2004]; Lucretius. (60–55 BCE) *De rerum natura*. Trans. William H. D. Rouse. Rev. Martin Ferguson Smith. Loeb Classical Library. Cambridge, Mass.: Harvard University Press, 1975; Marcadé, Jean. *Roma amor: Essay on Erotic Elements in Etruscan and Roman Art*. Geneva, Switz.: Nagel, 1961; Nussbaum, Martha C. "The Incomplete Feminism of Musonius Rufus, Platonist, Stoic, and Roman." In Martha C. Nussbaum and Juha Sihvola, eds., *The Sleep of Reason: Erotic Experience and Sexual Ethics in Ancient Greece and Rome*. Chicago, Ill.: University of Chicago Press, 2002, 283–326; Nussbaum, Martha C. *The Therapy of Desire: Theory and Practice in Hellenistic Ethics*. Princeton, N.J.: Princeton University Press, 1994; Ovid. (ca. 1 BCE) *Art of Love*. In *Ovid: The Erotic Poems*. Trans. Peter Green. New York: Penguin, 1982, 166–238; Petronius. *Satyrica*. Ed. and trans. Robert Bracht Branham and Daniel Kinney. Berkeley: University of California Press, 1996; Plautus. *Curculio* [*The Weevil*]. In *Plautus*, vol 2: *Casina. The Casket Comedy. Curculio. Epidicus. The Two Menaechmuses*. Trans. Paul Nixon. Loeb Classical Library. Cambridge, Mass.: Harvard University Press, 1917, 186–259. <artemis.austincollege.edu/acad/cml/rcape/comedy/> [accessed 1 October 2004]; Plutarch. *Fall of the Roman Republic. Six Lives: Marius, Sulla, Crassus, Pompey, Caesar, Cicero*. Trans. Rex Warner. Harmondsworth, U.K.: Penguin, 1972; Pomeroy, Sarah B. *Goddesses, Whores, Wives, and Slaves: Women in Classical Antiquity*. New York: Schocken, 1975; Richlin, Amy. (1983) *The Garden of Priapus: Sexuality and Aggression in Roman Humor*, rev. ed. New York: Oxford University Press, 1992; Richlin, Amy, ed. *Pornography and Representation in Greece and Rome*. New York: Oxford University Press, 1992; Suetonius Tranquillus, Gaius. *The Lives of the Twelve Caesars*. Trans. Robert Graves. Harmondsworth, U.K.: Penguin, 1979; Williams, Craig A. *Roman Homosexuality: Ideologies of Masculinity in Classical Antiquity*. New York: Oxford University Press, 1999.

Jørgen Mejer

ADDITIONAL READING

Benko, Stephen. *Pagan Rome and the Early Christians*. Bloomington: Indiana University Press, 1984; Boswell, John. *Christianity, Social Tolerance, and Homosexuality: Gay People in Western Europe from the Beginning of the Christian Era to the Fourteenth Century*. Chicago, Ill.: University of Chicago Press, 1980; Brendel, Otto. "The Scope and Temperament of Erotic Art in the Graeco-Roman World." In Theodore Bowie and Cornelia V. Christenson, eds., *Studies in Erotic Art*. New York: Basic Books, 1970, 3–107; Brisson, Luc. *Sexual Ambivalence: Androgyny and Hermaphrodism in Graeco-Roman Antiquity*. Trans. Janet Lloyd. Berkeley: University of California Press, 2002; Brunt, P. A. "'Amicitia' in the Late Roman Republic." In Robin Seager, ed., *The Crisis of the Roman Republic: Studies in Political and Social History*. Cambridge, U.K.: Heffer, 1969, 199–218; Bullough, Vern L. *Homosexuality: A History*. New York: New American Library, 1979; Cantarella, Eva. *Bisexuality in the Ancient World*. Trans. Cormac Ó Cuilleanáin. New Haven, Conn.: Yale University

Press, 1992; Cantarella, Eva. (1981) *Pandora's Daughters: The Role and Status of Women in Greek and Roman Antiquity*. Trans. Mauren K. Fant. Baltimore, Md.: Johns Hopkins University Press, 1987; Catullus. *The Complete Poems*. Trans. Guy Lee. New York: Oxford University Press, 1990; Dierichs, Angelika. *Erotik in der rümischen Kunst*. Mainz, Ger.: von Zabern, 1997; Engels, Frederick. (1884) "The Gens and the State in Rome." In *The Origin of the Family, Private Property, and the State*. Peking, China: Foreign Languages Press, 1978, 142–55; Epictetus. *The Discourses of Epictetus*. Trans. Christopher Gill and Robin Hard. London: Everyman's, 1995; Fantham, Elaine. "*Stuprum*: Public Attitudes and Penalties for Sexual Offences in Republican Rome." *Echos du Monde Classique/Classical Views* 35 (1991), 267–91; Gardner, Iain, and Samuel N. C. Lieu, eds. *Manichaean Texts from the Roman Empire*. New York: Cambridge University Press, 2004; Goldhill, Simon. *Love, Sex, and Tragedy: How the Ancient World Shapes Our Lives*. Chicago, Ill.: University of Chicago Press, 2004; Grimal, Pierre. *Love in Ancient Rome*. New York: Crown, 1967; Hallett, Judith P. "Roman Attitudes toward Sex." In Michael Grant and Rachel Kitzinger, eds., *Civilization of the Ancient Mediterranean: Greece and Rome*, vol. 2. New York: Scribner's, 1988, 1265–78; Hallett, Judith P., and Marilyn B. Skinner, eds. *Roman Sexualities*. Princeton, N.J.: Princeton University Press, 1997; Hubbard, Thomas K. *Homosexuality in Greece and Rome: A Sourcebook of Basic Documents*. Berkeley: University of California Press, 2003; Johns, Catharine. *Sex or Symbol? Erotic Images of Greece and Rome*. Austin: University of Texas Press, 1982; Konstan, David. *Sexual Symmetry: Love in the Ancient Novel and Related Genres*. Princeton, N.J.: Princeton University Press, 1994; Konstan, David, and Martha Nussbaum, eds. "The Construction of Sexuality in the Classical World." *differences: A Journal of Feminist Cultural Studies* [special issue] 2:1 (1990); Kraut, Richard. "Soul Doctors." [Review of *The Therapy of Desire: Theory and Practice in Hellenistic Ethics*, by Martha C. Nussbaum] *Ethics* 105 (April 1995), 613–25; Kuefler, Mathew. *The Manly Eunuch: Masculinity, Gender Ambiguity, and Christian Ideology in Late Antiquity*. Chicago, Ill.: University of Chicago Press, 2001; Lieu, Samuel N. C. (1985) *Manichaeism in the Later Roman Empire and Medieval China: A History Survey*, 2nd ed. Tübingen, Ger.: J.C.B. Mohr, 1992; Lilja, Saara. *Homosexuality in Republican and Augustan Rome*. Helsinki, Fin.: Societas Scientiarum Fennica, 1983; Lucretius. *On the Nature of Things: De rerum natura*. Trans. Anthony M. Esolen. Baltimore, Md.: Johns Hopkins University Press, 1995; Martial. *Epigrams*. Ed. and trans. David R. Shackleton Bailey. Loeb Classical Library. Cambridge, Mass.: Harvard University Press, 1993; McClure, Laura K. *Sexuality and Gender in the Classical World: Readings and Sources*. Malden, Mass.: Blackwell, 2002; McGinn, Thomas A. *Prostitution, Sexuality, and the Law in Ancient Rome*. New York: Oxford University Press, 1998; Musonius Rufus. "The Roman Socrates." Ed. and trans. Cora E. Lutz. Yale Classical Studies 10. New Haven, Conn.: Yale University Press, 1947, 3–147; Nussbaum, Martha C. "Eros and the Wise: The Stoic Response to a Cultural Dilemma." *Oxford Studies in Ancient Philosophy* 13 (1995), 231–67; Nussbaum, Martha C., and Juha Sihvola, eds. *The Sleep of Reason: Erotic Experience and Sexual Ethics in Ancient Greece and Rome*. Chicago, Ill.: University of Chicago Press, 2002; Oates, Whitney J., ed. *The Stoic and Epicurean Philosophers: The Complete Extant Writings of Epicurus, Epictetus, Lucretius, and Marcus Aurelius*, 9th pnt. New York: Random House, 1940; Rabinowitz, Nancy S., and Lisa Auanger, eds. *Among Women: From the Homosexual to the Homoerotic in the Ancient World*. Austin: University of Texas Press, 2002; Richlin, Amy. *The Garden of Priapus: Sexuality and Aggression in Roman Humor*. New Haven, Conn.: Yale University Press, 1983. Rev. ed., New York: Oxford University Press, 1992; Richlin, Amy. "Not Before Homosexuality: The Materiality of the *Cinaedus* and the Roman Law against Love between Men." *Journal of the History of Sexuality* 3:4 (1993), 523–73; Rousselle, Aline. (1983) *Porneia: On Desire and the Body in Antiquity*. Trans. Felicia Pheasant. Oxford, U.K.: Blackwell, 1988; Satlow, Michael L. "Rhetoric and Assumptions: Romans and Rabbis on Sex." In Martin Goodman, ed., *Jews in a Graeco-Roman World*. Oxford, U.K.: Clarendon Press, 1999, 135–44; Sextus Propertius. *The Poems*. Trans. Guy Lee. Oxford, U.K.: Oxford University Press, 1994; Singer, Irving. "Sex in Ovid and Lucretius." In *The Nature of Love*, vol. 1: *Plato to Luther*, 2nd ed. Chicago, Ill.: University of Chicago Press, 1984, 122–46; Smith, Mark. "Ancient Bisexuality and the Interpretation of Romans 1:26–27." *Journal of the American Academy of Religion* 64:2 (1996), 223–56; Sullivan, J. P. "Martial's

Sexual Attitudes." *Philologus: Zeitschrifte für Klassische Philologie* 123:2 (1979), 288–302; Tibullus. *Elegies.* Trans. Guy Lee. Leeds, U.K.: Francis Cairns, 1990; Treggiari, Susan. *Roman Marriage: Iusti Coniuges from the Time of Cicero to the Time of Ulpian.* New York: Oxford University Press, 1991.

ROUSSEAU, JEAN-JACQUES (1712–1778). The thought of Jean-Jacques Rousseau is often judged to be paradoxical if not contradictory, and that assessment seems particularly apt when applied to his understanding of sexuality. First, there is a glaring discrepancy between the life that he recommended to others, in his educational treatise *Emile* (1761) and his romantic novel *Julie* (1761), and the life that he lived himself, as recounted in his posthumously published autobiographical work, the *Confessions* (1782, 1789). In the former works Rousseau writes as an impassioned defender of conjugal and parental **love**, **marriage**, and the nuclear family. The latter work, however, makes it clear that Rousseau was anything but a contented spouse and good father: He was a man with strikingly unconventional sexual predilections; he fathered and then abandoned five children; and these were born to a woman to whom he was not then married.

Second, Rousseau's theoretical works about human sexuality appear to contradict themselves. In different places Rousseau provides opposing answers to questions like these: Is **sexual desire** a physical or a psychological need (prompted by the human imagination)? Is the family natural? Is female modesty natural? Ultimately, however, contradictions like these can be resolved. In fact, Rousseau's theoretical works offer a profound and complex but not contradictory view of human sexuality. He believed that human sexuality was different in the primordial state of nature than it is among civilized humans. He also maintained that conjugal and familial love are on the whole beneficial forces in the modern, bourgeois world, in which the praiseworthy citizenship that characterized ancient republics like Sparta and Rome is no longer an option: Only lovers are likely to overcome the calculated self-interest, despised by Rousseau, that in his view characterizes the modern world's inhabitants.

Our principal source for information about Rousseau's life is his *Confessions*, in which he recounts the often-embarrassing details of many of his sexual encounters with what, at the time, was unprecedented openness. In the *Confessions* Rousseau discusses masochistic, exhibitionist, and homosexual behavior in which he engaged, speaks of the *ménages à trois* in which he was involved, and acknowledges a proclivity for **masturbation**. He also confesses to having abandoned the five children of his who were born to his longtime companion Thérèse Levasseur (1721–1806), whom he met in 1745 and did not marry until 1768, long after the birth of the last of their children. He justified abandoning his children by claiming that in so doing he was acting like a "member of Plato's Republic": As a result of his action, his children, brought up in a foundling home, would become "workers and peasants rather than adventurers and fortune hunters" (*Confessions*, 299). Clearly the life that Rousseau lived differed strikingly from the life of conjugal fidelity and parental responsibility that he commended to others. Rousseau would have argued, though, that he was a "prodigy" (*Confessions*, 52), an extraordinary human being who was unable to live the life that he appropriately recommended to the mass of more ordinary people.

Rousseau was born in Geneva; his father was a watchmaker, and his mother died in childbirth. His father had to leave Geneva to avoid imprisonment, so Rousseau spent much of his boyhood raised by his mother's family. He himself fled from Geneva at age sixteen. While living in Savoy he encountered a benefactress, Louise Françoise de Warens

(1699–1762), who both tutored and seduced him. She enabled him to develop his philosophical, literary, and musical talents. Rousseau moved to Paris at age thirty; there he became one of the intellectuals involved in writing the *Encyclopédie* (Denis Diderot [1713–1784], Jean Le Rond D'Alembert [1717–1783], and Pierre Mouchon [1733–1797]) and also achieved notoriety by criticizing Enlightenment and civilization in seminal works like the *Discourse on the Sciences and the Arts* (1750) and the *Discourse on the Origin and Foundations of Inequality* (1755). Subsequent major works of Rousseau's, *Emile* and *The Social Contract* (1762), aroused further controversy, drawing criticism from both Catholic and Protestant theologians. As a result, Rousseau was unable to live in either Geneva or France.

Rousseau provides a speculative genetic account of the origin and development of human sexuality in the *Discourse on the Origin of Inequality* and his posthumously published *Essay on the Origin of Languages* (1781). He argues in the *Discourse* that sex was at first a physical need that was not particularly pressing and that humans originally lived isolated from and independent of one another, their occasional sexual encounters notwithstanding. Men and women copulated randomly, so there was a large supply of available sexual partners. As a result, men did not force themselves on women, and men did not dispute among themselves to win the favors of a particular woman. Women bore children infrequently and were able to raise them on their own. In short, sexual disputes did not occur in the peaceful state of nature, and the family did not exist there. That changed, though, after domiciles were invented, which led to the long-term cohabitation of men and women. The family then became natural, in that it was an appropriate response to the new situation that arose when particular men began to live with particular women for long periods in domiciles. Women then began to give birth to more children, hence to need men's assistance to provide for and look after their children. And men were willing to offer their assistance, because conjugal and paternal love, "the sweetest sentiments known to men" (*Discourse*, 146–47), naturally emerged in this new situation. Rousseau explicitly says that this period of human development, and not the earlier period prior to the invention of the family, was "the best for man" (*Discourse*, 150). The origin of love also had baleful consequences, though, as it led to the emergence of **jealousy** on the part of unsuccessful lovers and vanity on the part of successful ones.

Rousseau offers a completely different account of the nature of sex among civilized people, principally in *Emile*. The two accounts do not, however, contradict one another, he claims, because it is wrong "to confound what is natural in the savage state with what is natural in the civil state" (*Emile*, 406). He argues in *Emile*, quite remarkably, that sex is not a physical but a psychological need: "The senses are awakened by the imagination alone. Their need is not properly a physical need. It is not true that it is a true need" (333). In *Emile* Rousseau contends that male sexual arousal is hard to achieve but obviously necessary for successful heterosexual intercourse. He also asserts that women's sexual desire is stronger than men's. Women arouse men's desire (enabling men to satisfy women's desire) by masking their own desire. This masking of female desire constitutes women's sexual modesty, which is said here (unlike in the *Discourse*) to be natural. To be aroused, men must seem to themselves to have overcome their partners' reluctance. In other words, men are aroused by thinking that they triumph over their partners' reluctance. It is the self-esteem that this triumph generates (Rousseau's word for which is *amour-propre*) that accounts for male arousal. Thus men principally desire not their partners but their partners' esteem. Rousseau therefore understands sex among civilized people more as a product of human psychology than of human physiology. He also argues that modesty makes civilized sexual relations more pleasurable than the animal coupling that characterized the state of nature.

Concerning relations between the sexes and gender roles, Rousseau contends that good societies are based in part on heightening the sexual differentiation between men and women, so as to make each sex more dependent on the other. He claims that men and women have different but complementary strengths, so that the two sexes are effectively equal: "All the faculties common to the two sexes are not equally distributed between them; but taken together, they balance out" (*Emile*, 363). For example, men are superior in theoretical reason, but women are superior in practical reason. Men and women are not independent of one another; if they were, "they would live in eternal discord, and their partnership could not exist" (*Emile*, 377). Instead, the sexes are interdependent: "The social relation of the sexes . . . produces a moral person of which the woman is the eye and the man the arm" (*Emile*, 377). As a result, Rousseau denies the independent personhood of both men and women; neither a man nor a woman is an independent whole, because both men and women are instead complementary parts. In addition, though, he contends that men are less dependent on women than women are on men: "Woman and man are made for one another, but their mutual dependence is not equal. Men depend on women because of their desires; women depend on men because of both their desires and their needs. We would survive more easily without them than they would without us" (*Emile*, 364).

Rousseau's discussion of women in *Emile* is marred by occasional gross generalizations that have often been the subject of feminist critique. For example, "Almost all little girls learn to read and write with repugnance" (368). In addition, because maternity is certain but paternity an inference, Rousseau insists that women must do more than men to reassure their spouses of their sexual fidelity. Women must therefore care about their reputations, which means that, unlike men, they must be subject to public opinion: "Opinion is the grave of virtue among men and its throne among women" (365). Contentions like these, along with Rousseau's broader claim that women necessarily depend on men, have understandably aroused considerable feminist opposition. But at least with respect to the question of women's dependence, the dispute between Rousseau and his feminist critics arguably reveals agreement about a mutually shared end: equality between the sexes. Their chief disagreement concerns the appropriate means to that end. Thus Mary Wollstonecraft (1759–1797), Rousseau's first feminist critic, faults him in *A Vindication of the Rights of Woman* (1792) for trying to "make one moral being of a man and woman" (68). Since women depend on men, Rousseau maintains that women must differentiate themselves from men, so as to make men dependent on women: "The more women want to resemble [men], the less women will govern men, and then men will truly be the masters" (*Emile*, 363). Wollstonecraft does not want women "to have power over men" (107); she wants them to aim not for "empire—but equality" (162). Rousseau, like Wollstonecraft, supports equality between the sexes. But she believes that equality is possible because men and women need not depend on one another. By contrast, he believes that equality between the sexes is possible only because women can make men depend on them, just as women themselves depend on men.

Rousseau offers a qualified defense of romantic love, and an unqualified defense of conjugal love, as means of promoting morality in modern societies that in his view were suffused with selfishness. In his "Letter to D'Alembert" (1758), Rousseau observes that "the love of humanity and of one's country" are the loftiest sentiments but that when these are "extinguished," as is the case in corrupt modern times, "there remains only love, properly so called, to take their place, because its charm is more natural and is more difficult to erase from the heart than that of all the others" (117). "The most vicious of men is he who isolates himself the most, who most concentrates his heart in himself." Since selfishness of this sort is the characteristic vice of modern times, romantic love is an appropriate remedy for it: "It is much better to love a mistress than to love oneself alone in all the world." True lovers are morally superior to other modern men because only they can overcome their selfishness: "Where is the true lover who is not ready to immolate himself for his beloved, and where is the sensual and coarse passion in a man who is willing to die?" (*Emile*, 391). Furthermore, romantic love not only provides a basis for morality; combining "the union of the hearts" with "the attraction of the senses" also makes for "the supreme happiness of life" (*Emile*, 327). Interestingly, though, Rousseau makes it clear that the true lover's happiness and passionate overcoming of selfishness are themselves based on an untruth: "What is true love itself if it is not chimera, lie, and illusion? We love the image we make for ourselves far more than we love the object to which we apply it. If we saw what we love exactly as it is, there would be no more love on earth" (*Emile*, 329).

Notwithstanding this realistic debunking of romantic love, Rousseau still contends that heterosexual love provides the most natural basis for human sociability, because it offers the most natural route leading humans from self-absorption to involvement with and concern for others. Rousseau's fictional account of the romance between Emile and his beloved Sophie indicates that romantic love should culminate with marriage. The romantic love of newlyweds then evolves over time into the more stable if less passionate conjugal love of spouses, who ultimately become parents. Believing that "the attraction of domestic life is the best counterpoison for bad morals" (*Emile*, 46), Rousseau presents the nuclear family as the only practical solution to the selfish individualism that in his view runs rampant in modern bourgeois societies.

In his life and his works, Rousseau offers two radically different but fundamentally important visions of human sexuality. In many of his works Rousseau depicts harmonious heterosexual relationships as the basis of the greatest happiness available to us in modern times and as the source of a deep concern for the welfare of others that enables us to overcome the selfish individualism that he regards as the besetting moral failing of modern times. Rousseau's life, however, as recounted in his *Confessions*, tells a very different story. There Rousseau speaks openly of his flouting of sexual conventions, of the sexual perversities that attracted him, and of the radical individualism that led him to abandon the children whom he had fathered. Depending on whether one looks at his works or at his life, Rousseau can be said to have fostered the modern cult of bourgeois domesticity and romantic love but also the sexual revolution that arose in opposition to that cult. That remarkably ambivalent legacy surely testifies to Rousseau's incalculable influence on the sexual life of men and women in the nineteenth, twentieth, and now the twenty-first centuries.

See also Abstinence; Feminism, History of; Feminism, Liberal; Friendship; Hobbes, Thomas; Hume, David; Love; Masturbation; Schopenhauer, Arthur; Scruton, Roger; Utopianism; Westermarck, Edward

REFERENCES

Diderot, Denis, Jean Le Rond D'Alembert, and Pierre Mouchon. (1745–1780). *Encyclopedia [Encyclopédie ou Dictionnaire raisonné des sciences, des arts et des métiers]*. Selections translated by Nelly S. Hoyt and Thomas Cassirer. Indianapolis, Ind.: Bobbs-Merrill, 1965; Rousseau, Jean-Jacques. (1782, 1789) *Confessions*. In *The Confessions and Correspondence, Including the Letters to Malesherbe*. Ed. Christopher Kelly, Roger D. Masters, and Peter G. Stillman. Trans. Christopher

Kelly. Hanover, N.H.: University Press of New England, 1995, 1–550; Rousseau, Jean-Jacques. (1755) *Discourse on the Origin and Foundations of Inequality*. In *The First and Second Discourses*. Trans. Roger D. Masters and Judith R. Masters. New York: St. Martin's Press, 1978, 76–248; Rousseau, Jean-Jacques. (1761) *Emile, or On Education*. Trans. Allan Bloom. New York: Basic Books, 1979; Rousseau, Jean-Jacques. (1781) *Essay on the Origin of Languages*. In *The First and Second Discourses Together with the Replies to Critics and Essay on the Origin of Languages*. Trans. and ed. Victor Gourevitch. New York: Harper and Row, 1986, 239–95; Rousseau, Jean-Jacques. (1761) *Julie, or the New Heloise: Letters of Two Lovers Who Live in a Small Town at the Foot of the Alps*. Trans. Philip Stewart and Jean Vaché. Hanover, N.H.: University Press of New England, 1997; Rousseau, Jean-Jacques. (1758) "Letter to M. D'Alembert on the Theatre." In *Politics and the Arts*. Trans. Allan Bloom. Ithaca, N.Y.: Cornell University Press, 1960, 1–137; Rousseau, Jean-Jacques. (1762) *On the Social Contract*. In *On the Social Contract with Geneva Manuscript and Political Economy*. Trans. Judith R. Masters. Ed. Roger D. Masters. New York: St. Martin's Press, 1978, 41–155; Schwartz, Joel. *The Sexual Politics of Jean-Jacques Rousseau*. Chicago, Ill.: University of Chicago Press, 1984; Wollstonecraft, Mary. (1792) *A Vindication of the Rights of Woman*. Ed. Charles W. Hagelman. New York: Norton, 1976.

Joel Schwartz

ADDITIONAL READING

Baier, Glen. "A Proper Arbiter of Pleasure: Rousseau on the Control of Sexual Desire." *Philosophical Forum* 30:1 (1999), 249–68; Cranston, Maurice. *Jean-Jacques: The Early Life and Work of Jean-Jacques Rousseau 1712–1754*. New York: Norton, 1983; Cranston, Maurice. *The Noble Savage: Jean-Jacques Rousseau 1754–1762*. Chicago, Ill.: University of Chicago Press, 1991; Cranston, Maurice. *The Solitary Self: Jean-Jacques Rousseau in Exile and Adversity*. Chicago, Ill.: University of Chicago Press, 1997; Deleuze, Gilles. (1962) "Jean-Jacques Rousseau: Precursor of Kafka, Céline, and Ponge." In *Desert Islands and Other Texts 1953–1974*. Trans. Michael Taormina. Los Angeles, Calif.: Semiotext(e), 2004, 52–55; Elshtain, Jean Bethke. "Jean-Jacques Rousseau: Virtuous Families and Just Polities." In *Public Man, Private Woman: Women in Social and Political Thought*. Princeton, N.J.: Princeton University Press, 1981, 148–70; Fermon, Nicole. *Domesticating Passions: Rousseau, Women, and Nation*. Hanover, N.H.: University Press of New England, 1987; Hartle, Ann. "Augustine and Rousseau: Narrative and Self-Knowledge in the Two *Confessions*." In Gareth B. Matthews, ed., *The Augustinian Tradition*. Berkeley: University of California Press, 1999, 263–85; Hartle, Ann. *The Modern Self in Rousseau's Confessions: A Reply to St. Augustine*. Notre Dame, Ind.: University of Notre Dame Press, 1984; Keohane, Nannerl. " 'But for Her Sex . . . ': The Domestication of Sophie." *University of Ottawa Quarterly* 49 (July 1979), 390–400; Kofman, Sarah. "Rousseau's Phallocratic Ends." In Nancy Fraser and Sandra Lee Bartky, eds., *Revaluing French Feminism: Critical Essays on Difference, Agency, and Culture*. Bloomington: Indiana University Press, 1992, 46–59; Koppelman, Andrew. "Sex Equality and/or the Family: From Bloom vs. Okin to Rousseau vs. Hegel." *Yale Journal of Law and the Humanities* 4 (Summer 1992), 399–432; Lange, Lynda. "Rousseau and Modern Feminism." *Social Theory and Practice* 7 (Fall 1981), 245–77. Reprinted in Mary Lyndon Shanley and Carole Pateman, eds., *Feminist Interpretations and Political Theory*. University Park: Pennsylvania State University Press, 1991, 95–111; Lange, Lynda. "Rousseau: Women and the General Will." In Lorenne M. G. Clark and Lynda Lange, eds., *The Sexism of Social and Political Theory*. Toronto, Can.: University of Toronto Press, 1979, 41–52; Marso, Lori Jo. *(Un)Manly Citizens: Jean-Jacques Rousseau's and Germaine de Staël's Subversive Women*. Baltimore, Md.: Johns Hopkins University Press, 1999; Okin, Susan Moller. "Rousseau." In *Women in Western Political Thought*. Princeton, N.J.: Princeton University Press, 1979, 99–194; Okin, Susan Moller. "Rousseau's Natural Woman." *Journal of Politics* 41:2 (May 1979), 393–416; Paglia, Camille. "Return of the Great Mother: Rousseau vs. Sade." In *Sexual Personae: Art and Decadence from Nefertiti to Emily Dickinson*. New Haven, Conn.: Yale University Press, 1990, 230–47; Rapaport, Elizabeth. "On the Future of Love: Rousseau and the Radical Feminists." *Philosophical Forum*

5:1–2 (1973–1974), 185–205. Reprinted in POS1 (369–88); Singer, Irving. "Rousseau: The Attempt to Purify Passion." In *The Nature of Love*, vol. 2: *Courtly and Romantic*. Chicago, Ill.: University of Chicago Press, 1984, 303–43; Thomas, Paul. "Jean-Jacques Rousseau, Sexist?" *Feminist Studies* 17 (Summer 1991), 195–217; Weiss, Penny A. *Gendered Community: Rousseau, Sex, and Politics*. New York: New York University Press, 1993; Wexler, Victor. " 'Made for Man's Delight': Rousseau as Antifeminist." *American Historical Review* 81 (April 1976), 266–91; Wingrove, Elizabeth Rose. *Rousseau's Republican Romance*. Princeton, N.J.: Princeton University Press, 2000; Zerilli, Linda M. G. *Signifying Woman: Culture and Chaos in Rousseau, Burke, and Mill*. Ithaca, N.Y.: Cornell University Press, 1994.

RUDDICK, SARA. *See* Completeness, Sexual

RUSSELL, BERTRAND (1872–1970). Bertrand Arthur William Russell was one of the more unique, fascinating, and intelligent persons of the modern world. He was a mathematician (coauthoring *Principia mathematica* with Alfred North Whitehead), philosopher (see, for example, "The Philosophy of Logical Atomism" [1918] and *Human Knowledge: Its Scope and Limits* [1948]), educator, political activist, feminist, anticommunist, Lord of the British Empire, recipient of the Order of Merit, Nobel Laureate (for literature, 1950), and Honorary Fellow of the British Academy. He was married four times, siring his last child at age sixty-six. The fourth time he married he was eighty, and his bride was thirty years his junior. At eighty-eight, he still spoke at rallies for nuclear disarmament. Russell's positions on social issues were far ahead of their time.

Although Russell's family was part of the wealthy British aristocracy, his childhood was unhappy. His mother died when he was two. Two years later his father died, and Russell was sent to live with his grandparents. Because his grandfather died within another two years, Russell's early education was directed by his grandmother, who was religious, cold, and an unflinching disciplinarian. Life with her at Pembroke Lodge was filled with what Russell later referred to as "foolish prohibitions" (*Autobiography*, vol. 1, 43). Due to his grandmother's influence, Russell's early religious beliefs were typically Victorian. His inquisitive nature, intellectual gifts, and rebellious spirit, fueled by her groundless prohibitions, eventually caused Russell to reject organized religion and to carry out a frank campaign against the standard Victorian prohibitions. At a time when such views were unthinkable for most people, he defended euthanasia, abolishing the death penalty, and sexual freedom.

Russell outspokenly opposed many moral standards of the time. Because various clergymen intervened, including the Episcopal Bishop of New York, William Manning (1866–1949), he was denied in 1940 an academic post at the City University of New York (CUNY) (see Paul Edwards, "Appendix," *Why I Am Not a Christian*; and Conrad Russell, 24) on the grounds that his works were "lecherous, libidinous, lustful, venerous, erotomaniac, aphrodisiac, irreverent, narrow-minded, untruthful, and bereft of moral fiber" (*Autobiography*, vol. 2, 334). Russell refers to this incident as "a typical American witch-hunt." In a letter in response to encouragement from one of his supporters, Russell wrote that he was glad that CUNY students disagreed with Manning; otherwise, he would have had to "despair of the young" (348).

Russell and his second wife, Dora Winifred Black (1894–1986), had an open **marriage**. They agreed to allow one another to have sexual relations with others (which they did) and that if Dora became pregnant by someone else, they would divorce. Dora was impregnated by an American journalist, and she and Russell divorced. While they were together, motivated by the absence in England of a school progressive enough to meet their objectives, they started their own (Beacon Hill) in 1927. They offered students a very liberal education. They treated all religions as simply historical practices to be studied and contrasted with one another, without expressing any favoritism. They allowed the children considerable freedom of expression and permitted them to exercise nude. (Russell thought that childhood **masturbation** should not be forbidden or punished; *Marriage and Morals*, 277–81, "Sex Education," 115–16.) Another woman, Ottoline Morrell (1882–1946), had the greatest influence on Russell. He credits her with having rejuvenated him in 1911 (*Autobiography*, vol. 2, 3, 8). She was overwhelmed by his intellectual powers, and Russell was so taken with her that he tried for several years to persuade her to leave her husband and marry him. Although she never succumbed, they remained friends and confidants until her death. Lady Ottoline introduced Russell and D. H. Lawrence to each other (Moore, 3).

Throughout his life, Russell was a staunch feminist. He joined the National Union of Women's Suffrage Societies (NUWSS) in 1906 and was elected to its Executive Committee. In 1907, NUWSS asked him to run for a seat in Parliament under the banner of woman's suffrage, and he agreed to do so, but it was a forgone conclusion that the seat would go to the Conservative or Tory candidate. He was attacked both by men and, to Russell's surprise, by women. He stood his ground and received more votes than any non-Tory could have expected to receive. Throughout the remainder of his life he could always be depended upon to engage in debate on the behalf of women. He detested the idea (a "superstition") that men were superior to women, thinking it degrading not only to women but also to men (*Essays in Skepticism*, 16–18; *Unpopular Essays*, 157–59). Russell's moral position on **prostitution** and sexual relations in marriage reflected his **feminism**. For Russell, "The intrusion of the economic motive into sex is always . . . disastrous. Sexual relations should be a mutual delight, entered into solely from the spontaneous impulse of both parties." Partly on this basis, Russell condemned prostitution. He also (prophetically) condemned marital sexual relations entered into by wives economically dependent on their husbands: "[T]he total amount of undesired sex endured by women is probably greater in marriage than in prostitution" (*Marriage*, 153–55; *Why I Am Not a Christian*, 171–72; see Primoratz, "Prostitution," 173–74; Soble, 33–35).

In his autobiographical revelations, one often finds philosophical reflections on sexual morality. A particularly revealing passage describes his adulterous relationship in 1926 with Lady Constance Malleson (1895–1975). Russell relates that he was quite attracted to her and just happened to mention to her that he would be giving a speech on Baker Street. After the speech, he asked her to dine with him. Later they spent the night talking and making **love**. In Russell's reflections on this event (*Autobiography*, vol. 2, 19), he admits that most would consider his conduct imprudent but discounts this assessment on the grounds that, although they hardly knew each other, their encounter led to a relationship that was "profoundly serious," "profoundly important," both happy and painful, but worthwhile and never trivial. It did not bother Russell that she was very young and married. Nor did it bother him that he was married to Alys Pearsall Smith (1867–1951). Russell's actions and words spoke loudly in favor of a liberal view of **adultery**: So long as both participants benefit profoundly, adultery is justifiable. This view is reflected in his *Dictionary of Mind, Matter, and Morals*, where he claimed that sexual relations between consenting adults should not be grounds for criminal or civil prosecution, or for public disapproval, except when children are involved (236; see Primoratz, *Ethics and Sex*, 81). Even then, the authority of the state extends only to ensure that the children are cared for and properly educated and that the father financially supports them. Many of Russell's contemporaries judged his sexual affairs and philosophy to be sinful, but Russell rejected the very concept of sin, at least regarding what was commonly understood by the Victorians to be sinful. Russell thought the concept *sin* to be, except as an indication of what a society deigns blameworthy, a mistaken concept. When applied to others, "sin" is used to "justify cruelty and vindictiveness"; when it is applied to oneself, "it is morbid self-abasement" ("Sin," in Seckel, 278).

In *Marriage and Morals*, a work often cited by those opposing his CUNY appointment, Russell argued in favor of premarital sex (165–67). It helps prepare one for marriage. Further, it enables one to appreciate the difference between relationships established on the basis of sexual gratification and relationships based on intellectual or emotional compatibility (see *Why I Am Not a Christian*, 171), which basis has a better chance of sustaining marriage. He thought that the view that premarital sex was wrong to be only an ungrounded prejudice, having no rational basis. Russell argued against the Christian condemnation of premarital sex by claiming that it originated with **Saint Paul**'s (5–64?) disdain for sex (*Marriage and Morals*, 46–48) and that the Catholic Church promoted marriage only to prevent widespread fornication. (Russell did, however, admire **Saint Augustine** [354–430] as a philosopher; *Dictionary*, 14.) **Thomas Nagel** has written about *Marriage and Morals*, "So much of what he called for . . . has been achieved by the sexual revolution and the feminist movement that I suppose no one reads it any more" (*Concealment and Exposure*, 65).

In "Dogmatic and Scientific Ethics," Russell rejected the practice of lifetime monogamy (contrary to, for example, **Thomas Aquinas** [1224/25–1274], *Summa contra gentiles*, bk. 3, chaps. 122, 123) in favor of the freedom of people to follow their natural impulse to enjoy sexual relations based on mutual desire and nothing else (10; *Why I Am Not a Christian*, 69). Yet he also claimed, "Sex is at its best between a father and mother who love each other and their children" ("Sex Education," 118). Russell was no simplistic libertine. Although Russell personally found homosexual relations distasteful, he was strongly opposed to laws making it an offense for consenting adults. With regard to romantic love, Russell was skeptical. He claimed that for nine out of ten persons "a constant succession of partners is necessary" and that romantic love was an illusion incapable of resisting the exigencies of everyday life ("Institution of Marriage").

Although Russell's sexual views were shocking to the Victorians, and are today equally shocking for many faith-based conservatives, they were not said for their shock value. Russell's views were always founded on reason; he refused to accept anything on faith alone (this might be related to his empiricist epistemology). His views about sexual morality might be justifiable on the basis of the normative ethical theory he favored, utilitarianism, which judges the rightness of an action in terms of the ratio of its good and bad consequences. In an early essay, "The Elements of Ethics," Russell relied on G. E. Moore's (1873–1958) view that "goodness" was a nonnatural property and attempted to establish an objective basis for utilitarian principles. Eventually, Russell rejected Moore's view about goodness but not utilitarianism. In "Power and Moral Codes" (215–16) and *Human Society in Ethics and Politics* (92–98), he critically examined several varieties of utilitarianism, pointed out their weaknesses, and defended a form of act utilitarianism that judges the rightness and wrongness of an action in terms of what one expects will be, on balance, the best overall outcome (see Odell, 69–81).

From the perspective of only the primary parties involved in adultery, this utilitarianism was consistent with his actions. Russell felt confident that his affairs with Lady Constance and Ottoline Morrell would, on balance, have good consequences for both participants and, as far as he was concerned, they did. However, since Russell's theory judges our actions morally in terms of what are, on balance, their *overall* consequences, the pain and unhappiness experienced by the spouses affected must also be taken into account. About Russell's nearly cavalier morality of adultery, some philosophers would argue that both the damage caused to these third parties and the damage possibly done to the family institution and hence to society by widespread adultery far outweigh the advantages gained by the adulterous partners (**Richard Posner**, 183–86). Even from the moral philosophy he embraced, utilitarianism, it is unclear that Russell is fully able to justify adultery. (Note that part of Russell's criticism of prostitution in *Marriage and Morals* seems more indebted to **Immanuel Kant**'s [1724–1804] ethics than to utilitarianism: "Morality in sexual relations . . . consists essentially of respect for the other person, and unwillingness to use that person solely as a means of personal gratification." He asserted that "prostitution sins against this principle" [153].)

Russell would not, however, accept the broader utilitarian condemnation of his adulterous affairs. (This shows how difficult it can be to apply a utilitarian moral principle to actual behavior in a complex social context.) He would argue, I think, that monogamy is unrealistic; that most people need a variety of sexual partners; that sexual monogamy creates more unhappiness than would the practice of free love. Most people who have affairs lie to their spouses, and when they are found out (which is nearly inevitable), the pain their spouses experience is often greater than they would have experienced in an open marriage. Killing, stealing from, destroying the property of, and lying to others are recognized by Russell to be, under most circumstances, morally wrong. They do great harm. A society that does not prohibit such actions cannot survive. But a society founded on a candid acceptance of the human's natural appetite for sexual relations, one that rejects the judgment that this appetite is sinful, cannot help being, on Russell's view, a society in which widespread happiness would prevail.

See also Abstinence; Adultery; Augustine (Saint); Casual Sex; Consequentialism; Ellis, Albert; Ethics, Sexual; Feminism, Men's; Friendship; Jealousy; Kant, Immanuel; Love; Mandeville, Bernard; Marriage; Paul (Saint); Prostitution; Rimmer, Robert; Thomas Aquinas (Saint)

REFERENCES

Moore, Harry T. "Introduction." In Harry T. Moore, ed., *D. H. Lawrence's Letters to Bertrand Russell*. New York: Gotham Book Mart, 1948, 1–26; Nagel, Thomas. (2001) "Bertrand Russell: A Public Life." In *Concealment and Exposure and Other Essays*. Oxford, U.K.: Oxford University Press, 2002, 63–71; Odell, S. Jack. *On Russell*. Belmont, Calif.: Wadsworth, 2000; Posner, Richard A. *Sex and Reason*. Cambridge, Mass.: Harvard University Press, 1992; Primoratz, Igor. *Ethics and Sex*. London: Routledge, 1999; Primoratz, Igor. "What's Wrong with Prostitution?" *Philosophy* 68:264 (April 1993), 159–82; Russell, Bertrand. *The Autobiography of Bertrand Russell*. Vol. 1: *1872–1914*. Vol. 2: *1914–1944*. Boston, Mass.: Little, Brown, 1951; Russell, Bertrand. *Dictionary of Mind, Matter, and Morals*. Ed. Lester E. Denonn. New York: Philosophical Library, 1952; Russell, Bertrand. "Dogmatic and Scientific Ethics." *The Outlook* 53 (5 January 1924), 9–10; Russell, Bertrand. (1910) "The Elements of Ethics." In *Philosophical Essays*, rev. ed. London: Allen and Unwin, 1966, 13–59; Russell, Bertrand. *Essays in Skepticism*. New York: Philosophical Library, 1962; Russell, Bertrand. *Human Knowledge: Its Scope and Limits*. New York: Simon and Schuster, 1948; Russell, Bertrand. *Human Society in Ethics and Politics*. New York: Simon and Schuster, 1955; Russell, Bertrand. "The Institution of Marriage Is Here to Stay." *Jewish Daily Forward* (19 December 1926), E1; Russell, Bertrand. (1929) *Marriage and Morals*. New York: Liveright, 1970; Russell, Bertrand.

(1918) "The Philosophy of Logical Atomism." In Robert C. Marsh, ed., *Logic and Knowledge: Essays 1901–1950*. London: George Allen and Unwin, 1956, 177–281; Russell, Bertrand. (1938) "Power and Moral Codes." In Charles Pigden, ed., *Russell on Ethics: Selections from the Writings of Bertrand Russell*. London: Routledge, 1999, 202–20; Russell, Bertrand. (1926) "Sex Education." In *On Education, Especially in Early Childhood*. London: Unwin, 1973, 115–21; Russell, Bertrand. *Unpopular Essays*. New York: Simon and Schuster, 1950; Russell, Bertrand. *Why I Am Not a Christian and Other Essays on Religion and Related Subjects*. Ed. Paul Edwards. New York: Simon and Schuster, 1963; Russell, Conrad. *Academic Freedom*. London: Routledge, 1993; Seckel, Al, ed. *Bertrand Russell on God and Religion*. Buffalo, N.Y.: Prometheus, 1986; Soble, Alan. *Sexual Investigations*. New York: New York University Press, 1996; Thomas Aquinas. (1258–1264) *On the Truth of the Catholic Faith. Summa contra gentiles. Book Three: Providence. Part II*. Trans. Vernon J. Bourke. Garden City, N.Y.: Image Books, 1956; Whitehead, Alfred North, and Bertrand Russell. *Principia mathematica*, 3 vols. Cambridge: Cambridge University Press, 1910–1913.

S. Jack Odell

ADDITIONAL READING

Ayer, Alfred Jules. *Bertrand Russell*. New York: Viking, 1972; Brink, Andrew. *The Psychobiography of a Moralist*. Atlantic Highlands, N.J.: Humanities Press, 1989; Dewar, Lindsay. *Marriage without Morals: A Reply to Mr. Bertrand Russell*. London: Society for Promoting Christian Knowledge, 1931; Edwards, Paul. "Russell, Bertrand." In Lawrence C. Becker and Charlotte B. Becker, eds., *Encyclopedia of Ethics*, 2nd ed., vol. 3. New York: Routledge, 2001, 1526–28; Ellis, Albert. "Adultery: Pros and Cons." In *Sex without Guilt*. New York: Lyle Stuart, 1958, 51–65; Ellis, Albert. "Healthy and Disturbed Reasons for Having Extramarital Relations." In Gerhard Neubeck, ed., *Extramarital Relations*. Englewood Cliffs, N.J.: Prentice-Hall, 1969, 153–61; Fishman, Stephen M. "Marital Friendship: Toward a Reconception of Romance." In Alan Soble, ed., *Sex, Love, and Friendship*. Amsterdam, Holland: Rodopi, 1997, 421–27; Hampshire, Stuart. "He Had His Ups and Downs." [Review of *Bertrand Russell*, vol. 2, *1921–1970: The Ghost of Madness*, by Ray Monk] *New York Review of Books* (17 May 2001), 42–44; Klemke, E. D., ed. *Essays on Bertrand Russell*. Urbana: University of Illinois Press, 1970; Lawrence, D. H. *D. H. Lawrence's Letters to Bertrand Russell*. Ed. Harry T. Moore. New York: Gotham Book Mart, 1948; McMaster University. *The Bertrand Russell Archives*. <www.mcmaster.ca/russdocs/russell.htm> [accessed 8 September 2004]; Monk, Ray. *Bertrand Russell*, Vol. 1, *1872–1921: The Spirit of Solitude*. London: Jonathan Cape, 1996. *Bertrand Russell*, Vol. 2, *1921–1970: The Ghost of Madness*. New York: Free Press, 2001; Primoratz, Igor. "What's Wrong with Prostitution?" *Philosophy* 68:264 (April 1993), 159–82. Reprinted in HS (291–314); POS3 (339–61); POS4 (451–73). Expanded, revised as "Prostitution," in *Ethics and Sex*. London: Routledge, 1999, 88–109; Russell, Bertrand. *Marriage and Morals*. London: Allen and Unwin, 1929; Russell, Bertrand. "Marriage and the Population Question." *International Journal of Ethics* 26 (1916), 443–61; Russell, Bertrand. "My Own View of Marriage." *The Outlook* 48 (7 March 1928), 376–77; Russell, Bertrand. "Ostrich Code of Marriage." *Forum* 80 (1928), 7–10; Russell, Bertrand. (1918) "The Philosophy of Logical Atomism." In Robert C. Marsh, ed., *Logic and Knowledge: Essays 1901–1950*. London: George Allen and Unwin, 1956, 177–281. Reprinted, New York: Capricorn, 1971; Russell, Bertrand. *Power: A New Social Analysis*. London: Allen and Unwin, 1938. Reprinted, London: Routledge, 1995; Russell, Bertrand. (1930) "The Sense of Sin." In Louis Greenspan and Stefan Andersson, eds., *Russell on Religion: Selections from the Writings of Bertrand Russell*. London: Routledge, 1999, 186–204; Schilpp, Paul Arthur, ed. *The Philosophy of Bertrand Russell*. Evanston, Ill.: Northwestern University Press, 1944. La Salle, Ill.: Open Court, 1989; Weidlich, Thom. *Appointment Denied: The Inquisition of Bertrand Russell*. Amherst, N.Y.: Prometheus, 2000; Westermarck, Edward. *The Future of Marriage in Western Civilisation*. New York: Macmillan, 1936.

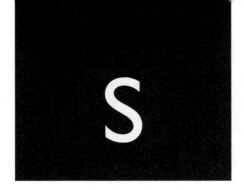

SACHER-MASOCH, LEOPOLD VON (1836–1895). Leopold Ritter von Sacher-Masoch was a German novelist known for his strange stories and way of life. His countryman Richard von Krafft-Ebing (1840–1902), a pioneer of **sexology**, named "masochism" after him (*Psychopathia Sexualis*, 105).

Masoch was born in Lemberg in Galicia (Lvov, Poland), the oldest son of the head of the police and a Russian woman of noble origin. His birth was dramatic and there were serious doubts that he would survive. In his literary development, the role of his childhood is emphasized (he enjoyed the beatings he received at home from his aunt Countess Zenobia). In 1848 the family moved to Prague, where Masoch learned German. They moved again, in 1854, to Graz, where he took a doctoral degree of law at the age of nineteen. In 1856, he attained the position of *Privatdozent* for German history at Graz. Masoch resigned in 1870 to concentrate on writing.

Though Masoch had a series of affairs, including a young novelist Emilie Mataja (1855–1938), he never was a Don Juan but more a Don Quixote. In 1873 he married Angelika Aurora Rümelin (1845–1908). The affair with Aurora, as many of Masoch's relationships, began with correspondence, and eventually she met the writer dressed as one of his heroines. Masoch tried to inject his fictional ideals into family life. Aurora changed her name to Wanda, in accordance with the heroine of Masoch's novel *Venus im Pelz*. A mixture of life and art was not new for Masoch: His novel *Die geschiedene Frau* (*The Divorced Woman*) was a side product of his affair with a doctor's wife who left her husband for Masoch. This tendency peaked with Wanda. Masoch, for example, urged his wife to infidelity. His instability, incompetence in practical matters, and continuous humiliation of her turned Wanda against him.

After separating from Wanda, Masoch formed a relationship with his secretary and translator, Hulda Meister (1856–1918). In 1886 they moved to Lindheim, Germany. In this village Masoch received a position of patron of some kind and became a local Tolstoy to the peasants. His health gradually declining, he died in 1895, probably insane. Wanda moved to Paris, where she published her memoir, *The Confessions*, and died in poverty in 1908.

Masoch is best known for his novel *Venus*, but eighty novels and around a hundred short stories are reported to have been written by him. Some of these resemble his principal work (*Master Masochist*), but his corpus also includes folk tales (*A Light for Others*), plays, and historical works. In literature, his influence remains marginal. Nevertheless, in the Europe of his time Masoch was a household name, even hailed as the new Turgenev. One may debate whether his fame came from his literary talent or his extraordinary life. Masoch is sometimes labeled a writer of scandals. One can imagine that his stories caused resentment among the petit bourgeois of the Habsburg empire, but his contemporaries did not find his work offensive. It was his life that made a splash.

Masoch represents the ideal of modern writer who seeks to mold his life after his art, and *vice versa*. Despite this avant-guardism, Masoch was not a first-rank writer. His plots are stereotypical. His style, if better than average, is pompous, even sentimental and sterile. He is aptly characterized as a romantic of the Goethean spirit and as annoyingly intimate.

The dominant position of *Venus* among Masoch's works is justified. It encompasses all the issues that figure into his art: domination, **sexual perversion**, the merging of the personal and the fictional, **fantasy**, and idealism. The novel was not originally an independent work but part of a planned six-part volume on the natural history of humanity, *The Heritage of Cain*. The themes of the parts were to be **love**, property, state, war, work, and death. Only the first and second parts were published. *Venus* is a love story that takes place in a luxurious atmosphere and concentrates on describing the decadent inner life. The book idealizes and romanticizes sexual perversion and questions institutionalized forms of sexuality, like **marriage**.

Masoch's reputation is based largely on his impact on the study of sexuality. Though masochism is a sexual behavior, to understand masochism (or any other form of sexual expression) only as a physical phenomenon is to miss much that is special about *human* sexuality (see **Thomas Nagel** and **Roger Scruton**). Masochism is not simply the reverse of sadism. If it is a perversion (or **paraphilia**), it is a mental perversion in which carnal gratification plays a minor role. Whether masochism is a perversion in some robust sense, as a deviation from what is "right" or "normal" in the sexual domain, is debatable.

There are, on one standard view, two major forms of masochism, the *material* and the *moral*. In these terms, masochism involves satisfaction acquired by suffering, either corporal (material) or mental (moral). This approach enables sadism and masochism to be assimilated under one phenomenon, **sadomasochism**. Their reciprocity is based on the idea that the object of the sadist's activity is a masochist. An alternative view is that the masochist is a genuine subject, not an object. Hence masochism is not the reverse of sadism but independent of it.

The predominance of the sexual aspect of masochism and the primacy of sadism are views derived from the studies of Krafft-Ebing, **Sigmund Freud** (1856–1939), and **Havelock Ellis** (1859–1939). The main weakness of the psychoanalytic account of masochism is that it overlooks the complexly staged character of masochism that Masoch's works make evident. A more balanced treatment was provided by the French philosopher Gilles Deleuze (1925–1995), who in 1967 published, with an extensive introduction, his translation of *Venus*. Deleuze studied masochism through Masoch and separately from the sadism of the **Marquis de Sade** (1740–1814).

Deleuze, partly following Theodor Reik's (1888–1969) *Masochism in Sex and Society*, enumerates five central features of masochism: fantasy, suspension, persuasion, provocative fear, and contract (*Coldness and Cruelty*, 74–76). In masochism, pleasure is abstract and intellectualized; in this way culture replaces nature in sexuality. *Fantasy* represents the reflective and planned nature of the pleasures of masochism, in which everything must be envisioned beforehand (see Reik, "Characteristics," 324–26). The ritualized and symbolic nature of masochistic fantasy exemplifies culture's replacement of nature. Masochistic pleasure is also conceived in terms of *suspension* ("suprasensualism"; *Venus*, 97–98): It is never immediate or carnal but the result of careful, delicate preparation. Suspension functions to raise anxiety and thereby excitement. Masochism does not aim at orgasm; it is hard to find descriptions of sexual acts, in this sense, in Masoch. He does not require Sadeian provocation. *Persuasion*, the masochist's expression of pain, humiliation, and embarrassment, acts as a signal to the mistress. His begging for punishment is not only submission but also a command that the mistress continue. *Provocative fear* has, in this ritualized "negotiation," a balancing role. Masochistic submission is aggressive, and by it the masochist aims to resolve anxiety, defuse pain, and allow the enjoyment of the forbidden. All this yields a refined, sterile form of sexuality.

Finally, *contracts* play a decisive role in masochism. Masoch made several contracts with his mistresses (Deleuze, app. 2). A contract is always made between equals, in this case between the masochist *qua* subject and his mistress, and in it the conditions of the relationship are articulated. The contract reveals the salient point that even though the masochist seems to be a slave, in reality he is bound by *his* words and decisions (see Vera). Often contracts are rewritten to incorporate more severe conditions. Usually they are actual documents, which reflects Masoch's questioning the institution of marriage and its suffocating sexual roles. Contracts also reflect the idealism in Masoch, because they represent the perfect form of a love relationship.

Idealism and idealization have other roles in Masoch. (Note that *Venus* begins with **G.W.F. Hegel** [1770–1831] and ends with **Plato** [427–347 BCE].) Masoch's aesthetic idealism can be seen in his characters, who are (unlike Sadeian villains) art lovers. The world created by Masoch is a still life. This aesthetics of the frozen is shown by the statues and paintings in his work, which are exemplars of ideal **beauty**. The political dimension of Masoch's idealism is found in his models of men and women (Deleuze, 66–67, 96–100, and chap. 4). For men, the models are Cain, history's first criminal; Christ, who represents spirituality and atonement; and the Greek, who is caught in masochistic triangles. The idealized models of women are the Grecian, representing paganism and nature; the sadistic mistress, acting as the puppet of the masochist (contrary to appearances); and the ideal woman of severe maternal power who has overcome sadism.

Masoch's relevance lies not so much in his descriptions of sexuality but is more political. Although he dislocated the traditional power roles of men and women, he did not overcome traditional gender roles. The subjects in his stories are always men. What is more important is that Masoch questioned the institution of marriage, depicted an alternative form of sexuality, and fully revealed the slavish aspects of mental life. One can find deep irony and sensitivity in his work, in which he made the most private issue, sexuality, a matter of public debate. One perhaps needs, however, to adopt a masochistic state of mind to reach these conclusions.

See also Bataille, Georges; Ellis, Havelock; Existentialism; Fantasy; Freud, Sigmund; Nagel, Thomas; Objectification, Sexual; Paraphilia; Perversion, Sexual; Poststructuralism; Sade, Marquis de; Sadomasochism; Scruton, Roger

REFERENCES

Deleuze, Gilles. (1967) *Coldness and Cruelty*. Trans. Jean McNeil. New York: Zone Books, 1989; Krafft-Ebing, Richard von. (1886) *Psychopathia Sexualis*. Munich, Ger.: Matthes and Seitz Verlag, 1984; Nagel, Thomas. "Sexual Perversion." *Journal of Philosophy* 66:1 (1969), 5–17; Reik, Theodor. "Characteristics of Masochism." In Margaret Ann Fitzpatrick-Hanly, ed., *Essential Papers on Masochism*. New York: New York University Press, 1995, 324–43; Reik, Theodor. *Masochism in Sex and Society*. Trans. M. H. Beigel and G. M. Kurth. New York: Grove Press, 1962; Sacher-Masoch, Leopold von. (1869) *Die geschiedene Frau: Passionsgeschichte eines Idealisten*. Ed. Michael Farin. Munich, Ger.: Belleville, 1985; Sacher-Masoch, Leopold von. *A Light for Others and Other Jewish Tales from Galicia*. Trans. Michael O. Pecko. Riverside, Calif.: Ariadne Press, 1994; Sacher-Masoch, Leopold von. *The Master Masochist: Tales of a Sadistic Mistress*. Trans. Eric

Lemuel Randall. London: Senate, 1996; Sacher-Masoch, Leopold von. (1870) *Venus in Furs and Selected Letters of Leopold von Sacher-Masoch*. Trans. Uwe Moeller and Laura Lindgren. New York: Blast Books, 1989; Sacher-Masoch, Wanda von. (1907) *The Confessions of Wanda von Sacher-Masoch*. Trans. Marian Phillips, Caroline Hébert, and V. Vale. Illustrated ed. San Francisco, Calif.: Re/Search, 1990; Scruton, Roger. *Sexual Desire: A Moral Philosophy of the Erotic*. New York: Free Press, 1986; Vera, Diane. "Temporary Consensual 'Slave Contract.'" In Pat Califia, ed., *The Lesbian S/M Safety Manual*. Boston, Mass.: Alyson Publications, 1988, 75–76.

Juhana Lemetti

ADDITIONAL READING

Cleugh, James. *The Marquis and the Chevalier: A Study in the Psychology of Sex as Illustrated by the Lives and Personalities of the Marquis de Sade (1740–1814) and the Chevalier von Sacher-Masoch (1836–1905)*. Boston, Mass.: Little and Brown, 1952. Westport, Conn.: Greenwood Press, 1972; Deleuze, Gilles. (1967) *Masochism. An Interpretation of Coldness and Cruelty. Together with the Entire Text of Venus in Furs by Leopold von Sacher-Masoch*. Trans. Jean McNeil and Aude Willm. New York: Braziller, 1971. Reprint, *Coldness and Cruelty*. Trans. Jean McNeil. New York: Zone Books, 1989; Deleuze, Gilles. (1967) "Mysticism and Masochism." In *Desert Islands and Other Texts 1953–1974*. Trans. Michael Taormina. Los Angeles, Calif.: Semiotext(e), 2004, 131–34; Ellis, Havelock. (1897) *Studies in the Psychology of Sex*, vol. 3: *Analysis of the Sexual Impulse. Love and Pain. The Sexual Impulse in Women*, 2nd ed. Philadelphia, Pa.: F. A. Davis, 1927; Fitzpatrick-Hanly, Margaret Ann, ed. *Essential Papers on Masochism*. New York: New York University Press, 1995; Freud, Sigmund. (1919) "A Child Is Being Beaten: A Contribution to the Study of the Origin of Sexual Perversion." Trans. James Strachey. In Margaret Ann Fitzpatrick-Hanly, ed., *Essential Papers on Masochism*. New York: New York University Press, 1995, 159–81; Freud, Sigmund. (1924) "The Economic Problem of Masochism." Trans. James Strachey. In Margaret Ann Fitzpatrick-Hanly, ed., *Essential Papers on Masochism*. New York: New York University Press, 1995, 274–85; Money, John. "Taking Your Punishment Like a Man: The Lovemap of Masochism." In *The Adam Principle. Genes, Genitals, Hormones, & Gender: Selected Readings in Sexology*. Buffalo, N.Y.: Prometheus, 1993, 300–304; Nagel, Thomas. "Sexual Perversion." *Journal of Philosophy* 66:1 (1969), 5–17. Reprinted in P&S1 (247–60); POS1 (76–88). Reprinted, revised, in Thomas Nagel, *Mortal Questions*. Cambridge: Cambridge University Press, 1979, 39–52; POS2 (39–51); POS3 (9–20); POS4 (9–20); STW (105–12); Noyes, John K. *The Mastery of Submission: Inventions of Masochism*. Ithaca, N.Y.: Cornell University Press, 1997; Olkowski, Dorothea. "Monstrous Reflection: Sade and Masoch—Rewriting the History of Reason." In Arleen Dallery and Charles E. Scott, eds., *Crisis in Continental Philosophy: Selected Studies in Phenomenology and Existential Philosophy*. Albany: State University of New York Press, 1990, 189–200; Sacher-Masoch, Leopold von. (1891) *Jewish Life: Tales from Nineteenth-Century Europe*. Trans. Virginia L. Lewis. Riverside, Calif.: Ariadne Press, 1991; Sartre, Jean-Paul. (1943) "First Attitude toward Others: Love, Language, Masochism." In *Being and Nothingness*. Trans. Hazel E. Barnes. New York: Philosophical Library, 1956, 478–91; Schlichtegroll, C. F. von. *Sacher-Masoch und der Masochismus*. Dresden, Ger.: H. R. Dohrn, 1901; Weinberg, Thomas S. "Sacher-Masoch, Leopold Ritter von." In Vern L. Bullough and Bonnie Bullough, eds., *Human Sexuality: An Encyclopedia*. New York: Garland, 1994, 525–26.

SADE, MARQUIS DE (1740–1814). Donatien Alphonse François de Sade is one of the most scandalous writers. His celebrated, clandestine novels deal with what is now called "sadism," causing pain to get sexual pleasure, but Sade deals comprehensively with the joys of vice, crime, and perverted sexuality. All these are somehow eroticized or understood from the point of view of a person's desire to attain sexual gratification. Sade is a pornographer and a philosopher of perverted sex. His novels have until recently been censored, yet his readership has been wide and his influence considerable. Sade's philosophy has been seen as either one of unlimited freedom or of moral and religious rebellion. In the first sense, Sade is seen as trying to break loose from all restrictions on one's fantasies, desires, thoughts, and acts. In this context he has been called the "Divine Marquis." But Sade can also be seen as promoting evil, as if to replace virtue with vice and life with destruction, as if his infinite rage would like to destroy all the world around him. Sade is, according to this view, the ultimate egoist. As the philosopher of liberty, Sade's aims are basically laudable or even ethical. As the morally rebellious thinker, he is unconditionally evil. Sade is either an Enlightenment thinker whose message is normative or a subversive thinker who describes the horrors of the human mind, in which case the value of his work is its exploration of the mind's darkest recesses.

Sade's life was colorful, adventurous, and tragic to an almost unparalleled degree. He was born in Paris to a noble family who could boast of Petrarch's (1304–1374) Laura among their ancestors. His early adulthood was spent in the French army, and not much is known about it. Later he divided his time between Paris and his chateau, La Coste in Provence, where he staged orgies that caused him trouble. He spent twenty-five years (one-third of his life) in prisons and asylums. He was imprisoned by a *lettre de cachet* acquired by Madame de Motreuil, his mother-in-law, who was angered by his financial irresponsibility and licentious sexual behavior. He seduced his sister-in-law. After the French revolution, Sade was a free man for a while, but spent his last days in the Charenton mental hospital. He was a revolutionary district judge (1793) but was arrested for being an aristocrat. He was going to be guillotined but miraculously avoided death. He had already in 1772 received a death sentence in Marseilles for poisoning prostitutes and sodomizing his servant. He was executed in effigy at Aix. Sade was a libertine whose private life, when he was free, was geared toward sexual pleasure in all its forms. Although it is not certain, it seems that he never killed anyone or caused serious bodily harm, beyond a whipping in an erotic context (see Weinberg, 526).

Sade's voluminous writings consist of pornographic novels, short stories, plays, and his letters (a major source of biographical information). His main novels are *Justine* (1791), *Juliette* (1797), *120 Days of Sodom* (1785–1789?), and *Philosophy in the Bedroom* (1796).

Justine is the story of a virtuous and innocent young woman who wanders through France from chateau to chateau, experiencing one misfortune after another. She is raped and abused repeatedly. Her innocent mind never learns from her bitter experiences; she remains unable to avoid danger but never becomes corrupted. Sade thereby wrote a parody of Voltaire's (1694–1778) *Candide* (1759).

Justine's sister Juliette is her opposite, a woman who quickly understands that virtue is a disastrous policy and therefore wants to be vicious. Sade's satire in *Juliette* is aimed at **Aristotle** (384–322 BC), who claimed that one becomes virtuous by doing virtuous deeds (*Nicomachean Ethics*, 1103a30–1103b, 1105a, 1179b25). Sade seems to reply that one becomes vicious by doing evil deeds. One's conscience dies, and one becomes able to enjoy vice. Juliette is a successful libertine whose life is as destructive as it is happy. *Justine* and *Juliette* thus mirror each other. This is true, too, in terms of their **language**. Justine's style is old-fashioned, flowery, decorative, and vain, which reflects Justine's thought—the source of her troubles. Juliette's language is straightforward and immodest and disguises nothing. On the contrary, it explains everything as it is. The reader gets a recipe for success in life. *Justine* is a pessimistic book, while *Juliette* is optimistic.

The greatest of Sade's works is *120 Days*, a massive compilation of all possible **sexual desire**s and activities, written like a medieval *Summa*. Four male friends gather in the Castle of Silling in the Black Forest in wintertime. There female prostitutes tell them stories of sexual pleasures and activities that the libertines, slaves to their perverted whims, subsequently try with their resident slaves. This remarkably comprehensive collection may be read as a textbook of perverted sexuality.

The publication history of Sade's works is complicated. *Justine* appeared in three different versions, of which the last, together with *Juliette*, formed a single edition that was confiscated by the police in 1801 from his publisher Nicolas Messé. Its author was arrested and eventually put into the Charenton lunatic asylum. Sade denied authorship. He was also assigned, wrongly, the authorship of the pamphlet *Zoloé*, which angered Napoleon. Sade was never released. *120 Days* was written in the Bastille just before the Parisians stormed and destroyed it. The manuscript was on a long scroll of paper that was lost when Sade was forced to leave his belongings in the cell. It was found in 1900 and published in 1904; a definitive edition by Maurice Heine (1884–1940) appeared in 1931–1935.

Sade had high ambitions of being a playwright and penned more than twenty plays. One, *Oxtiern*, was staged unsuccessfully in Paris in 1791. Later he directed plays in Charenton in which the inmates were actors. Peter Weiss's (1916–1982) play *The Persecution and Assassination of Jean-Paul Marat as Performed by the Inmates of the Asylum of Charenton under the Direction of the Marquis de Sade* (1964) depicts this stage of his life and provides an interpretation of Sade as a champion of liberty.

Sade's thought must be extrapolated from his novels, which can be read philosophically as part of the Enlightenment. (This is argued by Horkheimer [1895–1973] and Adorno [1903–1969] in *Dialectic of Enlightenment* [1944].) Sade is an atheist, materialist, and egoist who believes that the purpose of life is to maximize personal short-term pleasure. He wants to provide a rationale for the libertine lifestyle and advise his readers how it can be achieved. For Sade, all pleasure is erotic in nature—as if anticipating **Sigmund Freud**'s (1856–1939) idea of libidinal energy as the basic motivating factor in human behavior. In the possible world Sade describes, all action is directed toward sexual pleasure, regardless of its cost. He presupposes that libertines (Juliette) are not only happier than virtuous persons (Justine) but also more socially successful. To live out one's fantasies seems to promote one's power, social status, and financial success. This is the opposite of what is commonly believed, but Sade's texts are both ironic and subversive.

Influenced by Julien LaMettrie (1700–1751) and **Thomas Hobbes** (1588–1679), two famous materialists, Sade's world was materialistic and therefore without God. According to Sade's metaphysics, the world consists of dead atoms, which move around aimlessly, purposelessly, in infinite, otherwise empty space. In true Epicurean manner, these atoms form constellations that happen to be our world and its occupants. Matter exists, but the world is normatively empty: There are no objective moral laws or values, let alone a spiritual entity such as God. This universe creates and destroys busily and endlessly: Atoms form patterns that immediately dissolve. From this Sade infers his basic normative principles: Respect the natural order, admit that Nature creates and kills randomly, and do the same. It is a mistake to expect coherent logic here. What Sade provides is a parody of Natural Philosophy. For instance, for Sade the role of death is to dissolve the patterns of atoms so that they can form something else. Then he argues that if a person creates something (e.g., conceiving a baby), he acts against Nature, and nothing good can follow from this. He should instead destroy and not try to hamper the creative possibilities of Nature (see **Camille Paglia**, 14). Sade draws some practical consequences from these ideas. He recommends anal intercourse (homosexual and heterosexual) and condemns vaginal intercourse, because anal intercourse is not procreative. Then he moves on to a parody of utilitarian thinking, providing arguments in favor of anal sex: It is supremely pleasurable, it avoids venereal diseases such as syphilis, it preserves a girl's virginity, and it avoids pregnancy. It also has the interesting property of being consistent with sexual equality, because both men and women can (passively) practice it.

Because Nature creates and destroys, and people should not create, their destiny is to destroy. Hence Sade's norm of destructiveness: torture, maim, and kill as often and as much as possible. In this way one serves Nature. Juliette admires the Emperor Nero, who watched Rome burn in 64, playing his harp and enjoying the destruction. In its orgies of torture and killing, as well as furious and perverted sex, *Juliette* is an especially cruel book. Killing is the logical consequence of libertine action, as the final respectful gesture toward Nature and its mechanical and brutal laws. Keep in mind that Sade never talks about orgasm but always about "discharge." A modern reader easily misses this important philosophical fact. "Orgasm" is a psychological term that unifies emotion and **fantasy** with bodily feelings and entails satisfaction. Sade does not use this kind of mentalistic language. His "discharge" is a mechanistic term, borrowed from the military domain of guns and cannonballs, fire and smoke, bloody guts and loose body parts. This destructiveness is what he is interested in, not personal feelings of satisfaction.

Imagine a libertine in action, raping and torturing victims and enjoying the sexual pleasures derivable from doing so. Sade approaches this subject matter by creating a cyclic context in which the libertine's procedure becomes standardized, regulated, and comprehensible. This approach can be found clearly in *Juliette*. Initially, the stage is set for an orgy: the castle Silling in *120 Days*, a boudoir in *Philosophy in the Bedroom*, or a torture chamber. Here we meet the actors, often called friends or heroes. We also meet their victims, whose role is to provide pleasure to their masters and become thereby absolutely disposable; they are collections of atoms whose moment of dissolution is at hand. The environment is described in a sufficiently detailed way so that the reader knows where he or she is. Next, the heroes start talking, discussing philosophy, ethics, metaphysics, cultural anthropology, and history while sketching the reasons for their strange actions. They tend to be learned men and women interested in philosophy and other fields of study, as enlightened people are. Again and again, they convince themselves and their friends of the facts of the material, godless universe where pain, suffering, and death are the only significant sources of pleasure. These thoughts excite and stimulate them, driving them into a rage that resembles madness. They are ready for their pleasure, by merging fantasy and desire. What the heroes think and dream is important to them, not what and who is around them. They want to move from their present situation to a new one that exists in their crazed imaginations, so they proceed to act. Now follows a sexually loaded description of their trip to discharging, starting from caresses and ending with a violent act, perhaps murder. The libertine discharges, which is to say that he or she (women discharge, too) shoots his or her energy through a barrier into the void. The libertine explodes, empties himself or herself, and in a sense dies, ending up on the other side of space, time, reason, and language. This is, for Sade, the meaning of the ultimate pleasure, joining mighty Nature in the only way possible for a free person.

In this context, violence and destruction are symbolically symmetrical: Both the libertine hero and the victim are destroyed. But this symmetry is deceptive, which becomes clear when we think of the key features of the situation. The hero has instigated it, he or she is able to enjoy it, and only he or she can return to repeat the proceedings. He or she is indispensable, in contrast to the victim, who is spoiled, wasted, and then replaced with another. The hero recovers from the discharge-induced stupor and starts gathering strength to repeat the performance. For Sade, repetition is important. After rest, the philosophizing talk starts again, so that a circle of language is formed: philosophy, fantasy, desire, action, discharge, void, recovery, philosophy, fantasy, desire, . . . Here the void, or abyss, is essential. Because Nature is void, empty of meaning and value, a natural act leads the agent to the void. Lecherous acts reach toward the sudden abyss, into which the actor is thrown by means of discharge. This is, somehow, the ultimate pleasure. It is not easy for us to see why this should be so, since Sade is not referring to the common, modern idea of orgasm. For Sade, it seems, this pleasure is infinite and ultimate because discharge moves the actor through a barrier into empty space where he is free in his ecstasy.

Thus, an important concept and metaphor in Sade is that of a (moral and mental) barrier. On Sade's theory of sexual excitement and pleasure, it is required that the actor meets resistance that is overcome and leads him or her to discharge. Ecstasy is located in the void beyond the barrier. In Sade's dream world, the barrier is built on the language of fantasy, and the imagination brings about the feelings of pleasure that the hero desires. There are many barriers: atheistic language and its blasphemies, conventional moral norms, normal standards of virtue, positive law and natural laws that define crime, and of course the shocking cruelties of torture and death. In all these the libertine mind can experience the resistance it needs to discharge and reach the abyss. All the barriers are, in a sense, passive. They are objects that should be there to provide resistance but that should be destroyed by means of subversive acts. Sadeian heroes do not want active resistance from people who fight back and make them struggle against determined opponents. They want passive objects so that they alone can be active subjects and agents. This makes Sade's novels tedious and boring, because the heroes attack their helpless victims again and again with utterly predictable results. The heroes also subvert norms and break rules that are already meaningless and uninteresting. If not read theoretically and philosophically, their awful rages and furies become pointless.

Sade at least provides impressive examples of subversive action in an amusing way. **Incest** is a good example. Many heroes want to marry their own daughters. This is subversive because incest destroys the language of family relationships. When a father marries his own daughter, he is both her father and husband. If they have a child, he is both the child's father and grandfather. These examples can be multiplied, but the main point is that an incestuous man breaks the norms of kinship and thus adds sexual pleasure to his life. Some attempts to increase sexual enjoyment are interesting. Consider the hero who cuts off the head of a goose that he is penetrating anally. The contractions of the gut around the hero's penis are supremely enjoyable. Sade's work has its dark (and perhaps repellent) humor.

Sade is not an academic philosopher, so accusing him of logical inconsistencies is inappropriate. Yet one significant problem looms large in his novels, the problem of the lack of existence of objective, morally binding norms. If all norms are relative, as Sade argues, murder may be acceptable. Thus when a libertine fantasizes a delicious murder, he should realize that no norm against the planned action exists; hence, neither a barrier nor a void could be encountered. Thoughts of pleasure should vanish accordingly. Sade faces here the deontological paradox. If one must help the poor, and there are no poor, then one must create poverty; else one cannot do one's duty. Sadeian heroes need norms, laws, and canons of virtue to exist to be able to break them. So they need to pretend that these barriers are more robust than the merely relative, subjective conventions that Sade claims they are. It follows that libertine pleasure is impossible. Perhaps the anger, rage, and bitterness shown by many Sadeian heroes is a reaction to this impossibility. They cannot with equanimity accept the cruel fate imposed on them by this paradox.

There is one special Sadeian pleasure that must be mentioned: eating human excrement. *120 Days* dedicates an alarmingly large number of pages to descriptions of this delicacy. Young children are fed well, and the food is pleasantly spiced so that their feces are as appetizing as possible. Such is Sade's technique of attacking his readers. It is difficult to enjoy these pages, as even Gilbert Lély (1904–1985) admits (306–7). These dirty scenes also contain a wonderful parody of the culture of fine food and the values of gourmandism (à la Jean Anthelme Brillat-Savarin [1755–1826]). Such libertines are scavengers, whose enjoyment, hard fought, must lead them to feelings of revenge against Nature. As scavengers they cannot even discharge. They must become avengers who attack every norm, law, and virtue with all their might, aggressively seeking their cosmic revenge against Nature. These people rape, torture, and kill passive objects—only in this way can they discharge and reach the void. The final stage in this creation of a Sadeian hero is the free predator, a sovereign individual who has reached the stage of Stoic apathy and can simulate the mechanistic principles of destruction found in Nature. He is totally free, emotionless, capricious, a mechanical man, a perfect being, as described at the end of *120 Days*.

Scholarly interpretations of Sade's strange and frightening philosophy have come from, among others, Roland Barthes, **Georges Bataille** (1897–1962), **Jacques Lacan** (1901–1981), and Pierre Klossowski (1905–2001). Barthes's *Sade, Fourier, Loyola* is a study of three unreadable authors: "None of these three authors is bearable" (3). Barthes's Sade is the scientist of desire: He classifies, enumerates, defines, and analyzes all the possible passions, desires, and fantasies that have ever appeared under the rubric "sin." But his research methodology is borrowed from the theater. He arranges his heroes and their victims on the stage, in ritual postures that form artificial episodes, which dissolve after the possibilities of the display of fantasy or passion have been exhausted. In this way the philosophical cycle of talk-torture-discharge-void-recuperation-talk achieves its theatrical embodiment. Barthes is most imaginative when he describes the material circumstances surrounding the adventures of the heroes, such as the food, watered silk, the family, machines, colors, and so on. These are the words that make up Sadeian language and discourse, and Barthes maps them out in memorable fashion. After reading Barthes, it is difficult to read Sade without this new lexicon. For example, Barthes writes: "Among the tortures Sade imagines (a monotonous, scarcely terrifying list, since it is most often based on the butcher shop, i.e., on abstraction), only one is disturbing: that which consists in sewing the victim's anus or vagina . . . Why? Because at first sight sewing frustrates castration" (168–69). To sew is to mend and repair, but in this case it means mutilation and amputation. This is a typical example of Barthes's strategy of writing the meanings of Sade's words picked up from the theater of pain.

Bataille's works, such as *Madame Edwarda* (1941) and especially *Story of the Eye* (1928), might look like Sadeian novels, but the resemblance is misleading. Bataille's works need not be interpreted on the basis of his expertise about Sade. As Annie Le Brun has emphasized (91), "One looks vainly in Sade for anything resembling this 'fundamental fascination with death.' . . . How can Bataille write, in the preface to *Madame Edwarda*, that 'Nothing leads me to think that sensual pleasure is the essence of this life,' or even, in his introduction to *Erotism*, that 'eroticism opens onto death,' without realizing that such assertions contradict fundamental aspects of Sade's thought?" Le Brun seems right. Bataille's philosophy of eroticism must be distinguished from his influential interpretations of Sade's texts. In his "The Use Value of D.A.F. de Sade" (*Visions of Excess*), Bataille defends Sade against some surrealists who, according to Bataille, treat Sade like excrement, the release of which gives one fleeting pleasure without any need to look back to what has been produced. All this is related to Bataille's theory of waste, expenditure, and excretion as the opposite of useful work and the accumulation of property. He then reads Sade in terms of his own views, borrowing some descriptions from *120 Days* in which Verneuil eats feces and vomit, and concludes that "nothing can stop the movement that leads human beings toward an even more shameless awareness of the erotic bond that links them to death, to cadavers, and to horrible physical pain" (*Visions*, 101). Bataille wanted to transform Sade into the precursor of his philosophy of deadly eroticism.

Klossowski's *Sade, My Neighbor* has been very influential but is somewhat dated. His picture of a Sadeian hero is that of a scavenger who moves around restlessly without finding the true consummation of his passions (for Klossowski, Sade's world is masculine). He rebels against God, society, morality, and virtue, but because he is a rebel by nature he needs that against which he rebels. That is a constant source of despair, as he cannot annihilate God. If he could, he would loose everything, including his pleasure. So he can enjoy pleasure only as long as he is dissatisfied. This pessimistic view of Sadeian heroes does not recognize their ability to transform themselves into avengers and finally into free predators. Klossowski shows a certain sympathy toward the heroes, his neighbors, because they are ultimately weak and vulnerable victims themselves, victims of their own passion. This narrow interpretation does not do justice to Sade's scandalousness. Klossowski's Sade is a pseudorational system builder and protoliberal seeker of truth.

Lacan's essay "Kant with Sade" has an almost mythical image in the world of Sade interpretations, although it is only mentioned, not commented on. The reason is easy to decipher: The essay makes a valuable point, but the reasons behind it are another matter. They lie beneath a veil of words. Lacan's main point is that it pays to compare **Immanuel Kant**'s (1724–1804) *Critique of Practical Reason* (1788) and Sade's *Philosophy in the Bedroom* (where libertines instruct a young girl in the methods and pleasures of sex and vice). Both works teach their own version of ethics—but certainly from different perspectives. Lacan claims that Kant and Sade agree on something important, the existence of a Universal Law of Morality. In Kant's case the Fundamental Law of Pure Practical Reason, the Categorical Imperative, is: "So act that the maxim of your will could always hold at the same time as a principle in a giving of universal law" (28; Ak 5:30), while in Sade we find something like a Universal Imperative of Pleasure, which is, in Lacan's terms: "I have the right of enjoyment over your body . . . and I will exercise this right, without any limit stopping me in the capriciousness of the exactions that I might have the taste to satiate" (58). This looks more like Hobbes's statement of Natural Rights than Kant's Fundamental Law. Nevertheless, Lacan's thesis, that Sade's works accord with Kant's ethics and actually complete it, is challenging.

Sade has been one of the great, if hidden, influences behind the interest in sexuality and eroticism in all its forms since the beginning of the twentieth century. In this tradition it is important to liberate our thoughts from the constraints of the puritanical conventional moralism that has been part of Christian culture. The human mind and its fantasies are not as simple and well regulated as is often demanded. If we do not admit this and do not dive more deeply under the atavistic layers of the human mind, we will miss that which not only enlightens us but might even save us. In this sense Sade is the "Divine Marquis," the most radical thinker who ever lived.

See also Bataille, Georges; Coercion (by Sexually Aggressive Women); Hobbes, Thomas; Kant, Immanuel; Nietzsche, Friedrich; Objectification, Sexual; Perversion, Sexual; Poststructuralism; Rape; Sacher-Masoch, Leopold von; Sadomasochism; Tantrism; Violence, Sexual

REFERENCES

Airaksinen, Timo. *The Philosophy of the Marquis de Sade*. London: Routledge, 1995; Aristotle. (ca. 325 BCE?) *Nicomachean Ethics*. Trans. Terence Irwin. Indianapolis, Ind.: Hackett, 1985; Barthes, Roland. (1971) *Sade, Fourier, Loyola*. Trans. Richard Miller. London: Jonathan Cape, 1977; Bataille, Georges. *Erotism: Death and Sensuality*. Trans. Mary Dalwood. San Francisco, Calif.: City Lights Books, 1986; Bataille, Georges. *Visions of Excess: Selected Writings, 1927–1939*. Trans. Allan Stoekl, with Carl R. Lovitt and Donald M. Leslie. Minneapolis: University of Minnesota Press, 1985; Horkheimer, Max, and Theodor Adorno. (1944) *Dialectic of Enlightenment*. Trans. John Cumming. New York: Continuum, 1990; Kant, Immanuel. (1788) *Critique of Practical Reason*. Ed. and trans. Mary Gregor. Cambridge: Cambridge University Press, 1997; Klossowski, Pierre. (1967) *Sade, My Neighbor*. Trans. Alphonso Lingis. Evanston, Ill.: Northwestern University Press, 1991; Lacan, Jacques. (1966) "Kant with Sade." Trans. James B. Swenson, Jr. *October*, no. 51 (Winter 1989), 55–75; Le Brun, Annie. *Sade: A Sudden Abyss*. Trans. Camille Naish. San Francisco, Calif.: City Lights Books, 1990; Lély, Gilbert. *The Marquis de Sade: A Biography*. Trans. Alec Brown. London: Elek Books, 1961; Paglia, Camille. *Sexual Personae: Art and Decadence from Nefertiti to Emily Dickinson*. New Haven, Conn.: Yale University Press, 1990; Sade, The Marquis de. *Juliette*. Trans. Austryn Wainhouse. New York: Grove Press, 1968; Sade, The Marquis de. *The 120 Days of Sodom and Other Writings*. Comp. and trans. Austryn Wainhouse and Richard Seaver. New York: Grove Press, 1966; Sade, The Marquis de. *Three Complete Novels: Justine, Philosophy in the Bedroom, Eugenie de Franval, and Other Writings*. Trans. Austryn Wainhouse and Richard Seaver. New York: Grove Press, 1965; Weinberg, Thomas S. "Sade, Marquis de (Donatien-Alphonse-François, Comte de Sade." In Vern L. Bullough and Bonnie Bullough, eds., *Human Sexuality: An Encyclopedia*. New York: Garland, 1994, 526–27.

Timo Airaksinen

ADDITIONAL READING

Airaksinen, Timo. "The Style of Sade: Sex, Text and Cruelty." In Alan Soble, ed., *Sex, Love, and Friendship*. Amsterdam, Holland: Rodopi, 1997, 527–35; Barbone, Steven. "Sade, Donatien-Alphonse-François, Marquis de." In Timothy F. Murphy, ed., *Reader's Guide to Lesbian and Gay Studies*. Chicago, Ill.: Fitzroy Dearborn, 2000, 523–24; Beauvoir, Simone de. (1951–1952) "Must We Burn Sade?" Trans. Annette Michelson. In Austryn Wainhouse and Richard Seaver, comp., *The Marquis de Sade: The 120 Days of Sodom and Other Writings*. New York: Grove Press, 1966, 3–64; Bencivegna, Ermanno. "Kant's Sadism." *Philosophy and Literature* 20:1 (1996), 39–46; Blanchot, Maurice. (1949) *Lautréamont and Sade*. Trans. Stuart Kendall and Michelle Kendall. Stanford, Calif.: Stanford University Press, 2004; Bloch, Iwan. (1900) *Marquis de Sade: His Life and Works*. Trans. James Bruce. New York: Brittany, 1948; Bloch, Iwan. (1901) *Marquis de Sade: The Man and His Age. Studies in the History of the Culture and Morals of the 18th Century*. Trans. James Bruce. Newark, N.J.: Julian Press, 1931. New York: AMS, 1974; Carter, Angela. *The Sadeian Woman and the Ideology of Pornography*. New York: Pantheon Books, 1978; Cleugh, James. *The Marquis and the Chevalier: A Study in the Psychology of Sex as Illustrated by the Lives and Personalities of the Marquis de Sade (1740–1814) and the Chevalier von Sacher-Masoch (1836–1905)*. Boston, Mass.: Little and Brown, 1952. Westport, Conn.: Greenwood Press, 1972; Dworkin, Andrea. "The Marquis de Sade (1740–1814)." In *Pornography: Men Possessing Women*. New York: Perigee, 1981, 70–100; Ferguson, Frances. "Justine, or the Law of the Road." In *Pornography, the Theory: What Utilitarianism Did to Action*. Chicago, Ill.: University of Chicago Press, 2004, 57–74; Ferguson, Frances. "Sade and the Pornographic Legacy." *Representations* 36 (Autumn 1991), 1–21. Reprinted, with changes, as "Eugénie, or Sade and the Pornographic Legacy." In *Pornography, the Theory: What Utilitarianism*

Did to Action. Chicago, Ill.: University of Chicago Press, 2004, 75–95; Gallop, Jane. *Intersections: A Reading of Sade with Bataille, Blanchot, and Klossowski*. Lincoln: University of Nebraska Press, 1982; Gonzalez-Crussi, Frank. "The Divine Marquis." In *On the Nature of Things Erotic*. San Diego, Calif.: Harcourt Brace Jovanovich, 1988, 69–93; Gray, Francine du Plessix. *At Home with the Marquis de Sade: A Life*. New York: Simon and Schuster, 1998; Heumakers, Arnold. "De Sade, a Pessimistic Libertine." In Jan Bremmer, ed., *From Sappho to De Sade: Moments in the History of Sexuality*. London: Routledge, 1989, 108–22; Klossowski, Pierre. "Sade, or the Philosopher-Villain." Trans. Alphonso Lingis. *SubStance* 15:2 (1986), 5–25; Lacan, Jacques. "Kant avec Sade." In *Écrits*. Paris: Editions du Seuil, 1966, 765–90. "Kant with Sade." Trans. James Swenson. *October*, no. 51 (Winter 1989), 55–75; Lever, Maurice. *Sade: A Biography*. Trans. Arthur Goldhammer. New York: Farrar, Straus and Giroux, 1993; Marcus, Steven. (1966) "A Child Is Being Beaten." In *The Other Victorians: A Study of Sexuality and Pornography in Mid-Nineteenth-Century England*. New York: Bantam, 1977, 255–68; Olkowski, Dorothea. "Monstrous Reflection: Sade and Masoch—Rewriting the History of Reason." In Arleen Dallery and Charles E. Scott, eds., *Crisis in Continental Philosophy: Selected Studies in Phenomenology and Existential Philosophy*. Albany: State University of New York Press, 1990, 189–200; Olkowski, Dorothea. "Repetition and Revulsion in the Marquis de Sade." [Reply to Timo Airaksinen, "The Style of Sade: Sex, Text and Cruelty"] In Alan Soble, ed., *Sex, Love, and Friendship*. Amsterdam, Holland: Rodopi, 1997, 537–45; Paglia, Camille. "Return of the Great Mother: Rousseau vs. Sade." In *Sexual Personae: Art and Decadence from Nefertiti to Emily Dickinson*. New Haven, Conn.: Yale University Press, 1990, 230–47; Sade, The Marquis de. (1782) "Dialogue between a Priest and a Dying Man." Trans. Steven Barbone. *Philosophy and Theology* 12:2 (2000), 341–58; Shattuck, Roger. "The Divine Marquis." In *Forbidden Knowledge: From Prometheus to Pornography*. San Diego, Calif.: Harcourt Brace, 1996, 227–99; Singer, Irving. "Sade and Stendhal." In *The Nature of Love*, vol. 2: *Courtly and Romantic*. Chicago, Ill.: University of Chicago Press, 1984, 344–75; Sontag, Susan. (1965) "Marat/Sade/Artaud." In *Against Interpretation and Other Essays*. New York: Farrar, Straus and Giroux, 1966, 163–74; Sparshott, Francis. "Kant without Sade." *Philosophy and Literature* 21:1 (1997), 151–54; Žižek, Slavoj. "Kant and Sade: The Ideal Couple." *Lacanian Ink* 13 (Fall 1998), 12–25.

SADOMASOCHISM. Sadomasochism, a term combining "sadism" and "masochism," is the activity of deriving pleasure, gratification, or satisfaction, often physical and sexual, sometimes mental and emotional, from inflicting on others, or submitting to, painful beatings, bondage, humiliation, and similar abusive procedures. Sadism, the enjoyment of delivering pain to others, was named after the **Marquis de Sade** (1740–1814), the French author of *Justine* (1791) and many other works of **pornography** devoted to the topic. Masochism, the enjoyment of being hurt, humiliated, or abused by another, was named after the German **Leopold von Sacher-Masoch** (1836–1895), whose famous novel *Venus in Furs* was published in 1870. Sadomasochism is sometimes referred to, especially by advocates or practitioners, as "BDSM" (bondage, discipline, sadism, masochism). BDSM, along with many other sexual variations (some of which are **paraphilia**s or **sexual perversion**s), is often contrasted with "vanilla sex"—heterosexual intercourse unadorned by anything "kinky."

Many people, in particular political and sexual conservatives and some feminists, object to BDSM, while political and sexual liberals and libertarians, and again some feminists, defend or pardon it. The conservative objection to BDSM is usually merely an application or extension of its criticism of all nontraditional sexuality—for example, any **sexual activity** conducted outside a Christian **marriage**. A secular, conservative disciple of **Immanuel Kant** (1724–1804) would arrive at a similar conclusion: Sadomasochism, like all nonmarital sexual activity, is wrong because it violates the personhood of the participants, even if the acts are consensual. The liberal defense of sadomasochism is commonly grounded in the power of free and informed **consent** to legitimize any sexual acts in which adults wish to engage (see Primoratz). Some feminists, not only liberal feminists but also lesbian feminist (and male gay) practitioners of BDSM, defend sadomasochism as well as a host of other sexual variations. Lesbian advocates of sadomasochism use liberal or libertarian arguments in support of their practices, emphasizing personal freedom and **privacy** rights (see Samois Collective; contrast with Card, "Review"; Linden et al.).

There are also feminists who denounce sadomasochism while still accepting other types of nontraditional sexuality, such as **homosexuality** and sex outside marriage, on the grounds that it eroticizes, replicates, or reinforces patriarchal social patterns of dominance and submission in which women and others are subordinated (see Chancer, 15–42; Linden et al.; and the exchange between Hopkins and Vadas). Similar objections—that it eroticizes inequality—have been raised against pornography. Legal scholar and "unmodified feminist" **Catharine MacKinnon**, for one, finds the liberal defense of sadomasochism bankrupt:

> Tolerance is the solution liberalism offers. A very substantive sexual blackmail lies at the heart of this liberal tolerance. To not criticize anyone's sexuality [for example, that of various sexual minorities], it is women, specifically, who are used and abused by men, women who are sacrificed. . . . [T]he defense of lesbian sadomasochism would sacrifice all women's ability to walk down the street in safety for the freedom to torture a woman in the privacy of one's basement . . . in the name of everyone's freedom of [sexual] choice. (15)

And Sandra Bartky argues that sadomasochists who also claim to be feminists suffer from self-estrangement: "When the parts of the self are at war with one another, a person may be said to suffer from self-estrangement. That part of [a person] which is compelled to produce sexually charged scenarios of humiliation is radically at odds with the [person] who devotes much of her life to the struggle against oppression" (51). Women who want to entertain a sexual **fantasy** of dominating or being dominated should not act on these desires. To do so is to collude with women's subordination.

Sadomasochism is often a variant sexual practice in which dominating and submitting to the demands, sexual or otherwise, of another person are erotically arousing. Its practitioners claim that BDSM involves the voluntary and consensual temporary creation, through role-playing, of an imbalanced power relationship. In "scenes" or dramas negotiated and decided upon in advance by both participants, bondage, humiliation, and the infliction of pain are employed in expressing this power imbalance. A sadomasochistic subculture (or community) has constructed a **language** and rules for carrying out these activities. "Tops" (dominant persons) and "bottoms" (submissives) engage in activities involving the expression of power, and they rely on "safe" words to indicate that a scene should be stopped (say, if the masochist has reached his or her pain limit) or steered in another direction (if he or she wants to experience a different sort of pain). "Sadomasochism," declares Gayle Rubin, "is not a form of violence, but is rather a type of ritual and contractual sex play whose aficionados go to great lengths . . . to ensure the safety and enjoyment of one another" (22; see Califia). Many people not familiar with BDSM might imagine that it is nothing but "the tyrannical exercise of one will upon a helpless other," yet practitioners claim that "consensual S/M is typically collaborative, involving careful training, initiation rites, a scrupulous definition of limits, and a constant confirmation of reciprocity" (McClintock, 226).

One surprising thing is that sadomasochism has been embraced not only by some gay men but also by some lesbian women; the latter, goes one line of thought, should know better, since they are well versed in the oppressive power relations of the **heterosexism** of patriarchal culture. But insofar as sadomasochism is a matter of cooperation—the participants rely on the skills and determination of each other to produce mutual satisfaction—it is a locale for the assertiveness of both persons, not the genuine submission of one to the other. Hence even lesbian sadomasochism "constitutes a body of sexual practices in which woman is sexual agent through and through. . . . [T]he masochist acts out her sexuality, constructs scenarios, takes on roles, sets limits. The sadist also acts out her sexuality and takes on roles. . . . Lesbian S/M, then, is a matter of teamwork of female sexual agents" (O'Neill, 85). It is the *agency* of the participants that redeems what might seem just like more of the same subordination of women.

Playful sadomasochism, at least, seems to have come out of the closet into mainstream sexual culture. In research conducted by sociologist Lillian Rubin, she found that

> [a]bout a quarter of the study's population said they had experimented with some form of bondage, an activity more prominent in the under-35 groups. . . . Sometimes it was nothing more than one partner or the other being pinned down with hands over the head. . . . Sometimes people tied each other up, both men and women saying they enjoyed the dominance and submission side of the game equally well. "I can enjoy being tied up, and I like tying someone up," said 25-year-old Felicia, a New York editorial assistant. "It's part of the whole fantasy—sometimes to be the dominant one and then to turn it around into submission." (128)

Consider, too, Daphne Merkin's spanking confessional in the erudite pages of *The New Yorker* in 1996. Indeed, the American Psychiatric Association (APA) makes a distinction in the section of its *Diagnostic and Statistical Manual of Mental Disorders* devoted to sexual sadism and sexual masochism (529–30), asserting that "simulated" sadomasochism does not count as a paraphilia (as opposed to nonconsensual sadism). Perhaps the APA was responding to those, including the National Organization for Women, who argued that consensual BDSM did not constitute a mental disorder. Sadomasochism seems no longer to be "the last taboo" (see Greene and Greene).

American psychiatrists, among many others, had long considered a sexual interest in inflicting or receiving pain to be psychologically pathological. Richard von Krafft-Ebing (1840–1902) discussed both sadism and masochism, and provided detailed case studies, in his famous 1886 work on sexual perversion, *Psychopathia Sexualis*. In 1905, **Sigmund Freud** (1856–1939) took up Krafft-Ebing's terminology but theorized that sadism and masochism were actually one phenomenon. For Freud, "It can often be shown that masochism is nothing more than an extension of sadism turned round upon the subject's own self " (24). "The most remarkable feature of this perversion," he writes, is that sadism and masochism "occur together in the same individual" (25). Freud's view has been disputed by, for example, Gilles Deleuze (1925–1995). In his *Coldness and Cruelty*, one of the few genuinely philosophical works on masochism, Deleuze argues that it should not be fused with sadism as a single phenomenon "sadomasochism," since they differ in their techniques, concerns, and intentions.

Of course, sadomasochism is not free of faults. A top might become so overwhelmingly involved in the power she commands that she forgets to monitor her treatment of the "bottom." In this case, playful, controlled sadomasochism can become genuine abuse. When a "bottom" suffers from extremely low self-esteem and thinks he actually deserves the punishment and humiliation, he may no longer be an active participant but fully subordinate. BDSM can go wrong also when people take their sadomasochistic behaviors and attitudes into other facets of their lives, not keeping them within the confines of "scenes." In any event, the line between real abuse and innocuous sadomasochistic play is fine. Claudia Card has pointed out that "the only things distinguishing the behavior of [the top] from battery or other abuse may be the motivations of the parties and the consent of the [bottom]" (*Lesbian Choices*, 221). And, it can be argued, the mere presence of the top's motive to please the bottom (and the self) by soundly whipping the other and the consent of the bottom to be soundly whipped do not go very far in changing battery or physical abuse into *something else*. Indeed, the **law** may have difficulties distinguishing sadomasochistic play from a real attack (like the law often has difficulty distinguishing **date and acquaintance rape** from consensual sex). This may explain why in some jurisdictions the legal maxim *volenti non fit injuria* (one is not injured by acts to which one consents) is not applied to ostensibly consensual sadomasochism, and tops are sometimes charged with assault, **rape**, kidnapping, false imprisonment, or reckless endangerment.

Freud regarded sadomasochism (S/M) as the most common and significant of the perversions (23), and he suggested that masochism results as a way persons come to regulate, or psychologically handle, their primary desire to dominate others (24–25). Many people consider S/M perverted, wondering how a psychologically healthy person could derive pleasure from deliberately inflicting or receiving pain, brutality, or humiliation. Psychologists have explained the interest in BDSM in various ways: as an escape, as deviance, as a way to heal oneself after having been sexually abused, and as arising from childhood experiences. If, for example, a child is taught to feel ashamed of her body and **sexual desire**s, she might respond by disconnecting herself from them. As an adult, sadomasochistic play might allow her to reconnect with her body: "Lying naked on a bed bound to the bedposts with leather restraints, she is forced to be completely sexual. The restraint, the futility of the struggle, the pain . . . enable her body to fully connect with her sexual self in a way that has been difficult during traditional sex" (Apostolides, 62). For others, sadomasochism can be an escape from, or a way to ease, the anxieties and stresses associated with the demands and expectations of Western culture. In sadomasochistic play, the corporate CEO (chief executive officer) forgets himself and his weighty station, reduced to a purely physical, sexual creature while submitting, with the relief of delightful pleasure, to the infliction of pain and humiliation by his "Mistress" (a dominant woman). Others simply enjoy being "rebellious," going against society's taboos and sexual norms.

But some who engage in sadomasochism find it profoundly healing. For some women who have been sexually abused, acting out fantasies of their assault "in which crucial details, including the very meaning of the events, are changed," gives them a sense of control over that which was previously "uncontrollable" (Carol, 104). Note that sadomasochism might have all these (and other) purported benefits, in addition to being, for some, sexually gratifying, yet still replicate or reinforce the patriarchal subordination of women.

Jean-Paul Sartre's (1905–1980) discussion of "Concrete Relations with Others" in *Being and Nothingness* contains a philosophical anthropology of sadomasochism (361–430; see especially 404). According to Sartre, the experience of the Other gives rise to conflict. In particular, whether in **love** or sexual relationships or more generally, there is in my relation to the Other a failure of reciprocity or mutuality. We each attempt to preserve our freedom at the expense of the Other's freedom, leading to a battle of Wills. Thus relations with the Other become sadomasochistic, oscillating between the Other's being an object for me (sadism) and my being an object for the Other (masochism). Unity with the Other is perhaps an ideal state, but it is unrealizable. For Sartre, then, sadomasochism—even if not of a sexual sort—seems an essential part of the human condition, and his metaphysics might explain why sexual sadomasochism is so common. In more striking terms, this is the thesis of **Camille Paglia**, too, for whom sadomasochism is "a sacred cult, a pagan religion that reveals the dark secrets of nature. The bondage of sadomasochism expresses our own bondage by the body, our subservience to its brute laws, concealed by our myths of romantic love" (44–45).

On such views, sexuality is inherently sadomasochistic, even the vanilla sex variety of it engaged in by happily married loving couples. All that the practitioners of BDSM do is to acknowledge candidly, and to make obvious and clear, what is the case in any event, that all sexuality is sadomasochistic. (MacKinnon agrees but argues that this widespread sadomasochist sexuality is cultural and constructed, rather than either biological or metaphysical.) If we want confirmation of the idea of Sade's pornography that there could be "no sexual pleasure without the demonstration of power" (Ferguson, 26), we might find it in Philip Roth:

> [I]n sex there is no point of absolute stasis. There is no sexual equality . . . certainly not one where the allotments are equal, the male quotient and the female quotient in perfect balance. There's no way to negotiate metrically this wild thing. It's not fifty-fifty like a business transaction. It's the chaos of eros we're talking about. . . . What it is is trading dominance, perpetual imbalance. You're going to rule out dominance? You're going to rule out yielding? The dominating is the flint, it strikes the spark, it sets it going. (17–18)

See also Bataille, Georges; Casual Sex; Chinese Philosophy; Existentialism; Feminism, Lesbian; Genital Mutilation; Kant, Immanuel; Law, Sex and the; Liberalism; Love; Nietzsche, Friedrich; Objectification, Sexual; Paraphilia; Perversion, Sexual; Pornography; Rape; Sacher-Masoch, Leopold von; Sade, Marquis de; Violence, Sexual

REFERENCES

American Psychiatric Association. *Diagnostic and Statistical Manual of Mental Disorders*, 4th ed. [DSM-IV] Washington, D.C.: Author, 1994; Apostolides, Marianne. "The Pleasure of the Pain: Why Some People Need S&M." *Psychology Today* 32:5 (September–October 1999), 60–64; Bartky, Sandra Lee. *Femininity and Domination: Studies in the Phenomenology of Oppression*. New York: Routledge, 1990; Califia, Pat. "Feminism and Sadomasochism." *Heresies*, no. 12 ["Sex Issue"] 3:4 (1981), 30–34; Card, Claudia. *Lesbian Choices*. New York: Columbia University Press, 1995; Card, Claudia. "Review Essay: Sadomasochism and Sexual Preference." *Journal of Social Philosophy* 15:2 (1984), 42–52; Carol, Avedon. *Nudes, Prudes, and Attitudes: Pornography and Censorship*. Cheltenham, U.K.: New Clarion Press, 1994; Chancer, Lynn S. *Sadomasochism in Everyday Life: The Dynamics of Power and Powerlessness*. New Brunswick, N.J.: Rutgers University Press, 1992; Deleuze, Gilles. (1967) *Coldness and Cruelty*. Trans. Jean McNeil. New York: Zone Books, 1989; Ferguson, Frances. *Pornography, the Theory: What Utilitarianism Did to Action*. Chicago, Ill.: University of Chicago Press, 2004; Freud, Sigmund. (1905) *Three Essays on the Theory of Sexuality*. Trans. James Strachey. New York: Basic Books, 1975; Greene, Gerald, and Caroline Greene, eds. (1974) *SM: The Last Taboo*. New York: Blue Moon Books, 1995; Hopkins, Patrick D. "Rethinking Sadomasochism: Feminism, Interpretation, and Simulation." *Hypatia* 9:1 (1994), 116–41; Krafft-Ebing, Richard von. (1886, 1903) *Psychopathia Sexualis*, 12th ed. Trans. F. J. Rebman. New York: Paperback Library, 1965; Linden, Robin Ruth, Darlene R. Pagano, Diana E. H. Russell, and Susan Leigh Star, eds. *Against Sadomasochism: A Radical Feminist Analysis*. East Palo Alto, Calif.: Frog in the Well Press, 1982; MacKinnon, Catharine A. *Feminism Unmodified: Discourses on Life and Law.* Cambridge, Mass.: Harvard University Press, 1987; McClintock, Anne. "Maid to Order: Commercial S/M and Gender Power." In Pamela Church Gibson and Roma Gibson, eds., *Dirty Looks: Women, Pornography, Power.* London: BFI Publishing, 1993, 207–31; Merkin, Daphne. "Unlikely Obsession: Confronting a Taboo." *The New Yorker* (26 February and 4 March 1996), 98–115; National Organization for Women. "Testimony from Physicians and Psychiatrists for the S/M Policy Reform Statement" (22 March 1997). <members.aol.com/NOWSM/Psychiatrists.html> [accessed 30 August 2004]; O'Neill, Eileen. "(Re)presentations of Eros: Exploring Female Sexual Agency." In Alison M. Jaggar and Susan R. Bordo, eds., *Gender/Body/Knowledge: Feminist Reconstructions of Being and Knowing.* New Brunswick, N.J.: Rutgers University Press, 1989, 68–91; Paglia, Camille. *Sex, Art, and American Culture: Essays.* New York: Vintage, 1992; Primoratz, Igor. "Sexual Morality: Is Consent Enough?" *Ethical Theory and Moral Practice* 4:3 (2001), 201–18; Roth, Philip. *The Dying Animal.* Boston, Mass.: Houghton Mifflin, 2001; Rubin, Gayle. "Misguided, Dangerous and Wrong: An Analysis of Anti-Pornography Politics." In Alison Assiter and Avedon Carol, eds., *Bad Girls and Dirty Pictures: The Challenge to Reclaim Feminism.* London: Pluto Press, 1993, 18–40; Rubin, Lillian B. *Erotic Wars: What Happened to the Sexual Revolution?* New York: Farrar, Straus and Giroux, 1990; Sacher-Masoch, Leopold von. *Venus in Furs and Selected Letters of Leopold von Sacher-Masoch.* Trans. Uwe Moeller and Laura Lindgren. New York: Blast Books, 1989; Sade, The Marquis de. *Three Complete Novels: Justine, Philosophy in the Bedroom, Eugenie de Franval, and Other Writings.* Trans. Austryn Wainhouse and Richard Seaver. New York: Grove Press, 1965; Samois Collective, eds. *Coming to Power: Writings and Graphics on Lesbian S/M,* 1st ed. Palo Alto, Calif.: Up Press, 1981. Revised eds., Boston, Mass.: Alyson, 1982, 1987; Sartre, Jean-Paul. (1943) *Being and Nothingness: An Essay on Phenomenological Ontology.* Trans. Hazel E. Barnes. New York: Philosophical Library, 1956; Vadas, Melinda. "Reply to Patrick Hopkins." *Hypatia* 10:2 (1995), 159–61.

Carol V. Quinn

ADDITIONAL READING

Airaksinen, Timo. *The Philosophy of the Marquis de Sade.* London: Routledge, 1995; Alexander, Jonathan. "Bondage." In Timothy F. Murphy, ed., *Reader's Guide to Lesbian and Gay Studies.* Chicago, Ill.: Fitzroy Dearborn, 2000, 91–93; Apostolides, Marianne. "The Pleasure of the Pain: Why Some People Need S&M." *Psychology Today* 32:5 (September–October 1999), 60–64. <www.psychologytoday.com/htdocs/prod/ptoarticle/pto-19990901-000039.asp> and <www.findarticles.com/cf_dls/m1175/5_32/55625503/p1/article.jhtml> [accessed 31 August 2004]; Archard, David. "The Limits of Consensuality I: Incest, Prostitution, and Sadomasochism." In *Sexual Consent.* Boulder, Colo.: Westview, 1998, 98–115; Bartky, Sandra Lee. "Feminine Masochism and the Politics of Personal Transformation." *Women's Studies International Forum* 7:5 (1984), 323–34. Reprinted in *Femininity and Domination: Studies in the Phenomenology of Oppression.* New York: Routledge, 1990, 45–62; POS2 (219–42); Benjamin, Jessica. *The Bonds of Love: Psychoanalysis, Feminism, and the Problem of Domination.* New York: Pantheon, 1988; Benjamin, Jessica. "Master and Slave: The Fantasy of Erotic Domination." In Ann Snitow, Christine Stansell, and Sharon Thompson, eds., *Powers of Desire: The Politics of Sexuality.* New York: Monthly Review Press, 1983, 280–99; Bersani, Leo. *The Freudian Body: Psychoanalysis and Art.* New York: Columbia University Press, 1986; Braun, Walter. "Sadism and Bestiality." In *The Cruel and the Meek, Aspects of Sadism and Masochism: Being Pages from a Sexologist's Notebook.* Trans. N. Meyer. London: Luxor Press, 1967, 55–59; Brewis, Joanna, and Stephen Linstead. "Sadomasochism and Organization." In *Sex, Work and Sex Work: Eroticizing Organization.* London: Routledge, 2000, 126–50; Califia, Pat. "Feminism and Sadomasochism." *Heresies* #12 ["Sex Issue"] 3:4 (1981), 30–34. Reprinted in *Co-Evolution Quarterly* 33 (Spring 1982), 33–40; and Stevi Jackson and Sue Scott, eds., *Feminism and Sexuality: A Reader.* New York: Columbia University Press, 1996, 230–37; Califia, Pat. *Macho Sluts.* Los Angeles, Calif.: Alyson, 1988; Califia, Pat. *Public Sex: The Culture of Radical Sex.* Pittsburgh,

Pa.: Cleis Press, 1994; Califia, Pat, ed. *The Lesbian S/M Safety Manual*. Boston, Mass.: Alyson, 1988; Caplan, Paula J. *The Myth of Women's Masochism*, 1st ed. New York: Dutton, 1985. 2nd ed., Toronto, Can.: University of Toronto Press, 1993; Card, Claudia, ed. *Adventures in Lesbian Philosophy*. Bloomington: Indiana University Press, 1994; Deleuze, Gilles. (1967) "Mysticism and Masochism." In *Desert Islands and Other Texts 1953–1974*. Trans. Michael Taormina. Los Angeles, Calif.: Semiotext(e), 2004, 131–34; Deutsch, Helene. "The Significance of Masochism in the Mental Life of Women." *International Journal of Psychoanalysis* 11 (1930), 48–60; Fraker, Susan, and John Barnes. "California: Of Human Bondage." *Newsweek* (26 April 1976), 35; Freud, Sigmund. (1919) " 'A Child Is Being Beaten': A Contribution to the Study of the Origin of Sexual Perversions." In *The Standard Edition of the Complete Psychological Works of Sigmund Freud*, vol. 17. Trans. James Strachey. London: Hogarth Press, 1953–1974, 175–204; Freud, Sigmund. (1924) "The Economic Problem of Masochism." In *The Standard Edition of the Complete Psychological Works of Sigmund Freud*, vol. 19. Trans. James Strachey. London: Hogarth Press, 1953–1974, 159–70; Gearhart, Suzanne. "Foucault's Response to Freud: Sado-masochism and the Aestheticization of Power." *Style* 29 (Fall 1995), 389–403; Gebhardt, Paul. "Fetishism and Sadomasochism." In Martin S. Weinberg, ed., *Sex Research: Studies from the Kinsey Institute*. New York: Oxford University Press, 1976, 156–66; Gould, Carol C., ed. *Beyond Domination: New Perspectives on Women and Philosophy*. Totowa, N.J.: Rowman and Allanheld, 1984; Grimshaw, Jean. "Ethics, Fantasy, and Self-transformation." In A. Phillips Griffiths, ed., *Ethics* [*Philosophy* Supp. 35]. Cambridge: Cambridge University Press, 1993, 145–58. Reprinted in POS3 (175–87); Hanly, Margaret Ann Fitzpatrick, ed. *Essential Papers on Masochism*. New York: New York University Press, 1995; Hart, Lynda. *Between the Body and the Flesh: Performing Sadomasochism*. New York: Columbia University Press, 1998; Hopkins, Patrick D. "Rethinking Sadomasochism: Feminism, Interpretation, and Simulation." *Hypatia* 9:1 (1994), 116–41. Reprinted in POS3 (189–214); Hopkins, Patrick D. "Simulation and the Reproduction of Injustice: A Reply." *Hypatia* 10:2 (1995), 162–70; Kimball, Roger. "The Perversions of Michel Foucault." *The New Criterion* 11:7 (March 1993). <www.newcriterion.com/archive/11/mar93/foucault.htm> [accessed 8 June 2005]; Kipnis, Laura. *Bound and Gagged: Pornography and the Politics of Fantasy in America*. New York: Grove Press, 1996; Kittay, Eva Feder. "Pornography and the Erotics of Domination." In Carol C. Gould, ed., *Beyond Domination: New Perspectives on Women and Philosophy*. Totowa, N.J.: Rowman and Allanheld, 1984, 145–74; Lee, J. Roger. "Sadomasochism: An Ethical Analysis." In Robert M. Stewart, ed., *Philosophical Perspectives on Sex and Love*. New York: Oxford University Press, 1995, 125–37; MacKendrick, Karmen. *Counterpleasures*. Albany: State University of New York Press, 1999; Mann, Jay, and Natalie Shainess. "Sadistic Fantasies." *Medical Aspects of Human Sexuality* 8:2 (1974), 142–48; Marcus, Maria. *A Taste for Pain: On Masochism and Female Sexuality*. Trans. Joan Tate. New York: St. Martin's Press, 1981; Marcus, Steven. (1966) "A Child Is Being Beaten." In *The Other Victorians: A Study of Sexuality and Pornography in Mid-Nineteenth-Century England*. New York: Bantam, 1977, 255–68; McCosker, Anthony. "A Vision of Masochism in the Affective Pain of *Crash*." *Sexualities* 8:1 (2005), 30–48; Merck, Mandy. "The Feminist Ethics of Lesbian S/M." In *Perversions: Deviant Readings*. New York: Routledge, 1993, 236–66; Miller, Phillip, and Molly Devon. *Screw the Roses: Send Me the Thorns. The Romance and Sexual Sorcery of Sadomasochism*. Fairfield, Conn.: Mystic Rose Books, 1995; Moser, Charles. "Sadomasochism." *Journal of Psychology and Human Sexuality* 7 (1988), 43–56; Moser, Charles, and J. J. Madeson. *Bound to Be Free: The SM Experience*. New York: Continuum, 1996; Noyes, John K. *The Mastery of Submission: Inventions of Masochism*. Ithaca, N.Y.: Cornell University Press, 1997; Oaklander, L. Nathan. (1977) "Sartre on Sex." In Alan Soble, ed., *The Philosophy of Sex: Contemporary Readings*. Totowa, N.J.: Rowman and Littlefield, 1980, 190–206; Primoratz, Igor. *Ethics and Sex*. London: Routledge, 1999; Reeve, C.D.C. "Violence, Pornography, and Sadomasochism." In *Love's Confusions*. Cambridge, Mass.: Harvard University Press, 2005, 125–45; Reiersøl, Odd. "SM: Causes and Diagnoses" [in three parts]. *revisef65*. <www.revisef65.org/reiersol1.html> [accessed 30 August 2004]; Reik, Theodor. (1941) *Masochism in Sex and Society*. Trans. Margaret Beigel and Gertrud Kurth. New York: Grove Press, 1962; Ross,

John Munder. *Sadomasochism of Everyday Life: Why We Hurt Ourselves—and Others—and How to Stop*. New York: Simon and Schuster, 1997; Rubin, Gayle. "The Leather Menace: Comments on Politics and S/M." In Samois Collective, eds., *Coming to Power: Writings and Graphics on Lesbian S/M*, 1st ed. Palo Alto, Calif.: Up Press, 1981, 192–225; Sartre, Jean-Paul. (1946) *Anti-Semite and Jew*. Trans. George J. Becker. New York: Schocken, 1948; Segal, Lynne. "Sensual Uncertainty, or Why the Clitoris Is Not Enough." In Sue Cartledge and Joanna Ryan, eds., *Sex and Love: New Thoughts on Old Contradictions*. London: Women's Press, 1983, 30–47; Shattuck, Roger. "The Divine Marquis." In *Forbidden Knowledge: From Prometheus to Pornography*. San Diego, Calif.: Harcourt Brace, 1996, 227–99; Sircello, Guy. "Loving Pain." In *Love and Beauty*. Princeton, N.J.: Princeton University Press, 1989, 179–83; Soble, Alan. "Sadomasochism." In *Pornography, Sex, and Feminism*. Amherst, N.Y.: Prometheus, 2002, 32–39; Stekel, Wilhelm. (1925) *Sadism and Masochism: The Psychology of Hatred and Cruelty*, 2 vols. New York: Liveright, 1929; Stoller, Robert. *Pain and Passion: A Psychoanalyst Explores the World of S&M*. New York: Plenum, 1991; Stoltenberg, John. *Refusing to Be a Man: Essays on Sex and Justice*. Portland, Ore.: Breitenbush Books, 1989; Theroux, Paul. "Nurse Wolf." *The New Yorker* (15 June 1998), 50–63; Vadas, Melinda. "Reply to Patrick Hopkins." *Hypatia* 10:2 (1995), 159–61. Reprinted in POS3 (215–17); Vance, Carole S., ed. *Pleasure and Danger: Exploring Female Sexuality*. London: Routledge and Kegan Paul, 1984; Weinberg, Thomas S., ed. *S&M: Studies in Dominance and Submission*. Amherst, N.Y.: Prometheus, 1995.

SAINT AUGUSTINE. *See* Augustine (Saint)

SAINT PAUL. *See* Paul (Saint)

SAINT THOMAS AQUINAS. *See* Thomas Aquinas (Saint)

SAME-SEX MARRIAGE. *See* Marriage, Same-Sex

SARTRE, JEAN-PAUL. *See* Existentialism

SCHOPENHAUER, ARTHUR (1788–1860). Arthur Schopenhauer was the son of a wealthy Danzig merchant whose death, probably by suicide, in 1805 left him financially secure and free to pursue philosophy despite his failure to secure a permanent teaching post or, until late in life, find a wide audience for his writings. Although he never devoted a full-length work exclusively to human sexuality, Schopenhauer discusses it extensively in his major work, *The World as Will and Representation* (1818; revised and expanded, 1844, 1859 [*WWR*]), especially the essay "The Metaphysics of Sexual Love" (*WWR*, vol. 2, 531–67). His *On the Will in Nature* (1836 [*WN*]), *On the Basis of Morality* (1841 [*BM*]), and *Parerga and Paralipomena* (1851 [*PP*]) contain additional material related to human sexuality.

Schopenhauer's chief claim to originality as a theorist of human sexuality comes from the central place he gives it both in his account of human psychology, especially through his introduction of the concept of the Unconscious (if not the term), and in his larger metaphysical vision, which makes the sexual impulse the purest expression of the essence of the world, the Will. While his writings enjoyed great popularity from the 1850s until around World War I, his greatest impact on the philosophy of sex probably comes through his influence on **Friedrich Nietzsche** (1844–1900; see Higgins) and **Sigmund Freud** (1856–1939; see Gardner; Gupta).

Schopenhauer's philosophy constitutes both a continuation and a radical revision of the transcendental idealism of **Immanuel Kant** (1724–1804). Against the skepticism of **David Hume** (1711–1776), Kant attempted to preserve the necessity and universality of Newtonian physics while accepting the empiricist claim that all human knowledge arises from sense experience. To do so, he distinguished between *noumena* ("things-in-themselves"), which exist outside and independent of the mind, and *phenomena* ("appearances"), through which the external world is represented to consciousness. While agreeing with Hume that sense-data alone, and not the objects that cause them, are immediately present to consciousness, Kant argued that the mind situates these sense-impressions within a spatial and temporal framework that belongs not to them or their causes but rather to the knowing subject and that the mind orders and connects these discrete sense-impressions to produce a unified and lawful experience of the world. Thus, the laws of nature are guaranteed to be universal features of experience, since they are contributed not by the external world but by the knowing subject. The thing-in-itself, however, remains by definition forever inaccessible to experience, and its existence is defended by Kant in large part to avoid charges of repeating George Berkeley's (1685–1753) subjective idealism, which denied the existence of any extramental entities.

While accepting the division of the world into *phenomena* (called "representations" by Schopenhauer) and *noumena*, which division he considered "Kant's greatest merit" (*WWR*, vol. 1, 417), Schopenhauer in his doctoral dissertation (*On the Fourfold Root of the Principle of Sufficient Reason*, 1814; expanded, 1847) radically revised and simplified Kant's complex account of how the subject organizes sense-data. He argued that the category of causality alone serves to connect and integrate sense-data into a unified world of experience. Schopenhauer, as a result, denied the possibility of human freedom on the phenomenal level, where exceptionless physical and psychological laws govern all events, but permitted it on the noumenal level in the creative activity of the transcendental subject, which constitutes both the empirical subject (the phenomenal self composed of inner states and mental events) and the external world given in experience.

More important, Schopenhauer rejected Kant's agnosticism about *noumena*, arguing that the empirical subject, itself grounded in the transcendental subject, could acquire knowledge of the noumenal realm through introspection. (For a critical discussion of this move, see Atwell, 106–28; Janaway, *Self and World*, 188–207.) The most basic reality we perceive in ourselves, he claimed, is not the intellect that contemplates the world but the will that desires and strives to master it. The intellect, far from being the ruling faculty of the mind, is merely the creation of the more primitive will that operates on a preconscious or unconscious level to determine behavior. Extending this psychological insight to include the entire noumenal realm, Schopenhauer concluded that the whole of existence is in itself nothing but the expression of a single, undivided "Will" (or, more precisely, "Will-to-live") that manifests itself throughout the natural world, from the inorganic physical and chemical processes, through the countless species of plant and animal life, to its highest level of expression, the human species.

Whether Schopenhauer's metaphysical system is directed at a reductive materialist account of nature (albeit within a transcendental idealist framework) or demands a more sophisticated interpretation has been the subject of some dispute (see Janaway, "Will and Nature"; Schmidt). In any case, Schopenhauer, unlike thinkers such as **René Descartes** (1596–1650) and Kant, held that the human species, while expressing the Will-to-live in its most developed and complex manner, does not form an ontologically or morally separate level of reality distinct from the physical world:

> Although in man, as (Platonic) Idea, the will finds its most distinct and perfect objectification, this alone could not express its true being. In order to appear in its proper significance, the Idea of man would need to manifest itself, not alone and torn apart, but accompanied by all the forms of animals, through the plant kingdom to the inorganic. They all supplement one another for the complete objectification of the Will. (*WWR*, vol. 1, 153)

In this way, Schopenhauer's philosophy is as closely connected with the monistic naturalism of **Baruch Spinoza** (1632–1677; see Schulz) as it is with the idealism of Kant.

But while Schopenhauer's attempt to give a scientific and naturalistic account of the sexual impulse and the varieties of human sexual behavior may echo the earlier efforts of Spinoza, he considered all previous philosophical theories valueless for understanding sexuality: "I have no predecessors either to make use of or refute; the subject has forced itself on me objectively and has become connected of its own accord with my consideration of the world" (*WWR*, vol. 2, 533). Looking instead to his own theory of the self as expressing the Will-to-live (both objectively, as a material body subject to the laws of nature, and subjectively, as a self-conscious agent subject to psychological laws), Schopenhauer produced an original and in many respects quite contemporary philosophy of sex.

Schopenhauer's contribution to the current understanding of sex, on the biological and physiological levels, is limited by his transcendental idealism (but see Magee's defense, 73–104). Since, within this framework, the transcendental subject (that is, the Will-to-live) constitutes the external world, including its own body, as an object of experience for itself, he concludes that the human body is "nothing but the phenomenal appearance of the will, its becoming visible, the objectivity of the will; . . . teeth, gullet, and intestinal canal are objectified hunger; the genitals are objectified sexual impulse" (*WWR*, vol. 1, 108; see also *WN*, 26–47, *passim*). However useful such a symbolic approach to the sexual apparatus may be for psychoanalysis, its scientific value for understanding the biological foundations of human sexuality is minimal.

As a psychologist of sex, however, Schopenhauer's importance can hardly be overstated. Unlike many previous philosophers (essentially Platonic and Christian), Schopenhauer refused to distinguish between a higher psychological or spiritual ideal of **love** and a lower physical state of **sexual desire**. Rather, he reduced the former to a manifestation of the latter: "All amorousness is rooted in the sexual impulse alone, is in fact only a more closely determined, specialized, and, indeed, in the strictest sense, individualized sexual impulse" (*WWR*, vol. 2, 533). Schopenhauer then makes the sexual impulse (the satisfaction of which "is the ultimate goal of almost all human effort"; vol. 2, 533) the ubiquitous explanation of human behavior: "It is the cause of war and the aim and object of peace, the basis and the serious aim of the joke, the inexhaustible source of wit, the key to all hints and allusions, and the meaning of all secret signs and suggestions, all unexpressed proposals, and all stolen glances; . . . the hourly thought of the unchaste, and the constantly recurring reverie of the chaste even against their will" (vol. 2, 513).

The immense psychological significance Schopenhauer granted to the sex drive, in turn, rests on his unique metaphysical interpretation of it: "That which makes itself known to the individual consciousness as sexual impulse in general, and without direction to a definite individual of the other sex, is in itself, and apart from the phenomenon, simply the Will-to-live" (*WWR*, vol. 2, 535). Given this identification of the sexual impulse with the Will-to-live, "it is clear why sexual desire bears a character very different from that of any other; it is not only the strongest of desires, but is even specifically of a more powerful kind than all the others are. . . . For it is the desire that constitutes even the very nature of man. In conflict with it, no motive is so strong as to be certain of victory" (vol. 2, 512–13).

To explain its power, Schopenhauer carefully distinguished between the sexual impulse as it appears in consciousness (i.e., as a desire whose satisfaction is required for and directed toward individual happiness) and its metaphysical function in preserving the species (where the happiness of the individual is a matter of indifference). Unlike Spinoza, who rejected any explanation or moral evaluation of human sexuality in terms of a natural end toward which sex is directed, in favor of one given solely in terms of efficient mechanical causation, Schopenhauer's account of how the sexual impulse directs and determines human behavior is unapologetically teleological. The sexual impulse, which Schopenhauer considered to be "the most complete manifestation of the Will-to-live, its most distinctly expressed type" (*WWR*, vol. 2, 514), aims solely toward the preservation and continuation of the human species: "The vehemence of the sexual impulse . . . [is] evidence that, through the function that it serves, the animal belongs to that in which the true inner being really and mainly lies, namely, the *species*; whereas all the other functions and organs serve directly only the individual, whose existence is at bottom only secondary" (vol. 2, 511).

Since the ultimate goal of the sexual impulse is the survival of the species, not the satisfaction of the individual, the pleasure and happiness that individuals obtain from sex cannot belong to its end but must rather pertain to its means:

> Nature can attain her end only by implanting in the individual a certain *delusion*, and by virtue of this, that which in truth is merely a good thing for the species seems to him a good thing for himself, so that he serves the species, whereas he is under the delusion that he is serving himself. . . . This delusion is instinct. . . . Thus [consciousness] imagines it is pursuing individual ends, whereas in truth it is pursuing merely general ends. (vol. 2, 538)

Likewise, Schopenhauer's "eugenic conception" (Janaway, "Will and Nature," 152) of sexual attraction as expressing not aesthetic judgments but rather the suitability of a potential mate to compensate for an individual's deficiencies and thereby produce healthy offspring (he calls it "the sense of the species"; vol. 2, 539) reveals how, for Schopenhauer, even standards of physical **beauty** result from unconscious biological causes. In both cases, the conscious beliefs and desires of individuals serve to mask rather than reveal the true causes of their sexual behavior.

It is not surprising, then, that for Schopenhauer the standards that should govern sexual behavior are to be grounded not on the conscious desires and intentions of the individual but solely on their functional utility for reproduction and maintenance of offspring (as in evolutionary theory and its offspring, sociobiology and **evolutionary psychology**). For example, recognizing that men are able to produce far more offspring than women, he concludes that "conjugal fidelity for the man is artificial, for the woman natural; and so adultery on the part of the woman is much less pardonable than on the part of the man, both objectively on account of the consequences, and subjectively on account of its being unnatural" (*WWR*, vol. 2, 542). Likewise, since social institutions exist to further these natural ends, Schopenhauer quite consistently argues that "no valid reason can be given why a man should not have a second wife when his first is suffering from chronic illness, is barren, or has gradually become too old. . . . Polygamy is not a matter of dispute at all, but is to be taken as a fact that is met with everywhere; its mere regulation is the problem" (*PP*, vol. 2, 623–24). At no time does Schopenhauer appeal to romantic notions such as love or moral obligation to justify any sexual practices; he appeals only to reproductive utility. Curiously, this emphasis on reproductive utility places Schopenhauer well within the practical boundaries of traditional Christian (or at least Catholic) thought on the topic, which perhaps reveals his own somewhat bourgeois attitudes toward sexuality.

Schopenhauer had little to say about all the varieties of sexual behavior that do not fit into his teleological account, except to condemn them. But while he freely adopts the **language** of "unnaturality" and "vice" when discussing nonreproductive sexual acts, these terms are employed naturalistically rather than moralistically. For example, he regards **masturbation** as the sign of a physical ailment, "more a matter of diet than ethics; for this reason works against it are written by medical men . . . and not by moralists" (*BM*, 60). **Bestiality**, on the other hand, is condemned as "an offense against the species" (*BM*, 60) because it cannot result in children.

Pederasty, however, received more sustained treatment from Schopenhauer, returned to and expanded on in the third edition of *WWR*. (There is no evidence to support Magee's [346–49] accusation that Schopenhauer himself had inclinations toward pederasty; see Safranski, 135–39.) Unlike masturbation, which, like Freud, he considered mainly a childhood phenomenon, and unlike bestiality, which is exceedingly rare, pederasty is "frequently practiced at all times and in all countries of the world, in spite of its detestable nature" (vol. 2, 561). While in the first two editions of *WWR* he dismissed it as a "misguided instinct" (vol. 2, 560), the near universality of pederasty among cultures ultimately convinced him that "it arises in some way from human nature itself." But if so, pederasty would be a puzzle, the way **homosexuality** generally is a puzzle from the perspective of **evolution**. Schopenhauer recognizes this very well: "Now that something so thoroughly contrary to nature, indeed going against nature in a matter of the greatest importance and concern to her, should arise from nature herself is such an unheard-of-paradox that its explanation confronts us as a difficult problem" (vol. 2, 562). Following the (untenable) medical belief of the ancient Greeks that the sperm of old men and young boys produce weak offspring who diminish the vitality of the species, Schopenhauer explained pederasty as a subterfuge of nature to direct the male libido away from behaviors that would result in inferior offspring: "In consequence of her own laws, nature was hard pressed, and resorted to a makeshift, a stratagem, by a perversion of the instinct" (vol. 2, 566). One might also say that "kin selection," as the mechanism by which evolution perhaps produces or maintains homosexuality, looks similarly makeshift.

Apart from the exceptions just raised, discussions of homosexuality, fetishism, and other sexual phenomena are almost entirely absent from Schopenhauer's writings, probably due to the standards of propriety of his time as much as to their tangential relationship to reproduction. He makes only a passing reference to same-sex attraction as a lifelong feature of an individual's sexuality, where his explanation follows the same misguided logic of his discussion of pederasty (*WWR*, vol. 2, 565). Schopenhauer's reduction of homosexuality to pederasty and his description of both as a ruse of nature are obviously inadequate for understanding either phenomenon. Still, his attempt to explain nonheterosexual behavior naturalistically—"here there was no question of moral admonition against the vice, but of a proper understanding of the essential nature of the matter" (vol. 2, 566)—at least marks an advance in method over much of the philosophical tradition since **Saint Augustine** (354–430).

Nevertheless, those looking to Schopenhauer as a forerunner of the Sexual Revolution of the late twentieth century will be disappointed on a number of points. He neglects almost entirely the female's/woman's perspective in his explanation of sexual behavior and his prescriptions for it, entirely in keeping with the sexist attitudes of his era and his own misogyny (see especially his essay "On Women"; *PP*, vol. 2, 614–27). Moreover, consistently with his own philosophy but in sharp contrast to modern attitudes, Schopenhauer rejects all forms of **sexual activity**, *most especially those that are fecund*, as exercises in metaphysical futility: "[L]overs are traitors who secretly strive to perpetuate the whole trouble and toil that would otherwise rapidly come to an end. Such an ending they try to frustrate, as others like them have frustrated it previously" (*WWR*, vol. 2, 560). The proper attitude toward sexuality is renunciation and puritanical self-denial, not self-indulgence, as a means of abolishing the Will. Whether such radical metaphysical pessimism automatically turns into nihilism, as Nietzsche charged (see Young's defense, 135–52), Schopenhauer's conflicted attitudes toward the value and purpose of sex are unlikely to attract many adherents.

In the final analysis, Schopenhauer's enduring importance for the philosophy of sex lies not in his ontology of the evil of sex but in his insights as a psychologist of human sexuality. By recognizing, nearly a century before Freud, the primacy of sexuality in the formation of personality and the explanation of behavior, and in his willingness to look beneath the surface of consciousness to find the hidden energies and purposes that drive everyday human existence, Schopenhauer helped make possible the scientific study of human sexuality and reflecting on it apart from Western religious and cultural traditions. For that reason alone, his writings on sexuality merit continued examination and consideration.

See also Beauty; Evolution; Fichte, Johann Gottlieb; Freud, Sigmund; Homosexuality and Science; Marriage; Natural Law (New); Nietzsche, Friedrich; Paglia, Camille; Pedophilia; Psychology, Evolutionary; Thomas Aquinas (Saint)

REFERENCES

Atwell, John E. *Schopenhauer on the Character of the World: The Metaphysics of Will*. Berkeley: University of California Press, 1995; Gardner, Sebastian. "Schopenhauer, Will, and the Unconscious." In Christopher Janaway, ed., *The Cambridge Companion to Schopenhauer*. Cambridge: Cambridge University Press, 1999, 375–421; Gupta, R. K. "Freud and Schopenhauer." *Journal of the History of Ideas* 36:4 (1975), 721–28; Higgins, Kathleen Marie. "Schopenhauer and Nietzsche: Temperament and Temporality." In Christopher Janaway, ed., *Willing and Nothingness: Schopenhauer as Nietzsche's Educator*. Oxford, U.K.: Clarendon Press, 1998, 151–77; Janaway, Christopher. *Self and World in Schopenhauer's Philosophy*. Oxford, U.K.: Clarendon Press, 1989; Janaway, Christopher. "Will and Nature." In Christopher Janaway, ed., *The Cambridge Companion to Schopenhauer*. Cambridge: Cambridge University Press, 1999, 138–70; Magee, Bryan. (1983) *The Philosophy of Schopenhauer*, 2nd ed. Oxford, U.K.: Clarendon Press, 1997; Safranski, Rudiger. *Schopenhauer and the Wild Years of Philosophy*. Trans. Ewald Osers. Cambridge, Mass.: Harvard University Press, 1989; Schmidt, Alfred. "Schopenhauer und der Materialismus." *Schopenhauer-Jahrbuch* 58 (1977), 9–48; Schopenhauer, Arthur. (1814, 1847) *On the Fourfold Root of the Principle of Sufficient Reason*. Trans. E.F.J. Payne. LaSalle, Ill.: Open Court, 1974; Schopenhauer, Arthur. (1841) *On the Basis of Morality*. Trans. E.F.J. Payne. Indianapolis, Ind.: Hackett, 1995; Schopenhauer, Arthur. (1836) *On the Will in Nature*. Trans. E.F.J. Payne. New York: Berg, 1992; Schopenhauer, Arthur. (1851) *Parerga and Paralipomena*, 2 vols. Trans. E.F.J. Payne. Oxford, U.K.: Clarendon Press, 1974; Schopenhauer, Arthur. (1818, 1844, 1859) *The World as Will and Representation*, 2 vols. Trans. E.F.J. Payne. New

York: Dover, 1966; Schulz, Ortrun. "Schopenhauers spinozistische Grundansicht." *Schopenhauer-Jahrbuch* 74 (1993), 51–72; Young, Julian. *Willing and Unwilling: A Study in the Philosophy of Arthur Schopenhauer*. Dordrecht, Holland: Martinus Nijhoff, 1987.

Lance Byron Richey

ADDITIONAL READING

Alexander, W. M. "Philosophers Have Avoided Sex." *Diogenes* 72 (Winter 1970), 56–74; Atwell, John E. "Schopenhauer on Men, Women, and Sexual Love." *Midwest Quarterly* 38:2 (1997), 143–57; Baum, Günther. "Freundschaft und Liebe im Wiederstreit von Ideal und Leben." *Schopenhauer-Jahrbuch* 66 (1985), 103–14; Bilsker, Richard. "Freud and Schopenhauer: Consciousness, the Unconscious, and the Drive towards Death." *Idealistic Studies* 27:1–2 (1997), 79–90; Cyzyk, Mark. "Conscience, Sympathy, and Love: Ethical Strategies toward Confirmation of Metaphysical Assertions in Schopenhauer." *Dialogue* 32:1 (1989), 24–31; Gardiner, Patrick. *Schopenhauer*. New York: Penguin, 1967. Reprinted, Bristol, U.K.: Thoemmes Press, 1997; Green, Eleanor H. "Schopenhauer and D. H. Lawrence on Sex and Love." *D. H. Lawrence Review* 8 (1975), 329–45; Guéry, François. "Une découverte métaphysique de Schopenhauer: l'amour." In Jean Lefranc, ed., *Schopenhauer*. Paris: Éditions de l'Herne, 1997, 145–50; Janaway, Christopher, ed. *The Cambridge Companion to Schopenhauer*. Cambridge: Cambridge University Press, 1999; Kolenda, Konstantin. "Schopenhauer: Reality Is Blind Will." In *Philosophy's Journey: A Historical Introduction*. Prospect Heights, Ill.: Waveland, 1987, 147–53; Malter, Rudolf. "Schopenhauer und die Biologie: Metaphysik der Lebenskraft auf empirischer Grundlage." *Berichte zur Wissenschaftsgeschichte* 6 (1983), 41–58; Parrhysius, Kurt. "A Physician on Schopenhauer's Philosophy of the Will-to-Live." *Schopenhauer-Jahrbuch* 53 (1972), 427–29; Schopenhauer, Arthur. (1851) "On Women." In *Selections*. Ed. DeWitt H. Parker. New York: Charles Scribner's Sons, 1956, 434–47; Schopenhauer, Arthur. *Werke in zehn Bänden*. Ed. Arthur Hübscher. Zürich, Switz.: Diogenes, 1977; Simmel, Georg. (1907) *Schopenhauer and Nietzsche*. Trans. Helmut Loiskandle, Deena Weinstein, and Michael Weinstein. Urbana: University of Illinois Press, 1991; Singer, Irving. "The Morality of Compassion: Contra Kant and Schopenhauer." In *Explorations in Love and Sex*. Lanham, Md.: Rowman and Littlefield, 2001, 21–45; Singer, Irving. "Romantic Pessimism: Goethe, Novalis, Schopenhauer, Wagner." In *The Nature of Love*, vol. 2: *Courtly and Romantic*. Chicago, Ill.: University of Chicago Press, 1984, 432–81; Soll, Ivan. "The Hopelessness of Hedonism and the Will to Power." *International Studies in Philosophy* 18:2 (1986), 97–112; Taylor, Charles S. "Nietzsche's Schopenhauerianism." *Nietzsche-Studien* 17 (1988), 45–73; Welsen, Peter. *Schopenhauers Theories des Subjekts: Ihre tranzendental-philosophischen, anthropologischen und naturmetaphysischen Grundlagen*. Würzburg, Ger.: Königshausen und Neumann, 1995; Young, Christopher, and Andrew Brook. "Schopenhauer and Freud." *International Journal of Psychoanalysis* 75 (1994), 101–18. <www.carleton.ca/~abrook/SCHOPENY.htm> [accessed 18 October 2004].

SCIENCE, SEXUAL. *See* Sexology

SCRUTON, ROGER (1944–). Roger Vernon Scruton was born and raised in High Wycombe, Buckinghamshire. Educated at Jesus College, Cambridge, he taught for twenty-one years (1971–1992) at Birkbeck College, London, where he became professor of aesthetics in 1985. Between 1992 and 1995 Scruton held a chair in philosophy at Boston University. He also became a barrister-at-law in 1978. He now combines chasing foxes with the pursuit of knowledge. With about twenty philosophical and critical books as well as numerous articles and works of fiction to his credit, his output has been prolific. His career has been distinguished as much by controversy as by achievement. Never one to admire emperor's clothes or succumb to the tyranny of political correctness, Scruton's cultural, moral, and political conservatism has often put him at odds with the academic establishment in the English-speaking world. Before the collapse of communism in the early 1990s he was a champion of underground academic freedom in Eastern Europe.

Since Scruton is highly cultured and widely read, many scholars who disagree with aspects of his work nonetheless respect him (Johnson, 208). Martha Nussbaum, despite writing a critical review of *Sexual Desire* (*SD*), Scruton's treatise on sexuality, when it first appeared in 1986 ("Sex in the Head"), eventually commended the book as "certainly the most interesting philosophical attempt as yet to work through the moral issues involved in our treatment of persons as sex partners" ("Objectification," 261; see also 287n.64). Like other reviewers (e.g., Strawson), Nussbaum thought his treatment of sexuality excessively intellectualized. Many whose amatory lives are personally satisfactory and morally responsible would not describe their experience in Scrutonian terms. Indeed, they would probably find *Sexual Desire* incomprehensible or even unreadable (Strawson, 207). As Francis Hutcheson (1694–1746) observed, "[T]he natural Dispositions of Mankind will operate regularly in those who never reflected upon them, nor form'd just Notions about them" (vii). Scruton has certainly reflected long and hard upon them and supports his complex views by a carefully thought out philosophy of mind.

Sexual Desire reveals a wide-ranging but not uncritical eclecticism, **Immanuel Kant** (1724–1804) being the most mentioned philosopher and **Aristotle** (384–322 BCE) the one most approvingly referred to. The early chapters are pervaded by three kindred theses, which are made in varying degrees to appear as the basis of Scruton's argument: (1) the discontinuity of the personal and the animal aspects of humanity; (2) the immunity of the personal from scientific investigation; and, less prominently and not consistently, (3) a conception of reason as action guiding in an absolute way. All three theses are at variance with the British empiricist tradition. That our corporeal nature is not part of our essence as "thinking beings" is a doctrine conspicuous in the rationalist philosopher **René Descartes** (1596–1650; *Meditations on First Philosophy*, II) and characteristic of much contemporary and subsequent continental thought. Denigration of the material is, however, repudiated by English-speaking writers such as **Bernard Mandeville** (1670–1733), who places man firmly in the animal domain (*Fable of the Bees*, vol. 1, 41–42, 204–5), and **David Hume** (1711–1776), who argues that the passions of animals, though cruder, are analogous to human passions and should be similarly explained (*Treatise of Human Nature*, II.i.12, II.ii.12). **Edward Westermarck** (1862–1939) also maintained, in true evolutionary vein, a continuum between mankind and other animals (*History of Human Marriage*, chap. 1). What Charles Darwin (1809–1882) joined together, Scruton is keen to put asunder. He asserts, for example, that a wolf's remaining with his mate is not comparable to human marital fidelity, because animals are without "genuine individualising thoughts" (*SD*, 79). But does not a horse or a dog know his own master and a ewe her own lamb?

That human experience is not susceptible to scientific explanation is asserted early on (*SD*, 4), where the doctrine is said to have a genealogy going back to Kant or possibly Aristotle. This theme recurs in Scruton's discussion of sociobiology (chap. 7), where he contrasts two incompatible ways of understanding the world: the scientific and the intentional. Because humans have self-awareness and a capacity for self-criticism that animals lack, our conduct can never be appraised purely in scientific terms. Sociobiologists err in assimilating human behavior to animal behavior, which has no underlying intentional structure (181–88). For this reason, Scruton castigates as "pseudo-scientific" mid-twentieth-century American sexologists (mostly William Masters [1915–2001] and Virginia Johnson, but Alfred Kinsey

[1894–1956] as well) for their "repeated references to the 'effective functioning', 'adequacy' and 'frequency' of 'sexual performance' "—descriptions whose depersonalizing neutrality and reductionism misrepresent the phenomena to which they refer (viii, 74).

At times Scruton imposes unduly narrow limits on human understanding, as when he condemns as a perversion of reason the spirit of the Enlightenment that sought to explain what had been previously accepted as mysterious (SD, 70–71). This resolve accords with his romantic, Wagnerian temperament but is unsupported by cogent argument. It is a reasonable proposition that the scope of empirical enquiry is a contentious issue. Yet Scruton castigates **Michel Foucault** (1926–1984) for supposing that our moral preoccupation with the sexual can be historically explained (34, 362–63) and maintains, instead, that it is an *a priori* truth about human nature. His conviction about this might have been less secure had his acquaintance with sexual experience included primitive races rather than being confined to the most polite classes of "civilised" societies (see 363). The issues that he claims are *a priori* have been thought suitable for empirical investigation by writers less controversial than Foucault. The project of adumbrating the natural history of human sexuality, also undertaken by Westermarck, seems legitimate, but on Scruton's view it is ruled out *a priori*.

The intellectual foundations of Scruton's thought are ambiguous but remote from the neutrality and detachment he claims at the end of the book (SD, 361). He proposes "to sketch a sexual morality, whose basis will be located, not in religious belief, but in human nature," yet on the same page (14) he asserts that "religious experience provides the securest everyday background to sexual morality." A sort of Manichaean conflict between the physical and the spiritual pervades the book. His lugubrious phrases—"the pain of incarnation," "this confrontation with our embodiment" (137), and "the sin of existence itself " (228)—reveal Scruton to be a man acutely ill at ease with our status as creatures of flesh and blood (see Johnson, 215–17). However, unlike **Plato** (427–347 BCE), whose formulation of the "question" he rejects (216–19), and unlike Kant, whom he rebukes for his "failure to see that our animal nature is not just conjoined with, but also entirely transformed by . . . a transcendental self" (84), Scruton finds in erotic **love** a realm in which the conflicts allegedly generated by our embodiment are resolved (251; see 337).

Scruton's central doctrine—that the most developed form of **sexual desire** is characterized by its intentionality, the quality of mental states that have *conceptual* and not merely *perceptual* objects—can be maintained without the aforementioned commitments. This point is exemplified by work earlier than his (**Thomas Nagel**'s 1969 essay "Sexual Perversion"; Stafford's 1977 "On Distinguishing between Love and Lust") and also by later writers (e.g., Morgan, "Sex in the Head"). Scruton, however, defends the stronger thesis that intentionality is definitive of *all* sexual desire and arousal, properly so-called. These are idiosyncratic definitions of "sexual desire" and "sexual arousal," for they entail the peculiar proposition that "[a]nimals are never sexually aroused; they do not feel sexual desire, nor do they have sexual fulfilment" (SD, 36; see 59). Scruton does not, of course, deny that animals experience physiological excitation but reserves the term "arousal" to denote the mental state that, he maintains, is exclusive to rational beings. Unlike mere appetites (such as for food), sexual desire and arousal are individualizing: They are always "a response to a particular person" (29, 78–82) and are "not transferable to another" (30, 76). Hence his definitions also seem to have the odd implication that we cannot experience desire or arousal with **pornography**, for in viewing pornography sexual interest is easily transferable from object to object and "individualizing intentionality" is absent. (Blackburn makes the same point about couples who hook up in a singles bar and sailors returning to shore;

106–7.) Scruton, however, sometimes lapses into inconsistency, as when he speaks of desire roaming freely (309) and of "the element of generality [in desire] which tempts us always to experiment" (339; see 359).

The concept of **sexual perversion** deployed by Scruton (which is closely akin to Nagel's) follows naturally from his thesis that sexual desire is the exclusive prerogative of a rational being, someone "characterized not only by his ability to reason but also by his possession of a first-person perspective, responsibility and the rich interpersonal emotional life which those entail" (*SD*, 288). "Sexual desire involves the marshalling and directing of animal urges towards an interpersonal aim, and an interpersonal fulfilment" (289). Perversion consists in the separation of these animal and interpersonal elements—as in, for example, fetishism and pornography, but not **homosexuality**, which Scruton acknowledges (albeit with reservations; 305) to be capable of interpersonal intentionality comparable to that of heterosexuality. "The complete or partial failure to recognise, in and through desire, the personal existence of the other is . . . an affront both to him and to oneself. Moreover, in so divorcing sexual conduct from the impulse of accountability and care, we remove from the sphere of personal relations the major force which compels us to unite with others, to accept them and to compromise our lives on their account" (289; see 343). Scruton's concept of obscenity is similarly derivative. Obscenity involves "a 'depersonalised' perception of human sexuality, in which the body and its sexual function are uppermost in our thoughts and all-obliterating" (138). This is the essence of pornography. By contrast, a genuine *erotic* work "is one which invites the reader to re-create in imagination the first-person point of view of someone party to an erotic encounter" (139; for doubts about this distinction, see Soble, 101–2). **Prostitution** is discountenanced because it reduces an experience that should be deeply personal to a commercial transaction (156–60). Both pornography and prostitution are linked to sexual **fantasy**, an anarchic world governed by "monstrous myths" in which "human reality has been poisoned by the expendability and replaceability of the other" (346).

The penultimate chapter of *Sexual Desire*, which insists that virtue is linked to personal flourishing, is strongly reminiscent of Aristotle. Scruton finds his ethical theory preferable to Kant's, whose attribution of motivating force to reason is dubious. Aristotle obviates this problem by invoking the notion of a long-term point of view whose realization is antecedently desired (*SD*, 325). Scruton proceeds to address the scope and purpose of sexual morality and the aims of moral education. These should include the cultivation of appropriate feelings and the disposition to see as desirable only what will bring long-term fulfillment, in favor of which immediate gratifications must be postponed or sacrificed. Because (as in **G.W.F. Hegel** [1770–1831]) the capacity to give and receive erotic love is incomparably valuable in attaining self-fulfillment (337), we have reason to acquire it and to eschew those sexual habits (want of chastity; **adultery**) that are vicious because they militate against it (338). "The task of sexual morality is to unite [the personal and the sexual], to sustain thereby the intentionality of desire, and prepare the individual for erotic love" (343). "The ideal of virtue remains one of 'sexual integrity': of a sexuality that is entirely integrated into the life of personal affection, and in which the self and its responsibility are centrally involved and indissolubly linked to the pleasures and passions of the body" (346).

The final chapter of *Sexual Desire*, "The Politics of Sex," is a vindication of existing institutions in the face of the liberationist ideology that arose late in the twentieth century—fantasies akin to those of **Jean-Jacques Rousseau** (1712–1778), who believed that shaking off conventions would restore mankind to a state of innocence and freedom (*SD*,

348). Against such claims, Scruton argues that sexual desire itself, being largely a social artifact, could not exist in a state of nature. Moreover, some kind of social structure involving a public morality is necessary to nourish a long-term view of things. Conservative thinkers from the time of Aristotle have sought to base political order on domestic relations and the erotic bond that underlies them (350–51). No social order is spontaneously self-sustaining, but requires the support of institutions (354). Like Hegel, Scruton maintains that civil society is nothing without the state, which is its realized form (355). The chapter closes with a eulogy of **marriage** and the family (356–61). Scruton shrouds these favored institutions with a veil of quasi-religious mystification. But he does not state clearly whether the concept of "the sacred" he invokes is a social artifact, useful because it supports the social order, or an independent reality warranted by a real god. He seems to vacillate between these two views (349, 352–53). A promised sequel volume (355) in which the themes of this chapter would be developed has never appeared, although early in 2004 he published a book (*Death-Devoted Heart*) on sexuality and the sacred in Richard Wagner (1813–1883).

Most controversial is Scruton's treatment of homosexuality. Since 1986 his attitude has gravitated from ambivalence (*SD*, 305–11) to outright hostility. In *Sexual Desire* he admits (as does Nagel) that since homosexual relations are just as capable of interpersonal intentionality as heterosexual relations, same-sex sexuality is not intrinsically obscene or perverted (though it may exist in perverted forms). He suggests, however, that for reasons related to the sameness or difference of gender between two sexually interacting parties, and the vulnerability or lack of it implied by that sameness or difference, the intentionality of homosexual desire and heterosexual desire might diverge in morally significant ways. At the same time, he does concede that the arguments he adduces to support this claim are not very cogent. (See Nussbaum ["Sex in the Head," 51–52] and Johnson [213], both of whom highlight the weakness of his argument.) For Scruton, gender is partly a cultural artifact, but one based on "the deep division between man and woman," which is part of "the inward constitution of reality" (*SD*, 260)—a thesis supported by sociobiology (264) and anthropology (266–67). Given his contempt for sociobiology, it is surprising that he should mention this here.

Shortly after the publication of *Sexual Desire*, an article in a professional journal argued that Scruton's admission that homosexual desire is spontaneous and not necessarily perverted, along with his persuasive views about the constructive purposes of moral education, committed him to the positive treatment of homosexuality by moral educators (Stafford, "Love and Lust Revisited"). Scruton was invited by this journal to respond but declined to do so (Stafford, *Essays*, ix). Two years later, perhaps in an attempt to obviate this unwelcome corollary of *Sexual Desire*, Scruton enunciated a new doctrine defending both **heterosexism** and homophobia—first in a lecture, reprinted as an essay ("Sexual Morality and the Liberal Consensus"), then in a more demotic newspaper article ("Why Heterosexism Is Not a Vice"). He offered the argument that since homosexuals tend not have children, they have no interest in the well-being of society or in its future and therefore indulge their carnal appetites without restraint. Only by sublimating their sexuality in useful work could homosexuals acquire a stake in the community and a sense of social responsibility. Therefore "we should continue to instil in our children feelings of revulsion" toward homosexuality ("Heterosexism").

Scruton's new argument is original, being unrelated to either the weak, gender-based argument advanced in *Sexual Desire* or the perversion-based (or Natural Law) sallies generally deployed by conservative moralists. However, it is both logically and factually flawed and incongruous with the abundant humane insights that he had previously expressed. These inconsistencies have been exposed, and the evil consequences to which his homophobic prescriptions give rise have been displayed (Stafford, "The Two Minds of Roger Scruton"). Scruton has not been persuaded to recant. Indeed, in an essay published as the second of a three-part exchange with Martha Nussbaum (see her "Lesbian and Gay Rights"), he maintained that the perpetuation of revulsion to homosexuality is "a human good" ("Gay Reservations," 121). His justification for reviling gay men is that "[t]here is in homosexual union between men a vector which tends to promiscuity" and that any society that is accommodating toward gay relationships must "school itself to regard promiscuity—with all that it means by way of social breakdown, impermanence and the loss of care—as morally neutral" (122).

This argument may be countered by two criticisms, both of which (ironically) are found in Scruton's own work. First, promiscuity is to some extent a *consequence* of the hostility to which gays have been subjected and hence cannot justify that hostility (see Thomas and Levin, 31–32, 129–30, 173–74). As he once remarked, "The fate of persons is inseparable from the history of the institutions which form and nurture them" (*SD*, 350). The homophobic society that he endorses has done nothing to foster in homosexuals a disposition toward stable and responsible relationships. Instead, it has encouraged self-loathing and furtiveness, thereby sustaining the evils that he deplores (Sullivan, *Love Undetectable*, 141; *Virtually Normal*, 107). Second, a gay-friendly society need not condone promiscuity (or **casual sex**) and so would not be susceptible to the problems that this might cause. As Scruton himself has pointed out, promiscuity is "something that the wiser proponents of [homosexual love] have . . . always condemned" ("Sexual Morality," 264). Instead of joining forces with these wise people, he recommends religiously based indoctrination to "endarken" minds with revulsion at homosexuality ("Sexual Morality," 271). This strategy, which requires the propagation of prejudice and the psychological maiming of male homosexuals, is incompatible with Scruton's assertion that "the child ought to be happy," to have what he needs to flourish (*SD*, 326), and to be encouraged in "the successful employment of those capacities that are integral to his being" (*SD*, 327). His policy has baneful consequences precisely for children, including the irreparable damage wrought when they become alienated from their own sexuality (Sullivan, *Love Undetectable*, 141). It is with some justification, then, that Scruton has been charged with "intellectual schizophrenia" (Stafford, "Two Minds," 192).

See also Activity, Sexual; Animal Sexuality; Anscombe, G.E.M.; Aristotle; Communication Model; Completeness, Sexual; Desire, Sexual; Ethics, Sexual; Ethics, Virtue; Existentialism; Heterosexism; Homosexuality, Ethics of; Kant, Immanuel; Leibniz, Gottfried; Nagel, Thomas; Phenomenology; Sex Education; Sexology

REFERENCES

Blackburn, Simon. *Lust: The Seven Deadly Sins*. New York: New York Public Library/Oxford University Press, 2004; Descartes, René. (1641) *Meditations on First Philosophy, with Selections from the Objections and Replies*, revised ed. Trans. and ed. John Cottingham. Cambridge: Cambridge University Press, 1996; Hume, David. (1739–1740) *A Treatise of Human Nature*. Ed. David Fate Norton and Mary J. Norton. Oxford, U.K.: Oxford University Press, 2000; Hutcheson, Francis. (1728) *An Essay on the Nature and Conduct of the Passions and Affections*. Hildesheim, Ger.: Georg Olms, 1971; Johnson, Edward. "Inscrutable Desires." *Philosophy of the Social Sciences* 20:2 (1990), 208–21; Mandeville, Bernard. (1714, 1729) *The Fable of the Bees*, 2 vols. Ed. F. B. Kaye. Oxford, U.K.: Clarendon Press, 1924; Morgan, Seiriol. "Sex in the Head." *Journal of Applied Philosophy*

20:1 (2003), 1–16; Nagel, Thomas. "Sexual Perversion." *Journal of Philosophy* 66:1 (1969), 5–17; Nussbaum, Martha C. "Lesbian and Gay Rights: Pro." In Michael Leahy and Dan Cohn-Sherbok, eds., *The Liberation Debate: Rights at Issue*. London: Routledge, 1996, 89–107; Nussbaum, Martha C. "Nussbaum's Reply" [to Roger Scruton]. In Michael Leahy and Dan Cohn-Sherbok, eds., *The Liberation Debate: Rights at Issue*. London: Routledge, 1996, 122–29; Nussbaum, Martha C. "Objectification." *Philosophy and Public Affairs* 24:4 (1995), 249–91; Nussbaum, Martha C. "Sex in the Head." *New York Review of Books* (18 December 1986), 49–52; Scruton, Roger. *Death-Devoted Heart: Sex and the Sacred in Wagner's Tristan and Isolde*. New York: Oxford University Press, 2004; Scruton, Roger. "Gay Reservations." In Michael Leahy and Dan Cohn-Sherbok, eds., *The Liberation Debate: Rights at Issue*. London: Routledge, 1996, 108–24; Scruton, Roger. *Sexual Desire: A Philosophical Investigation*. London: Weidenfeld and Nicolson, 1986. *Sexual Desire: A Moral Philosophy of the Erotic*. New York: Free Press, 1986; Scruton, Roger. "Sexual Morality and the Liberal Consensus." In *The Philosopher on Dover Beach—Essays*. Manchester, U.K.: Carcanet, 1990, 261–72; Scruton, Roger. "Why Heterosexism Is Not a Vice." *The Sunday Telegraph* (24 September 1989), 20; Soble, Alan. *Pornography, Sex, and Feminism*. Amherst, N.Y.: Prometheus, 2002; Stafford, J. Martin. *Essays on Sexuality and Ethics*. Solihull, U.K.: Ismeron, 1995; Stafford, J. Martin. "Love and Lust Revisited: Intentionality, Homosexuality and Moral Education." *Journal of Applied Philosophy* 5:1 (1988), 87–100; Stafford, J. Martin. "On Distinguishing between Love and Lust." *Journal of Value Inquiry* 11:4 (1977), 292–303; Stafford, J. Martin. "The Two Minds of Roger Scruton." *Studies in Philosophy and Education* 11:2 (1991), 187–93; Strawson, Galen. "Ideal Coitions." *The Times Literary Supplement* (28 February 1986), 207–8; Sullivan, Andrew. *Love Undetectable: Reflections on Friendship, Sex, and Survival*. New York: Knopf, 1998; Sullivan, Andrew. *Virtually Normal: An Argument about Homosexuality*. New York: Knopf, 1995; Thomas, Laurence M., and Michael E. Levin. *Sexual Orientation and Human Rights*. Lanham, Md.: Rowman and Littlefield, 1999; Westermarck, Edward. (1891) *The History of Human Marriage*, 2nd ed. London: Macmillan, 1894. 5th ed., 3 vols. London: Macmillan, 1921; New York: Allerton, 1922.

J. Martin Stafford

ADDITIONAL READING

Belliotti, Raymond. "Roger Scruton." In *Good Sex: Perspectives on Sexual Ethics*. Lawrence: University Press of Kansas, 1993, 77–84; Hamilton, Christopher. "Sex." In *Living Philosophy: Reflections on Life, Meaning and Morality*. Edinburgh, Scot.: Edinburgh University Press, 2001, 125–41; Hegel, G.W.F. (1821) *Elements of the Philosophy of Right*. Ed. Allen W. Wood. Trans. Hugh B. Nisbet. Cambridge: Cambridge University Press, 1995; Johnson, Edward. "Inscrutable Desires." [Essay review of *Sexual Desire: A Moral Philosophy of the Erotic*, by Roger Scruton] *Philosophy of the Social Sciences* 20:2 (1990), 208–21. Reprinted in HS (53–66); Jung, Patricia Beattie, and Ralph F. Smith. *Heterosexism: An Ethical Challenge*. Albany: State University of New York Press, 1993; Langton, Rae. "Love and Solipsism." In Roger Lamb, ed., *Love Analyzed*. Boulder, Colo.: Westview, 1997, 123–52; Langton, Rae. "Sexual Solipsism." *Philosophical Topics* 23:2 (1995), 149–87; Lilla, Mark. "Sex and the Conservative Body." *The Public Interest*, no. 85 (Fall 1986), 86–94; Morgan, Seiriol. "Dark Desires." *Ethical Theory and Moral Practice* 6:4 (2003), 377–410; Nagel, Thomas. "Sexual Perversion." *Journal of Philosophy* 66:1 (1969), 5–17. Reprinted in P&S1 (247–60); POS1 (76–88). Reprinted, revised, in Thomas Nagel, *Mortal Questions*. Cambridge: Cambridge University Press, 1979, 39–52; and POS2 (39–51); POS3 (9–20); POS4 (9–20); STW (105–12); Nussbaum, Martha C. "Objectification." *Philosophy and Public Affairs* 24:4 (1995), 249–91. Reprinted in POS3 (283–321); POS4 (381–419). Reprinted, revised, in *Sex and Social Justice*. New York: Oxford University Press, 1999, 213–39; Nussbaum, Martha C. "Sex in the Head." *New York Review of Books* (18 December 1986), 49–52. [Letters by Martha Nussbaum and Roger Scruton, *New York Review of Books* (29 January 1987), 49; (7 May 1987), 46–47]; Pateman, Carole. Review of *Sexual Desire: A Moral Philosophy of the Erotic*, by Roger Scruton. *Ethics* 97:4 (1987), 881–82; Rorty, Richard. "Sex and the Single Thinker." *The New Republic* (2 June 1986), 34–37; Scruton, Roger. "Attitudes, Beliefs and Reasons." In John Casey, ed., *Morality and Moral Reasoning*. London: Methuen, 1971, 25–100; Scruton, Roger. "Kiss Me, Cate." [Review of *Only Words*, by Catharine A. MacKinnon] *National Review* (1 November 1993), 61–62; Scruton, Roger. "Sex for Sale." *National Review* (8 June 1992), 47–49; Scruton, Roger. "Sexual Arousal." In A. Phillips Griffiths, ed., *Philosophy and Practice*. Cambridge: Cambridge University Press, 1985, 255–73; Soble, Alan. "Ex Post Facto Reasons" and "Irreplaceability by Individuation." In *The Structure of Love*. New Haven, Conn.: Yale University Press, 1990, 153–57, 293–98; Soble, Alan. "Transcendental Illusions." In *Sexual Investigations*. New York: New York University Press, 1996, 102–6; Stafford, J. Martin. "Love and Lust Revisited: Intentionality, Homosexuality and Moral Education." *Journal of Applied Philosophy* 5:1 (1988), 87–100. Reprinted in *Essays on Sexuality and Ethics*. Solihull, U.K.: Ismeron, 1995, 65–78; HS (177–90); Stafford, J. Martin. "On Distinguishing between Love and Lust." *Journal of Value Inquiry* 11:4 (1977), 292–303. Reprinted in *Essays on Sexuality and Ethics*. Solihull, U.K.: Ismeron, 1995, 53–64; Stafford, J. Martin. "The Two Minds of Roger Scruton." *Studies in Philosophy and Education* 11:2 (1991), 187–93. Reprinted in *Essays on Sexuality and Ethics*. Solihull, U.K.: Ismeron, 1995, 93–99.

SEDUCTION. To seduce is to lead a person from a right or intended course of action into something wrong or unintended. Seduction occurs in many contexts: Hearing the game on the television in the next room might pull me away from my work. Eve was seduced by the serpent into thinking she could attain greater powers. People can be seduced sexually, of course. (Perhaps this is how Eve persuaded Adam to eat the forbidden fruit.) Two sorts of philosophical questions arise about sexual seduction: the conceptual question of what seduction is and the moral question about its permissibility.

Sexual seduction can be minimally characterized as one person's attempting to get another person, initially unwilling, to engage in sex. Without initial unwillingness, **sexual activity** might be routine, acquiescence, or celebration, among other things, but not seduction. Further, the morally interesting cases of seduction must be intentional and not, say, accidental. If a person has sex with another but never tried to arrange it, no seduction occurred.

But this initial definition must be refined, because it conflates **rape** and seduction. (The analytic culprit is "to get.") The rapist uses force or its threat to engage in sex with the other or does so without, or contrary to, the other's **consent**. By contrast, what the seducer tries to do, without force or threat, is to bring about that consent. In rape, the person acted upon is initially unwilling and remains so, whereas in seduction this person's psychology changes from initial unwillingness to willingness. The minimal conception, to keep rape and seduction distinct, must be refined by stipulating that the "getting" is not done by force or its threat and that the initially unwilling person eventually does become willing.

That getting someone to engage in sexual relations by using force, its threat, or other coercive tactics must be distinguished from seduction can be illustrated by considering **sexual harassment** and **date** or **acquaintance rape**. Sexual harassment and date rape are both difficult concepts, but for the purpose of discussion let them include (among other things) threatening to inflict costs short of bodily injury on a person if he or she persists in declining sexual activity (see Reitan, 102–3). Bob might threaten to discredit Mary at their workplace if she does not engage in sex with him. He might convey to her that he will be sulky, out of temper, and uncooperative unless Mary capitulates, in circumstances where Mary must depend on him. Or he might aggressively and repeatedly press himself on Mary during a date, refusing to take "no" for an answer. Whether or not these are paradigm cases of sexual harassment or date rape, no one would be inclined to characterize them as instances of seduction. Even if Bob did succeed in getting Mary to engage in sex with him by employing these tactics, he has not been successful in changing an initially unwilling Mary into a willing Mary.

A variant of the minimal conception of seduction has been suggested by Jean-Paul Sartre, who proposes that to seduce another person is to make oneself into a fascinating object for the other, an object that then captures the other's attention (*Being and Nothingness*, 484–85). This "capturing" by making oneself attractive is one way to understand the "getting" of the minimal conception. Sartre is not thinking exclusively about erotic seduction. Still, on this "fascination" conception of seduction, sexual seduction could be characterized as attempting to get an initially unwilling other to engage in sexual activity by presenting oneself in a way designed to "capture" (without, of course, employing force or its threat) the erotic attention of the other person. The seducer, in this case, will have to know what the unwilling other would be "captured" by and present himself or herself accordingly. This will involve knowledge of the other's erotic likes and perhaps her psychosexual weaknesses. There is not much to be said for trying to capture the other by making oneself into Sherlock Holmes when the other prefers, indeed swoons over, Spiderman.

The fascination conception of seduction, even if it keeps rape and seduction distinct by insisting that the "capturing" not be accomplished by force or its threat, still falls into conflating rape and seduction in a different and more subtle way and so requires refinement. This view counts as seduction cases in which one person gets an initially unwilling person to engage in sexual activity by lying, which can be an especially effective means of presenting oneself in such a fascinating way as to "capture" the other. There are, of course, strong moral reasons for objecting to obtaining sex by employing lies (see Mappes), but the issue is whether lying to obtain sex counts as rape or, as on the fascination model, only seduction. In the **law**, "fraud in the inducement," which includes obtaining sex through lying, generally does not count as rape (see, for example, the American Law Institute's Model Penal Code, art. 213.3), although some jurists and philosophers think it should, depending on the circumstances (for discussion, see **Richard Posner**, 81–82, 392–94; Doniger; Muehlenhard and Schrag; Murphy). A lie that presents oneself as the savior of the other, who is in a desperate situation, might be a "capturing" by fascination that amounts to rape. Other lies (say, the use of cosmetics, which present oneself as fascinating while concealing wrinkles, scars, and warts) seem too innocuous to be considered rape. So the fascination conception of seduction must be refined; it must include a criterion by which it can be determined when presenting oneself as fascinating by lying is seduction and when presenting oneself as fascinating goes too far and thereby amounts to rape.

An interesting question is whether the fascination model muddles the distinction between seduction and "winning over," in which one person shows another that he or she already has some quality that the other is seeking in an erotic partner. Suppose Joe, who is a rock musician, would like to engage in sex with Connie. She is initially unwilling but does not know his vocation. When declining Joe's overture, Connie tells him that she is fascinated by rock stars, so much so that she makes a hobby of increasing her tally of rock star conquests. Joe then tells her truthfully that he plays lead guitar in a well-known rock band and produces evidence: his photograph on a concert advertisement. Connie immediately adds him to her tally. Must the fascination conception say that Joe has seduced Connie by making himself irresistibly attractive to her? After all, Joe *did* something to present himself as fascinating: He *told the truth*. Ordinarily, however, we would say that Joe has simply won Connie over, and without much effort. He would have similarly just "won her over" if, having found out her sexual preferences, he became a rock musician (quitting his job at the post office).

Søren Kierkegaard (1813–1855) alerts us to another quality of seduction: "Whoever is unable to captivate a girl to such an extent that she loses sight of everything he does not wish her to see, whoever is unable to pervade a girl's being to such an extent that it is from her that everything emanates as he wishes it, he is and remains a bungler" ("Diary of the Seducer," 363). What distinguishes seduction from both winning over and obtaining sexual relations by lying, on Kierkegaard's view, is this: The seducer attempts to capture the other's attention not by engaging or appealing to any of the other's existing sexual motives but by causing the other to develop a new motive, a previously absent inclination, urge, or desire to engage in sexual relations with the seducer. And the seducer creates this new motive in the other without employing force or deception. Call this the "narrow motivational" conception of seduction.

The narrow motivational conception retains the plausible idea that seduction operates by contriving to capture another's sexual attention. Consider, however, a case in which an initially unwilling other has a nascent urge to have sex with the aspiring seducer but also a much stronger contrary motivation, a desire to avoid a potentially entangling attachment. Suppose, now, that the aspiring seducer successfully stokes this nascent sexual urge into dominance. According to the narrow motivational conception, no seduction has occurred, for the aspiring seducer did not cause the intended target to develop a previously absent desire to engage in sex with the seducer. But stoking a person's nascent urge to engage in sex to the point where it takes over is a paradigm case of seduction. So the narrow motivational conception is too restrictive.

On a "broad motivational" conception of seduction one person gets an initially unwilling other to engage in sexual relations either by contriving to induce in the target a new inclination or urge to have sex with him or her or by rendering effective an existing inclination or urge to have sex with him or her that is currently inhibited by some other motive. This conception of seduction preserves the aspects of the minimal, fascination, and narrow motivational conceptions that are worth preserving. It can therefore distinguish seduction from rape, from sex obtained by deception, and from winning over. Is this conception also able to distinguish seduction from other related sexual phenomena?

Consider an attempt to get an initially unwilling other to engage in sexual activity by the offer of money, or goods, or reciprocal sexual favors. Hugh offers Divine a hundred dollars for her to engage in sex with him, or a ring, or he promises to do for her in bed an act of which she is especially fond. Divine, finding the proposed transaction agreeable, accepts. It is not obviously true that we would call all or many of these cases "seduction" (and certainly not in those cases that are **prostitution**). Like winning another over, the behavior engages a target's existing motives as they are. On the broad motivational conception, seduction involves either multiplying the motives of the target or altering the relative capacities of the target's motives to determine action. Hence the broad motivational conception seems to yield the right answer in these cases. Suppose, now, that Hugh's offering Divine the money, the jewel, or her favorite sexual act did create in her a previously absent motive to engage in sex with him or decreased her reluctance to engage in sex with him (based, perhaps, on moral considerations), thereby allowing her embryonic desire to have sex with him to grow and become determinative. In such a case, Divine has been seduced, and this is what the broad motivational conception would say.

Assuming, at least provisionally, that the broad motivational conception of seduction is on the right track, we turn to the question of the moral status of seduction. On the least permissive view, seduction is never morally right; on the most permissive, it is never morally wrong; and there are views that fall between these extremes.

Of course, most if not all seduction would be morally rejected by any **sexual ethics** that is already in general impermissive, for example, the sexual ethics of Roman Catholicism (indeed, all the major religions) and various conservative, secular ethical views. Sexual seduction takes place largely outside **marriage**, and these impermissive sexual ethics all contend that nonmarital sexual conduct is morally wrong. (Even so, **Thomas Aquinas** [1224/25–1274] came up with special reasons for objecting to certain types of seduction; see *Summa theologiae*, vol. 43, 2a2ae, ques. 154, art. 1, 207.) Whether these impermissive sexual ethics would also prohibit seduction *within* marriage likely varies. To the extent that an impermissive sexual ethics emphasizes the procreative purpose of marital sex and rebukes the pursuit of sexual pleasure for its own sake in marriage (for example, **Augustine** [354–430]), not even seduction in marriage would be morally acceptable.

But even if a generally impermissive sexual ethics at least allowed seduction when and only when practiced by a married couple, such a moral view about seduction is not very easy to maintain (or as difficult to maintain as any impermissive sexual ethics is difficult to maintain). For sometimes seduction carried out by and on unmarried adults seems to be permissible. Jane Gallop, perhaps somewhat flamboyantly, argues that seducing male professors could be empowering for female graduate students and thus make a positive contribution to their development (39–43). Less controversially, imagine an unmarried couple that has a long, mutually rewarding sexual history, but one partner is recently rendered sexually reticent by worries about his or her sexual capacity or attractiveness. Were the other partner to respond by mounting a successful seduction, restoring the first partner's confidence, that would seem to be morally permissible, if not laudable. At least from a nontraditional and nonreligious perspective, human flourishing has been advanced without any loss.

The most permissive view about seduction is that even though seduction might have a bad reputation, there is truly nothing wrong with it. Consider, for example, a common type of sexual **liberalism**, according to which the valid consent by all participants is sufficient to render any given sexual activity morally legitimate (Primoratz, 201–2). Sexual liberals typically regard as valid consent any token of consent that is given by a mentally competent adult in the absence of force, threat of force, unwarranted pressure, or deception. Depending on how strict one is about what constitutes valid consent, some instances of seduction might be disallowed by sexual liberalism. But as long as seduction does not interfere with a person's providing "free and informed" consent, seduction must be regarded as morally innocuous.

To be sure, the principle of free and informed consent has been central to biomedical ethics for some time (see Faden and Beauchamp). But *autonomy* is another value to take into account. Autonomy is the capacity of an agent to form, revise, and pursue a set of goals by his or her own lights. According to a "principle of autonomy," individuals must refrain from performing actions that are likely to interfere with others' exercising this capacity. Championed by John Stuart Mill (1806–1873) in his classic work *On Liberty* (58–69), this principle is a focus of agreement among diverse moral theories, including those that derive from **Immanuel Kant** (1724–1804). Like the principle of free and informed consent, the principle of autonomy is a mainstay of biomedical ethics (Beauchamp and Walters, 22) and is embraced widely by ordinary folk. A case can be made that seduction, as defined by the broad motivational conception, violates the principle of autonomy, for any attempt to tamper with the goals and motivational structure of another person is likely to interfere with his or her capacity to be autonomous (see Cave, 7–8). Creating new inclinations and goals in other persons or altering the relative importance of their goals, thereby changing initial unwillingness into willingness, appears to interfere with autonomy. Thus seduction seems to be *prima facie* immoral and, as with other *prima facie* wrongs, could be justified only by fairly weighty considerations. To take just two examples: Pursuing *my own* sexual pleasure does not seem to be significant enough to justify reducing your autonomy; however, promoting *your sexual confidence* (and perhaps your autonomy at the same time) in the context of a long-standing relationship may be acceptable. The view that sits between the two extreme views, that seduction is either always right or always wrong, thus seems to be vindicated. Seduction has an immoral element in it, but in some cases it can turn out to be on balance permissible.

Other views about the morality of seduction have been proposed. One position, based on the work of Harry Frankfurt, is that seduction may be wrong when it interferes with the target's freedom of the will: Seduction may induce a person to act on a first-order desire (to have sex) that is in conflict with a second-order desire (not to have sex) that the person also has (Bigelow et al.). Another position suggests that seduction is morally suspicious because it embodies an attitude of dominance (McBride, 257–61). Yet another argument is that seduction is immoral, even in the presence of valid consent of the target, when it aims malevolently at the target's abasement or humiliation (Morgan, 398–404). Each of these lines of thought is similar in its own way to the critique of seduction that is based on the principle of autonomy. This may be a sign that moral philosophy is moving in the right direction about this issue.

See also Consent; Existentialism; Flirting; Harassment, Sexual; Hobbes, Thomas; Kierkegaard, Søren; Liberalism; Rape; Rape, Acquaintance and Date

REFERENCES

American Law Institute. (1962) *Model Penal Code: Official Draft and Explanatory Notes*. Philadelphia, Pa.: Author, 1985; Beauchamp, Tom L., and Leroy Walters, eds. *Contemporary Issues in Bioethics*, 6th ed. Belmont, Calif.: Wadsworth, 2003; Bigelow, John, Ian Gold, and Robert Pargetter. "Seduction." Unpublished manuscript, Philosophy Department, Monash University, Australia; Cave, Eric M. "Sexual Liberalism and Seduction." Paper presented to the Society for the Philosophy of Sex and Love, Central Division meetings of the American Philosophical Association (24 April 2003), Cleveland, Ohio; Doniger, Wendy. "Sex, Lies, and Tall Tales." *Social Research* 63:3 (1996), 663–99; Faden, Ruth R., and Tom L. Beauchamp. *A History and Theory of Informed Consent*. New York: Oxford University Press, 1986; Frankfurt, Harry G. "Freedom of the Will and the Concept of a Person." *Journal of Philosophy* 68:1 (1971), 5–20; Gallop, Jane. *Feminist Accused of Sexual Harassment*. Durham, N.C.: Duke University Press, 1997; Kierkegaard, Søren. (1843) "Diary of the Seducer." In *Either/Or*, vol. 1. Trans. David F. Swenson and Lillian M. Swenson (1944). Rev. Howard A. Johnson. Princeton, N.J.: Princeton University Press, 1959, 297–440; Mappes, Thomas A. "Sexual Morality and the Concept of Using Another Person." In Thomas A. Mappes and Jane S. Zembaty, eds., *Social Ethics*, 4th ed. New York: McGraw-Hill, 1992, 203–16; McBride, William L. "Sexual Harassment, Seduction, and Mutual Respect: An Attempt at Sorting It Out." In Linda Fisher and Lester Embree, eds., *Feminist Phenomenology*. Dordrecht, Holland: Kluwer, 2000, 249–66; Mill, John Stuart. (1859) *On Liberty*. Ed. Alburey Castell. New York: F. S. Crofts, 1947; Morgan, Seiriol. "Dark Desires." *Ethical Theory and Moral Practice* 6:4 (2003), 377–410; Muehlenhard, Charlene L., and Jennifer L. Schrag. "Nonviolent Sexual Coercion." In Andrea Parrot and Laurie Bechhofer, eds., *Acquaintance Rape: The Hidden Crime*. New York: Wiley, 1991, 115–28; Murphy, Jeffrie G. "Some Ruminations on Women, Violence, and the Criminal Law." In Jules Coleman and Allen Buchanan, eds., *In Harm's Way: Essays in Honor of Joel Feinberg*. Cambridge: Cambridge University Press, 1994, 209–30; Posner, Richard A. *Sex and Reason*. Cambridge, Mass.: Harvard University Press, 1992; Primoratz, Igor. "Sexual Morality: Is Consent Enough?" *Ethical Theory and Moral Practice* 4:3 (2001), 201–18; Reitan, Eric. "Date Rape and Seduction: Towards a Defense of Pineau's Definition of 'Date Rape.'"

Southwest Philosophy Review 20:1 (2004), 99–106; Sartre, Jean-Paul. (1943) *Being and Nothingness.* Trans. Hazel E. Barnes. New York: Simon and Schuster, 1966; Thomas Aquinas. (1265–1273) *Summa theologiae*, 60 vols. Trans. Blackfriars. Cambridge, U.K.: Blackfriars, 1964–1976.

Eric M. Cave

ADDITIONAL READING

Baudrillard, Jean. *Seduction*. Trans. Brian Singer. New York: St. Martin's Press, 1990; Becker-Theye, Betty. *The Seducer as Mythic Figure in Richardson, Laclos, and Kierkegaard.* New York: Garland, 1988; Ben-Ze'ev, Aaron. "The Seductive Space." In *Love Online: Emotions on the Internet.* Cambridge: Cambridge University Press, 2004, 1–25; Capellanus, Andreas. (ca. 1174–1186) *The Art of Courtly Love.* Trans. John Jay Parry. New York: Columbia University Press, 1990; Casanova, Jacques. *The Memoirs of Jacques Casanova: Venetian Years* (1826–32), 6 vols. Trans. Arthur Machen. New York: Putnam's Sons, 1959; Cave, Eric M. *Preferring Justice: Rationality, Self-Transformation, and the Sense of Justice.* Boulder, Colo.: Westview, 1998; Ellis, Albert, and Robert O. Conway. *The Art of Erotic Seduction.* New York: Lyle Stuart, 1969; Fletcher, John. "Gender, Sexuality, and the Theory of Seduction." *Women* 11:1–2 (2000), 95–108; Gallop, Jane. *The Daughter's Seduction: Feminism and Psychoanalysis.* Ithaca, N.Y.: Lyle Stuart, 1969; Giroud, Françoise, and Bernard-Henri Lévy. (1993) "On Seduction and Its Games." In *Women and Men: A Philosophical Conversation.* Trans. Richard Miller. Boston, Mass.: Little, Brown, 1995, 185–211; Gonzalez-Crussi, Frank. "The Conditions for Seduction, According to an Old Chinese Text." In *On the Nature of Things Erotic.* San Diego, Calif.: Harcourt Brace Jovanovich, 1988, 119–39; Greene, Robert. *The Art of Seduction.* New York: Viking, 2001; Gross, Nicolas P. *Amatory Persuasion in Antiquity: Studies in Theory and Practice.* Newark: University of Delaware Press, 1985; Hershfield, Jeffrey. "The Threat of Acquaintance Rape: A Reply to Reitan." *Southwest Philosophy Review* 20:2 (2004), 171–73; Kelley, William G., Jr. "Rhetoric as Seduction." *Philosophy and Rhetoric* 6:2 (1969), 69–80; Kierkegaard, Søren. (1844) "The Consequence of the Relationship of Generation." In *The Concept of Anxiety: A Simple Psychologically Orienting Deliberation on the Dogmatic Issue of Hereditary Sin.* Trans. Reidar Thomte, with Albert B. Anderson. Princeton, N.J.: Princeton University Press, 1980, 62–73; Kierkegaard, Søren. (1845) "Quidam's Diary." In *Stages on Life's Way.* Trans. Walter Lowrie. Princeton, N.J.: Princeton University Press, 1945, 188–362; King, C. Richard. "Siren Scream of Telesex: Speech, Seduction, and Simulation." *Journal of Popular Culture* 30:3 (1996), 91–101; Lefkowitz, Mary R. "Seduction and Rape in Greek Myth." In Angeliki E. Laiou, ed., *Consent and Coercion to Sex and Marriage in Ancient and Medieval Societies.* Washington, D.C.: Dumbarton Oaks, 1993, 17–37; MacLeod, Mary. "Comments on Eric M. Cave's 'Sexual Liberalism and Seduction.'" Paper presented to the Society for the Philosophy of Sex and Love, Central Division meetings of the American Philosophical Association (24 April 2003), Cleveland, Ohio; Mappes, Thomas A. (1985) "Sexual Morality and the Concept of Using Another Person." In Thomas A. Mappes and Jane S. Zembaty, eds., *Social Ethics: Morality and Social Policy*, 4th ed. New York: McGraw-Hill, 1992, 203–16. 5th ed., 1997, 163–76. 6th ed., 2002, 170–83. Reprinted in POS4 (207–23); Miller, Geoffrey. "Arts of Seduction." In *The Mating Mind: How Sexual Choice Shaped the Evolution of Human Nature.* New York: Doubleday, 2000, 258–91; Moulton, Janice. "Sexual Behavior: Another Position." *Journal of Philosophy* 73:16 (1976), 537–46. Reprinted in HS (91–100); POS1 (110–18); POS2 (63–71); POS3 (31–38); POS4 (31–38); Ovid. (ca. 1 BCE) *Art of Love.* In *Ovid: The Erotic Poems.* Trans. Peter Green. New York: Penguin, 1982, 166–238; Pineau, Lois. "Date Rape: A Feminist Analysis." *Law and Philosophy* 8:2 (1989), 217–43. Reprinted in Hugh LaFollette, ed., *Ethics in Practice: An Anthology*, 1st ed. Cambridge, Mass.: Blackwell, 1997, 418–28. 2nd ed., 2002, 410–17; in Leslie P. Francis, ed., *Date Rape: Feminism, Philosophy, and the Law.* State College: Pennsylvania State University Press, 1996, 1–26; HS (483–509); Pybus, Cassandra. *Seduction and Consent: A Case of Gross Moral Turpitude.* Port Melbourne, Vic.: Mandarin, 1994; Roussel, Roy. *The Conversation of the Sexes: Seduction and Equality in Selected 17th and 18th Century Texts.* New York: Oxford University Press, 1982; Shattuck, Roger. "Milton in the Garden of Eden." In *Forbidden*

Knowledge: From Prometheus to Pornography. San Diego, Calif.: Harcourt Brace, 1966, 49–76; VanderVelde, Lea. "The Legal Ways of Seduction." *Stanford Law Review* 48:4 (1996), 817–901; Vroon, Piet, Anton van Amerongen, and Hans de Vries. *Smell: The Secret Seducer.* New York: Farrar, Straus and Giroux, 1994; Walsh, Sylvia. "Desire and Love in Kierkegaard's *Either/Or.*" In Alan Soble, ed., *Sex, Love, and Friendship.* Amsterdam, Holland: Rodopi, 1997, 610–22; Watson, Richard. "The Seducer and the Seduced." *Georgia Review* 39:2 (1985), 353–66.

SEX AND THE ARTS. *See* Arts, Sex and the

SEX AND THE BIBLE. *See* Bible, Sex and the

SEX AND THE LAW. *See* Law, Sex and the

SEX AND THE MILITARY. *See* Military, Sex and the

SEX EDUCATION. Sex education has been controversial since its origins in the social hygiene and moral purity movements of the late nineteenth and early twentieth century (McKay, *Sexual Ideology*, 1–2; Moran, *Teaching Sex*, 26 ff.). It has been deployed, historically, as a prophylactic against the dangerous consequences of adolescent **sexual activity**, including **sexually transmitted diseases**, pregnancy, and moral degradation (Allen, 154; Diorio and Munro, 347; Harrison and Hillier, 279; Irvine, *Sexuality Education*, 65; Moran, "Modernism," 481; Whatley and Trudell). It exemplifies an instrumentalist use of the curriculum to solve social problems (Bay-Cheng, 64) rather than to convey knowledge or promote critical understanding. As expressed in an influential report in 1918, this instrumentalist approach requires that "subject values and teaching methods must be tested in terms of the laws of learning and the application of knowledge to the activities of life, rather than primarily in terms of the demands of any subject as a logically organized science" (Commission on the Reorganization, 2–3). Schooling increasingly focused on behavioral objectives, and predetermined behavioral solutions to extrascholastic problems define the content of teaching and obscure epistemological differences within fields of study (Kliebard). The sex education curriculum is not defined by diverse scholarly inquiry about sexual phenomena but by social problems associated with adolescent sexual activity (Diorio, "Contraception," 239).

Conspiracy of Silence. The late-nineteenth- and early-twentieth-century belief that sex should not be discussed publicly precluded school-based sex education (Burnham, 150–51; Imber, 353; Moran, "Modernism," 494). This "conspiracy of silence" (Burnham, 278n.2) reflected not only euphemistic sensibilities but a psychology (derived from John Locke; 1632–1704) that viewed children as *tabulae rasae* whose innocence should not be spoiled by providing them with sexual information (Moran, "Modernism," 494, 502). Sex, idealized as a procreative function reserved for married heterosexual couples, was the source of children and parental **love** and constituted the family as the fundamental social unit and wellspring of personal virtue (Strong, 130–31). Children were expected to learn sexual virtue through direct involvement in their families. Sex was private, and public talk threatened to open it to licentious pursuit for its own sake.

Public acceptance that talking about sex in schools could be educational, not corrupting, was promoted by two social movements. One was the antiprostitution or purity campaign that attacked the double standard whereby society expected sexual purity from women but overlooked men's recourse to commercial sex. **Prostitution** took sex out of the home and challenged the family ideal; to attack it, however, purity crusaders had to speak publicly about sex (Burnham, 159; Luker, "Sex," 607–8). The second movement that introduced sex into public discourse involved the promulgation by physicians of new medical knowledge about venereal disease. Doctors such as Prince A. Morrow (1846–1913), who founded the American Society for Sanitary and Moral Prophylaxis in 1905, drew attention to European studies of the seriousness of syphilis and gonorrhea, including their transmission to monogamous spouses by infected partners and then to fetuses and neonates by infected mothers (Brandt, 12–16, 24; Burnham, 153–54; Moran, "Modernism," 485). These mothers presumably caught the disease from husbands who got it from prostitutes. Prostitution and venereal disease together threatened not only family virtue but social health.

The conspiracy of silence inhibited physicians from speaking publicly about venereal disease, while the purity campaigners—laypersons and mostly women (Luker, "Sex," 609)—lacked prestige. In 1913 these movements united to create the American Social Hygiene Association (Brandt, 38; Imber, 345–46), fused by a belief that medicine lent authority and purity provided moral legitimacy to sex talk and by a commitment that both aspects of the problem should be addressed through sex education (Burnham, 158–59; Imber, 346; Moran, *Teaching Sex*, chap. 2).

Physicians adopted the purity crusaders' message that sexual **abstinence** before **marriage** and fidelity within it ensured protection against infection (Burnham, 159–60). They attacked as unscientific the "doctrine of necessity," which held that men needed to release semen regularly (Carter, 218; Imber, 346; Moran, *Teaching Sex*, 35) and which purity campaigners condemned as a self-serving justification for male profligacy (Luker, "Sex," 607). This alliance between purity and medicine bestowed on the sex education movement a presumption of congruence between moral and scientific teachings about sex. As belief in male sexual necessity faded, the movement adopted the alternative but equally unscientific doctrine that sexual restraint was essential to health and social flourishing. Sex educators in the decades preceding World War II orchestrated a theory of human sexual development that drew on a particular reading of the theory of **evolution** and a selective deployment of information about the reproductive processes of plants, birds, and animals to demonstrate that the monogamous procreative family was the pinnacle of natural development (Carter, 233–48).

Inciting Sex. The boundary between sexual speech and action can be obscure (Irvine, 2002, 132–33; MacKinnon, chap. 1), and sex educators continue to grapple with the problem of how to teach about sex without encouraging students to engage in it (Carter, 225; Imber, 349–50; McKay, *Sexual Ideology*, 1, 67). Some opponents never fully accepted that this problem could be solved and continue to see sex education as evil. A Philadelphia newspaper in 1913 condemned sex education as "teaching vice to little children" (Burnham, 163), and in 1968 the Christian Crusade issued a popular anti-sex-education booklet, *Is the Schoolhouse the Place to Teach Raw Sex?* (Moran, *Teaching Sex*, 179–80).

Scientific knowledge protects talking about sex in schools because scientific knowledge is supposedly inherently chaste. Science also provides shelter for sex educators because medical evidence about venereal disease generates legitimate fear, which together with chaste knowledge was assumed to yield effective control of sexual behavior (Brandt, 25; Carter, 215–16, 247–48; Imber, 347; Moran, "Modernism," 493; *Teaching Sex*, 190). Fear of venereal disease was joined in the mid-twentieth century by fear of adolescent pregnancy and, still later, of HIV/AIDS (human immunodeficiency virus/acquired immunodeficiency syndrome). Many sex educators worry, however, about the immoral impact of any medical developments that might lessen fear on the part of students, such as penicillin to treat venereal disease or contraceptives for preventing pregnancy, because such developments could make the pursuit of pleasure appear safe.

Writings in sex education stress negativity. Irvine notes that "escalating cultural anxiety about the 'epidemic' of teenage pregnancy has prompted a range of strategies to deter sexual activity or postpone reproduction among adolescents" (*Sexuality Education*, 65), the more so because of the perceived "obvious peril and enormous costs of teen pregnancy" (Banks and Wilson, 233). Sex educators still lack a "discourse of desire" (Fine), largely because procreation is inappropriate for adolescents and nonprocreative, nonmarital sex is questionably moral at best. Sex thus has no legitimate place in adolescent lives (Allen, 151; Harrison and Hillier, 279; Irvine, *Talk*, 13).

Essentialism and Constructionism. Sex education curricula commonly assume that sexual interest occurs naturally in adolescent bodies: "[O]ur [educational] interventions . . . in the field of adolescent sexuality are grounded on the drive reductionist belief that unless actively stopped, teens will have sex at every opportunity" (Bay-Cheng, 66). Sexuality is seen as something students bring with them into school. Schools must react to sex, but they do not influence what it is (Irvine, *Sexuality Education*, 3; Whatley). This understanding is embedded in a contentious biological essentialism. Seen as a biologically determined phenomenon, sex constitutes "an overpowering force which the social/moral/medical has to control" (Weeks, 8). This essentialism has been widely challenged, by many feminists and others, who argue that sex is a sociocultural construction (see Diorio, "Conceptions," 5436). According to **Michel Foucault** (1926–1984), one of the most influential social constructionist theorists, "sexuality must not be thought of as a kind of natural given which power tries to hold in check. . . . It is the name that can be given to a historical construct" (105). **Social constructionism** addresses the variable ways in which behaviors are imbued with erotic meanings. Male and female gamete combination constitutes sexual reproduction, but the coital behaviors by which this combination usually is achieved would not be experienced as sexual if they had not been eroticized socially; *in vitro* fertilization is a reproductive process, but it is not a sexual activity. Reproduction may be sex biologically, but it is not erotically sexual unless it is made so by society.

According to constructionist theories, sexual behavior and **sexual desire** have to be learned (Gagnon and Simon, 8–9), which raises new issues for sex education. Rather than just teaching about and controlling natural instincts, schools must account for the social variability of sexual phenomena and their own role as agents in constructing these phenomena; schools are implicated in the making of sexuality (Johnson, 184; see Epstein; Harrison and Hillier; Haywood; Mac an Ghaill). Traditional understandings, which took heterosexual genital intercourse as an inherently erotic activity toward which people were instinctively impelled, generated standard moral problems: Who should engage in coitus and why? Does pleasure legitimize **contraception**? How should noncoital activities be judged? Sexuality itself was not a moral problem. Constructionism, particularly as deployed by feminist writers, problematizes sexuality more fundamentally by politicizing it. In feminist eyes, sexuality is constructed in an inequitable society exhibiting oppressive power differentials between genders and across various **sexual orientation**s. Socially constructed sexuality reflects oppression, which cannot be regarded educationally as a benign natural phenomenon. By accepting as natural the contingent and inequitable patterns of socially produced sexuality, and by overlooking the fluidity of students' sexual identities and the school's role in their construction, sex educators reproduce oppressive sexual understandings and practices, including **heterosexism** and homophobia (Diorio, "Feminist-Constructionist," 27–29; "Sexuality," 293). Constructionist perspectives have not been exploited widely by sex educators, however (Diorio, "Contraception," 245; "Sexuality," 278–79; Irvine, *Sexuality*, 1–2; Pollis, 89–96).

Teenage Pregnancy. Sex education disputes are epitomized in the contemporary campaign against adolescent pregnancy. Teenage pregnancy was identified in 1995 by President William Jefferson Clinton as an epidemic constituting the United States' "most serious social problem" (Schultz, 594). No one supports adolescent childbearing (Luker, *Dubious Conceptions*, 135), and numerous sources repeat a litany of problems that are supposedly generated by it:

> [A] million teenage girls [in the United States] each year find themselves pregnant. . . . Teenage motherhood—usually unwed motherhood . . . has monumental social consequences. . . . If one wanted to spawn a generation of vulnerable families, one would seek to increase the number of families headed by fifteen- and sixteen-year-old mothers. A single teenage mother is less likely to complete high school or to be employed than her peers, and her child is at greater risk than other children for a host of health and developmental problems, and also for physical and sexual abuse. Both mother and child are likely to experience poverty and its predictable consequence, chronic welfare dependency. (Whitehead, 73)

This passage elides together as "teenage girls" two distinct groups: eighteen- and nineteen-year-olds, who are more likely to be married or cohabiting with a partner than younger girls, and all teenagers; and it then speaks negatively of families headed by fifteen- and sixteen-year-old mothers. The birthrates between younger and older adolescents in the United States in the mid-1990s were substantially different, being 34 and 86 per 1,000, respectively (American Academy of Pediatrics, 516; Singh and Darroch, 19). The percentage of births to adolescents of all ages, out of the total births to all women in the United States in 1995, was 12.6 percent—a drop of 18 percent from 1990 (Singh and Darroch, 20). This is many, but not a whole "vulnerable" generation, especially given the fact that within the 1 million annual births to adolescents in the United States, the birthrate in eighteen- and nineteen-year-olds is 2.5 times larger than that in younger girls.

Adolescent childbearing is associated with negative effects (American Academy, 518; Cocca, 64; Hayward et al., 750). One approach to the problem holds that teenage childbearing is caused by a breakdown in moral self-control, the appropriate cure for which is sex education that teaches young people to "just say no" (Geronimus, 405–6, 408). Indulgence in sexual pleasure presumably leads to the poverty and deprivation described by Barbara Whitehead. Adolescent childbearing arguably is more an effect than a cause of social and economic deprivation, however (Mabray and Labauve, 32; Young et al., 364). Eighty-three percent of childbearing adolescents in the United States live in low-income families, whereas only 38 percent of all adolescents live in such families (American Academy, 517). Either poverty contributes to adolescent pregnancy or poor teenagers are much more susceptible to sexual pleasure than richer ones. Poor adolescents who bear a child are poor before, rather than because of, the pregnancy. Poor and richer adolescents face different life chances and life expectancies. Poor teenagers (and their parents) die younger than their better-off peers. In a society in which social support for mothers is limited, potential mothers must consider the availability of help from their parents in caring for offspring, especially when their own wage-earning potential is limited. In a low life-span community, the earlier a girl has a child, the greater the chances that her parents will be able to help with its care. In a society in which social support for child care is weak, parental vigor can be an important consideration in timing a pregnancy. Early childbearing in poor communities may not be an abandonment of the values of responsible parenting but an expression of them under adverse conditions (Geronimus, 424). Early childbearing can be a rational choice (Haywood et al., 752), since the consequences could be even worse were childbearing delayed.

The negative consequences of teen childbearing do not accrue directly as a result of the age of the mother. Mortality rates are lower among infants born to fifteen-year-old mothers in some of the poorest communities in the United States than among those birthed by women in the same communities who are twenty-five to thirty-five (Geronimus, 414–15). While negative life consequences for offspring are associated with low birth weights, these weights do not consistently correlate with the mother's age. Insofar as poverty generates the negative life consequences accruing to children born to adolescent mothers, and to the extent that the socioeconomic situation of poor teenagers is unlikely to change substantially over the coming two decades of their lives ("Ever Higher Society"), employing sex education to induce poor teenagers to delay pregnancy will not improve the life chances of their offspring and may actually diminish them.

In addition to poverty, factors contributing to teenage pregnancy include adolescents' perceptions of their control over their destiny; extent of parental, especially maternal, education; parental expectations about the educational achievements of their children; and parenting styles within teenagers' families (Hayward et al., 770; Young et al., 362–64, 369–71). With the possible exception of young people's perceived abilities to control their lives, these factors exert influence before teenagers encounter sex education programs, and none can be changed by such programs.

Dropping out of secondary school has a negative impact on life chances. Many writers (Lewis et al., 1573–75; Young et al., 370–71) assume that a sense of personal control over one's life is necessary for success. Dropping out of school impacts negatively on a person's sense of control (Lewis et al., 1589). A low sense of personal control is a significant predictor of youthful pregnancy (Young et al., 370). Nonmarital adolescent pregnancy "has a negative but statistically insignificant effect on later adulthood sense of control" (Lewis et al., 1589). Low personal perceptions of control have little effect on whether a student completes school, but "nonmarital pregnancy increases the odds of later dropping out by 72%" (Lewis et al., 1591, 1593–94). Failing to complete secondary school impacts negatively on a person's life chances, and getting pregnant while in school seriously diminishes an adolescent's chances to complete. Thus getting pregnant does not in itself damage a teenager's life chances, but leaving school does, and getting pregnant increases the chances of leaving school. The message for education seems clear: Since pregnancy and parenthood damage adolescents' chances of staying in school, encourage young people not to get pregnant, but if they do, enable them to continue their schooling.

Attending school while parenting a child is difficult, since public approval is lacking and support services minimal. If the public was really concerned about the negative life expectations of the offspring of teenage mothers, one might expect public provision of easy-access health and child-care facilities for adolescent parents and their children, and academic support for parents to continue their schooling. "Just say no" education programs take no account of these issues.

Approaches to Pregnancy. Disagreement continues over how best to limit teen pregnancies, between the abstinence-only approach and what has come to be known as "comprehensive" sex education. Abstinence advocates previously opposed sex education, for fear of inducing sexual activity, but since 1970 they have actively promoted abstinence-only programs (McKay, *Sexual Ideology*, 28, 67; Moran, *Teaching Sex*, 210). Abstinence approaches have been supported in the United States by federal legislation, which provides funds for any program that "teaches that a mutually faithful monogamous relationship in the context of marriage is the expected standard of human sexual activity" and that "bearing children out of wedlock is likely to have harmful consequences for the child, the child's parents, and society," and stresses "the importance of attaining self-sufficiency before engaging in sexual activity" (Cocca, 65). Abstinence-only programs are criticized for not accepting that "sexual expression is an essential component of healthy human development for individuals of all ages" (see Planned Parenthood) and for failing to assist students in understanding and negotiating sexual situations and to make decisions about sexual behavior (McKay, "Common Questions," 132). These critics favor a comprehensive approach that emphasizes "acquiring information and forming attitudes, beliefs, and values about identity, relationships . . . sexual development, reproductive health, interpersonal relationships, affection, intimacy, body image, and gender" and that "respects the diversity of values and beliefs" (National Guidelines, 6).

The comprehensive approach accepts human sexual variability and unpredictability in the behavior of students. It is precisely these open-ended qualities to which abstinence advocates object. They argue that comprehensive sex education does not eliminate teenage pregnancy and venereal disease—despite substantial evidence to the contrary from European countries (Lewis and Knijn; Lottes)—and that even if it did, it would be unacceptable because it legitimates immorality. Adolescents should be told what to think and do: "[S]ex education works best when it combines clear messages about behavior with strong moral . . . support for the behavior sought. . . . It is . . . normative. It establishes and reinforces a socially desirable behavior" (Whitehead, 69). Another critic accused comprehensive educators of contributing to "the debasement of sexuality and the corruption of young people's character" and claimed that sex is "out of control" in our society and that students must "develop sexual self-control and the ability to apply core ethical values" (Lickona, 84).

By understanding sex as a naturally generated force that young people must resist (Tapia, 26), abstinence-only curricula are essentialist, and abstinence advocates denounce attempts to broaden students' conceptions of sexual activity beyond heterosexual coitus. Whitehead criticizes comprehensive sex educators for drawing teenagers' attention to mutual **masturbation** as a risk-free sexual activity (e.g., see Cobb). Such activity, she believes, is an inevitable step on the way to genital coitus (64). Noncopulative sexual activity, or "outercourse," is, for Whitehead, "a precursor of intercourse. But do we need studies to tell us this? Is it not graven in our memory that getting to third base vastly increases the chances of scoring a run?" Indeed, "teaching noncoital sex techniques as a way of reducing the risks of coitus comes close to educational malpractice" (68).

Many comprehensive sex educators have retreated to offering an abstinence message qualified by acknowledgment that some students inevitably will be sexually active and hence should be taught about safe sex (Irvine, *Talk*, 188). Even this limited approach is rejected by abstinence advocates because it creates space for students themselves to decide how to behave. Abstinence educators do not overtly oppose personal choice by students, but in their view choosing is legitimated not by the adequacy of decision-making processes but by the accuracy of the outcome—good choosing is making the right choice (McKay, *Sexual Ideology*, 67).

Education and Health. One way to understand sexual health is as the absence of venereal diseases and sexual dysfunction. This leaves open what constitutes healthy sexual *activity*. If venereal disease is spread by men visiting prostitutes, for example, which is the proper public health response? To regulate commercial sex so that only noninfected prostitutes practice it, or ban prostitution because even if all prostitutes were healthy, their activities are immoral? Enforcing the presumptive moral standard would serve medical objectives but also might impede the legitimate sexual expression of those who believe that extramarital sexual activity is not wrong and that it may contribute to psychological health. Sex educators cannot avoid issues about sexual morality by restricting their attention to health (see Soble). This is illustrated by the controversial history of the Sexuality Information and Education Council of the United States, founded in 1954, and the attacks on its cofounder, Mary Calderone (1904–1998). Calderone believed that sex education should be approached in scientific rather than religious terms (McKay, *Sexual Ideology*, 79; Somerville, 21 ff.). She was attacked viciously on religious and moral grounds. Even if sex educators promote sexual health, however, they must consider whether extramarital, nonreproductive, noncoital, gay, lesbian, bisexual, and transsexual activities, adolescent childbearing, and masturbation are "healthy."

The concept of health was broadened beyond somatic conditions in the last half of the twentieth century to include psychological, social, and environmental factors. It has been identified as a right of individuals and communities (Giami, 8). By linking sexuality to this broader conception of health, some educators have argued that students have a right to comprehensive sex education, because young people are entitled to make their own sexual decisions, which requires appropriate information and interpersonal skills (Landry et al., 261; Scales, 563). Abstinence-only programs thus infringe students' rights. Alexander McKay claims that "abstinence-only . . . programmes . . . are clearly deficient" ("Common Questions," 132), and Debby Mabray and Bill Labauve assert that "all young people deserve access to the information and skills required to aid them in developing responsible decisions about sexuality" (31). Appealing to the United Nations Convention on the Rights of the Child, Peter Aggleton and Cathy Campbell argue that young people should be treated "as sentient beings, meaning givers and construers of their own reality . . . [and] health programmes [should] more genuinely work for the young people whose needs they purport to meet" (285). While supportive of comprehensive sex education, claims about the needs and rights of young people no more provide an objective basis for resolving disputes over the content of sex education than do appeals to sexual morality or the notion of sexual health.

Sex Education Curricula. Even if young people do have a right to comprehensive sex education, it still must be determined who is responsible for fulfilling this right. McKay states that "sexual health educators have a duty to meet the sexual health needs of all their students, including those who have chosen or will choose to become sexually active"

("Common Questions," 133). This suggests that all sex educators, regardless of their views about whether young people are entitled to be sexually active, need to recognize that adolescents have a right to make this choice and hence that all educators are responsible for providing students with the information and skills to do so. McKay's view apparently demands that abstinence proponents overrule their own beliefs about what students should know and do and, instead, follow a comprehensive perspective. This imposes a moral burden on sex educators who honestly believe that adolescent sexual activity is wrong. Similarly, when school authorities impose an abstinence-only policy on sex education teaching, they impose an opposite burden on educators who believe in adolescent sexual freedom.

Such moral standoffs intensify public conflict over curriculum policy. Democratic ideals often have been deployed to support the view that when opinion about the curriculum is divided, decisions about the content of teaching should be made through a majoritarian political procedure. Students within any jurisdiction, whether a school district, state, province, or nation, should all be taught the views of the party that wins this contest. This results in a uniform curriculum, the disgruntlement of part of the population, and the disablement of some teachers from acting on their own moral commitments.

One possible way to avoid this moral disablement of teachers is to adopt a pluralistic approach and link it to a definition of education that holds that an appropriate function of schooling is to give students as accurate a picture as possible of what the world is like. Just what such a picture contains, with respect to sexuality, is contested, and it arguably should not be the role either of the political process or an educational system to make a final determination. Both politics and education, however, should recognize that different versions of the picture exist, and both domains of public action need mechanisms for accommodating epistemological diversity. A pluralist approach to the sex education curriculum within any school system can accommodate both the comprehensive and the abstinence-only perspectives by enabling teachers to adhere to their own commitments. Some teachers will promote abstinence, while others will take a comprehensive approach. No one teacher will necessarily provide students with a complete picture of the contested understanding of sexuality, but an overall diversity of views will exist in the system as a whole. As long as the system remains open to teachers' holding varying viewpoints, students will be able to encounter advocates of different perspectives. They will thereby come to see the contested nature of the subject and the presence of differing individual commitments.

We can agree with McKay that students have a right to comprehensive sex education, if we add the proviso that this duty is carried by the educational system as a whole, not by each individual teacher. Otherwise we would morally disable teachers who believe honestly in one perspective or another. We can fulfill our duty to students by providing them with as complete a picture as possible of our overall understanding of sexuality at the system level, while respecting the moral integrity of individual teachers. Moral absolutists will reject this pluralist approach, however, because while they wish to be enabled to do what they believe is right, they also feel a responsibility to stop other people from doing what they think is wrong (see Diorio, "Consequentialism," "Rights").

From the point of view of promoting critical understanding, much sex education is of questionable value. The content of teaching is driven by social problems outside the school and, as these problems are differently defined and their causes differently identified, disagreements arise over what should be taught. Much contemporary scholarship about sex and sexuality is ignored in sex education curricula, and teachers and schools remain largely unaware of their own role in making, rather than in merely controlling, young people's sexuality.

See also Abstinence; Adultery; Contraception; Diseases, Sexually Transmitted; Ellis, Albert; Ethics, Sexual; Feminism, History of; Philosophy of Sex, Teaching the; Rimmer, Robert; Russell, Bertrand; Scruton, Roger; Thomas Aquinas (Saint); Westermarck, Edward

REFERENCES

Aggleton, Peter, and Cathy Campbell. "Working with Young People—Towards an Agenda for Sexual Health." *Sexual and Relationship Therapy* 15:3 (2000), 283–96; Allen, Louisa. "Beyond the Birds and the Bees: Constituting a Discourse of Erotics in Sexuality Education." *Gender and Education* 16:2 (2004), 151–67; American Academy of Pediatrics Committee on Adolescence. "Adolescent Pregnancy—Current Trends and Issues: 1998." *Pediatrics* 103:2 (1999), 516–20; Banks, Ivan W., and Patricia I. Wilson. "Appropriate Sex Education for Black Teens." *Adolescence* 24 (Spring 1989), 233–45; Bay-Cheng, Laina Y. "The Trouble of Teen Sex: The Construction of Adolescent Sexuality through School-Based Sexuality Education." *Sex Education* 3:1 (2003), 61–74; Brandt, Allan M. *No Magic Bullet: A Social History of Venereal Diseases in the United States since 1880.* New York: Oxford University Press, 1985; Burnham, John C. *Paths into American Culture.* Philadelphia, Pa.: Temple University Press, 1988; Carter, Julian B. "Birds, Bees, and Venereal Disease: Toward an Intellectual History of Sex Education." *Journal of the History of Sexuality* 10:2 (2001), 213–49; Cobb, John C. "Outercourse as a Safe and Sensible Alternative to Contraceptives." *American Journal of Public Health* 87:8 (1997), 1380–81; Cocca, Carolyn E. "From 'Welfare Queen' to 'Exploited Teen': Welfare Dependency, Statutory Rape, and Moral Panic." *NWSA Journal* (National Women's Studies Association) 14:2 (2002), 56–79; Commission on the Reorganization of Secondary Education. *Cardinal Principles of Secondary Education.* Washington, D.C.: Government Printing Office, 1918; Diorio, Joseph A. "Conceptions of Sex Education." In T. Torston and T. N. Postlewaite, eds., *International Encyclopedia of Education.* Oxford, U.K.: Pergamon Press, 1994, 5435–41; Diorio, Joseph A. "Consequentialism and Peace Education." *New Zealand Journal of Educational Studies* 24:1 (1989), 19–33; Diorio, Joseph A. "Contraception, Copulation Domination, and the Theoretical Barrenness of Sex Education Literature." *Educational Theory* 35:3 (1985), 239–54; Diorio, Joseph A. "Feminist-Constructionist Theories of Sexuality and the Definition of Sex Education." *Educational Philosophy and Theory* 21:2 (1989), 23–31; Diorio, Joseph A. "Rights, Equality, and the Ethics of School Policy." *Curriculum Inquiry* 16:2 (1986), 147–78; Diorio, Joseph A. "Sexuality, Difference, and the Ethics of Sex Education." *Journal of Social Philosophy* 32:3 (2001), 277–300; Diorio, Joseph A., and Jennifer A. Munro. "Doing Harm in the Name of Protection: Menstruation as a Topic for Sex Education." *Gender and Education* 12:3 (2000), 347–65; Epstein, Debbie. "Practising Heterosexuality." *Curriculum Studies* 1:2 (1993), 275–86; "Ever Higher Society, Ever Harder to Ascend." *The Economist* (1 January 2005), 28–30; Fine, Michelle. "Sexuality, Schooling, and Adolescent Females: The Missing Discourse of Desire." *Harvard Educational Review* 58:1 (1988), 29–53; Foucault, Michel. *The History of Sexuality*, vol. 1: *An Introduction.* Trans. Robert Hurley. New York: Vintage, 1980; Gagnon, John H., and William Simon. *Sexual Conduct: The Social Sources of Human Sexuality.* London: Hutchinson, 1973; Geronimus, Arline T. "Teenage Childbearing and Personal Responsibility: An Alternative View." *Political Science Quarterly* 112:3 (1997), 405–30; Giami, Alain. "Sexual Health: The Emergence, Development, and Diversity of a Concept." *Annual Review of Sex Research* 13 (2002), 1–35; Harrison, Lyn, and Lynne Hillier. "What Should Be the 'Subject' of Sex Education?" *Discourse: Studies in the Cultural Politics of Education* 20:2 (1999), 279–88; Hayward, Mark D., William R. Grady, and John O. G. Billy. "The Influence of Socioeconomic Status on Adolescent Pregnancy." *Social Science Quarterly* 73:4 (1992), 750–72; Haywood, Chris. " 'Out of the Curriculum': Sex Talking, Talking Sex." *Curriculum Studies* 4:2 (1996), 229–49; Imber, Michael. "Toward a Theory of Curriculum Reform: An Analysis of the First Campaign for Sex Education." *Curriculum Inquiry* 12:4 (1982), 339–62; Irvine, Janice M. *Sexuality Education across Cultures: Working with Differences.* San Francisco, Calif.: Jossey-Bass, 1995; Irvine, Janice

M. *Talk about Sex. The Battles over Sex Education in the United States.* Berkeley: University of California Press, 2002; Johnson, Richard. "Sexual Dissonances: Or the 'Impossibility' of Sexuality Education." *Curriculum Studies* 4:2 (1996), 163–89; Kliebard, Herbert M. *The Struggle for the American Curriculum, 1893–1958.* Boston, Mass.: Routledge and Kegan Paul, 1986; Landry, David J., Jacqueline E. Darroch, Susheela Singh, and Jenny Higgins. "Factors Associated with the Content of Sex Education in U.S. Public Secondary Schools." *Perspectives on Sexual and Reproductive Health* 35:6 (2003), 261–69; Lewis, Jane, and Trudie Knijn. "Sex Education Materials in The Netherlands and in England and Wales: A Comparison of Content, Use and Teaching Practice." *Oxford Review of Education* 29:1 (2003), 113–32; Lewis, Susan K., Catherine E. Ross, and John Murowsky. "Establishing a Sense of Personal Control in the Transition to Adulthood." *Social Forces* 77:4 (1991), 1573–99; Lickona, Thomas. "Where Sex Education Went Wrong." *Educational Leadership* (November 1993), 84–89; Lottes, Ilsa L. "Sexual Health Policies in Other Industrialized Countries: Are There Lessons for the United States?" *Journal of Sex Research* 39:1 (2002), 79–83; Luker, Kristin. *Dubious Conceptions: The Politics of Teenage Pregnancy.* Cambridge, Mass.: Harvard University Press, 1996; Luker, Kristin. "Sex, Social Hygiene, and the State: The Double-edged Sword of Social Reform." *Theory and Society* 27:5 (1998), 601–34; Mabray, Debbie, and Bill J. Labauve. "A Multidimensional Approach to Sexual Education." *Sex Education* 2:1 (2002), 31–44; Mac an Ghaill, Máirtín. "Towards a Reconceptualised Sex/Sexuality Education Policy: Theory and Cultural Change." *Journal of Education Policy* 11:3 (1996), 289–302; MacKinnon, Catharine A. *Only Words.* Cambridge, Mass.: Harvard University Press, 1993; McKay, Alexander. "Common Questions about Sexual Health Education." *Canadian Journal of Human Sexuality* 9:2 (2000), 129–37; McKay, Alexander. *Sexual Ideology and Schooling: Towards Democratic Sexuality Education.* Albany: State University of New York Press, 1999; Moran, Jeffrey P. " 'Modernism Gone Mad': Sex Education Comes to Chicago, 1913." *Journal of American History* 83:2 (1996), 481–513; Moran, Jeffrey P. *Teaching Sex: The Shaping of Adolescence in the 20th Century.* Cambridge, Mass.: Harvard University Press, 2000; National Guidelines Task Force. *Guidelines for Comprehensive Sexuality Education,* 2nd ed. New York: Sexuality Information and Education Council of the United States, 1996; Planned Parenthood Federation of America. "Reducing Teenage Pregnancy." <www.plannedparenthood.org/library/TEEN-PREGNANCY/Reducing.html> [accessed 12 December 2004]; Pollis, Carol A. "An Assessment of the Impact of Feminism on Sexual Science." *Journal of Sex Research* 25:1 (1988), 85–105; Scales, Peter. "Sex Education in the '70s and '80s: Accomplishments, Obstacles, and Emerging Issues." *Family Relations* 30:4 (1981), 557–66; Schultz, Katherine. "Constructing Failure, Narrating Success: Rethinking the 'Problem' of Teen Pregnancy." *Teachers College Record* 103:4 (2001), 582–607; Singh, Susheela, and Jacqueline E. Darroch. "Adolescent Pregnancy and Childbearing: Levels and Trends in Developed Countries." *Family Planning Perspectives* 32:1 (2000), 14–23; Soble, Alan. "Health." In *Sexual Investigations.* New York: New York University Press, 1996, 143–74; Somerville, Rose. "Family Life and Sex Education in the Turbulent Sixties." *Journal of Marriage and the Family* 33:1 (1971), 11–35; Strong, Bryan. "Ideas of the Early Sex Education Movement in America, 1890–1920." *History of Education Quarterly* 12 (Summer 1972), 129–61; Tapia, Andres. "Abstinence: The Radical Choice for Sex Education." *Christianity Today* 37:2 (1993), 24–29; Weeks, Jeffrey. *Sexuality and Its Discontents: Meanings, Myths, and Modern Sexualities.* London: Routledge and Kegan Paul, 1985; Whatley, Mariamne H. "Raging Hormones and Powerful Cars: The Construction of Men's Sexuality in School Sex Education and Popular Adolescent Films." *Journal of Education* 170:3 (1988), 100–121; Whatley, Mariamne, and Bonnie Trudell. "Sexual Abuse Prevention and Sexuality Education: Interconnecting Issues." *Theory into Practice* 28:3 (1989), 177–82; Whitehead, Barbara Dafoe. "The Failure of Sex Education." *Atlantic Monthly* 274:4 (October 1994), 55–80; Young, Tamera M., Jean Turner, George Denny, and Michael E. Young. "Examining External and Internal Poverty as Antecedents of Teen Pregnancy." *American Journal of Health Behavior* 28:4 (2004), 361–73.

Joseph A. Diorio

ADDITIONAL READING

Archard, David. "How Should We Teach Sex?" *Journal of the Philosophy of Education* 32:3 (1998), 437–49; Balanko, Shelley L. "Good Sex? A Critical Review of School Sex Education." *Guidance and Counseling* 17:4 (2002), 117–23; Bloodsworth, Mary K. "Teachers." In Timothy F. Murphy, ed., *Reader's Guide to Lesbian and Gay Studies*. Chicago, Ill.: Fitzroy Dearborn, 2000, 578–80; Calderone, Mary S. "The Case for Chastity." In Henry Anatole Grunwald, ed., *Sex in America*. New York: Bantam, 1964, 140–51; Carpenter, Laura M. "The Ambiguity of 'Having Sex': The Subjective Experience of Virginity Loss in the United States." *Journal of Sex Research* 38:2 (2001), 127–39; Carr, David. "Between the Rock and the Hard Place: The Contemporary Dilemma of Sex Education." In Michael J. Reiss and S. Abdul Mabud, eds., *Sex Education and Religion*. Cambridge, U.K.: The Islamic Society, 1998, 168–85; Diorio, Joseph A. "Sex, Love, and Justice: A Problem in Moral Education." *Educational Theory* 31:3–4 (1982), 225–35. Reprinted in Alan Soble, ed., *Eros, Agape, and Philia: Readings in the Philosophy of Love*. New York: Paragon House, 1989, 273–88; Diorio, Joseph A., and Jenny Munro. "What Does Puberty Mean to Adolescents? Teaching and Learning about Bodily Development." *Sex Education* 3:2 (2003), 119–31; Elia, John P. "Democratic Sexuality Education: A Departure from Sexual Ideologies and Traditional Schooling." *Journal of Sex Education and Therapy* 25:2–3 (2000), 122–29; Halstead, J. Mark, and Michael J. Reiss. *Values in Sex Education: From Principles to Practice*. London: Routledge/Falmer, 2003; Hoffman, Saul D. "Teenage Childbearing Is Not So Bad After All . . . Or Is It? A Review of the New Literature." *Family Planning Perspectives* 30:5 (1998), 236–40; Hottois, James, and Neal A. Milner. *The Sex Education Controversy: A Study of Politics, Education, and Morality*. Lexington, Mass.: D. C. Heath, 1975; Irvine, Janice M. "Doing It with Words: Discourse and the Sex Education Culture Wars." *Critical Inquiry* 27:1 (2000), 58–76; Irvine, Janice M. "Sex Education." In Bonnie Zimmerman, ed., *Lesbian Histories and Cultures*. New York: Garland, 2000, 679–80; Kant, Immanuel. (1803) *Education*. Trans. Annette Churton. London: Kegan Paul, Trench, Trubner, 1899; Kirby, Douglas. "Effective Approaches to Reducing Adolescent Unprotected Sex, Pregnancy, and Childbearing." *Journal of Sex Research* 39:1 (2002), 51–57; Lenskyj, Helen. "Beyond Plumbing and Prevention: Feminist Approaches to Sex Education." *Gender and Education* 2:2 (1990), 217–30; Macgillivray, Ian K. *Sexual Orientation and School Policy*. Lanham, Md.: Rowman and Littlefield, 2003; Mayo, Chris. *Disputing the Subject of Sex: Sexuality and the Public School Controversies*. Lanham, Md.: Rowman and Littlefield, 2004; Meredith, Peter. *Sex Education: Political Issues in Britain and Europe*. London: Routledge, 1989; Müller, Rudolf. "Sex Education." In John Money and Herman Musaph, eds., *Handbook of Sexology*. Amsterdam, Holland: Excerpta Medica, 1977, 297–310; Randall, Hilary E., and E. Sandra Byers. "What Is Sex? Students' Definitions of Having Sex, Sexual Partner, and Unfaithful Sexual Behaviour." *Canadian Journal of Human Sexuality* 12:2 (2003), 87–96; Reiss, Michael. "Conflicting Philosophies of School Sex Education." *Journal of Moral Education* 24:4 (1995), 371–82; Remez, Lisa. "Oral Sex among Adolescents: Is It Sex or Is It Abstinence?" *Family Planning Perspectives* 32:6 (2000), 298–304; Rimmer, Robert H. *Let's Really Make Love: Sex, the Family, and Education in the Twenty-First Century*. Amherst, N.Y.: Prometheus, 1995; Rosenberg, Debra. "The Battle over Abstinence." *Newsweek* (9 December 2002), 67–71; Rousseau, Jean-Jacques. (1761) *Emile, or On Education*. Trans. Allan Bloom. New York: Basic Books, 1979; Russell, Bertrand. (1926) "Sex Education." In *On Education, Especially in Early Childhood*. London: Unwin, 1973, 115–21; Samson, Jean-Marc. "The Objectives of Sex Education in the Schools." *Journal of Moral Education* 3 (1974), 207–22; Sattler, H. V. "Sex Education." In *New Catholic Encyclopedia*, vol. 13. New York: McGraw-Hill, 1967, 151–52; Sears, James T., ed. *Sexuality and the Curriculum: The Politics and Practices of Sexuality Education*. New York: Teachers College Press, Columbia University, 1992; Stafford, J. Martin. "In Defence of Gay Lessons." *Journal of Moral Education* 17:1 (1988), 11–20; Stafford, J. Martin. "Love and Lust Revisited: Intentionality, Homosexuality and Moral Education." *Journal of Applied Philosophy* 5:1 (1988), 87–100. Reprinted in *Essays on Sexuality and Ethics*. Solihull, U.K.: Ismeron, 1995, 65–78; HS (177–90); Thomson, Rachel. "Diversity, Values and Social Change: Renegotiating a Consensus on Sex Education." *Journal of Moral Education* 26:3 (1997), 257–71; Young,

Tamera M., Sue S. Martin, Michael E. Young, and Ling Ting. "Internal Poverty and Teen Pregnancy." *Adolescence* 36 (Summer 2001), 289–304; Weekes, Debbie. "Get Your Freak On: How Black Girls Sexualize Identity." *Sex Education* 2:3 (2002), 251–62.

SEX WORK. In 1978, prostitute/activist Carol Leigh (more recently known professionally as Scarlot Harlot) coined the term "sex work" (*Unrepentant Whore*, 69). Twenty years later, she explained: "This invention was motivated by my desire to reconcile my feminist goals with the reality of my life and the lives of the women I knew. I wanted to create an atmosphere of tolerance within and outside the women's movement for women working in the sex industry" ("Inventing Sex Work," 223).

Whatever the rhetorical or political advantages (or drawbacks; see Quan) of "sex work," it is thoroughly inclusive. It puts into the same category all those, both male and female, who earn money from sex-related employment: erotic dancers in clubs or bars, peep show strippers, lingerie models, lap dancers, telephone sex providers, Internet "live cam" performers, erotic masseurs, pornographic film and video actors, pornographic paperback writers, therapeutic sex surrogates (Redlich, 164), subjects in sex research (Masters and Johnson, 10–11), professional dominatrices (see Juliette; Kenney; McClintock), and prostitutes, from inexpensive streetwalkers to pricy call girls. Some of these workers resist being classified with prostitutes, citing moral or legal lines they do not cross. Others might cite special skills called on by their vocation (e.g., the dominatrix well versed in the techniques of psychological humiliation) that prostitutes do not need or have.

It could be argued that performing in pornographic films, erotic dancing, and providing telephone sex require and utilize dramatic skills absent in **prostitution**. However narrow these skills, these workers have or develop communicative expertise that enables them to arouse their audiences in part through appearing to be aroused (see **Thomas Nagel**; Soble, 73–74) and by playing to the fantasies of their customers. But these abilities are often also essential for and employed by the prostitute, at least the successful ones (let alone many wives). While pretense and delicately contrived **fantasy** might play a larger role in other sex work, they are often part of the prostitute's toolbox. Indeed, a prostitute's psychological acumen might be formidable, and many learn the subtle tricks of the trade as well as car salesmen learn theirs. In comparing the prostitute not with the pornographic film actor but the college professor, Martha Nussbaum observes, "Both performances involve skill. It might plausibly be argued that the professor's involves a more developed skill . . . but we should be cautious here. Our culture is all too ready to think that sex involves no skill and is simply 'natural,' a view that is surely false" (284; see Shrage, "Exotic Erotica," 159).

There might also be differences of degree or type of physical contact between prostitution and other sex services, which might provide substance to the claim of some sex workers that they do not cross certain moral or legal lines. Actors in pornographic films often have sexual contact with others, leading to orgasm, with the purpose of arousing eventual viewers of the product. But even though peep shows (see Christina; Funari), telephone sex (see Flowers), and advanced Internet technology allow indirect physical interaction, often to orgasm, between sex workers and customers, barriers or spatial distance preclude actual physical contact (Ben-Ze'ev, 4–5). Lap dancers routinely engage in physical contact, often to orgasm for the customer (Beasley; Lewis), but erotic dancers may or may not allow their customers to touch them and may or may not touch their customers. Professional dominatrices may beat or humiliate their clients, whose thrill is to be subservient, yet they do not necessarily service their clients sexually. (Advertisements placed by some dominatrices state explicitly that they do not engage in prostitution, i.e., coital sex; see Highleyman, 146.) Prostitutes, even though they commonly refrain from kissing customers on the mouth (unlike, say, girls in a county fair kissing booth), typically engage in intimate copulatory **sexual activity**. But lingerie models merely pose while their clients, at a safe distance across the room, masturbate. In all these activities, however, some people are paid to behave in sexual ways for someone else's sexual pleasure or to satisfy other interests, that is, to engage in sexual activity, construed broadly, for compensation. It is not clear why the absence of direct contact or even orgasm makes a moral difference, unless one attaches special significance to oral, anal, or vaginal copulation. Perhaps, then, the entire sex industry could be condemned *or* vindicated with one fell swoop (see Garb; Shrage, "Prostitution," 44).

Although it is common in our culture to draw moral distinctions between levels of sexual contact, individuals and communities have disagreed widely about the meaning of different acts, ranging from holding hands and kissing to various forms of copulation. (Recall the controversy over what to call the subcoital physical encounters between Bill Clinton and Monica Lewinsky.) Utilitarian and religious explanations can often be found for why in some societies the lines are drawn in certain ways, but it is doubtful that an objective basis exists for drawing the lines in one particular way. For example, anthropologists tell us about the preadolescent homosexual fellatio insemination carried out by the Sambia, which in that Melanesian culture might not be conceived as sexual at all (Herdt; Shrage, "Should Feminists," 350–51; Soble, 124–26, 154–55). In some cultures, mouth kissing "is considered dangerous, unhealthy, or disgusting" (Tiefer, 80) and hence to be avoided. It is, for them, more "intimate" than copulation.

Nussbaum finds little moral difference between a prostitute and a woman paid to undergo anal probing (a "colonoscopy artist") for the edification of medical students (285). Both can be legitimate "bodily services." (Consider, also, Ford's analogy between prostitution and the work of hospital aides and orderlies.) If no principled grounds for morally distinguishing among various kinds of sex work exist, or for distinguishing sex work from work in general, other than personally subjective or socially conventional standards (but see Pateman, 562; Wartofsky, 193), then why not tolerate or even respect all its forms? The strongest arguments defending prostitution, whether utilitarian or libertarian, are applicable to other sex work. Commercial sex services provide outlets for people who would otherwise experience frustration, sometimes to the point, on the one hand, of extreme psychological distress or, on the other, of being tempted to violate the rights of others. Further, a free society allows people to make a living any way they choose, if their choices are sufficiently autonomous and they do not harm or violate the rights of others. One might disapprove of such choices when they conflict with one's ideals, but these personal standards, even if widely held, seem inadequate for establishing that sex workers lack self-respect or disregard their moral obligations (see Primoratz, 30–33, 170–72).

Opposing arguments often invoke broadly utilitarian, feminist, or liberal concerns. The entire sex industry can be condemned for promoting the sexual abuse and exploitation of girls and women (including some of the most vulnerable members of society) and for harming women outside the industry. Girls and women are coerced into making **pornography** and stripping, both of which often lead to prostitution. The sex industry is organized in such a way that these activities are economically interdependent (see **Catharine MacKinnon** and **Andrea Dworkin** [1946–2005]; also *Final Report of the Attorney General's Commission on Pornography*). That girls and women are sometimes coerced or emotionally manipulated into exhibiting their bodies does not, however, provide sufficient reason for condemning the industry in principle, at least if we consider how sex work might be organized in a society that permitted it legally (see Califia; Shrage, "Exotic Erotica," 158–61; "Should Feminists," 358–59). Further, even some feminists argue that women often make autonomous decisions to engage in sex work in present nonideal circumstances (**Camille Paglia**, *Vamps and Tramps*, 59–61). Whatever harms women suffer, on this view, are a consequence of voluntary **consent** and something for which they must take responsibility.

Camille Paglia considers stripping to be an art form, "a sacred dance of pagan origins," which she traces back to the temple prostitution of ancient Babylon (*Sexual Personae*, 22–23). The *danse orientale* or "belly dancing" involves voluptuous movements of the hips and breasts with the purpose of inciting male desire. Salome's "Dance of the Seven Veils" represents what the Judeo-Christian tradition (in contrast to the Hindu) fears and attempts to suppress: female sexual allure and power. In this tradition, men are weak and vulnerable, and women's sexuality is a threat to order and virtue. Their erotic power is nowhere more openly displayed than in erotic dance. It is therefore myopic to insist that female strippers are entirely or only exploited. Performing in strip clubs "provide[s] women with the opportunity to invert, caricature, tease, manipulate, and exploit those who use their bodies. . . . The fact that most bar patrons are unaware of the insult only adds to its power" (Manderson, 314).

At least to some extent, then, erotic dancers are not victims of male lust and power but autonomous artists in control of their work environment and their relationships with customers, who are often shy and awkward in their presence, at least when not in groups. Paglia describes stripping as an art form for the masses, a slice of popular culture. Men who go to clubs that offer erotic dancing pay tribute to female **beauty**, just as ancient Mesopotamian men made offerings, worshipped goddesses, and interacted with their priestesses in the temples. The mystery of the generally aloof female does not dissipate with her clothes. It is always there, for the male gaze cannot penetrate the inner secrets of the female's body or her soul (see Wells). Women, we know, also patronize strip clubs in which men dance erotically. The women typically go there in groups, often as a novelty, and perhaps experience something akin to male bonding. By contrast, men seek in strip clubs and especially from lap dancing a sexual and even emotional experience, hoping to connect at some personal level with the performers.

The significance of imagination and fantasy in erotic dancing, as in telephone sex and encounters with professional dominatrices, is clear. The professional and the client create a dreamlike experience in which the client's needs or desires are fulfilled in the context of a temporary fantasy world. A lap dance or a telephone sex conversation is often a joint artistic endeavor. (In Nicholson Baker's novel *Vox*, two conversants on a hotline sketch elaborate scenarios for each other, accomplishing remarkably clever feats.) The fact that such "intercourse" is anonymous and not to be repeated with the same person might enhance its expressiveness, for one might feel extraordinarily free to be oneself or, alternatively, to take on another persona. This can be true for both client and provider. It might also hold for noncommercial **casual sex**. Pure sensuality, devoid of encumbrances, responsibilities, and consequences, can be liberating and stress-relieving, a safe escape from the dull realities and moral limits of ordinary life (Paglia, *Sex, Art, and American Culture*, 24–25).

It is possible that services provided by sex workers, ranging from prostitution to telephone conversations, can be addictive for some men, and perhaps the sex industry threatens existing marriages or relationships. For one thing, wives might have difficulty competing with or living up to the glamorized images created by professional seductresses or photographic models. (Chesler claims that pornography "hampers men's abilities to relate in intimate and nourishing ways, particularly when they marry.") But these fears might underrate the capacity of men to distinguish fantasy from reality, and they underestimate the ubiquitous and similar threats that exist at the workplace, in the supermarket, and in the apartment next door. Men's need for sexual variety and novelty (which is apparently greater than women's, as claimed by evolutionists; Symons, 23–25) can often be safely satisfied by sex workers, and men's ability to compartmentalize can often isolate or minimize its effects.

See also Activity, Sexual; Addiction, Sexual; Adultery; Casual Sex; Communication Model; Consent; Cybersex; Dworkin, Andrea; Ethics, Sexual; Fantasy; Hinduism; Feminism, Lesbian; Indian Erotology; Law, Sex and the; MacKinnon, Catharine; Objectification, Sexual; Paglia, Camille; Pornography; Privacy; Prostitution; Psychology, Evolutionary; Sacher-Masoch, Leopold von; Sadomasochism; Social Constructionism

REFERENCES

Baker, Nicholson. *Vox.* New York: Random House, 1993; Beasley, Juliana. *Lapdancer.* New York: PowerHouse Books, 2003; Ben-Ze'ev, Aaron. *Love Online: Emotions on the Internet.* Cambridge: Cambridge University Press, 2004; Califia, Pat. "Whoring in Utopia." In *Public Sex: The Culture of Radical Sex.* Pittsburgh, Pa.: Cleis Press, 1994, 242–48; Chesler, Phyllis. "Letter, December 7, 1983" (Exhibit 13 [44] in The Minneapolis Hearings). In Catharine A. MacKinnon and Andrea Dworkin, eds., *In Harm's Way: The Pornography Civil Rights Hearings.* Cambridge, Mass.: Harvard University Press, 1997, 228; Christina, Greta. "Are We Having Sex Now or What?" In David Steinberg, ed., *The Erotic Impulse: Honoring the Sensual Self.* New York: Jeremy P. Tarcher, 1992, 24–29; *Final Report of the Attorney General's Commission on Pornography.* Nashville, Tenn.: Rutledge Hill, 1986; Flowers, Amy. "Research from Within: Participant Observation in the Phone-Sex Workplace." In James E. Elias, Vern L. Bullough, Veronica Elias, and Gwen Brewer, eds., *Prostitution: On Whores, Hustlers, and Johns.* Amherst, N.Y.: Prometheus, 1998, 390–95; Ford, Kimberly-Anne. "Evaluating Prostitution as a Human Service Occupation." In James E. Elias, Vern L. Bullough, Veronica Elias, and Gwen Brewer, eds., *Prostitution: On Whores, Hustlers, and Johns.* Amherst, N.Y.: Prometheus, 1998, 420–34; Funari, Vicki. "Naked, Naughty, Nasty: Peep Show Reflections." In Jill Nagle, ed., *Whores and Other Feminists.* New York: Routledge, 1997, 19–35; Garb, Sarah H. "Sex for Money Is Sex for Money: The Illegality of Pornographic Film as Prostitution." *Law and Inequality* 13:2 (1995), 281–301; Herdt, Gilbert. *Sambia Sexual Culture: Essays from the Field.* Chicago, Ill.: University of Chicago Press, 1999; Highleyman, Liz. "Professional Dominance: Power, Money, and Identity." In Jill Nagle, ed., *Whores and Other Feminists.* New York: Routledge, 1997, 145–55; Juliette. "Autobiography of a Dominatrix." In Thomas S. Weinberg, ed., *S&M: Studies in Dominance and Submission.* Amherst, N.Y.: Prometheus, 1995, 61–70; Kenney, Shawna. *I Was a Teenage Dominatrix: A Memoir.* New York: Retro Systems Press, 1999; Leigh, Carol. "Inventing Sex Work." In Jill Nagle, ed., *Whores and Other Feminists.* New York: Routledge, 1997, 223–31; Leigh, Carol. *Unrepentant Whore: Collected Works of Scarlot Harlot.* San Francisco, Calif.: Last Gasp, 2004; Lewis, Jacqueline. "Lap Dancing: Personal and Legal Implications for Exotic Dancers." In James E. Elias, Vern L. Bullough, Veronica Elias, and Gwen Brewer, eds., *Prostitution: On Whores, Hustlers, and Johns.* Amherst, N.Y.: Prometheus, 1998, 376–89; MacKinnon, Catharine A., and Andrea Dworkin, eds. *In Harm's Way: The Pornography Civil Rights Hearings.* Cambridge, Mass.: Harvard University Press, 1997; Manderson, Leonore. "The Pursuit of Pleasure and the Sale of Sex." In Paul R. Abramson and Steven D. Pinkerton, eds., *Sexual Nature Sexual Culture.* Chicago, Ill.: University of Chicago Press, 1995, 305–29; Masters, William H., and Virginia E. Johnson. *Human Sexual Response.* Boston, Mass.: Little, Brown, 1966; McClintock, Anne. "Maid to Order: Commercial S/M and Gender Power." In Pamela Church Gibson and Roma Gibson, eds., *Dirty Looks: Women, Pornography, Power.* London, U.K.: BFI Publishing, 1993, 207–31; Nagel, Thomas. "Sexual Perversion."

Journal of Philosophy 66:1 (1969), 5–17; Nussbaum, Martha C. " 'Whether from Reason or Prejudice.' Taking Money for Bodily Services." In *Sex and Social Justice*. New York: Oxford University Press, 1999, 276–98; Paglia, Camille. *Sex, Art, and American Culture: Essays*. New York: Vintage, 1992; Paglia, Camille. *Sexual Personae: Art and Decadence from Nefertiti to Emily Dickinson*. New York: Yale University Press, 1990; Paglia, Camille. *Vamps and Tramps: New Essays*. New York: Vintage Books, 1994; Pateman, Carole. "Defending Prostitution: Charges against Ericsson." *Ethics* 93:4 (1983), 561–65; Primoratz, Igor. *Ethics and Sex*. London: Routledge, 1999; Quan, Tracy. " 'Sex Work'?" [Letter] *New York Review of Books* 39:18 (5 November 1992), 61; Redlich, Fritz. "The Ethics of Sex Therapy." In William H. Masters, Virginia E. Johnson, and Robert C. Kolodny, eds., *Ethical Issues in Sex Therapy and Research*. Boston, Mass.: Little, Brown, 1977, 143–57; Shrage, Laurie. "Exotic Erotica and Erotic Exotica: Sex Commerce in Some Contemporary Urban Centers." In *Moral Dilemmas of Feminism: Prostitution, Adultery, and Abortion*. New York: Routledge, 1994, 120–61; Shrage, Laurie. "Prostitution and the Case for Decriminalization." *Dissent* (Spring 1996), 41–45; Shrage, Laurie. "Should Feminists Oppose Prostitution?" *Ethics* 99:2 (1989), 347–61; Soble, Alan. *Sexual Investigations*. New York: New York University Press, 1996; Symons, Donald. *The Evolution of Human Sexuality*. Oxford, U.K.: Oxford University Press, 1979; Tiefer, Leonore. (1995) "The Kiss." In *Sex Is Not a Natural Act and Other Essays*, 2nd ed. Boulder, Colo.: Westview, 2004, 77–84; Wartofsky, Marx. "On Doing It for Money." In Thomas A. Mappes and Jane S. Zembaty, eds., *Biomedical Ethics*. New York: McGraw-Hill, 1981, 186–95; Wells, Melanie. "Woman as Goddess: Camille Paglia Tours Strip Clubs." *Penthouse* (October 1994), 56–61, 132.

Robert M. Stewart

ADDITIONAL READING

Allison, Anne. *Nightwork: Sexuality, Pleasure, and Corporate Masculinity in a Tokyo Hostess Club*. Chicago, Ill.: University of Chicago Press, 1994; Austin, Miranda. *Phone Sex*. Emeryville, Calif.: Greenery Press, 2002; Bell, Laurie, ed. *Good Girls/Bad Girls: Feminists and Sex Trade Workers Face to Face*. Seattle, Wash.: Seal Press, 1987; Brewis, Joanna, and Stephen Linstead. *Sex, Work and Sex Work: Eroticizing Organization*. London: Routledge, 2000; Califia, Pat. "Whoring in Utopia." In *Public Sex: The Culture of Radical Sex*. Pittsburgh, Pa.: Cleis Press, 1994, 242–48. Reprinted in POS4 (475–81); Chapkis, Wendy. *Live Sex Acts: Women Performing Erotic Labor*. New York: Routledge, 1997; Chernoff, John M. *Exchange Is Not Robbery: More Stories of an African Bar Girl*. Chicago, Ill.: University of Chicago Press, 2005; Chernoff, John M. *Hustling Is Not Stealing: Stories of an African Bar Girl*. Chicago, Ill.: University of Chicago Press, 2004; Christina, Greta. "Are We Having Sex Now or What?" In David Steinberg, ed., *The Erotic Impulse: Honoring the Sensual Self*. New York: Jeremy P. Tarcher, 1992, 24–29. Reprinted in POS3 (3–8); POS4 (3–8); Dank, Barry M., and Roberto Refinetti, eds. *Sex Work and Sex Workers*. New Brunswick, N.J.: Transaction Publishers, 1999; Delacoste, Frédérique, and Priscilla Alexander, eds. *Sex Work: Writings by Women in the Sex Industry*, 1st ed. Pittsburgh, Pa.: Cleis Press, 1987. 2nd ed., San Francisco, Calif.: Cleis Press, 1998; Eaves, Elisabeth. *Bare: On Women, Dancing, Sex, and Power*. New York: Knopf, 2002; Elias, James E., Vern L. Bullough, Veronica Elias, and Gwen Brewer, eds. *Prostitution: On Whores, Hustlers, and Johns*. Amherst, N.Y.: Prometheus, 1998; Faludi, Susan. "The Money Shot." *The New Yorker* (30 October 1995), 64–87. (Letters: 11 December 1995, 10); Frank, Katherine. *G-Strings and Sympathy: Strip Club Regulars and Male Desire*. Durham, N.C.: Duke University Press, 2002; Frank, Katherine. "Stripping, Starving, and the Politics of Ambiguous Pleasure." In Merri Lisa Johnson, ed., *Jane Sexes It Up*. New York: Four Walls/Eight Windows, 2002, 171–206; Friend, Tad. "Naked Profits: The Employees Take Over a Strip Club." *The New Yorker* (12 and 19 July 2004), 56–61; Goldman, Emma. (1910) "The Traffic in Women." In *Anarchism and Other Essays*. New York: Dover, 1969, 177–94; Hughes, Donna M. "The Internet and Sex Industries: Partners in Global Sexual Exploitation." *IEEE Technology and Society Magazine* (Spring 2000), 35–42. <www.uri.edu/artsci/wms/hughes> [accessed 14 October 2004]; Hughes, Donna M. "Sex Tours via the Internet." *Agenda: A Journal about Women and Gender*, no. 28 (1996), 71–76; Jackson, Stevi, and Sue Scott, eds. "Commercial Sex"

[Part Four] In *Feminism and Sexuality: A Reader*. New York: Columbia University Press, 1996, 289–378; Leigh, Carol. (Scarlot Harlot) "Thanks, Ma." In Rodney Sappington and Tyler Stallings, eds., *Uncontrollable Bodies: Testimonies of Identity and Culture*. Seattle, Wash.: Bay Press, 1994, 243–61; LeMoncheck, Linda. "I Only Do It for the Money: Pornography, Prostitution, and the Business of Sex." In *Loose Women, Lecherous Men: A Feminist Philosophy of Sex*. New York: Oxford University Press, 1997, 110–54; Lewis, Jacqueline. "Controlling Lap Dancing: Law, Morality, and Sex Work." In Ronald Weitzer, ed., *Sex for Sale: Prostitution, Pornography, and the Sex Industry*. New York: Routledge, 2000, 203–16; Liepe-Levinson, Katherine. *Strip Show: Performances of Gender and Desire*. London: Routledge, 2002; McNair, Brian. *Striptease Culture: Sex, Media and the Democratisation of Desire*. London: Routledge, 2002; Nagel, Thomas. "Sexual Perversion." *Journal of Philosophy* 66:1 (1969), 5–17. Reprinted in P&S1 (247–60); POS1 (76–88). Reprinted, revised, in Thomas Nagel, *Mortal Questions*. Cambridge: Cambridge University Press, 1979, 39–52; and POS2 (39–51); POS3 (9–20); POS4 (9–20); STW (105–12); Nagle, Jill, ed. *Whores and Other Feminists*. New York: Routledge, 1997; Overall, Christine. "What's Wrong with Prostitution? Evaluating Sex Work." *Signs* 17:4 (1992), 705–24; Quan, Tracy. " 'Sex Work'?" [Letter] *The New York Review of Books* 39:18 (5 November 1992), 61. <www.nybooks.com/articles/2769> [accessed 5 April 2004]; Richards, David A. J. "Commercial Sex and the Rights of the Person." In *Sex, Drugs, Death, and the Law: An Essay in Human Rights and Overcriminalization*. Totowa, N.J.: Rowman and Littlefield, 1982, 84–153; Scarlot Harlot. (Web site) <bayswan.org/Scarlot.html> [accessed 14 April 2004]; Shrage, Laurie. "Feminist Perspectives on Sex Markets." In Edward Zalta, ed., *The Stanford Encyclopedia of Philosophy* (18 February 2004). <plato.stanford.edu/entries/feminist-sex-markets/> [accessed 24 August 2004]; Shrage, Laurie. "Should Feminists Oppose Prostitution?" *Ethics* 99:2 (1989), 347–61. Reprinted in HS (275–89); POS3 (323–38); POS4 (435–50); STW (71–80); Tewksbury, Richard. "Male Strippers: Men Objectifying Men." In Christine L. Williams, ed., *Doing "Women's Work": Men in Nontraditional Occupations*. Newbury Park, Calif.: Sage, 1993, 168–81; Theroux, Paul. "Nurse Wolf." *The New Yorker* (15 June 1998), 50–63; Tiefer, Leonore. "The Kiss." In *Sex Is Not a Natural Act and Other Essays*, 1st ed. Boulder, Colo.: Westview, 1995, 77–81. 2nd ed., 2004, 77–84. "The Kiss," 50th Anniversary Lecture, The Kinsey Institute for Research in Sex, Gender, and Reproduction (24 October 1998). <www.kinseyinstitute.org/originalsite/tiefer-talk.html> [accessed 13 October 2004]; Truong, Thanh-Dan. "Serving the Tourist Market: Female Labour in International Tourism." In Stevi Jackson and Sue Scott, eds., *Feminism and Sexuality: A Reader*. New York: Columbia University Press, 1996, 373–78; Uebel, Michael. "Strip Culture." *Journal for the Psychoanalysis of Culture and Society* 4 (Fall 1999), 322–25; Weitzer, Ronald, ed. *Sex for Sale: Prostitution, Pornography, and the Sex Industry*. New York: Routledge, 2000; Williams, Linda. "A Provoking Agent: The Pornography and Performance Art of Annie Sprinkle." In Pamela Church Gibson and Roma Gibson, eds., *Dirty Looks: Women, Pornography, Power*. London: BFI Publishing, 1993, 176–91; Zillmann, Dolf, and Jennings Bryant. "Pornography's Impact on Sexual Satisfaction." *Journal of Applied Social Psychology* 18:5 (1988), 438–53.

SEXOLOGY. "Sexology," the English-language term for the scientific study of **sexual desire** and behavior, first appeared in Elizabeth Willard's *Sexology as the Philosophy of Life* (1867). A subproject of the broader medicalization of modern societies, the theorization and empirical scrutiny of sexuality emerged largely throughout western Europe, particularly Germany, in the late nineteenth century. German physician Iwan Bloch (1872–1922) coined the term "*Sexualwissenschaft*" for this area (Hoenig, 38). The taxonomic practices and medical languages associated with the scientific study of sexuality arose concomitantly with the social sciences, psychiatry, and evolutionary theory. Sexology's main challenge has been to establish and legitimize itself as both a science and a viable clinical profession with cultural authority over issues of sexuality and gender.

Early European sexologists were a disparate group with diverse sexual theories, methods, and politics. Erotic practices and preferences became an object of medical study by scientists such as Károly Mária Benkert (1824–1882), Richard von Krafft-Ebing (1840–1902), **Havelock Ellis** (1859–1939), Albert Moll (1862–1939), and Magnus Hirschfeld (1868–1935), all of whom contributed to the construction of new methodologies, languages, and classifications of bodies and pleasures (see Gay, 223–28; Hoenig; Robinson, *Modernization*). Early sexology was strained by the tension between viewing sexuality as an innate, biological force and seeing it as socially and culturally mediated. In general, however, sexologists theorized sex as primarily instinctual and congenital. They produced new classificatory systems of sexual health and deviance in which "**sexual perversion**" was an inherent, biological characteristic (**Michel Foucault** [1926–1984], 42–44). Although some sexologists thought that individuals could also acquire unnatural desires (e.g., by excessive **masturbation**), they believed this was most likely if individuals were already constitutionally predisposed. This medicalization of sex proliferated new sexual categories while effecting an evaluative shift from "badness" to "sickness" (Conrad and Schneider), a judgment often just as socially negative (see Irvine, "Reinventing," 433; Szasz, 170).

In the United States, sexology was an umbrella term for a multidisciplinary group of researchers, clinicians, and educators. Although the field was composed of diverse theoretical perspectives, empirical practices, and practitioners, many sexology professionals emphasized biomedical science as both a methodology and a legitimation for the study of sex. Among early U.S. sexologists, such as physician and sex surveyer Clelia Mosher (1863–1940) and gynecologist Robert Latou Dickinson (1861–1950), it was biologist Alfred Kinsey's (1894–1956) research that garnered the most visibility for the young field. Kinsey ranks as one of the most influential sex researchers of the twentieth century. He and his associates at the Institute for Sex Research, Indiana University (now the Kinsey Institute for Research in Sex, Gender, and Reproduction), are best known for *Sexual Behavior in the Human Male* (1948) and *Sexual Behavior in the Human Female* (1953). These "Kinsey reports" gave the postwar nation a glimpse into American sexual lives, underscoring the chasm between sexual norms and actual behavior. Kinsey's pioneering research aided the transition in the States from religious to scientific authority over sexual matters.

Kinsey's research was a significant departure from earlier sex research, particularly from the psychoanalytic case study method. Kinsey's books were based on sex histories collected from almost 12,000 white women and men. (Interviews conducted with Afro-Americans were excluded from the reports because that sample was not large enough.) Subjects were often members of institutions Kinsey visited, including prisons, schools, and workplaces. On the average, interviews lasted 90 to 120 minutes and covered hundreds of items. Although based on a large number of adults, Kinsey's findings could not be safely generalized; he used volunteers rather than a representative random sample (see Cochran et al.; Robinson, *Modernization*, 43–49).

In contrast to the sexologists Krafft-Ebing and Ellis, who categorized sexual behaviors as "abnormal" or "perversion," Kinsey eschewed both the moralism of religion and the pathologizing gaze of psychiatry. He viewed sexual behavior as resulting from an interplay of biological, social, and psychological influences. Although he studied how factors such as class, gender, and religion shaped someone's sexual life, he viewed these as constraints on a natural human sexuality derived from our mammalian heritage. He challenged the notion of fixed sexual identities that nineteenth- and early-twentieth-century sexologists had advanced (e.g., "homosexual"), arguing that "the world is not to be divided into sheep and goats" (*Male*, 639). The Kinsey Scale located persons on a 0–6 continuum, ranging from exclusively heterosexual (0) to exclusively homosexual (6) in **sexual activity** and interest.

Although unsuccessful as a research tool, the scale destabilized the cultural presupposition of rigid sexual types. Kinsey believed everyone had a capacity for **homosexuality**. Hence he spoke only of homosexual behavior, not about a distinct **sexual orientation**, sexual identity, or type of person.

The media coverage of Kinsey's revelatory research along with an escalating sexualization of the culture increased public acceptance of sex research. Like Kinsey, William Masters (1915–2001) and Virginia Johnson helped consolidate scientific sexology in the United States. Trained as a gynecologist, Masters began his physiological sex research in 1954. In 1955, he established the Reproductive Biology Research Foundation (now the Masters and Johnson Institute) under the auspices of St. Louis's Washington University School of Medicine. Political expedience led him to invite psychologist Johnson into the project in 1957, after one of Masters's early subjects, a prostitute, advised him that a woman should join him in the laboratory work.

While Kinsey studied the heterogeneity of sexual behavior, Masters and Johnson studied sexual physiology. In their research, sexology and medicine were successfully aligned. Reflecting broad changes in the sexual culture of the 1960s, the public greeted the publication of *Human Sexual Response* (1966) with enthusiasm. Its first printing sold out within three days, and it soared to number two on the *New York Times* nonfiction bestseller list. Based on 10,000 "complete cycles of sexual response" (orgasms) in 694 subjects (15), *Human Sexual Response* developed a four-stage physiological model of sexual activity—excitement, plateau, orgasm, and resolution (but see Robinson, *Modernization*, 126–33; Tiefer, 41–61). This scheme was foundational for much later sex research and therapy. Masters and Johnson also wrote the innovatory *Human Sexual Inadequacy* (1970), a comprehensive textbook of sexual problems and treatment. Masters estimated that less than five years after its publication, 3,500 to 5,000 clinics devoted to sexual problems were established in the States. *Inadequacy* indicated a number of major sexual problems. For men, these were premature ejaculation, primary and secondary impotence, and ejaculatory incompetence. For women, they included dyspareunia (painful intercourse), vaginismus (tightening of the vaginal muscles that prohibits penetration), and several orgasmic difficulties. Masters and Johnson developed clinical treatment protocols for each sexual problem. Eventually these "inadequacies" were adopted by the American Psychiatric Association as "mental disorders" (see the third edition of its *Diagnostic and Statistical Manual*, 275–81, and the expanded characterization in the 4th edition, 493–518). The clinical therapy of Masters and Johnson was primary behavioral. Later therapists, such as Helen Singer Kaplan (1929–1995), expanded this to include psychoanalysis. In *The New Sex Therapy*, Kaplan altered Masters and Johnson's sexual cycle to include also a "desire" phase.

Twentieth-century sexology has experienced internal disagreements. By the late 1960s, some practitioners departed from the scientific poise of Kinsey, Masters and Johnson, and Singer. This wing, "humanistic sexology," was an alternative to the rigid biomedicine that focused more on the mechanics of sexual functioning than on sexual pleasure. Representative groups are the National Sex Forum, the Institute for the Advanced Study of Human Sexuality (founded by Ted McIlvenna), and the Center for Marital and Sexual Studies in Long Beach, California (William Hartman and Marilyn Fithian). This sexology is grounded in humanistic psychology, the clinical and theoretical work of Wilhelm Reich (1897–1957; see Robinson, *Freudian Left*, 9–73), and the human potential movement. The human potential movement influenced sexology through its promotion of sexual fulfillment, its emphasis on feeling over intellect, and its use of techniques such as encounter groups, massage, bodywork, and sensory awareness. In the 1970s and early 1980s, conflicts between scientific and humanistic sexologists arose over the therapeutic utility of nudity (see Hartman and Fithian), the use of sexual surrogates in therapy (Redlich, 154), touch between therapist and patient (Redlich, 149–53), and the effectiveness of sexual films in education and therapy.

By the late twentieth century, biomedical sexology prevailed over the humanistic. Advances in neuroscience and genetic research (e.g., the Human Genome Project) and the proliferation of new "enhancement technologies" contributed to the ongoing medicalization of life (see Elliott). In particular, the development of sex-enhancing drugs (Viagra was approved by the Food and Drug Administration in 1998 and soon after extolled by Bob Dole) helped ensure the triumph of scientific sexology and the intensification of the medicalization of sexuality (Tiefer, 107–12, 219–42).

The history of sexology has been one of controversy. Sex is a stigmatized subject casting suspicion on those who study it, and sexologists, both researchers and educators, are particularly vulnerable. Many have been, in effect, censored. After controversy over its initial publication, sales of the 1909 edition of Bloch's *Sexual Life of Our Time* were restricted to lawyers and physicians. A British court labeled Ellis's *Sexual Inversion* scandalous and obscene during the trial of a man prosecuted in 1898 for selling it to a policeman. The Rockefeller Foundation terminated the funding of Kinsey in 1954 after congressional investigation prompted by public outrage over *Human Female*. The laboratory of Masters and Johnson was once vandalized. When Masters wanted to publish data in 1960, his work was rejected as pornographic by a psychiatric journal, and he was banned for life from publishing in two obstetrics and gynecology journals. Mary Calderone, who founded the Sexuality Information and Education Council of the United States to advocate sex research and education, was denounced as a communist and a pervert. Calderone and other sex educators were not infrequently spit on and threatened (Irvine, *Talk*, 43–60). Those who study sex have also been subject to speculation about and attack on their own sexuality. After their children were continually teased that their parents were "sex mongers," Masters and Johnson sent them to boarding school (Irvine, *Disorders*, 69). A biographer of Kinsey sparked controversy by alleging that his scholarly pursuits were motivated by sexual kinkiness (Jones).

Attacks on sex research increased in the late twentieth century with the rise in social influence and political power of right-wing and religious groups (Concerned Women for America; Traditional Values Coalition). Kinsey remained a target of conservatives. Judith Reisman and Edward Eichel (*Kinsey, Sex, and Fraud*) alleged that Kinsey and his colleagues were closet homosexuals and pedophiles who championed child molestation. Although the Kinsey Institute publicly refuted these charges, they encouraged representative Steve Stockman to introduce House Resolution 2749 (1995), which called for investigating fraud or other criminality in Kinsey's research. Although the bill died in committee, other attacks succeeded. In the early 1990s, Senator Jesse Helms (1921–), Congressman William Dannemeyer, and the Family Research Council helped block federal funding for sex research: the Survey of Health and AIDS-Related Practices (Laumann et al., 39–44) and the American Teenage Study (Ericksen, 176–208). Controversy continued into the twenty-first century. In 2003, Congress ordered the National Institutes of Health to justify its grants to over 160 research projects, most of which investigated sexual behavior and HIV (human immunodeficiency virus) transmission, after some conservative congressmen complained that the studies were improper and wasteful (see Brainard). Its ongoing vulnerability to attack accentuates that the legitimacy of sexology as a field of inquiry is inextricably bound to the anxieties, pleasures, ambivalence, and stigmas attached to sex itself.

Sexology's legacy is complex. By establishing sex as an appropriate subject of scientific scrutiny, it contributed to the acceptability of sex. At the same time, some sexological discourses pathologized sexuality through the invention of new categories of deviant people and practices. Moreover, these categories reinforced sexual regulation and hierarchies. But they also permitted people to organize resistance to social control. Sexology consolidated the modernization of sex, locating sexuality—a point well pressed by Michel Foucault—as the deepest truth of the modern subject.

See also Addiction, Sexual; Bisexuality; Bullough, Vern L.; Dysfunction, Sexual; Ellis, Albert; Ellis, Havelock; Foucault, Michel; Freud, Sigmund; Freudian Left, The; Herdt, Gilbert; Homosexuality and Science; Money, John; Orientation, Sexual; Paraphilia; Perversion, Sexual; Psychology, Evolutionary; Psychology, Twentieth- and Twenty-First-Century; Sherfey, Mary Jane; Singer, Irving

REFERENCES

American Psychiatric Association. *Diagnostic and Statistical Manual of Mental Disorders*, 3rd ed. Washington, D.C.: Author, 1980. 4th ed., 1994; Bloch, Iwan. (1907) *The Sexual Life of Our Time in Its Relations to Modern Civilization.* Trans. Eden Paul. (1908) New York: Allied, 1928; Brainard, Jeffrey. "Congress Asks NIH to Justify More Than 160 Research Projects." *Chronicle of Higher Education* (27 October 2003), A24; Cochran, William G., Frederick Mosteller, and John W. Tukey. *Statistical Problems of the Kinsey Report on Sexual Behavior in the Human Male; A Report of the American Statistical Association, Committee to Advise the National Research Council, Committee for Research in Problems of Sex.* Washington, D.C.: American Statistical Association, 1954; Conrad, Peter, and Joseph W. Schneider. *Deviance and Medicalization: From Badness to Sickness*, exp. ed. Philadelphia, Pa.: Temple University Press, 1992; Elliott, Carl. *Better Than Well: American Medicine Meets the American Dream.* New York: Norton, 2003; Ellis, Havelock. (1896/1897) *Studies in the Psychology of Sex*, vol. 2: *Sexual Inversion*, 3rd ed. Philadelphia, Pa.: F. A. Davis, 1915; Ericksen, Julia. *Kiss and Tell: Surveying Sex in the Twentieth Century.* Cambridge, Mass.: Harvard University Press, 1999; Foucault, Michel. (1976) *The History of Sexuality*, vol. 1: *An Introduction.* Trans. Robert Hurley. New York: Vintage, 1978; Gay, Peter. "Problematic Attachments." In *The Bourgeois Experience: Victoria to Freud*, vol. 2: *The Tender Passion.* New York: Oxford University Press, 1986, 198–254; Hartman, William E., and Marilyn A. Fithian. "Enhancing Sexuality Through Nudism." In Herbert A. Otto, ed., *The New Sexuality.* Palo Alto, Calif.: Science and Behavior Books, 1971, 122–39; Hoenig, J. "Dramatis Personae: Selected Biographical Sketches of 19th Century Pioneers in Sexology." In John Money and Herman Musaph, eds., *Handbook of Sexology.* Amsterdam, Holland: Excerpta Medica, 1977, 21–43; Irvine, Janice M. *Disorders of Desire: Sex and Gender in Modern American Sexology.* Philadelphia, Pa.: Temple University Press, 1990; Irvine, Janice M. "Reinventing Perversion: Sex Addiction and Cultural Anxieties." *Journal of the History of Sexuality* 5:3 (1995), 429–50; Irvine, Janice M. *Talk about Sex: The Battles over Sex Education in the United States.* Berkeley: University of California Press, 2002; Jones, James H. *Alfred C. Kinsey: A Public/Private Life.* New York: Norton, 1997; Kaplan, Helen Singer. *The New Sex Therapy: Active Treatment of Sexual Dysfunction.* New York: Brunner/Mazel, 1974; Kinsey, Alfred, Wardell Pomeroy, and Clyde Martin. *Sexual Behavior in the Human Male.* Philadelphia, Pa.: W. B. Saunders, 1948; Kinsey, Alfred, Wardell Pomeroy, Clyde Martin, and Paul Gebhard. *Sexual Behavior in the Human Female.* Philadelphia, Pa.: W. B. Saunders, 1953; Laumann, Edward O., John H. Gagnon, Robert T. Michael, and Stuart Michaels. *The Social Organization of Sexuality: Sexual Practices in the United States.* Chicago, Ill.: University of Chicago Press, 1994; Masters, William H., and Virginia E. Johnson. *Human Sexual Inadequacy.* Boston, Mass.: Little, Brown, 1970; Masters, William H., and Virginia E. Johnson. *Human Sexual Response.* Boston, Mass.: Little, Brown, 1966; Redlich, Fritz. "The Ethics of Sex Therapy." In William H. Masters, Virginia E. Johnson, and Robert C. Kolodny, eds., *Ethical Issues in Sex Therapy and Research.* Boston, Mass.: Little, Brown, 1977, 143–57; Reisman, Judith A., and Edward W. Eichel. *Kinsey, Sex, and Fraud: The Indoctrination of a*

People. Ed. J. Gordon Muir and John H. Court. Lafayette, La.: Huntington House, 1990; Robinson, Paul. *The Freudian Left: Wilhelm Reich, Geza Roheim, Herbert Marcuse*. New York: Harper and Row, 1969; Robinson, Paul. *The Modernization of Sex: Havelock Ellis, Alfred Kinsey, William Masters and Virginia Johnson*. New York: Harper and Row, 1976; Szasz, Thomas S. "The Product Conversion—From Heresy to Illness." In *The Manufacture of Madness: A Comparative Study of the Inquisition and the Mental Health Movement*. New York: Harper and Row, 1970, 160–79; Tiefer, Leonore. (1995) *Sex Is Not a Natural Act and Other Essays*, 2nd ed. Boulder, Colo.: Westview, 2004; Willard, Elizabeth Osgood Goodrich. *Sexology as the Philosophy of Life: Implying Social Organization and Government*. Chicago, Ill.: Walsh, 1867.

Janice M. Irvine

ADDITIONAL READING

Béjin, André. "The Decline of the Psycho-Analyst and the Rise of the Sexologist." In Philippe Ariès and André Béjin, eds., *Western Sexuality: Practice and Precept in Past and Present Times*. Trans. Anthony Forster. New York: Blackwell, 1985, 181–99; Bland, Lucy, and Laura Doan, eds. *Sexology in Culture: Labelling Bodies and Desires*. Chicago, Ill.: University of Chicago Press, 1998; Bland, Lucy, and Laura Doan, eds. *Sexology Uncensored: The Documents of Sexual Science*. Chicago, Ill.: University of Chicago Press, 1998; Bloch, Iwan. (1900) *Marquis de Sade: His Life and Works*. Trans. James Bruce. New York: Brittany, 1948; Bloch, Iwan. *Odoratus Sexualis: A Scientific and Literary Study of Sexual Scents and Erotic Perfumes*. New York: Panurge Press, 1934. Reprint, New York: AMS Press, 1976; Bloch, Iwan. *Die Prostitution*. Berlin, Ger.: L. Marcus, 1912; Brecher, Edward M. *The Sex Researchers*. Boston, Mass.: Little, Brown, 1969; Brecher, Ruth, and Edward Brecher. "The Work of Masters and Johnson." In Ruth Brecher and Edward Brecher, eds., *An Analysis of* Human Sexual Response. New York: New American Library, 1966, 16–107; Bullough, Vern L. *Science in the Bedroom: A History of Sex Research*. New York: Basic Books, 1994; Calderone, Mary S. "The Case for Chastity." In Henry Anatole Grunwald, ed., *Sex in America*. New York: Bantam, 1964, 140–51; Calderone, Mary S. *Release from Sexual Tensions*. New York: Random House, 1960; Calderone, Mary S., ed. *Manual of Contraceptive Practice*. Baltimore, Md.: Williams and Wilkins, 1964; Calderone, Mary S., and Eric W. Johnson. *The Family Book about Sexuality*. New York: Harper and Row, 1981; Cameron, J. M. "Sex in the Head." *New York Review of Books* (13 May 1976), 19–28; Carnes, Patrick. (1983, 1992) *Out of the Shadows: Understanding Sexual Addiction*, 3rd ed. Center City, Minn.: Hazelden, 2001; Chauncey, George, Jr. (1983) "From Sexual Inversion to Homosexuality: The Changing Medical Conceptualization of Female Deviance." In Kathy Peiss and Christina Simmons, eds., *Passion and Power: Sexuality in History*. Philadelphia, Pa.: Temple University Press, 1989, 87–117; Citizens Commission on Human Rights. "Psychiatric Diagnosis: Manufacturing Madness." In *Psychiatry: Destroying Religion*. Los Angeles, Calif.: Author, 1997, 44–47; Conrad, Peter, and Joseph W. Schneider. *Deviance and Medicalization: From Badness to Sickness*. St. Louis, Mo.: C. V. Mosby, 1980. Expanded edition, Philadelphia, Pa.: Temple University Press, 1992; Davidson, Arnold I. "Sex and the Emergence of Sexuality." *Critical Inquiry* 14:1 (1987), 16–48. Reprinted in Edward Stein, ed., *Forms of Desire: Sexual Orientation and the Social Constructionist Controversy*. New York: Routledge, 1992, 89–132; and *The Emergence of Sexuality: Historical Epistemology and the Formation of Concepts*. Cambridge, Mass.: Harvard University Press, 2001, 30–65; Davidson, Arnold I. "Styles of Reasoning, Conceptual History, and the Emergence of Psychiatry." In Peter Galison and David J. Strump, eds., *The Disunity of Science: Boundaries, Contexts, and Power*. Stanford, Calif.: Stanford University Press, 1996, 75–100. Reprinted, edited and abridged, as "Conceptual History and Conceptions of Perversions," in P&S2 (476–86); Davis, Katherine Bement. *Factors in the Sex Life of Twenty-Two Hundred Women*. New York: Harper and Brothers, 1929; De Cecco, John. "Sex and More Sex: A Critique of the Kinsey Conception of Human Sexuality." In David P. McWhirter, Stephanie A. Sanders, and June M. Reinisch, eds., *Homosexuality/Heterosexuality: Concepts of Sexual Orientation*. New York: Oxford University Press, 1990, 367–86; Devereux, George. "The Irrational in Sexual Research." In *From Anxiety to Method in the Behavioral Sciences*.

The Hague: Mouton, 1967, 103–17; Dickinson, Robert L. (1933) *Atlas of Human Sexual Anatomy*, 2nd ed. Baltimore, Md.: Williams and Wilkins, 1949; Dickinson, Robert L., and Lura Beam. *The Single Woman*. Baltimore, Md.: Williams and Wilkins, 1934; Dickinson, Robert L., and Lura Beam. *A Thousand Marriages: A Medical Study of Sex Adjustment*. Baltimore, Md.: Williams and Wilkins, 1931; Dreger, Alice Domurat. *Hermaphrodites and the Medical Invention of Sex*. Cambridge, Mass.: Harvard University Press, 1998; Ellis, Havelock. *Studies in the Psychology of Sex*, 4 vols. New York: Random House, 1936; Foucault, Michel. (1976/1984/1984) *The History of Sexuality*. Vol. 1: *An Introduction*. Trans. Robert Hurley. New York: Vintage, 1978. Vol. 2: *The Use of Pleasure*. Trans. Robert Hurley. New York: Pantheon, 1985. Vol. 3: *The Care of the Self*. Trans. Robert Hurley. New York: Vintage, 1986; Francouer, Robert T., Timothy Perper, and Norman A. Scherzer, eds. *A Descriptive Dictionary and Atlas of Sexology*. New York: Greenwood Press, 1991; Gathorne-Hardy, Jonathan. *Sex, the Measure of All Things: A Life of Alfred C. Kinsey*. Bloomington: Indiana University Press, 1998; Hall, Marny. "Not Tonight, Dear, I'm Deconstructing a Headache: Confessions of a Lesbian Sex Therapist." In Karla Jay, ed., *Lesbian Erotics*. New York: New York University Press, 1995, 15–27; Hartman, William E., and Marilyn A. Fithian. *Treatment of Sexual Dysfunction: A Bio-Psycho-Social Approach*. Long Beach, Calif.: Center for Marital and Sexual Studies, 1972; Hartman, William E., Marilyn A. Fithian, and Donald Johnson. (1970) *Nudist Society: The Controversial Study of the Clothes-Free Naturist Movement in America*. Rev. I. Bancroft. Los Angeles, Calif.: Elysium Growth Press, 1991; Hirschfeld, Magnus. *Sex in Human Relationships*. Trans. John Rodker. London: John Lane, 1935. Reprint, New York: AMS, 1975; Hirschfeld, Magnus. (1910) *Transvestites: The Erotic Drive to Cross-Dress*. Trans. Michael A. Lombardi-Nash. Buffalo, N.Y.: Prometheus, 1991; Horowitz, Helen. *Rereading Sex: Battles over Sexual Knowledge and Suppression in Nineteenth-Century America*. New York: Knopf, 2002; Hunt, Morton M. *The Natural History of Love*. New York: Knopf, 1959; Illich, Ivan. (1975) *Medical Nemesis: The Expropriation of Health*. New York: Pantheon, 1976; Irvine, Janice M. "The Kinsey Institute." In Bonnie Zimmerman, ed., *Lesbian Histories and Cultures*. New York: Garland, 2000, 426–27; Irvine, Janice M. " 'The Sociologist as Voyeur': Social Theory and Sexuality Research, 1910–1978." *Qualitative Sociology* 26:4 (2003), 429–56; Kaplan, Helen Singer. *Disorders of Sexual Desire and Other New Concepts and Techniques in Sex Therapy*. New York: Brunner/Mazel, 1979; Klein, Fritz, Barry Sepekoff, and Timothy Wolf. "Sexual Orientation: A Multi-Variable Dynamic Process." *Journal of Homosexuality* 11:1–2 (1985), 35–49; Kleinplatz, Peggy J., ed. *New Directions in Sex Therapy: Innovations and Alternatives*. Philadelphia, Pa.: Brunner-Routledge, 2001; Krafft-Ebing, Richard von. (1886, 1903) *Psychopathia Sexualis*, 12th ed. Trans. F. J. Rebman. New York: Paperback Library, 1965; Krivacska, James J., and John Money, eds. *The Handbook of Forensic Sexology: Biomedical and Criminological Perspectives*. Amherst, N.Y.: Prometheus, 1994; Laqueur, Thomas W. *Making Sex: Body and Gender from the Greeks to Freud*. Cambridge, Mass.: Harvard University Press, 1990; Laqueur, Thomas W. *Solitary Sex: A Cultural History of Masturbation*. New York: Zone Books, 2003; LeVay, Simon. "Hirschfeld and the Third Sex." In *Queer Science: The Use and Abuse of Research on Homosexuality*. Cambridge, Mass.: MIT Press, 1996, 11–40; LoPiccolo, Joseph. "The Evolution of Sex Therapy." *Sexual and Marital Therapy* 9:1 (1994), 5–7; Lotringer, Sylvère. *Overexposed: Treating Sexual Perversion in America*. New York: Pantheon, 1988; Magnus Hirschfeld Archive for Sexology, Humboldt University of Berlin. (Web site) <www2.rz.hu-berlin.de/sexology> [accessed 10 February 2005]; Maines, Rachel P. *The Technology of Orgasm, "Hysteria," the Vibrator, and Women's Sexual Satisfaction*. Baltimore, Md.: Johns Hopkins University Press, 1999; Mass, Lawrence. *Homosexuality and Sexuality: Dialogues of the Sexual Revolution*, vol. 1. New York: Haworth, 1990; Masson, Jeffrey Moussaieff. *A Dark Science: Women, Sexuality, and Psychiatry in the Nineteenth Century*. New York: Farrar, Straus and Giroux, 1986; Masters, William H., Virginia E. Johnson, and Robert C. Kolodny, eds. *Ethical Issues in Sex Therapy and Research*. Boston, Mass.: Little, Brown, 1977; McIlvenna, Ted, ed. *The Complete Guide to Safer Sex*. Fort Lee, N.J.: Barricade Books, 1992; Meyerowitz, Joanne. *How Sex Changed: A History of Transsexuality in the United States*. Cambridge, Mass.: Harvard University Press, 2002; Michael, Robert T., John H. Gagnon, Edward O. Laumann, and Gina Kolata. *Sex in America: A Definitive Survey*. Boston, Mass.: Little, Brown, 1994; Moll, Albert. (1931)

Perversions of the Sex Instinct. New York: AMS Press, 1976; Moll, Albert. (1909) *The Sexual Life of the Child*. Trans. Eden Paul. New York: Macmillan, 1912. New York: AMS, 1975; Money, John. *The Adam Principle. Genes, Genitals, Hormones, & Gender: Selected Readings in Sexology*. Buffalo, N.Y.: Prometheus, 1993; Money, John. *Lovemaps: Clinical Concepts of Sexual/Erotic Health and Pathology, Paraphilia, and Gender Transposition in Childhood, Adolescence, and Maturity*. New York: Irvington, 1986. Buffalo, N.Y.: Prometheus, 1988; Money, John, ed. *Sex Research: New Developments*. New York: Holt, 1965; Money, John, and Herman Musaph, eds. *Handbook of Sexology*. Amsterdam, Holland: Excerpta Medica, 1977; Mosher, Clelia D. *The Mosher Survey: Sexual Attitudes of 45 Victorian Women*. Ed. James Mahood and Kristine Wenburg. New York: Arno Press, 1980; Oosterhuis, Harry. *Stepchildren of Nature: Krafft-Ebing, Psychiatry, and the Making of Sexual Identity*. Chicago, Ill.: University of Chicago Press, 2000; Poovey, Mary. "Sex in America." *Critical Inquiry* 24:2 (1998), 366–92; Reich, Wilhelm. (1942) *The Discovery of the Orgone*, vol. 1: *The Function of the Orgasm. The Sex-Economic Problems of Biological Energy*. Trans. Vincent R. Carfagno. Oxford, U.K.: Touchstone, 1973; Reich, Wilhelm. (1930) *The Sexual Revolution: Toward a Self-Governing Character Structure*, 4th ed., rev. [*Die Sexualität im Kulturkampf*] Trans. Theodore P. Wolfe. New York: Noonday, 1969; Reisman, Judith A. *Kinsey: Crimes and Consequences. The Red Queen and the Grand Scheme*. Arlington, Va.: Institute for Media Education, 1998; Reiss, Ira L. *Journey into Sexuality: An Exploratory Voyage*. Englewood Cliffs, N.J.: Prentice-Hall, 1986; Reiss, Ira L. "Science and Sexology." In Vern L. Bullough and Bonnie Bullough, eds., *Human Sexuality: An Encyclopedia*. New York: Garland, 1994, 530–37; Robinson, Victor, ed. *Encyclopaedia Sexualis: A Comprehensive Encyclopaedia-Dictionary of the Sexual Sciences*. New York: Dingwall-Rock, 1936; Rosen, Raymond C., and Sandra R. Leiblum, eds. *Case Studies in Sex Therapy*. New York: Guilford, 1995; Schwartz, Mark F., and William H. Masters. "The Masters and Johnson Treatment Program for Dissatisfied Homosexual Men." *American Journal of Psychiatry* 141:2 (1984), 173–81; Simon, William. *Postmodern Sexualities*. New York: Routledge, 1996; Singer, Irving. *The Goals of Human Sexuality*. New York: Norton, 1973. New York: Schocken, 1974; Soble, Alan. "Health." In *Sexual Investigations*. New York: New York University Press, 1996, 143–74; Stoller, Robert J. "Impact of New Advances in Sex Research on Psychoanalytic Theory." In *Perversion: The Erotic Form of Hatred*. New York: Dell, 1975, 12–45; Stopes, Marie Carmichael. (1928) *Enduring Passion: Further New Contributions to the Solution of Sex Difficulties, Being the Continuation of Married Love*, 4th ed. New York: Putnam, 1931; Terry, Jennifer. *An American Obsession: Science, Medicine, and Homosexuality in Modern Society*. Chicago, Ill.: University of Chicago Press, 1999; Thurber, James, and E. B. White. (1929) *Is Sex Necessary? Or Why You Feel the Way You Do*. New York: Harper and Row, 1975; Tiefer, Leonore. "Historical, Scientific, Clinical, and Feminist Criticisms of 'The Human Sexual Response Cycle' Model." In *Sex Is Not a Natural Act and Other Essays*, 2nd ed. Boulder, Colo.: Westview, 2004, 41–61; Ulrichs, Karl Heinrich. (1864–1880) *The Riddle of "Man-Manly" Love: The Pioneering Work on Male Homosexuality*, 2 vols. Trans. Michael A. Lombardi-Nash. Buffalo, N.Y.: Prometheus, 1994; Updike, John. "Libido Lite." [Review of *Is Sex Necessary?* by James Thurber and E. B. White] *New York Review of Books* (18 November 2004), 30–31; Weeks, Jeffrey. *Invented Moralities: Sexual Values in an Age of Uncertainty*. New York: Columbia University Press, 1995; Weeks, Jeffrey. (1981) *Sex, Politics, and Society: The Regulation of Sexuality since 1800*, rev. ed. New York: Longman, 1989; Weeks, Jeffrey. *Sexuality and Its Discontents: Meanings, Myths, and Modern Sexualities*. London: Routledge and Kegan Paul, 1985; Weinberg, Martin S., ed. *Sex Research: Studies from the Kinsey Institute*. New York: Oxford University Press, 1976; Wiederman, Michael W., and Bernard E. Whitley, Jr., eds. *Handbook for Conducting Research on Human Sexuality*. Mahwah, N.J.: Erlbaum, 2002.

SEXUAL ACTIVITY. *See* Activity, Sexual

SEXUAL ADDICTION. *See* Addiction, Sexual

SEXUAL DESIRE. *See* Desire, Sexual

SEXUAL DYSFUNCTION. *See* Dysfunction, Sexual

SEXUAL ETHICS. *See* Ethics, Sexual

SEXUAL HARASSMENT. *See* Harassment, Sexual

SEXUAL OBJECTIFICATION. *See* Objectification, Sexual

SEXUAL ORIENTATION. *See* Orientation, Sexual

SEXUAL PERSONIFICATION. *See* Personification, Sexual

SEXUAL PERVERSION. *See* Paraphilia; Perversion, Sexual

SEXUAL USE. *See* Kant, Immanuel; Objectification, Sexual

SEXUAL VIOLENCE. *See* Violence, Sexual

SEXUALITY, DIMENSIONS OF. In its most rudimentary form, sexuality is the mixing of gametes. But especially in humans, sexuality is complex. On the evolutionary journey from "gametes" to "masculine/feminine," there are numerous way stations, whose connections with one another are contingent and, so far, only sketchily mapped. Edward Wilson locates the source of this complexity in **evolution**: "The growth in intelligence that accompanied" the enlargement of the human brain changed "even the most basic primate social qualities into nearly unrecognizable forms.... [I]n man the scales have become multidimensional, culturally adjustable, and almost endlessly subtle" (*Sociobiology*, 548). Human sexuality is thus the confluence of two mighty streams: biological ancestry and cultural heritage. The result is whirlpools, backwaters, white-water rapids, and a meandering river that threatens to overflow its banks.

Human biology affects human culture since the purpose of many social arrangements is to structure sexual development and familial relationships. And culture affects biology. Historical and cultural differences "enter so deeply into people's experience of sexual desire and activity that we may conclude that even this desire itself is not a 'natural' extra-historical constant, but, to some extent at least, an artifact of social arrangements" (Nussbaum, 1695). As a result of this dialectical interplay of biology and culture, "sexuality will remain an enigma. It would be naive, ahistorical, and self-aggrandizing to think that we might achieve an unassailable or even unique formulation of the problem of sexuality and its ethical resolution" (Cahill, 21). Nevertheless, we might be able to understand it more fully.

There is a family resemblance among sexuality's numerous forms. Whether a form is "normal" or "abnormal" depends on how distant it is from a paradigmatic type. Thus a woman's sexual body is "normal" if she has no penis but "abnormal" if she has no ovaries. Societies decide whether these differences are "anomalies" or merely "variations." There has been extensive debate about whether, for example, **homosexuality** is a "defect" or a valuable alternative.

Sexuality is not *essential* to our humanity but merely contingently *universal* (Fletcher, 3; cf. Grenz, 22–30). Someday, in a brave new world, we will reproduce in laboratories. At that time, a plausible case could be made for deleting the genes for our sexual organs to eliminate diseases such as ovarian cancer as well as the mania, betrayals, and violence that flow from lust. If this were to occur, we would still be human beings. But just as few of us now would choose feeding tubes over chewing a chocolate bar, few of us would choose to be asexual. (Some possible exceptions come to mind, e.g., Ti-Grace Atkinson [20].)

We are sexual in our chromosomes, gonads, hormones, internal and external sex organs, brains, upbringing, procreating, behaving, and social interacting. Each of these, far from being automatically determined, has variations and abnormalities (Sapp, 79–91; Symons, 43). A man's sex chromosomes may be the normal XY but also, much less frequently, XYY, XXY, or XXYY (Siann, 43–52). In "**intersexuality**," some people are born with ambiguous genitalia. Other people have a medically or socially "assigned sex" different from their chromosomal sex. Some individuals are reared as being of one sex (or gender) but experience themselves to be of the other sex. Drastic measures such as the surgical removal of the penis illustrate the possibility of great distance from the "normal" or paradigmatic type.

Human **sexual desire** and **sexual activity** are not altogether biologically hardwired. This plasticity emerged already in our subhuman precursors. **Masturbation**, cunnilingus, and **rape** are found in other animals (Hrdy, 158; Symons, 276–85). Human sexual behavior lies on a continuum with similar behavior in other primates. "Even the smile and the kiss, staple gestures of flirtation and foreplay among humans, have precursors among primate expressions" (Hrdy, 137). Few human sexual tendencies are absolutely out of our control, but many resist control. It is possible (but difficult) for a man to impregnate his wife, undergo sex-change surgery and hormone treatment, and then breast-feed his/her child. **Sexual orientation**—whether one is heterosexual, gay or lesbian, bisexual, or asexual—may be strongly resistant to change.

Unresolved questions about the origins of homosexuality point to the complexity and variability of sexuality. Not even by the twenty-first century has anyone provided a widely accepted explanation for the existence of homosexuality (Gilbert, 559–61; Zuk, 168–83). From one sort of evolutionary perspective, it should not exist, because homosexuals do not procreate (or not as often as heterosexuals). The strong discrimination cultures practice against homosexuality would seem to work toward eliminating it as well. But homosexuality exists, and persists. Whatever the reason, this orientation—not just homosexual acts but the disposition and preference—demonstrates (along with other socially scorned variations) the diversity of human sexuality.

For biologists, "sex" refers to the mixing of two or more different genetic materials into a new organism: "reproduction." This sex is not about pleasure (or **love**), because many animals "perform the sexual act mechanically and with minimal foreplay" (Wilson, *Human*,

121). An act's being reproductive in form or potential is ordinarily a sufficient condition for the act to be sexual (Soble, 136–37). A reproductive desire—a desire to become pregnant or to have children—is a sexual desire, but it is not the *same* desire as the desire for genital intercourse, for some people practice **contraception** and others "endure" intercourse to bear a child. Since sexuality is centrally about reproduction, being pregnant and giving birth are part of sexuality. Breast-feeding might also be considered part of sexuality, but bottle feeding is rather distant from the paradigm.

Scientific advances complicate this picture. A technician who mixes sperm and ova in a petri dish does not spend his or her day engaged in "sex." Nevertheless, this activity is part of the realm of sexuality since it results directly in new life. Nature itself sometimes separates human reproduction and "sex." The birth of identical twins is part of reproduction. Biologically, the second embryo is not the product of "sex," of combining genes, but rather of the asexual cloning of a second embryo from the first (Genetic Science Learning Center).

To say that going through pregnancy or a fertilized egg's twinning are part of the realm of sexuality is not to say that they are "sexual acts," at least as we ordinarily use that term. "Sexual acts" are, in general, acts that include the distinctive feelings a person has when genitally or otherwise physically aroused (for discussion, see Soble, chap. 3). These feelings are in great part bodily, but they often involve the whole self. They are often pleasurable but need not be. Instead, the feelings may be an ache in the loins or the rawness of insufficiently lubricated sex. (In some invertebrates, the "feeling" might be only that of the female's freezing in a receptive posture and the male's impulsive thrusting.) Sexual feelings can be desirable when they are pleasurable, or lead to orgasm, or result in birth. Their intensity ranges from a mild buzz to an earthshaking ecstasy. They often arise as part of the sexual attraction between persons. These feelings become intrinsically desirable and so are enjoyed in contexts that are only remotely related, if at all, to procreation—for example, when contraception is employed by a couple or when a solitary person employs **pornography** during masturbation.

One criterion for whether an activity is sexual is whether it typically involves these sexual feelings. One person may get aroused by a glimpse of a woman's gray sweater, while another may be unmoved by seeing her naked body. The first look is sexual; the second— say, during a pelvic exam by a doctor—is not. Most activities, of course, are not sexual activities; they do not evoke such feelings. Ordinarily, writing a philosophy essay, even an essay on sexuality, is not a sexual activity. Still, most activities may become sexual (Soble, 123–24, 142). Writing or lecturing about sex or the philosophy of sex might, in the proper frame of mind, produce these feelings.

Our feelings are usually "cognitive," not merely bodily sensations. They include memories and imaginings (or **fantasy**) as well. Through these other human capacities, we can feel not only the presence but also the absence of a friend; similarly, we can feel not only sexual pleasure but also the absence of sexual pleasure, as might occur in intercourse carried out merely from a sense of duty. Likewise, we can feel the distance between what is and what could or ought to be. The horror felt by a woman who is raped is a distinct sexual feeling, a feeling of **sexual violence**, not just generic bodily violence. This is why rape can be far more damaging than other kinds of attack. Further, we can feel another's feelings; doing so may be an important part of mutual sex (see Ruddick, 87–90).

The paradigmatic form of human "sexual activity" and the most popular use of the term "sex" is the activity by which a man and a woman join their genitals together in such a way that semen is ejaculated in the vagina. Nevertheless, sexual activity includes many other acts that are in varying degrees distant from this paradigm but still resemble them in a "family" way. Thus, if a man does not deposit semen into the vagina, as in *coitus interruptus*, he still engages in sexual activity. If his partner does not have an orgasm, they have still engaged in sex. They can engage in sex if they stimulate each other with their mouths or by clitoral and other touches. There are many forms of sex, including homosexual sex, that do not involve the central case of penis-vagina coupling.

In fact, most human sexual activity is not reproductive (even when it is penile-vaginal). Both biology and the human mind have made nonprocreative sex not only possible but probable. Several biological changes in the evolution of humans contributed to the high frequency of nonprocreative sex. Female estrus disappeared, and as a result, sexual activity is desired and engaged in at any time, even when fertilization cannot occur. Further (and related), ovulation became concealed, which made it difficult for a couple to plan their sexual activity to take place only when fertilization could occur. And female sexual pleasure and orgasm, which are strictly speaking unnecessary for fertilization and reproduction, contributed to sexual activity becoming intrinsically valuable and not merely instrumentally valuable as a tool for procreation.

Richard Posner has wondered, "If human beings, like other animals, are reproduction machines, as the evolutionary biologist considers them to be, their tendency to reproduce less when they can afford to reproduce more is deeply puzzling" (345). But it is not really puzzling, since our enlarged brains have made us more than reproductive machines. Our expansive minds enable us to engage in an extraordinary variety of nonsexual activities. And our expansive minds have similarly made it possible for us to engage in sexual activities for a wide variety of reasons other than procreation, for example, to exchange pleasure, express love, relieve boredom, prove maturity, prepare oneself for a good night's sleep, satisfy curiosity, make someone jealous, quiet a nagging spouse, procrastinate grading exams, and give gifts for anniversaries (see Sprinkle).

Broadly speaking, human sexuality can be defined as "the way of being in, and relating to, the world as a *male* or *female* person" (Kosnik et al., 82). In this context, "sexuality" and "sex" refer to classifying people as male or female. Biologically, "female" and "male" refer, respectively, to who contributes the larger and the smaller gamete to the reproductive process (Wilson, *Sociobiology*, 324). Male and female organisms do not otherwise universally have any sex-specific qualities or roles. Among lower animals (and humans), sometimes males and sometimes females are the soldiers, the hunters, or the caretakers. Among different animals, fertilization may take place inside or outside the body, and males or females may be pregnant (Zuk, 38–40, 51–53, 135).

The human sexual body is not just socially constructed (Soble, 142; cf. Plummer, 29–30). Women's bodies differ from men's bodies not only in their reproductive organs but also in other organs such as skin, heart, and brain. Similarly, the waxing and waning of sexual desire is a process only quasi-independent from biology. While the significance of developing hips or facial hair varies according to culture, these physical events occur no matter how a culture understands them. To be sure, sexual maturation also requires acceptance and affirmation of one's sexuality (Hotvedt, 159–62), but even that is often only loosely guided by culture. For example, men engage in masturbation as part of maturing in sexual embodiment but often do so without instruction.

The sexual body is also relational. Its directedness is primarily to persons as male or female; only secondarily is it directed toward their distinctively sexual body parts. We are attracted to sexual parts because they belong to the sexual whole, not vice versa. The sexual body as relational develops an outer-directed tendency. The often noted difference between solitary masturbation and genital intercourse indicates that other-directed sex is another dimension of sexual maturation. Of course, these relational aspects of human sexuality are not universal, even if common. Further, just as we are attracted to food because (and when) we are hungry, we are attracted to males and females because we have sexual bodies. If we try to encounter others as "just people," we must set aside or repress our sexual perceptivity. Usually, however, we immediately recognize whether someone is a male or a man or a female or a woman. We do so by observing their body, but also by noting their gendered—masculine or feminine—behavior. Still, gender can become quite distant from biological sex. Some women are said to be very feminine, others not, and others are described as masculine. But none of this has to do with their fertility or "sex" in the gamete sense. Feminine characteristics are, similarly, often predicated of men.

Because our bodies are male or female and we learn masculine and feminine (gendered) ways of behaving, it might be claimed, "*Sexuality* affects all aspects of the human person" (*Catechism*, #2332). Still, not all acts of a sexual person are sexual acts. When two women (or a man and a woman) discuss quantum physics, their encounter is not itself a sexual encounter. Of course, sex and gender can be relevant in some social and interpersonal contexts. Hiring a female lawyer in an all-male firm is a significant event. Holding hands with a male or a female, depending on the culture, has very different meanings. The symbolic significance of sex is an important yet variable aspect of it.

Humans communicate through symbols, most obviously in written or spoken **language**. But humans also communicate through their bodies. Many of our bodily gestures are conventional (waving goodbye), and in some contexts various sexual gestures have taken on conventionally symbolic meanings. But some bodily movements, although culturally molded, can be understood as natural symbols (Solomon). A sexual caress is a natural symbol of union just as a slap in the face is a natural symbol of disunion, though each can be culturally overlain with contrary meanings. Unlike less embodied communications such as writing letters or talking on the phone, sexual activities are ways that people meet in the flesh. In sexual embodiment, "we 'become' our bodies; our consciousness becomes bodily experience of bodily activity"(Ruddick, 88).

Because it can be symbolic and carry meanings, sexual union is often (perhaps somewhat misleadingly) described as a language (Guindon, 83–95; Nelson, 25–36). Sometimes uttering the words "I love you" or "I want you" is a more clear way to communicate what one is feeling than is bodily union (Vannoy, 11). But the distinctive power of mutual sexual sharing is the way it unites people through their embodiment. Shared sexual activity binds people not only through making one's partner a source or occasion of pleasure but more so through two basic forms of human presence: the union of carrying out a common activity together and the union of mutual touch. Shared sexual activities are not just about satisfying a desire for one's own pleasure (Abramson and Pinkerton, 34) but also about the enjoyment of one's own and another's embodied company. In this sense, "sex is . . . closer in meaning to hugging and kissing than to baby-making intercourse" (29). The ancient religious idea from Genesis that "two become one flesh" reappears in evolutionary biology as "pair-bonding" and in human language as "sexual love."

See also Abortion; Activity, Sexual; African Philosophy; Animal Sexuality; Catholicism, Twentieth- and Twenty-First-Century; Dysfunction, Sexual; Ethics, Sexual; Evolution; Firestone, Shulamith; Genital Mutilation; Intersexuality; Money, John; Orientation, Sexual; Phenomenology; Philosophy of Sex, Overview of; Philosophy of Sex, Teaching the; Psychology, Evolutionary; Reproductive Technology; Scruton, Roger; Social Constructionism; Utopianism; Westermarck, Edward

REFERENCES

Abramson, Paul R., and Steven D. Pinkerton. (1995) *With Pleasure: Thoughts on the Nature of Human Sexuality*, rev. ed. New York: Oxford University Press, 2002; Atkinson, Ti-Grace. *Amazon Odyssey*. New York: Links Books, 1974; Cahill, Lisa Sowle. "Sexuality and Christian Ethics: How to Proceed." In James B. Nelson and Sandra P. Longfellow, eds., *Sexuality and the Sacred: Sources for Theological Reflection*. Louisville, Ky.: Westminster John Knox, 1994, 19–27; *Catechism of the Catholic Church*, 2nd ed. Washington, D.C.: United States Catholic Conference, 2000; Fletcher, Joseph. "Indicators of Humanhood: A Tentative Profile of Man." *Hastings Center Report* 2 (November 1972), 1–4; Genetic Science Learning Center at the Eccles Institute of Human Genetics, University of Utah. "What Is Cloning?" <gslc.genetics.utah.edu/units/cloning/whatiscloning/> [accessed 30 August 2004]; Gilbert, Scott F. (1985) *Developmental Biology*, 7th ed. Sunderland, Mass.: Sinauer Associates, 2003; Grenz, Stanley J. *Sexual Ethics: An Evangelical Perspective*. Louisville, Ky.: Westminster John Knox, 1997; Guindon, André. *The Sexual Language: An Essay in Moral Theology*. Ottawa, Can.: University of Ottawa Press, 1977; Hotvedt, Mary. "Gender Identity and Sexual Orientation: The Anthropological Perspective." In Mark Schwartz, Albert Moraczewski, and James Monteleone, eds., *Sex and Gender: A Theological and Scientific Inquiry*. St. Louis, Mo.: Pope John Center, 1983, 144–76; Hrdy, Sarah Blaffer. *The Woman That Never Evolved*. Cambridge, Mass.: Harvard University Press, 1983; Kosnik, Anthony, William Carroll, Agnes Cunningham, Ronald Modras, and James Schulte. *Human Sexuality: New Directions in American Catholic Thought*. New York: Paulist Press, 1977; Nelson, James B. *Embodiment: An Approach to Sexuality and Christian Theology*. Minneapolis, Minn.: Augsburg, 1978; Nussbaum, Martha C. " 'Only Grey Matter'? Richard Posner's Cost-Benefit Analysis of Sex." *University of Chicago Law Review* 59:4 (1992), 1689–1734; Plummer, Ken. "Symbolic Interactionism and Sexual Conduct: An Emergent Perspective." In Christine Williams and Arlene Stein, eds., *Sexuality and Gender*. Malden, Mass.: Blackwell, 2002, 20–32; Posner, Richard. *Overcoming Law*. Cambridge, Mass.: Harvard University Press, 1995; Ruddick, Sara. (1971) "Better Sex." In Robert B. Baker and Frederick A. Elliston, eds., *Philosophy and Sex*, 1st ed. Buffalo, N.Y.: 1975, 83–104; Sapp, Stephen. *Sexuality, the Bible, and Science*. Philadelphia, Pa.: Fortress, 1977; Siann, Gerda. *Gender, Sex, and Sexuality: Contemporary Psychological Perspectives*. Bristol, Pa.: Taylor and Francis, 1994; Soble, Alan. *Sexual Investigations*. New York: New York University Press, 1996; Solomon, Robert. "Sexual Paradigms." *Journal of Philosophy* 71:11 (1974), 336–45; Sprinkle, Annie. "The Benefits of Sex." <www.anniesprinkle.org/html/writings/101_uses.html> [accessed 30 August 2004]; Symons, Donald. *The Evolution of Human Sexuality*. New York: Oxford University Press, 1979; Vannoy, Russell. *Sex without Love: A Philosophical Exploration*. Buffalo, N.Y.: Prometheus, 1980; Wilson, Edward O. "Sex." In *On Human Nature*. Cambridge, Mass.: Harvard University Press, 1978, 125–54; Wilson, Edward O. (1975) *Sociobiology: The New Synthesis*. [25th Anniversary edition] Cambridge, Mass.: Harvard University Press, 2000; Zuk, Marlene. *Sexual Selections: What We Can and Can't Learn about Sex from Animals*. Berkeley: University of California Press, 2002.

Edward Collins Vacek

ADDITIONAL READING

Angelides, Steven. *A History of Bisexuality*. Chicago, Ill.: University of Chicago Press, 2001; Archer, John, and Barbara Lloyd. (1982) *Sex and Gender*, 2nd ed. New York: Cambridge University Press, 2002; Breidenthal, Thomas. "Sanctifying Nearness." In Eugene F. Rogers, Jr., ed., *Theology and Sexuality: Classic and Contemporary Readings*. Malden, Mass.: Blackwell, 2002, 343–55; Burlew, Larry D., and David Capuzzi. "Sexuality Counseling: Introduction, Definitions, Ethics, and Professional Issues." In *Sexuality Counseling*. New York: Nova Science, 2002, 3–16; de Sousa, Ronald, and Kathryn Pauly Morgan. "Philosophy, Sex, and Feminism." <www.chass.utoronto.ca/~sousa/sexphil.html> [accessed 14 October 2004]; Duss-von Werdt, Josef. "The Polyvalent Nature of Sexuality." In Franz Böckle and Jacques-Marie Pohier, eds., *Sexuality in Contemporary Catholicism*. New York: Seabury,

1976, 93–102; Hefner, Philip J. "Sex, for God's Sake: Theological Perspectives." In Robert Bellig and George Stevens, eds., *The Evolution of Sex*. San Francisco, Calif.: Harper and Row, 1987, 139–54; Jeanniere, Abel. *The Anthropology of Sex*. New York: Harper and Row, 1967; John Paul II. *On the Family: Apostolic Exhortation Familiaris Consortio*. Washington, D.C.: United States Catholic Conference, 1982; Keane, Philip S. *Sexual Morality: A Catholic Perspective*. New York: Paulist Press, 1977; Kimura, Doreen. "Sex Differences in the Brain." <www.mermaids.freeuk.com/differ.html> [accessed 30 August 2004]; Milligan, Don. *Sex-Life: A Critical Commentary on the History of Sexuality*. London: Pluto Press, 1993; Mohr, Anne, and David Jessel. *Brain Sex: The Real Difference between Men and Women*. New York: Dell, 1989; Moore, Gareth. "Sexual Needs and Sexual Pleasures." *International Philosophical Quarterly* 35:2 (1995), 193–204; Nathanielsz, Peter W. *Life before Birth: The Challenges of Fetal Development*. New York: W. H. Freeman, 1996; Phillips, Larr. "Sex and Gender Identity across the Life Span." In Larry D. Burlew and David Capuzzi, eds., *Sexuality Counseling*. New York: Nova Science, 2002, 17–39; Ruddick, Sara. "On Sexual Morality." In James Rachels, ed., *Moral Problems: A Collection of Philosophical Essays*, 2nd ed. New York: Harper and Row, 1971, 16–34. Reprinted, revised, as "Better Sex," in Robert B. Baker and Frederick A. Elliston, eds., *Philosophy and Sex*, 1st ed. Buffalo, N.Y.: Prometheus, 1975, 83–104; P&S2 (280–99); and, abridged, in Judith A. Boss, ed., *Analyzing Moral Issues*, 3rd ed. New York: McGraw Hill, 2005, 368–77; Singer, Irving. "Criteria of Sexual Goodness." In *Sex: A Philosophical Primer*. Lanham, Md.: Rowman and Littlefield, 2001, 65–101; Solomon, Robert. "Sexual Paradigms." *Journal of Philosophy* 71:11 (1974), 336–45. Reprinted in HS (81–90); POS1 (89–98); POS2 (53–62); POS3 (21–29); POS4 (21–29); Sprinkle, Annie. "The Hazards of Sex." <www.anniesprinkle.org/html/writings/101_hazards.html> [accessed 15 February 2005]; Vacek, Edward Collins. *Love, Human and Divine: The Heart of Christian Ethics*. Washington, D.C.: Georgetown University Press, 1994; Whitehead, Evelyn Eaton, and James D. Whitehead. *A Sense of Sexuality: Christian Love and Intimacy*. New York: Doubleday, 1989.

SEXUALLY TRANSMITTED DISEASES (STDs). *See* Diseases, Sexually Transmitted

SHERFEY, MARY JANE (1918–1983). Mary Jane Sherfey, a physician and psychiatrist, explored the culturally explosive question of the nature of female sexuality. Her theories were first published in 1966 in the *Journal of the American Psychoanalytic Association* and then later as a provocative book, *The Nature and Evolution of Female Sexuality* (1972). This was intended to be the first of two volumes, but the second volume was never published.

Sherfey was born in Brazil, Indiana, and received her B.A. from the University of Indiana, studying with Alfred Kinsey (1894–1956). She then obtained the M.D. from the University of Indiana Medical School. Initially taking her residency in pediatrics, she switched to psychiatry, joining the staff at the Payne Whitney Clinic of the University of Cornell Medical School in New York. In 1955, Sherfey was appointed assistant professor of psychiatry at Cornell Medical School. She "was working in the very belly of the Freudian beast during the 1960s, when the term 'feminist psychoanalyst' was considered an oxymoron" (Chalker, 88). Sherfey subsequently entered private practice in New York to pursue research in the developmental physiology of human female sexuality. At the time of her death she was resident psychiatrist at Rusk State Hospital in Texas.

Sherfey questioned **Sigmund Freud**'s (1856–1939) theory of female sexual development, because that theory did not tally with her clinical experience with female patients. Freud's work, popularized by later psychoanalytic interpretations (for this history, see

Irving Singer, *The Goals of Human Sexuality*, 83–104), postulated distinct female orgasms: an "immature" clitoral orgasm and a "mature" vaginal orgasm. In attaining sexual maturity, a normal woman transfers erogenous allegiance from purely clitoral stimulation to vaginal intercourse. On this view, clitoral fixation was seen as abnormally masculine; normal development of femininity required penis-vagina sexuality. ("When erotogenic susceptibility to stimulation has been successfully transferred by a woman from the clitoris to the vaginal orifice, it implies that she has adopted a new leading zone for the purposes of later sexual activity" [Freud, *Three Essays on the Theory of Sexuality*, 87].) A woman's consistent failure to attain vaginal orgasm, or her having only orgasms through clitoral manipulation, was labeled frigidity and indicated psychological problems (Sherfey, *Nature*, 15). But many women have difficulty achieving orgasm by coitus alone (Hite, 229). Sherfey argued that natural physiological mechanisms were involved in this pattern instead of women's failing to be psychosexually mature. As Anne Koedt wrote in her famous 1970 essay, "Rather than tracing female frigidity to the false assumptions about female anatomy, our 'experts' have declared frigidity a psychological problem" (311).

According to the laboratory research of William Masters (1915–2001) and Virginia Johnson, on which Sherfey drew, there is no difference between clitoral and vaginal orgasm. Whether the clitoris is stimulated by direct manipulation or indirectly by traction on the clitoral tissues from penile thrusting during coitus, the orgasmic response is the same (*Human Sexual Response*, 66–67; see **Albert Ellis**; Alix Shulman). Orgasm consists of the rhythmic contractions of the extravaginal musculature against the greatly distended circumvaginal venous plexi and vestibular bulbs surrounding the lower third of the vagina, and contractions are experienced throughout the whole pelvic complex. Masters and Johnson also found that for female orgasm to occur there must be high sexual excitation with considerable engorgement of vestibular, labial, and preputial tissues due to continuous and appropriate stimulation. Their research explained why many women do not achieve orgasm with vaginal stimulation alone and why some women cannot achieve orgasm even with direct stimulation of the clitoral area: there is insufficient pelvic vasocongestion. Eastern tantric sexual practices over 5,000 years old stressed the necessity for males to perfect ejaculatory prevention techniques to prolong female sexual stimulation. Masters and Johnson advocated some of these techniques.

In male sexual anatomy, sexual pleasure through orgasm is tightly linked with the penis's reproductive function in ejaculating sperm into the vagina. By contrast, the female genitalia are anatomically diverse, incorporating not only the vagina with its reproductive function but also the clitoris, which is only a pleasure-producing organ (Gudorf, 65; Hrdy, *Woman*, 167; Stayton, 335). It is an interesting biological question why women, unlike men, possess a portion of sexual anatomy that is apparently distinct from the reproductive function of the genitalia. Human female sexuality apparently evolved to permit women to experience pleasure and orgasm without coitus. Why is the clitoris not *inside* the vagina, if Nature, either by evolution or Divine design, wanted to link reproduction and pleasure as tightly in the female as they are in the male? This difference suggests that there are possibly more fundamental biological differences between males and females. The psychoanalytic view of the psychologically healthy vaginal orgasm achieved by penile thrusting alone—justified by an assumed connection between pleasure and reproductive coitus—is perhaps only a political construction that in part serves to perpetuate women's social status (see Atkinson, 5–7, 13–23; **Andrea Dworkin** [1946–2005], 121–43). For that matter, why did female orgasm, no matter how induced, evolve at all? Biologists have debated this, because female orgasm may not be required for females to reproduce reliably and so might not have adaptive significance (see Hrdy, "Evolution," 312; *Woman*, 165, 227n.14, 237–39n.32; Singer, *Goals*, 159–97; Symons, *Evolution*, 86–95).

The science of human sexual biology has often claimed that sexual libido is "male" and that female sexual differentiation occurs from essentially "male" tissues. For example, the clitoris and, on some views, even the vagina, was the "inferior" or "lesser" homologue of the penis. (For the history of some of this biology of sexuality, see Laqueur; Soble.) Sherfey was attracted, instead, to what endocrinologists call the "inductor theory of primary sexual differentiation," according to which maleness in mammals is derived from the primacy of female morphology. Inductor theory asserts that mammalian embryos of either chromosomal sex are anatomically female during early fetal life. In male development, increasing levels of fetal androgen are required developmentally to prevail over circulating maternal estrogens to modify the intrinsic embryonic female anatomy. In humans, differentiation of the male external genitalia by the action of fetal androgens is completed by the end of the third fetal month. The female form does not require hormonally induced differentiation; without the androgen bath the embryo develops automatically into an anatomical female. Because fetal androgen is necessary to induce male development, male morphology is a derivation from the basic female pattern. (See Stephen Jay Gould [1941–2002], 153–54; **John Money**, "Eve before Adam.") This endocrinology was, for Sherfey, a "breathtaking, history-making" discovery; "[it] would strike a body blow at the Freudian concepts of female sexual development" (*Nature*, 14). The female's sexual anatomy and libido are not pale and ineffectual versions of the male's.

Sherfey hypothesized that the estrogenic uterine environment and lack of differentiating hormones during embryonic life give rise to primate females' sensitivity to hormonal conditioning, especially to the effect of androgens at puberty. Androgen-sensitive structures evolved that enhanced female sexual capacity, in particular a marked development of the clitoral system, skin erotism, and perineal sexual edema. These combine to yield an aggressive female sex drive with great desire and capacity for multiple copulations with multiple partners during estrus. Human females are endowed anatomically with massive systems of androgen-sensitive vascular tissues underlying the clitoral, preputial, glandular, and vestibular networks. It takes longer (than in men) to fill this huge network with blood during sexual excitation and, more significantly, longer for fluids to dissipate from engorged tissues, with or without orgasm. Without orgasmic contractions releasing the engorgement, a female might be edemous for hours or even days. Alternatively, if orgasm is reached, a woman might continue to have orgasms, due to the still-engorged vascular tissues, until she is physically exhausted. Sherfey called this phenomenon "satiation-in-insatiation" (*Nature*, 112).

When female primates manifest an insistent desire for **sexual activity** with numerous partners, females with the greatest pelvic edema and sexual drive obtain the breeding premium. Early hominid females, evolved from primate females with high androgen sensitivity, were also sexually insatiable, in that they would have coitus with as many males as desired until sexually satiated or exhausted. Human females, however, have concealed ("hidden") ovulatory cycles (see Diamond, 79) and are able to engage in sexual activity independently of estrus cycles. With adequate excitation, pelvic engorgement leading to orgasm may happen at any time, although the highest levels of pelvic vasocongestion occur in the last half of the human female's menstrual cycle. Human females retained estruslike cyclic vasocongestion but not external genital display.

Sherfey speculates that in virtue of their primate heritage ancestral human female promiscuity was normal and adaptive. If it is not now, it is because human females have been subjected to over 5,000 years of cultural repression of their sex drive to ensure prolonged maternal care of offspring, paternity, kinship, and property rights, which made possible modern civilization as we know it (*Nature*, 138). With the rise of settled agricultural economies, families of known genealogy and parentage could not exist unless the inordinate sexual demands of women were tamed. According to Sherfey, "Our myth of the female's relative asexuality is a biological absurdity. . . . [T]hroughout historic time—and even today—it could well be that women have indulged in so-called 'orgiastic parties,' having relations with one man after another, for precisely the purpose of gratifying this capacity for numerous, successive orgasms with coition" (*Nature*, 113–14).

British writer Brigid Brophy (1929–1995), in her iconoclastic essay "Monogamy" (29), offered a Sherfeyan picture of women's sexual biology and on that basis concluded (reversing received wisdom) that "higamus hogamus, it is man who is monogamous and, hogamus higamus, woman who is, by her biological nature, polygamous." Anthropologist Sarah Blaffer Hrdy acknowledged Sherfey's ideas of primate female promiscuity ("Evolution," 311–12) but cautioned that she would only "follow [Sherfey] at a safe distance." "Insatiability," wrote Hrdy, "is probably too strong a word, but an inclination . . . to solicit males could serve an important adaptive purpose in the lives of female primates" (*Woman*, 174; see 146). Donald Symons has replied that "the sexually insatiable woman is to be found primarily . . . in the ideology of feminism, the hopes of boys, and the fears of men" (*Evolution*, 92; see also "Another Woman," 299). The question of women's orgasms has been a political hot potato (see Lydon).

Sherfey's work has come under some criticism. The American Psychoanalytic Association, at its 1967 annual meeting, convened a panel on female sexuality that addressed Sherfey's 1966 article and Masters and Johnson's research (see Barker), and the papers were published in the July 1968 issue of the *Journal of the American Psychoanalytic Association* (see Heiman). In 1972, philosopher Irving Singer reviewed her book ("Anti-Climax"), claiming that "one would be hard-put to name a primatologist who believes that any female primate other than the human has recognizable orgasms as a usual concomitant of coital behavior." More recent studies of primate sexuality, however, contradict his opinion (Dixson, 126–37; Waal, 99–108). Singer has also argued, based on physiological evidence, that human females can experience three types of orgasm and that there is, after all, a difference between "vulval" (induced by clitoral stimulation) and "uterine" (induced by coitus) orgasms (*Goals*, 72–73); women who experience Sherfey's "satiation-in-insatiation" are those who "experience nothing but vulval orgasms" (*Goals*, 79). Singer bemoans that the "new orthodoxy" of a single, clitoris-based orgasm "is as tyrannical as the one [the Freudian] that preceded it" (*Goals*, 29; see *Explorations*, 67–68). Also to be acknowledged is the erotic sensitivity associated with the "G [Graefenberg]-spot" (see Tavris, 232–42; Whipple). Of course, any part of Sherfey's work on female sexuality that depends on the research of Masters and Johnson is vulnerable to the objection that their studies were methodologically flawed. Historian Paul Robinson, for example, claims that Masters and Johnson did not find "vaginal" orgasm because there was "a clitoral bias in [their] sample" (136).

See also Dysfunction, Sexual; Ellis, Albert; Evolution; Feminism, Lesbian; Feminism, Liberal; Firestone, Shulamith; Freud, Sigmund; Money, John; Psychology, Evolutionary; Singer, Irving; Thomas Aquinas (Saint)

REFERENCES

Atkinson, Ti-Grace. *Amazon Odyssey*. New York: Links, 1974; Barker, Warren J. "Female Sexuality." *Journal of the American Psychoanalytic Association* 16:1 (1968), 123–45; Brophy, Brigid.

"Monogamy." In *Don't Never Forget: Collected Views and Reviews*. London: Jonathan Cape, 1966, 28–31; Chalker, Rebecca. *The Clitoral Truth: The Secret World at Your Fingertips*. New York: Seven Stories Press, 2000; Diamond, Jared M. *The Third Chimpanzee: The Evolution and Future of the Human Animal*. New York: HarperCollins, 1992; Dixson, Alan F. *Primate Sexuality: Comparative Studies of the Prosimians, Monkeys, Apes, and Human Beings*. New York: Oxford University Press, 1998; Dworkin, Andrea. *Intercourse*. New York: Free Press, 1987; Ellis, Albert. "Is the Vaginal Orgasm a Myth?" In A. P. Pillay and Albert Ellis, eds., *Sex, Society, and the Individual*. Bombay, India: International Journal of Sexology Press, 1953, 155–62; Freud, Sigmund. (1905) *Three Essays on the Theory of Sexuality*. Trans. and ed. James Strachey. New York: Basic Books, 1975; Gould, Stephen Jay. *Hen's Teeth and Horse's Toes*. New York: Norton, 1983; Gudorf, Christine E. *Body, Sex, and Pleasure: Reconstructing Christian Sexual Ethics*. Cleveland, Ohio: Pilgrim Press, 1994; Heiman, Marcel. "Discussion of Sherfey's Paper on Female Sexuality." *Journal of the American Psychoanalytic Association* 16:3 (1968), 406–16; Hite, Shere. *The Hite Report: A Nationwide Study of Female Sexuality*. New York: Dell, 1976; Hrdy, Sarah Blaffer. "The Evolution of Human Sexuality: The Latest Word and the Last." *Quarterly Review of Biology* 54:3 (1979), 309–14; Hrdy, Sarah Blaffer. *The Woman That Never Evolved*. Cambridge, Mass.: Harvard University Press, 1981; Koedt, Anne. (1970) "The Myth of the Vaginal Orgasm." In Deborah Babcox and Madeline Belkin, eds., *Liberation Now! Writings from the Women's Liberation Movement*. New York: Dell, 1971, 311–20; Laqueur, Thomas. *Making Sex: Body and Gender from the Greeks to Freud*. Cambridge, Mass.: Harvard University Press, 1990; Lydon, Susan. "The Politics of Orgasm." In Robin Morgan, ed., *Sisterhood is Powerful: An Anthology of Writings from the Women's Liberation Movement*. New York: Vintage, 1970, 197–205; Masters, William H., and Virginia E. Johnson. *Human Sexual Response*. Boston, Mass.: Little, Brown, 1966; Money, John. "Eve before Adam Is the New Law of Genesis." In *The Adam Principle. Genes, Genitals, Hormones, & Gender: Selected Readings in Sexology*. Buffalo, N.Y.: Prometheus, 1993, 56–69; Robinson, Paul. *The Modernization of Sex: Havelock Ellis, Alfred Kinsey, William Masters and Virginia Johnson*. New York: Harper and Row, 1976; Sherfey, Mary Jane. "The Evolution and Nature of Female Sexuality in Relation to Psychoanalytic Theory." *Journal of the American Psychoanalytic Association* 14:1 (1966), 28–128; Sherfey, Mary Jane. (1972) *The Nature and Evolution of Female Sexuality*. New York: Vintage Books, 1973; Shulman, Alix. "Organs and Orgasms." In Vivian Gornick and Barbara K. Moran, eds., *Woman in Sexist Society: Studies in Power and Powerlessness*. New York: Basic Books, 1971, 198–206; Singer, Irving. "Anti-Climax." *New York Review of Books* (30 November 1972), 29–31; Singer, Irving. *Explorations in Love and Sex*. Lanham, Md.: Rowman and Littlefield, 2001; Singer, Irving. (1973) *The Goals of Human Sexuality*. New York: Schocken, 1974; Soble, Alan. "The History of Sexual Anatomy and Self-Referential Philosophy of Science." *Metaphilosophy* 34:3 (2003), 229–49; Stayton, William R. "A Theology of Sexual Pleasure." In Elizabeth Stuart and Adrian Thatcher, eds., *Christian Perspectives on Sexuality and Gender*. Grand Rapids, Mich.: Eerdmans, 1996, 332–46; Symons, Donald. "Another Woman That Never Existed." *Quarterly Review of Biology* 57:3 (1982), 297–300; Symons, Donald. *The Evolution of Human Sexuality*. New York: Oxford University Press, 1979; Tavris, Carol. *The Mismeasure of Woman*. New York: Simon and Schuster, 1992; Waal, Frans B. M. de. *Bonobo: The Forgotten Ape*. Berkeley: University of California Press, 1997; Whipple, Beverly. "G Spot and Female Pleasure." In Vern L. Bullough and Bonnie Bullough, eds., *Human Sexuality: An Encyclopedia*. New York: Garland, 1994, 229–32.

I. L. Coulter

ADDITIONAL READING

Barbach, Lonnie Garfield. *For Yourself: The Fulfillment of Female Sexuality*. New York: New American Library, 1975; Barnett, Marjorie. "I Can't Versus He Won't." *Journal of the American Psychoanalytic Association* 16:3 (1968), 588–600; Benda, Clemens E. "Come, Come Now." [Reply to Irving Singer, "Anti-Climax"] *New York Review of Books* (8 March 1973). <www.nybooks.com/articles/ 9923> [accessed 28 June 2005]; Benedek, Therese. "Discussion of Sherfey's Paper on Female

Sexuality." *Journal of the American Psychoanalytic Association* 16:3 (1968), 424–48; Blackledge, Catherine. *The Story of V: Opening Pandora's Box.* London: Wiedenfeld and Nicolson, 2003; Brecher, Edward M. "Women Rediscover Their Own Sexuality." In *The Sex Researchers.* Boston, Mass.: Little, Brown, 1969, 142–97; Brown, Ric[hard]. "Irving Singer and *The Goals of Human Sexuality.*" In David Goicoechea, ed., *The Nature and Pursuit of Love: The Philosophy of Irving Singer.* Amherst, N.Y.: Prometheus, 1995, 295–311; Ellis, Albert. "Is the Vaginal Orgasm a Myth?" In A. P. Pillay and Albert Ellis, eds., *Sex, Society, and the Individual.* Bombay, India: International Journal of Sexology Press, 1953, 155–62. Reprinted in Manfred F. DeMartino, ed., *Sexual Behavior and Personality Characteristics.* New York: Grove Press, 1963, 348–60; Fisher, Helen E. *The Sex Contract: The Evolution of Human Behavior.* New York: Morrow, 1982; Fisher, Seymour. *The Female Orgasm: Psychology, Physiology, Fantasy.* New York: Basic Books, 1973; Friedman, David. *A Mind of Its Own: A Cultural History of the Penis.* New York: Free Press, 2002; Geertz, Clifford. "Sociosexology." [Review of *The Evolution of Human Sexuality*, by Donald Symons] *New York Review of Books* (24 January 1980), 3–4; Glenn, Jules. "Types of Orgasm in Women. A Critical Review and Redefinition." *Journal of the American Psychoanalytic Association* 16:3 (1968), 549–64; Gould, Stephen Jay. "Freudian Slip." *Natural History* 96:2 (1987), 14–21; Gould, Stephen Jay. "Male Nipples and Clitoral Ripples." In *Bully for Brontosaurus: Reflections in Natural History.* New York: Norton, 1991, 124–38; Heiman, Marcel. "Female Sexuality. Introduction." *Journal of the American Psychoanalytic Association* 16:3 (1968), 565–68; Hrdy, Sarah Blaffer. "Empathy, Polyandry, and the Myth of the Coy Female." In Ruth Bleier, ed., *Feminist Approaches to Science.* New York: Pergamon, 1986, 119–46; Hrdy, Sarah Blaffer. "Female Reproductive Strategies." In Meredith F. Small, ed., *Female Primates: Studies by Women Primatologists.* New York: Alan R. Liss, 1984, 103–9; Keiser, Sylvan. "Discussion of Sherfey's Paper on Female Sexuality." *Journal of the American Psychoanalytic Association* 16:3 (1968), 449–56; Kestenberg, Judith S. "Discussion of Sherfey's Paper on Female Sexuality." *Journal of the American Psychoanalytic Association* 16:3 (1968), 417–23; Koedt, Anne. (1970) "The Myth of the Vaginal Orgasm." In Deborah Babcox and Madeline Belkin, eds., *Liberation Now! Writings from the Women's Liberation Movement.* New York: Dell, 1971, 311–20. <www.cwluherstory.com/CWLUArchive/vaginalmyth.html> [accessed 16 February 2005]; Lehrman, Sally. "The Virtues of Promiscuity." *AlterNet* (22 July 2002). <www.alternet.org/story .html?StoryID=13648> [accessed 16 February 2005]; Lowry, Thomas Power, ed. *The Classic Clitoris: Contributions to Scientific Sexuality.* Chicago, Ill.: Nelson-Hall, 1978; Lydon, Susan. (1968) "Understanding Orgasm." In Betty Roszak and Theodore Roszak, eds., *Masculine/Feminine: Readings in Sexual Mythology and the Liberation of Women.* New York: Harper and Row, 1969, 201–8; Mead, Margaret. "On Freud's View of Female Psychology." In Jean Strouse, ed., *Women and Analysis: Dialogues on Psychoanalytic Views of Femininity.* New York: Grossman, 1974, 95–106; Mitchell, Juliet. "The Clitoris and the Vagina." In *Psychoanalysis and Feminism: Freud, Reich, Laing, and Women.* New York: Vintage, 1975, 105–8; Moore, Burness. "Psychoanalytic Reflections on the Implications of Recent Physiological Studies of Female Orgasm." *Journal of the American Psychoanalytic Association* 16:3 (1968), 569–87; Nicholson, Paula. "Feminism and the Debate about Female Sexual Dysfunction: Do Women Really Know What They Want?" *Sexualities, Evolution, and Gender* 5:1 (2003), 37–39; Odier, Charles. (1948) *Anxiety and Magic Thinking.* Trans. Mary-Louise Schoelly and Mary Jane Sherfey. New York: International Universities Press, 1956; Orr, Douglas. "Anthropological and Historical Notes on the Female Sexual Role." *Journal of the American Psychoanalytic Association* 16:3 (1968), 601–12; Robertiello, R. C. "The 'Clitoral versus Vaginal Orgasm' Controversy and Some of Its Ramifications." *Journal of Sex Research* 6 (1970), 307–11; Seaman, Barbara. "Is Woman Insatiable?" In *Free and Female: The Sex Life of the Contemporary Woman.* New York: Coward, McCann, and Geoghegan, 1972, 25–47; Segal, Lynne. "Sensual Uncertainty, or Why the Clitoris Is Not Enough." In Sue Cartledge and Joanna Ryan, eds., *Sex and Love: New Thoughts on Old Contradictions.* London: Women's Press, 1983, 30–47; Sherfey, Mary Jane. "On the Nature of Female Sexuality." In Jean Baker Miller, ed., *Psychoanalysis and Women.* Harmondsworth, U.K.: Penguin, 1973, 136–53; Sherfey, Mary Jane. "Some Biology of Sexuality." *Journal of Sex and Marital Therapy* 1:2 (1974), 97–109; Singer, Irving. "Reply to Clemens E.

Benda." *New York Review of Books* (8 March 1973). <www.nybooks.com/articles/9923> [accessed 28 June 2005]; Small, Meredith F. *Female Choices: Sexual Behavior of Female Primates.* Ithaca, N.Y.: Cornell University Press, 1993; Stoller, Robert J. "Impact of New Advances in Sex Research on Psychoanalytic Theory." In *Perversion: The Erotic Form of Hatred.* New York: Dell, 1975, 12–45; Wallen, Kim. "The Evolution of Female Sexual Desire." In Paul R. Abramson and Steven D. Pinkerton, eds., *Sexual Nature Sexual Culture.* Chicago, Ill.: University of Chicago Press, 1995, 57–79.

SINGER, IRVING (1925–   ). Irving Singer, one of the most prolific philosophers of sex and **love** in the last third of the twentieth century and the beginning of the twenty-first, has devoted a good deal of his writings to examining two notable distinctions: the difference between "sensuous" and "passionate" sexuality, and another between the "appraisal" and "bestowal" components of love.

Born in Brooklyn, New York, Singer attended Brooklyn College (1941–1943), during the early involvement of the United States in World War II, and then served in the U.S. Army until 1946, having been in combat in Germany. He later earned his three degrees from Harvard University (A.B., 1948; M.A., 1949; Ph.D., 1952). In 1953 he began teaching at Cornell University, moving on to the University of Michigan (1956) and, finally, to the Massachusetts Institute of Technology in 1959, where he became professor of philosophy.

Singer has written around twenty books, not only on human love and sexuality but also on meaning in life, aesthetics, the Spanish American philosopher George Santayana (1863–1952), the films of Alfred Hitchcock (1899–1980) and other directors, and the operas of Wolfgang Amadeus Mozart (1756–1791) and Ludwig van Beethoven (1770–1827). He has also written many articles and reviews. His earliest piece on love, a discussion of the Spanish *existentialiste* philosopher José Ortega y Gasset (1883–1955), appeared in 1958 in the *Hudson Review.* His first book on sex, *The Goals of Human Sexuality*, a palatable mix of philosophy and **sexology**, came out in 1973.

Among Singer's philosophical writings, the three-volume *The Nature of Love* stands out as a magnificent, majestic achievement, a trilogy that combines Singer's own philosophical reflections on love with an exploration—comprehensive, detailed, clear, rigorous, insightful—of the history of the idea of love in Western philosophy as well as the arts and humanities more generally. In 1,300 or so pages, Singer educates us about and critically assesses the views of (to name a small number of his protagonists) **Plato, Aristotle**, Plotinus, Ovid, Lucretius, **Augustine, Aquinas**, and Luther (in volume 1); Capellanus, Dante, Shakespeare, **Rousseau, Sade**, Stendhal, **Kant**, Schlegel, **Hegel**, Shelley, Byron, Goethe, **Schopenhauer**, and Wagner (in volume 2, the longest); and **Kierkegaard, Nietzsche, Freud**, Proust, D. H. Lawrence, George Bernard Shaw, Jean-Paul Sartre, and Simone de Beauvoir (in volume 3). Along the way, Singer spends many pages on sexuality, a pleasantly unavoidable task when discussing the likes of Plato, the medieval Christians, **Hume**, Kant, Sade, Schopenhauer, Tolstoy, Lawrence, and Freud, if not nearly everyone else listed in the indices. The trilogy could have been faithfully titled, were it not so cumbersome, *The Natures of Love and Sex and Their Relationship or Lack of Same: A Philosophical History from Plato to Ti-Grace Atkinson, or 350 BCE to 1980.* This is explanation enough why, if there is one work in the philosophy of sex and love that is a must read for serious students of the subject, it is *The Nature of Love.* But not only the content will be found agreeable. In speaking about what the profoundly unromantic, unmasking Freud incisively detected in human love relationships, Singer elegantly expresses his underlying thought: "Flying into each other's arms in the hope of escaping the pain and ugliness of the ordinary world, they merely create a microcosm that includes the hatred and hostility which belong to the very being of intimacy" (*Nature*, vol. 3, 115).

It is in *Nature* that Singer lays out the distinction between appraisal and bestowal (vol. 1, "Appraisal and Bestowal," 3–22; vol. 3, "Toward a Modern Theory of Love," 369–437). If X likes, is attracted to, or desires Y in virtue of perceiving value in Y or in Y's traits or features, value that exists independently of X's feelings about and attitudes toward Y, then X has appraised Y. Appraisals of all kinds occur in various contexts and are everyday events. There is no formal difference between X's appraising a house or car before buying it and X's appraising Y. The idea that appraisal figures prominently in love might be attributable to Plato (427–347 BCE), for something like the formula *love is the desire for the perpetual possession of the beautiful and good* (vol. 1, 68) seems extractable from the *Symposium* (starting with the elenchus of Agathon, near 200e, and continuing through the instruction of Socrates by Diotima, e.g., 205e). Bestowal, or the conferring, imparting, or *giving* of value, is quite different from *responding* to value. "[L]ove creates a new value, one that is not reducible to the individual or objective value that something [or someone] may also have. This further type of valuing I call bestowal" (vol. 1, 5). On Singer's view, genuine human love is a combination of appraisal and bestowal: "Love is related to both; they interweave in it. Unless we appraised we could not bestow a value that goes beyond appraisal; and without bestowal there would be no love" (vol. 1, 9). If Plato's *eros* is an ancient model for an appraising type of love, Christian *agape* may be an appropriate model for love as the bestowal of value (vol. 1, chap. 13). "God does not love that which is already in itself worthy of love, but . . . that which in itself has no worth acquires worth just by becoming the object of God's love," wrote Anders Nygren ([1890–1978]; *Agape and Eros*, 78). Singer's distinction between appraisal and bestowal is not new, of course. At the very least, we should acknowledge Nygren's monumental treatise from the 1930s. His focus was theological. Singer, by contrast, not only used the distinction between appraisal and bestowal in exploring the history of the idea of love but also extensively applied it to the cases that are most interesting from a secular perspective, human-human romantic, erotic, and marital loves. (Beyond *Nature*, Singer's elaborations of appraisal and bestowal can be found in *The Pursuit of Love* and "Reply.")

Singer's writings on sex and love cover a wide spectrum of issues and topics, from those of perennial interest—Plato's heady discourses on *eros* in the *Symposium* and *Phaedrus*; Immanuel Kant's (1724–1804) anal-retentive sketch of human sexuality and his equally constipated sexual prohibitions; Sigmund Freud (1856–1939) on everything that ails us, or why we should be happy that we are not too unhappy; William Masters (1915–2001) and Virginia Johnson's much praised but monodimensional characterization of the orgasm of the human female—to questions of more recent vintage: whether **same-sex marriage** is altogether commendable; the future of sexual, loving relations between men and women in a world slouching ever more closely to complete sexual equality; and the implications of an ethical and social philosophy of sexual pluralism.

Singer first considered the distinction between sensuous and passionate sexuality in *The Goals of Human Sexuality* (chap. 2, 41–65). That material was rewritten and published nearly thirty years later in *Sex: A Philosophical Primer* (chap. 2, 17–63). More on the sensuous and the passionate can be found in Singer's book on the operas of Mozart and Beethoven, in *Explorations in Love and Sex*, and in his omnibus "Reply" to critics and commentators, those who convened for a three-day weekend colloquium in 1991 at Brock University specifically to read papers and converse about, principally but not exclusively, Singer's *Nature of Love*. According to Singer,

> In sexual behavior, men and women may concentrate upon sensory fulfillment and even seek to prolong it indefinitely. . . . For some people, sexuality amounts to little more than the sensuous, and even the end-pleasure of orgasmic relief becomes subordinate to the delights of intervening sensory enjoyment. (*Primer*, 19; cf. *Goals*, 41)

Here Singer is describing sensuous sexuality. In the passionate style, by contrast,

> sex is charged . . . with emotions of yearning, craving, anticipation, hopefulness, or trepidation, and possibly a sense of joyful oneness with another person. In this mode sexuality includes . . . [a] dissipation of sexual drive through a powerful release of pent-up energy. (*Primer*, 19; cf. *Goals*, 41–42)

So "the sensuous appears in our search for sensory gratification, the passionate in the goodness of emotional fulfillment" (*Explorations*, 65–66). Singer takes us on a compact walk through the history of the philosophy of sex, starting with Plato and ending with Freud, with many stops in between, illustrating how the sensuous and the passionate and the relationship between them are treated by various thinkers. Being a sexual pluralist, Singer is not about to judge one style better than the other (*Goals*, 79), although he does lay out the pros and cons of each type.

What sensuous sexuality has going for it is that its "consummations" (orgasms) may be easier to attain than in the passionate mode and that it provides an "immediate gratification" that "afford[s] moments of exquisite, even excruciating, sensory pleasure." What the passionate does is to "yield . . . a sense of importance that cannot come from the sensuous alone"; sensuousness seems "mindless and superficial." But passionate sexuality "runs the risk of being painful or mad" and is sometimes disruptive, destroying families and starting wars (*Primer*, 29–32; cf. *Goals*, 49–51). Further,

> In the passionate mode, orgasms can be overwhelming [*Goals*, 51: "tend to be emotionally very powerful"]. Nevertheless, they may not be more satisfying, and often are less enjoyable, than the pleasures of the sensuous. (*Primer*, 31)

In the central sexological chapter of *Goals*, Singer ties together the distinction between the sensuous and the passionate and the physiology and anatomy of female sexuality. His conclusion is either gratifying or annoying, depending on one's social and political attitudes: "There is reason to believe that *vulval* orgasms [commonly induced by clitoral manipulation] are consummations in which the sensuous predominates while *uterine* orgasms [commonly induced by penis-vagina intercourse] have a special dependency upon the passionate" (79, italics added).

Singer was not, back then, one to worry about offending politically correct sensibilities. He stood up to the Church of the Clitoral Orgasm, whose high priest and priestess were Masters and Johnson and whose missionaries were legions of phalloliberated feminists. But his "radical" thesis of the early 1970s, the association of sensuousness with "clitoral" orgasms and passionate sexuality with the "vaginal," with its supposition that these orgasms are physiologically and psychologically distinct entities, is missing from the section of *Explorations* (2001) where we expect to find it (60–68). In volume 3 of *Nature*, published in 1987, Singer mentions his thesis from *Goals* but is extremely cautious. He asks us to "leav[e] aside questions about the accuracy of my psychological and physiological speculations, which must be subject to the findings of empirical investigators" (376). A few years later, at the conference held in his honor, he gracefully admitted that "some of the physiological and biological details on which *The Goals* relied have now been shown to be mistaken" ("Reply," *Nature and Pursuit*, 346; *Explorations*, 143). It is far from unusual, however, for a piece of philosophy or science to go astray, yet in being bold and provocative instigates others to productive intellectual activity. "Investigators in the field began to sense the possibility of scientific, experimental work that had not been allowed previously. An exciting new approach to understanding human response in this area seemed to be opening up as never before" ("Reply," *Nature and Pursuit*, 345; *Explorations*, 142).

See also Ethics, Sexual; Friendship; Hobbes, Thomas; Love; Marriage; Marriage, Same-Sex; Philosophy of Sex, Overview of; Philosophy of Sex, Teaching the; Plato; Sexology; Sherfey, Mary Jane

REFERENCES

Nygren, Anders. *Den kristna kärlekstanken genom tiderna* (Part I, 1930; Part II, 1936). *Agape and Eros.* Trans. Philip S. Watson. Chicago, Ill.: University of Chicago Press, 1982; Plato. (ca. 380 BCE) *Symposium.* Trans. Alexander Nehamas and Paul Woodruff. Indianapolis, Ind.: Hackett, 1989; Singer, Irving. *Explorations in Love and Sex.* Lanham, Md.: Rowman and Littlefield, 2001; Singer, Irving. *George Santayana: Literary Philosopher.* New Haven, Conn.: Yale University Press, 2000; Singer, Irving. *The Goals of Human Sexuality.* New York: Norton, 1973. New York: Schocken, 1974; Singer, Irving. "Marriage: Same-Sex and Opposite-Sex." In *Sex: A Philosophical Primer*, exp. ed. Lanham, Md.: Rowman and Littlefield, 2004, ix–xxxii; Singer, Irving. *Meaning in Life: The Creation of Value.* New York: Free Press, 1992; Singer, Irving. "The Morality of Sex: Contra Kant." *Critical Horizons* 1:2 (2000), 175–91; Singer, Irving. *Mozart and Beethoven: The Concept of Love in Their Operas.* Baltimore, Md.: Johns Hopkins University Press, 1977; Singer, Irving. *The Nature of Love.* Vol. 1: *Plato to Luther* [1st ed., 1966], 2nd ed. Chicago, Ill.: University of Chicago Press, 1984. Vol. 2: *Courtly and Romantic*, 1984. Vol. 3: *The Modern World*, 1987; Singer, Irving. (1958) "Ortega on Love." In *Explorations in Love and Sex.* Lanham, Md.: Rowman and Littlefield, 2001, 199–216; Singer, Irving. *The Pursuit of Love.* Baltimore, Md.: Johns Hopkins University Press, 1994; Singer, Irving. "A Reply to My Critics and Friendly Commentators." In David Goicoechea, ed., *The Nature and Pursuit of Love: The Philosophy of Irving Singer.* Amherst, N.Y.: Prometheus, 1995, 323–61. Revised, reprinted as "The Nature and Pursuit of Love Revisited," in *Explorations in Love and Sex.* Lanham, Md.: Rowman and Littlefield, 2001, 105–67; Singer, Irving. *Sex: A Philosophical Primer.* Lanham, Md.: Rowman and Littlefield, 2001. Expanded edition, 2004; Singer, Irving. *Three Philosophical Filmmakers: Hitchcock, Welles, Renoir.* Cambridge, Mass.: MIT Press, 2004.

Alan Soble

ADDITIONAL READING

Benda, Clemens E. "Come, Come Now." [Reply to Irving Singer, "Anti-Climax"] *New York Review of Books* (8 March 1973). <www.nybooks.com/articles/9923> [accessed 28 June 2005]; Brown, Ric[hard]. "Irving Singer and *The Goals of Human Sexuality*." In David Goicoechea, ed., *The Nature and Pursuit of Love: The Philosophy of Irving Singer.* Amherst, N.Y.: Prometheus, 1995, 295–311. (Singer's reply: *The Nature and Pursuit of Love*, 345–48; *Explorations*, 141–46); Goicoechea, David, ed. *The Nature and Pursuit of Love: The Philosophy of Irving Singer.* Amherst, N.Y.: Prometheus, 1995; Koedt, Anne. (1970) "The Myth of the Vaginal Orgasm." In Deborah Babcox and Madeline Belkin, eds., *Liberation Now! Writings from the Women's Liberation Movement.* New York: Dell, 1971, 311–20. <www.cwluherstory.com/CWLUArchive/vaginalmyth.html> [accessed 16 February 2005]; Outka, Gene. *Agape: An Ethical Analysis.* New Haven, Conn.: Yale University Press, 1972; Robinson, Paul. *Sex, Opera, and Other Vital Matters.* Ithaca, N.Y.: Cornell University Press, 1995; Singer, Irving. "Anti-Climax." *New York Review of Books* (30 November 1972), 29–31; Singer, Irving. *The Creation of Value.* Baltimore, Md.: Johns Hopkins University Press, 1996; Singer, Irving. *Feeling and*

Imagination: The Vibrant Flux of Our Existence. Lanham, Md.: Rowman and Littlefield, 2001; Singer, Irving. *The Harmony of Nature and Spirit.* Baltimore, Md.: Johns Hopkins University Press, 1996; Singer, Irving. "The Morality of Sex: Contra Kant." *Critical Horizons* 1:2 (2000), 175–91. Reprinted in *Explorations in Love and Sex.* Lanham, Md.: Rowman and Littlefield, 2001, 1–20; POS4 (259–72); Singer, Irving. "Ortega on Love." *Hudson Review* 11:1 (1958), 145–54; Singer, Irving. *Reality Transformed: Film as Meaning and Technique.* Cambridge, Mass.: MIT Press, 1998; Singer, Irving. "Reply to Clemens E. Benda." *New York Review of Books* (8 March 1973). <www.nybooks.com/articles/9923> [accessed 28 June 2005]; Singer, Irving. *Santayana's Aesthetics.* Cambridge, Mass.: Harvard University Press, 1957. Reissued, *Santayana's Aesthetics: A Critical Introduction.* Westport, Conn.: Greenwood Press, 1973; Singer, Irving. "The Sensuous and the Passionate." In *The Goals of Human Sexuality.* New York: Norton, 1973. New York: Schocken, 1974, 41–65. Reprinted in POS1 (209–31); Singer, Irving. "Talking to the Doctor about Sex." [Review of *On the Nature of Things Erotic,* by F. Gonzalez-Crussi] *Los Angeles Times Book Review* (27 March 1988), 6; Singer, Irving. "Words and Music." *New York Review of Books* (20 April 1978). <www.nybooks.com/articles/8200> [accessed 14 February 2005]; Singer, Irving, ed. *Essays in Literary Criticism by George Santayana.* New York: Scribner's, 1956; Singer, Irving, and Josephine Singer. "Periodicity of Sexual Desire in Relation to Time of Ovulation in Women." *Journal of Biosocial Science* 4 (November 1972), 471–81; Soble, Alan. "Love and Value, Yet *Again.*" [Review essay of *The Reasons of Love,* by Harry G. Frankfurt] *Essays in Philosophy* 6:1 (2005). <www.humboldt .edu/~essays/soble2rev.html> [accessed 26 December 2004]; Soble, Alan. "Reconciling Eros and Agape." In *The Structure of Love.* New Haven, Conn.: Yale University Press, 1990, 23–28. Reprinted in STW (227–30); Soble, Alan. Review of *The Nature of Love,* vol. 3: *The Modern World,* by Irving Singer. *Canadian Philosophical Reviews* 8:2 (1988), 74–76; Vlastos, Gregory. "The Individual as an Object of Love in Plato." In *Platonic Studies.* Princeton, N.J.: Princeton University Press, 1973, 3–34. Reprinted in Alan Soble, ed., *Eros, Agape, and Philia: Readings in the Philosophy of Love.* New York: Paragon House, 1989, 96–124. Corrected reprint, 1999. Also, "Appendix II: Sex in Platonic Love," 38–42 (in Soble, 124–28); Žižek, Slavoj. *The Metastases of Enjoyment: Six Essays on Woman and Causality.* London: Verso, 1994.

SOCIAL CONSTRUCTIONISM. Social constructionists claim that **sexual orientation** is a cultural and historical, rather than natural, feature of persons. According to constructionists, the categories "homosexual" and "heterosexual" are relatively recent inventions: Prior to the late nineteenth century, there were no homosexuals or heterosexuals. Constructionists do not thereby claim that no one engaged in same-sex or other-sex acts back then but, rather, that those people who performed these sexual acts should not be labeled homosexuals and heterosexuals, since that mode of personal and cultural identity simply did not exist before the nineteenth century. (The same could be said for bisexuals.) According to constructionists, people are no more naturally divided into sexual orientations than the globe is naturally divided into various countries. Instead, history and culture invent the categories, and various cultures have drawn the sexual (or geographical) lines in various ways. Thus, constructionists think of differences in sexual orientation like differences in social class: People are not "naturally" lords or serfs, for example; they are lords or serfs only given a particular cultural and historical context. For constructionists, the same is true of sexual orientation.

Constructionism is typically contrasted with *essentialism,* which holds that sexual orientation is an objective, intrinsic, and culturally independent property of persons. According to essentialists, the categories of sexual orientation are transcultural and transhistorical, even though sexual orientations may manifest themselves in different ways in different places and times. Thus, an ancient Athenian male who sexually desired boys but not women would "count" as a gay male, according to essentialists, even though the age-hierarchy in his desires, which was typical in ancient Greece, does not correspond to the experience of most gay men today. **John Boswell** (1947–1994), widely considered a para-digmatic essentialist, has noted that "no one involved in [the essentialist-constructionist] debate actually identifies him- or herself as an 'essentialist,' although constructionists (of whom, in contrast, there are many) sometimes so label other writers" (34–35).

Some have compared the essentialist-constructionist debate to the philosophical debate between realists and nominalists (Boswell, 18 ff.). Essentialists are realists about sexual orientation: They believe that the categories of sexual orientation are real categories that are there to be discovered, despite whether anyone recognizes them. Constructionists, by contrast, are nominalists: They believe that the categories of sexual orientation are in-vented, not discovered.

Because there is much popular confusion about the precise boundaries of the essentialist-constructionist debate, as well as controversy among the participants themselves, it is useful to detail what the debate is *not* about. First, the essentialist-constructionist debate is some-times confused with the nature-nurture debate. The nature-nurture debate involves the cause or origin (aetiology) of sexual orientation; more precisely, it attempts to trace the factors, biological and environmental, that influence its development. Those who support the "nature" view claim that sexual orientation is innate (the result of genetic or other bio-logical factors); those who support the "nurture" view claim that it is learned or acquired. But the nature/nurture debate does not line up with the essentialist-constructionist debate in any straightforward way.

Many people mistakenly believe that essentialists must support the "nature" view and constructionists must support the "nurture" view. But although a biological marker for sex-ual orientation would support essentialism—since it would provide an objective, transhis-torical property grounding sexual orientation—the converse does not hold. It is possible to be an essentialist and yet to hold that the objective property of sexual orientation is not in-nate but acquired (perhaps in early childhood). Thus essentialists need not support the "nature" view, although those who support the "nature" view must be essentialists if they believe that biological factors are the *whole* aetiological story behind sexual orientation.

Constructionists must deny that sexual orientation is innate. After all, a biological marker for sexual orientation would be precisely the kind of transcultural objective prop-erty that constructionists reject and essentialists support. So if sexual orientation is not in-nate, it would seem to follow that it is acquired, as the "nurture" view claims. However, the idea that there is a genetic or other biological marker that exhaustively determines sexual orientation is simplistic. A more plausible view is that genes influence brain development and resulting psychological dispositions, including **sexual desire**s. These desires may or may not result in heterosexual or homosexual identity—that is, self-identification or public recognition as "straight" or "gay"—depending on various cultural circumstances. Thus, a constructionist could grant that genes strongly influence sexual desire, a concession that sounds closer to the "nature" view than the "nurture" view, but still deny that a person with these genetically influenced desires automatically "counts" as having a particular sexual orientation if the appropriate developmental context and resulting social identity are ab-sent. In that way, a constructionist could support something like the "nature" view without abandoning constructionism.

Another debate that is often confused with both the nature-nurture and essentialist-constructionist debates is what we might call the "voluntarist-involuntarist" debate. The voluntarist-involuntarist debate involves whether sexual orientation can be changed (perhaps through therapy). Although many people seem to believe that essentialists must be involuntarists and constructionists must be voluntarists, neither belief is correct.

Holding that sexual orientation is an objective and transcultural property is not tantamount to holding that it is immutable. For there is a difference between a property's being objective, in the relevant sense, and its being impervious to change. For example, being pregnant is objective and transcultural but not immutable; birth, miscarriage, and **abortion** cause it to change. Therefore, essentialists need not be involuntarists. Nor must constructionists be voluntarists, for holding that sexual orientation is socially constructed is not tantamount to holding that it is changeable. As David Halperin, a prominent constructionist, writes,

> Just because my sexuality is an artefact of cultural processes doesn't mean I'm not stuck with it. Particular cultures are contingent, but the personal identities and forms of erotic life that take shape within the horizons of those cultures are not. To say that sexuality is learned is not to say that it can be unlearned— any more than to say that culture changes is to say that it is malleable. (*One Hundred Years*, 51–52)

So there is no necessary connection between essentialism and involuntarism or between constructionism and voluntarism. Similarly, there is no necessary connection between involuntarism and "nature" or voluntarism and "nurture." That a trait is innate ("nature") does not mean that it cannot be changed: Genetics determine hair color, for example, but people can dye their hair. Nor does a trait's being learned ("nurture") mean that it cannot be unlearned. Consider the happy changeability of some of the bad habits we pick up at some point from friends or siblings. So if the essentialist-constructionist debate is not about the aetiology of orientation or about its changeability, what is it about?

One way of capturing the debate is to ask whether sexual orientation is *transhistorical* and *transcultural*, as essentialists claim, rather than culture-bound, as constructionists claim. Jonathan Katz, a prominent constructionist, claims that sexual orientation is "given meaning and character by its location in time and social space" (7), though this claim is somewhat ambiguous, for even essentialists concede that historical circumstances can influence the way sexual orientation is expressed and in that sense give sexual orientation some of its "meaning and character." The constructionists, however, assert a stronger claim: Without the appropriate social context, there is no **homosexuality** or heterosexuality but only homosexual and heterosexual acts and desires. As Robert Padgug writes, the categories of homosexuality and heterosexuality

> in fact take what are no more than a group of more or less closely related acts ("homosexual"/"heterosexual" behavior) and convert them into case studies of people ("homosexuals"/"heterosexuals"). This conversion of acts into roles/personalities, and ultimately into entire subcultures, cannot be said to have been accomplished before at least the seventeenth century, and, as a firm belief and more or less close approximation of reality, the late nineteenth century. What we call "homosexuality" (in the sense of the distinguishing traits of "homosexuals"), for example, was not considered a unified set of acts, much less a set of qualities defining particular persons, in pre-capitalist societies. (57)

Padgug emphasizes that "homosexuality" and "heterosexuality" (as well as, presumably, other orientations such as "**bisexuality**") refer to more than merely behaviors or desires: They delineate *kinds* of persons. Here Padgug echoes the thought of **Michel Foucault**

(1926–1984). In his *History of Sexuality,* writing of the nineteenth-century shift to which Padgug alludes, Foucault observes, "The sodomite had been a temporary aberration; the homosexual was now a species" (43).

Some anticonstructionists have argued that while premodern societies may not have used the *words* "homosexual" and "heterosexual," they certainly had the concepts. They often point to ancient texts, such as Aristophanes's speech at the banquet in **Plato**'s (427–347 BCE) *Symposium*, to support this point. Plato portrays the comic poet Aristophanes as relating a myth of three primordial "gender" types, each consisting of a double body: male-male, female-female, and male-female (the androgyne or hermaphrodite). After being split in two by Zeus (as punishment for not sufficiently respecting the gods), the resulting halves desperately sought to cling to their former counterparts. Plato's Aristophanes claims that the differences in sexual interest among his "postlapsarian" contemporaries can be explained by their having descended from different original types (*Symp.* 189e–93d).

Boswell (often cited as an essentialist, though he eschewed the label) argued that the myth's "manifest and stated purpose is to explain why humans are divided into groups of predominately homosexual or heterosexual interest. It is strongly implied that these interests are both exclusive and innate" (25). Halperin, along with other constructionists, disagrees, noting that on Aristophanes's account, male homosexuality and lesbianism are treated as distinct, separate categories, while male and female heterosexuality are lumped together into a shared third category. Moreover, the male homosexual category is further divided into boys who are attracted to men and men who are lovers of boys; it does not comprise male homosexuals *simpliciter* (that is, males who are attracted to males of any age or social status). On this basis, Halperin argues that the "conclusions that [Aristophanes] draws from his own myth help to illustrate the lengths to which classical Athenians were willing to go to avoid conceptualizing sexual behaviors according to a binary opposition between different- and same-sex sexual contacts" ("Sex before Sexuality," 44).

A *caveat*: While the presence of sexual orientation concepts in other cultures provides some evidence for sexual orientation's being a "natural" or "essential" rather than a "constructed" characteristic, such evidence is not conclusive. Ancient Romans and contemporary Americans have the concept of "senator," but the role of senator is clearly socially constructed. Conversely, the fact that a given society lacks a concept does not prove, by itself, that the thing to which the concept refers is constructed. It is possible for properties to exist without people recognizing them at a given time; humans had blood types before they had the concept "blood type." Further, even if a society lacks any particular incidence of a property (and not just the concept of that property), it does not follow that the property is socially constructed. The fact that a property is "natural" and objective does not entail that it is instantiated in every human culture; it is easy to imagine a culture's lacking persons with type AB blood, but blood type is "natural," as opposed to socially constructed, if anything is. (Some constructionists claim that *all* reality is socially constructed, but if they are right, constructionism about sexual orientation loses any interesting point of contrast; see Stein, 108–9.)

Richard Mohr has accused some constructionists of understanding the categories of sexual orientation so narrowly that it is trivially true that the categories are historically and culturally bound. He draws an analogy between sexual orientation concepts and "yuppie," an apparently culturally specific concept:

> If one defines "yuppie" in such a way that in the very definition there is an essential reference to Volvos or VCRs or [the television drama] "thirtysomething,"

> then necessarily the term can apply only to the modern era. On this account, it is question-beggingly true that yuppies did not exist in Attic Greece. If, however, one defines yuppies as middle-aged, effete, money-grubbing conspicuous consumers, then we have something that at least in theory could apply to other eras and places; it has at least the possibility of being instantiated in different cultures because definitionally it is culturally neutral. (237)

Similarly, if we define "homosexual" to include only those homosexuals with a modern sensibility, it is trivially true that no homosexuals existed in ancient Greece: On such a narrow definition, a premodern homosexual is impossible. Mohr thinks, however, that such a definition is clearly too narrow, and so he rejects this constructionist approach. If social constructionists wanted to rebut Mohr, they would need to formulate a definition of "homosexual" that is broad enough to be applicable in theory to pre-nineteenth-century persons, but that does not in fact apply to any such persons.

Still another way of construing the essentialist-constructionist debate is to ask whether sexual orientations are what philosophers call "natural kinds." One philosopher who adopts this approach is Edward Stein. Stein defines natural kinds as nonarbitrary groups that "play a role in scientific laws and explanations"; he defines natural human kinds as natural kinds that apply to people (81, 84). Natural human kinds include such categories as hemophiliacs, people with XY chromosomes, and biological mothers. They do not include the categories people named Ethel, registered Democrats, or readers of this paragraph. The latter are social, nominal, or "artifactual" kinds: categories that exist only in virtue of human intentions. Unlike natural kinds, social kinds do not "cut nature at its joints" or reveal some fundamental underlying structure in the members of the kind. (Note that the debate about natural kinds is not the nature-nurture debate.)

Are sexual orientations natural kinds? Essentialists seem to think so. Yet according to Stein (a moderate constructionist), that is a mistake. Stein illustrates the problem by developing an analogy. In (the fictional land) Zomnia, residents are especially concerned with one another's sleep habits. Most Zomnians sleep "oriented" on their stomachs ("fronters"), and until recently there has been pervasive discrimination against the minority who sleep on their backs ("backers.") But backer-rights-groups have begun to form, and an interest among Zomnians in the study of sleep orientation has emerged. So Zomnians treat sleep orientation much as we treat sexual orientation.

Stein contends that the Zomnians mistakenly treat the categories of sleep orientation as natural kinds. "Implicit in the Zomnian use of the terms 'backer' and 'fronter' is a view of human nature according to which a person's sleep orientation is a deep and important fact. . . . [But] it is a mistake to think that there are groups of these people that fit into these categories in virtue of natural and objective facts" (Stein, 74). Rather, "backer" and "fronter" should be viewed as social or "artifactual" kinds. Essentialists about sexual orientation, according to Stein, make a similar mistake, assuming that members of a given sexual orientation share an objective underlying trait, such as a genetic marker, that is amenable to scientific investigation, and investing that supposed trait with excessive importance.

The Zomnian analogy usefully illustrates the difference between natural and social kinds as applied to human traits. But it may also suggest a problem with characterizing the essentialist-constructionist debate as a debate about natural kinds. For there are at least two separate issues here: first, whether sleep orientations (or sexual orientations) are nonarbitrary categories that play a role in scientific explanations (that is, whether they are natural kinds), and second, whether those categories have, or should have, significance in social and political life. These issues vary independently. Some natural kinds (people with type AB blood) have little significance; some merely social kinds (convicted felons) have a great deal. The essentialist-constructionist debate seems to be primarily a debate about significance, in particular, about how differences in sexual attraction and behavior are important to self-concept and public identity. At least, those are the issues that constructionists typically focus on, and settling these issues of significance will not settle the issue of whether sexual orientations are natural kinds.

Such problems tend to confirm the widespread belief that participants in the essentialist-constructionist debate may be arguing past each other. Perhaps, for example, essentialists and constructionists are interested in different issues: Essentialists are primarily concerned with sexual *desire*, whereas constructionists are primarily concerned about sexual *identity* (Halwani). Some even believe that "essentialism" is largely a strawman created by constructionists, a point that is supported by the widespread eschewing of the essentialist label. Perhaps it would be fruitful to move beyond the essentialist-constructionist debate to formulate new questions about sexual orientation, its origins, contours, and significance. Note, too, that while we have focused here on the social construction of sexual orientation, one might also explore the social construction of sex itself, or of gender, or a variety of other things connected with sexuality.

See also Beauty; Bisexuality; Boswell, John; Evolution; Foucault, Michel; Homosexuality and Science; Intersexuality; MacKinnon, Catharine; Mead, Margaret; Money, John; Orientation, Sexual; Psychology, Evolutionary; Psychology, Twentieth- and Twenty-First-Century; Queer Theory; Sex Education; Sexology

REFERENCES

Boswell, John. "Revolutions, Universals, and Sexual Categories." In Martin Duberman, Martha Vicinus, and George Chauncey, Jr., eds., *Hidden from History: Reclaiming the Gay and Lesbian Past*. New York: Meridian, 1990, 17–36; Foucault, Michel. (1976) *The History of Sexuality*, vol. 1: *An Introduction*. Trans. Robert Hurley. New York: Vintage, 1978; Halperin, David M. *One Hundred Years of Homosexuality: And Other Essays on Greek Love*. New York: Routledge, 1990; Halperin, David M. "Sex before Sexuality: Pederasty, Politics, and Power in Classical Athens." In Martin Duberman, Martha Vicinus, and George Chauncey, Jr., eds. *Hidden from History: Reclaiming the Gay and Lesbian Past*. New York: Meridian, 1990, 37–53; Halwani, Raja. "Prolegomena to Any Future Metaphysics of Sexual Identity: Recasting the Essentialism and Social Constructionism Debate." In Linda Alcoff, Michael Hames-Garcia, Satya Mohanty, and Paula Moya, eds., *Redefining Identity Politics*. New York: Palgrave, 2005; Katz, Jonathan. *Gay American History*. New York: Crowell, 1976; Mohr, Richard D. "The Thing of It Is: Some Problems with Models for the Social Construction of Homosexuality." In *Gay Ideas: Outing and Other Controversies*. Boston, Mass.: Beacon Press, 1992, 221–42; Padgug, Robert. "Sexual Matters: On Conceptualizing Sexuality in History." In Edward Stein, ed., *Forms of Desire: Sexual Orientation and the Social Constructionist Controversy*. New York: Routledge, 1992, 43–67; Plato. (ca. 380 BCE) *Symposium*. Trans. Alexander Nehamas and Paul Woodruff. Indianapolis, Ind.: Hackett, 1989; Stein, Edward. *The Mismeasure of Desire: The Science, Theory, and Ethics of Sexual Orientation*. New York: Oxford University Press, 1999.

John Corvino

ADDITIONAL READING

Abelove, Henry, Michèle Aina Barale, and David M. Halperin, eds. *The Lesbian and Gay Studies Reader*. New York: Routledge, 1993; Boswell, John. "Revolutions, Universals, and Sexual Categories." *Salmagundi*, nos. 58–59 (Fall 1982–Winter 1983), 89–113. Reprinted, with "Postscript" (1988), in Martin Duberman, Martha Vicinus, and George Chauncey, Jr., eds., *Hidden from History:*

Reclaiming the Gay and Lesbian Past. New York: New American Library, 1989, 17–36; and John Corvino, ed., *Same Sex: Debating the Ethics, Science, and Culture of Homosexuality*. Lanham, Md.: Rowman and Littlefield, 1997, 185–202; Calhoun, Cheshire. "Making Up Emotional People: The Case of Romantic Love." In Susan A. Bandes, ed., *The Passions of Law*. New York: New York University Press, 1999, 217–40; Church, Jennifer. "Social Constructionist Models: Making Order Out of Disorder—On the Social Construction of Madness." In Jennifer Radden, ed., *The Philosophy of Psychiatry: A Companion*. New York: Oxford University Press, 2004, 393–406; Corvino, John, ed. "Identity and History." Part III of *Same Sex: Debating the Ethics, Science, and Culture of Homosexuality*. Lanham, Md.: Rowman and Littlefield, 1997, 177–263; Davidson, Arnold I. "Sex and the Emergence of Sexuality." *Critical Inquiry* 14:1 (1987), 16–48. Reprinted in *The Emergence of Sexuality: Historical Epistemology and the Formation of Concepts*. Cambridge, Mass.: Harvard University Press, 2001, 30–65; and Edward Stein, ed., *Forms of Desire: Sexual Orientation and the Social Constructionist Controversy*. New York: Routledge, 1992, 89–132; Davidson, Arnold I. "Styles of Reasoning, Conceptual History, and the Emergence of Psychiatry." In Peter Galison and David J. Strump, eds., *The Disunity of Science: Boundaries, Contexts, and Power*. Stanford, Calif.: Stanford University Press, 1996, 75–100. Reprinted, abridged, as "Conceptual History and Conceptions of Perversions," in P&S2 (476–86); DeLamater, John, and Janet Hyde. "Essentialism vs. Social Constructionism in the Study of Human Sexuality." *Journal of Sex Research* 35:1 (1998), 10–18; Diorio, Joseph A. "Feminist-Constructionist Theories of Sexuality and the Definition of Sex Education." *Educational Philosophy and Theory* 21:2 (1989), 23–31; Duberman, Martin, Martha Vicinus, and George Chauncey, Jr., eds. *Hidden from History: Reclaiming the Gay and Lesbian Past*. New York: Meridian, 1990; Dynes, Wayne R. "Wrestling with the Social Boa Constructor." In Edward Stein, ed., *Forms of Desire: Sexual Orientation and the Social Constructionist Controversy*. New York: Routledge, 1992, 209–38; Fausto-Sterling, Anne. *Sexing the Body: Gender Politics and the Construction of Sexuality*. New York: Basic Books, 2000; Fine, Arthur. "Science Made Up: Constructivist Sociology of Scientific Knowledge." In Peter Galison and David J. Strump, eds., *The Disunity of Science: Boundaries, Contexts, and Power*. Stanford, Calif.: Stanford University Press, 1996, 231–54; Foucault, Michel. (1976, 1984, 1984) *The History of Sexuality*, 3 vols. Trans. Robert Hurley. New York: Vintage, 1988–1990; Greenberg, David F. *The Construction of Homosexuality*. Chicago, Ill.: University of Chicago Press, 1988; Groenhout, Ruth. "Essentialist Challenges to Liberal Feminism." *Social Theory and Practice* 28:1 (2002), 51–75. Reprinted in Judith A. Boss, ed., *Analyzing Moral Issues*, 3rd ed. New York: McGraw-Hill, 2005, 581–89; Halperin, David M. "Sex before Sexuality: Pederasty, Politics, and Power in Classical Athens." In Martin Duberman, Martha Vicinus, and George Chauncey, Jr., eds., *Hidden from History: Reclaiming the Gay and Lesbian Past*. New York: New American Library, 1989, 37–53. Reprinted in John Corvino, ed., *Same Sex: Debating the Ethics, Science, and Culture of Homosexuality*. Lanham, Md.: Rowman and Littlefield, 1997, 203–19; Halwani, Raja. "Essentialism, Social Constructionism, and the History of Homosexuality." *Journal of Homosexuality* 35:1 (1998), 25–51; Harding, Jennifer. "Sexual Investigations—Essentialism and Constructionism." In *Sex Acts: Practices of Femininity and Masculinity*. London: Sage, 1998, 8–22; Jackson, Stevi, and Sue Scott, eds. "Essentialism and Social Constructionism." [Part One] In *Feminism and Sexuality: A Reader*. New York: Columbia University Press, 1996, 35–109; Jordan, Mark D. *The Invention of Sodomy in Christian Theology*. Chicago, Ill.: University of Chicago Press, 1997; Katz, Jonathan Ned. *The Invention of Heterosexuality*. New York: Dutton, 1995; Kennedy, Elizabeth Lapovsky, and Madeline Davis. (1987) "The Reproduction of Butch-Fem Roles: A Social Constructionist Approach." In Kathy Peiss and Christina Simmons, eds., *Passion and Power: Sexuality in History*. Philadelphia, Pa.: Temple University Press, 1989, 241–56; Koertge, Noretta. "Constructing Concepts of Sexuality: A Philosophical Commentary." In David P. McWhirter, Stephanie A. Sanders, and June M. Reinisch, eds., *Homosexuality/Heterosexuality: Concepts of Sexual Orientation*. New York: Oxford University Press, 1990, 387–97; Koertge, Noretta. "The Fallacy of Misplaced Precision." *Journal of Homosexuality* 10 (1984), 15–21; MacKinnon, Catharine A. (1997) "Keeping It Real: On Anti-'Essentialism.'" In *Women's Lives, Men's Laws*. Cambridge, Mass.: Harvard University Press, 2005, 84–90; Mondschein, Ken. "Surpassing the Love of Women: Male Homosexuality in the Pre-Modern World." *Renaissance* 9:6, no. 40 (2004), 43–50; Murray, Stephen O. *Homosexualities*. Chicago, Ill.: University of Chicago Press, 2000; Murray, Stephen O. *Social Theory, Homosexual Realities*. New York: Gay Academic Union, 1984; Nussbaum, Martha C. "Constructing Love, Desire, and Care." In David M. Estlund and Martha C. Nussbaum, eds., *Sex, Preference, and Family: Essays on Law and Nature*. New York: Oxford University Press, 1997, 17–43; Padgug, Robert A. "Gay Villain, Gay Hero: Homosexuality and the Social Construction of AIDS." In Kathy Peiss and Christina Simmons, eds., *Passion and Power: Sexuality in History*. Philadelphia, Pa.: Temple University Press, 1989, 293–313; Padgug, Robert A. "Sexual Matters: On Conceptualizing Sexuality in History." *Radical History Review* 20 (Spring–Summer 1979), 3–23. Reprinted in Edward Stein, ed., *Forms of Desire: Sexual Orientation and the Social Constructionist Controversy*. New York: Routledge, 1992; Posner, Richard A. "Social Constructionism." In *Sex and Reason*. Cambridge, Mass.: Harvard University Press, 1992, 23–30; Réaume, Denise G. "The Social Construction of Women and the Possibility of Change: Unmodified Feminism Revisited." *Canadian Journal of Women and the Law* 5:2 (1992), 463–83; Reynaud, Emmanuel. "Holy Virility: The Social Construction of Masculinity." In Peter F. Murphy, ed., *Feminism and Masculinities*. New York: Oxford University Press, 2004, 136–48; Simson, Rennie. "The Afro-American Female: The Historical Context of the Construction of Sexual Identity." In Ann Snitow, Christine Stansell, and Sharon Thompson, eds., *Powers of Desire: The Politics of Sexuality*. New York: Monthly Review Press, 1983, 229–35; Stein, Edward. "Essentialism and Constructionism about Sexual Orientation." In David L. Hull and Michael Ruse, eds., *The Philosophy of Biology*. Oxford, U.K.: Oxford University Press, 1998, 427–42. Also "Essentialism and Constructionism in Sexual Orientation." In Robert B. Baker, Kathleen J. Wininger, and Frederick A. Elliston, eds., *Philosophy and Sex*, 3rd ed. Amherst, N.Y.: Prometheus, 1998, 383–96; Stein, Edward, ed. *Forms of Desire: Sexual Orientation and the Social Constructionist Controversy*. New York: Garland, 1990. New York: Routledge, 1992; Thornton, Bruce S. "Social Constructionism and Ancient Greek Sex." *Helios* 18 (1991), 181–93; Thorp, John. "The Social Construction of Homosexuality." *Phoenix* 46:1 (1992), 54–65. <www.fordham.edu/halsall/med/thorp.html> [accessed 14 October 2004]; Tiefer, Leonore. (1995) *Sex Is Not a Natural Act and Other Essays*, 2nd ed. Boulder, Colo.: Westview, 2004; Udry, J. Richard. "Sociology and Biology: What Biology Do Sociologists Need to Know?" *Social Forces* 73:4 (1995), 1267–78; Williams, Craig A. "Sexual Roles and Identities." In *Roman Homosexuality: Ideologies of Masculinity in Classical Antiquity*. New York: Oxford University Press, 1999, 160–224; Wilson, Fiona. "The Social Construction of Sexual Harassment and Assault of University Students." *Journal of Gender Studies* 9:2 (2000), 171–88.

SOCIOBIOLOGY. *See* Evolution; Psychology, Evolutionary

SOLOMON, ROBERT C. *See* Communication Model

SPENCER, HERBERT (1820–1903). As a boy in England, Herbert Spencer was taught by his father and uncle. After working as an engineer on the construction of railways (1837–1841), he served as subeditor of *The Economist* (1848–1853), a London weekly that advocated free trade, a position that accorded with his lifelong antipathy to all but the most circumscribed of governmental activity. The rest of his life was spent writing and studying. He was largely self-taught and had no affiliation with any educational institution, apart from three months of school teaching (1837). More than half his literary output comprises the ten-volume *System of Synthetic Philosophy* (1862–1896), which includes biology, psychology, sociology, and ethics: a series of subjects that involves a temporal and logical progression and whose study, on his view, depends on some understanding of earlier members of the series. There must be life before there is thought and feeling; thought and feeling before social organization; and social organization before moral awareness or ethical institutions. Spencer's treatment of human sexuality accords with this evolutionary scheme.

Individuals die, whence the need for replacement by reproduction. The conflicting interests of different generations are subordinated or reconciled in various ways. The course of **evolution** involves a decrease in the sacrifice of individual life to that of the species, as is apparent from the extreme cases of protozoa, whose parents disappear completely in the life of progeny, and (by contrast) mammals, where the interests of parents and offspring are better reconciled. In mammals, the lives of adults are minimally subordinated to the rearing of children, as a result of four processes: (1) the elongation of the period that precedes reproduction, (2) fewer offspring being born, (3) an increase of the pleasure parents take in the care of them, and (4) the parents' longevity after cessation of reproduction.

Spencer's developed treatment of human sexuality is in volume 1 of *Principles of Ethics*, which includes chapters on chastity, **marriage**, and parenthood. He acknowledged that levels of chastity and social development are imperfectly correlated (§183). He believed, nevertheless, that there are general causal relationships exhibited by extreme types of society (§185). Attitudes toward chastity are likely to be more lax when or where food is plentiful and the mischief of leaving a child solely to its mother's care is less than in a harsher environment. Also, high rates of fecundity are likely to be esteemed in unsettled societies, where mortality from violence is great. Moreover, in militant societies where women are acquired as spoils of war or are exchanged commercially, the unrestrained egoism of men limits the growth of chastity (§186). However, a good social state cannot, for the following reasons, arise or be maintained without chastity: (1) Lack of paternal support must leave a mother overtaxed and entails inadequate nutrition of progeny; (2) promiscuity is inconsistent with the higher sentiments of affection, admiration, and sympathy, which have grown out of the sexual instinct and prompt people to establish monogamous relationships (§187). Moreover, (3) since social altruism grows out of altruism within the family, it is unlikely to develop without the context in which it is first nurtured by the practice of subordinating self to others (§76). And (4), much fiction, drama, poetry, and music are inspired by romantic **love**. Without chastity these art forms and the aesthetic pleasures they foster would be undermined (§187).

Celibacy, denying as it does the gratification of natural instincts, has unwelcome mental and physiological consequences. The married state, however, provides an opportunity for their fulfillment and brings into play the altruistic emotions that pertain to partnership and parenthood. Stable marriage, with its attendant responsibilities, is also an incentive to more assiduous application in the other business of life. These beneficial effects come about only if the marriage is based on the appropriate emotions, not if it is contracted for mercenary or dynastic reasons (§231). Marriages not based on affection are "reversions to those of earlier types, such as those found among the rudest savages" (§233).

Children are best born to women in the full vigor of their early years. If people marry too young, they are likely to be improvident, but if they wait too long, they will be past the time when they are most fit for childbearing and child rearing. The reconciliation of these two conflicting considerations involves elements of risk and compromise (§232). Spencer would surely have recoiled in horror at the way fertility is now artificially induced in women well past the biologically optimal age of childbearing.

Although spontaneous affection is necessary for a happy marriage, it is not sufficient for a suitably fruitful one, for which reason due care should be taken in the choice of a partner. Sickly, feebleminded, and ill-natured people make bad breeding stock who will bequeath defective constitutions to their progeny. (See similar ideas in the First Wave feminist Victoria Woodhull; 1838–1927.) Also, both children and parents will suffer if parents beget more than for which they can adequately provide (§234). Moreover, "in large [i.e., densely populated] nations, where multiplication is rather an evil than a benefit, the obligation [to reproduce] lapses; and the individual may . . . fitly discharge his or her indebtedness in some other way than by adding to the population" (§230).

The tendency toward state aid to parents (only incipient in Spencer's lifetime in the provision of publicly funded education) was one that he castigated with implacable vehemence, believing that parenthood is part of a natural mechanism that cannot be tampered with beneficially.

> Agitators and legislators have united in spreading a theory which, logically followed out, ends in the monstrous conclusion that it is for parents to beget children and for society to take care of them. . . . A system under which parental duties are performed wholesale by those who are not the parents, under the plea that many parents cannot or will not perform their duties—a system which thus fosters the inferior children of inferior parents at the necessary cost of superior parents and consequent injury of superior children—a system which thus helps incapables to multiply and hinders the multiplication of capables, or diminishes their capability, must bring decay and eventual extinction. (§236)

This is consonant with the thesis of the "survival of the fittest"—a phrase Spencer coined in 1864 (*Principles of Biology*, §165). A rigorous version of this principle pervades his first book *Social Statics* (1851), where he maintained, eight years before Charles Darwin's (1809–1882) *Origin of Species*, that nature constantly weeds out the physically, intellectually, and morally unfit and government should not intervene to preserve them (378–80).

Since the middle of the last century, sexuality has been discussed with increasing candor, and in Western democracies tolerance has been extended to a much wider range of lifestyles than would once have seemed conceivable. This new freedom is, however, accompanied by an acute malaise. In a recent book, Cheshire Calhoun writes: "Cultural conservatives charge liberalism with breeding an excessive emphasis on personal choice, self-expression, and lifestyle experimentation. The consequence is that we now live in a 'sex-riddled, divorce-prone' culture that militates against the development of such personal and civic virtues as self-sacrifice, self-discipline, planning for the future, concern for others, responsible conduct, and loyalty" (111). These charges are not easily refuted. The evils that now beset us are entirely consistent with a failure to live up to the conditions that Spencer specified as necessary for personal fulfillment and social well-being, which vindicates him as a thinker of great penetration and foresight. He held strong, coherent, and cogently argued opinions on issues of perennial interest, that is, the adverse personal and social consequences of sexual promiscuity; the proper emotional and economic foundations of sexual relationships; and the circumstances under which children should be born and raised. That much of what he wrote is now thought controversial and "politically incorrect" does not disqualify him as a subject for serious study.

See also Casual Sex; Evolution; Marriage; Psychology, Evolutionary

REFERENCES

Calhoun, Cheshire. *Feminism, the Family, and the Politics of the Closet: Lesbian and Gay Displacement.* New York: Oxford University Press, 2000. Chapter 5, "Defending Marriage," 107–31. Reprinted in POS4, 147–73; Darwin, Charles. *On the Origin of Species.* London: John Murray,

1859; Hudson, William Henry. *An Introduction to the Philosophy of Herbert Spencer*, 2nd ed. London: Watts, 1904; Kennedy, James G. *Herbert Spencer*. Boston, Mass.: Twayne's English Authors Series, no. 219, 1978; Spencer, Herbert. "The Ethics of Kant." In *Essays: Scientific, Political and Speculative*, vol. 3. London: Williams and Norgate, 1901, 192–216; Spencer, Herbert. (1864, 1867) *The Principles of Biology*, vols. 2 and 3 of *A System of Synthetic Philosophy*, 10 vols. London: Williams and Norgate; New York: Appleton, 1862–1896; Spencer, Herbert. (1893) *The Principles of Ethics*, vols. 9 and 10 of *A System of Synthetic Philosophy*, 10 vols. London: Williams and Norgate; New York: Appleton, 1862–1896; Spencer, Herbert. *Social Statics: or, The Conditions Essential to Human Happiness*. London: John Chapman, 1851. Reprinted, Farnborough, Hants, U.K.: Gregg International Publishers, 1970; Woodhull, Victoria C. (1874) "Tried as by Fire." In Madeleine B. Stern, ed., *The Victoria Woodhull Reader*. Weston, Mass.: M & S Press, 1974.

J. Martin Stafford

SPINOZA, BARUCH (1632–1677). Baruch (Benedict) Spinoza was the son of a merchant from Amsterdam whose family had fled Spain during the Inquisition. Though trained in the rabbinical tradition, he was excommunicated from the Portuguese Synagogue in 1656 for heresy. He thereafter devoted his life to philosophy and the new science (he learned the trade of lens grinding for telescopes). Spinoza wrote nothing explicitly on human sexuality. His major work, the *Ethics*, published posthumously in 1677, contains only two brief remarks on the topic, while the two works published during his lifetime, *Principles of Cartesian Philosophy* (1663) and *Theologico-Political Treatise* (1670), offer nothing on sexuality.

Nevertheless, later thinkers who thought much about sexuality credited him with many of the seminal insights about which they fashioned their own systematic reflections: two examples are **Arthur Schopenhauer** (1788–1860; see Birnbacher; Schulz) and **Sigmund Freud** (1856–1939; see Bertrand). Three central aspects of Spinoza's thought account for its revolutionary impact on views of sexuality: his program for the elimination of teleological explanation from science, his efforts to forge a new account of human affectivity, and his thoroughgoing naturalism.

Spinoza was known to his contemporaries as an acute critic of **René Descartes**'s (1596–1650) philosophy, in the *Principles*, and as a revolutionary political thinker: The *Theologico-Political Treatise*, though published anonymously, was recognized as his. The *Principles*, though it offers a faithful interpretation of the Cartesian system, alerts readers at many points to central areas where Spinoza disagrees with Descartes. The *Ethics* develops these themes extensively.

The Cartesian system is a radical dualism. Descartes and Galileo (1564–1642) are widely recognized as the founders of modern science with its mathematical methods and deterministic view of causal explanation, a program that seventeenth century thinkers called "the mechanical philosophy" and which represented a break from Aristotelian science with its emphasis on the qualitative features of reality, purpose and teleological explanation in science, and the presence of contingency throughout the natural order. In his defense and elaboration of the new method, however, Descartes exempted human behavior from its scope. Mind and body were conceived as radically distinct substances. In the world of body (*res extensa*) the laws of nature, mathematically codified and exceptionless, reigned supreme, whereas mind (*res cogitans*) was conceived as operating with free will and outside scientific explanation. Descartes argues (*Meditations*, V) that the human mind has limited access to the mind of God, an infinite thinking being, concluding that the material world, as a creation of God, contains purpose throughout, but the human mind has no access to God's purposes in making the world as he has. This banishes purpose from the range of explanations that the scientist may utilize to understand nature, leaving mechanical explanation unchallenged for the material world.

In the appendix to the first part of the *Ethics*, Spinoza inveighs heavily against the claim that purpose, known or unknown, figures in natural events. His extensive critique of teleology concludes with the remark that "nature has no fixed goal, and final causes are only figments of human imagination. . . . The doctrine of final causes turns nature completely upside down, regarding as an effect that which is a cause and vice versa" (all translations by LCR). Two consequences of this are developed at length in the next two parts of the *Ethics*: Human behavior and mental features are as subject to scientific causal explanation as anything else in nature, and purpose, whose biological analog is "function," plays no role in the explanation of either.

It follows that it is as frivolous to explain **sexual desire** in terms of a "procreative function" as it is to explain the flight of an arrow in terms of where it is trying to go—its "natural place" in **Aristotle**'s (384–322 BCE) physics (*De generatione et corruptione*, II.4, 330b30–332a). Spinoza's definition of sexuality exploits this nonfunctional element: "Sexual drive [*libido*] is the desire and love of the commingling of bodies" (def. 48, appendix, *Ethics* 3; see Rice, "Spinoza's Account"). It is worth noting that Freud chose Spinoza's Latin term, *libido*, in his own account of sexual drive.

To understand the implications of rejecting teleology and Spinoza's definition of sexual drive, we need to understand his notions of "desire" and "**love**," which in turn takes us into his account of affectivity—another departure from Descartes, who had viewed the passions as essentially bodily and somehow interacting with the mind. Spinoza uses "affect" (*affectus*) to avoid the Cartesian and Stoic view of passions as detrimental to human welfare. Affects for Spinoza are expressions of a single underlying force, which he calls "*conatus*": the drive of an organism to maintain itself within a given state, often translated "self-preservation." The theory of *conatus* is developed extensively in part 3 of the *Ethics* (see Fóti; Mistura; Nails; Rice, "Emotion"). Spinoza says that *conatus* may be called "will" if related to mind, "appetite" if related to mind/body, or "desire" if we are conscious of it (scholium to proposition 9 of *Ethics* 3). It is a dynamic principle (Bickel; Burbage and Chouchan) whose causal efficacy has nothing to do with whether we are conscious of it. There is perhaps some anticipation here of Freud's notion of the unconscious, though the differences between Freud and Spinoza are many (Hessing; Kaplan; Rice, "Freud"). Conational drive is also cast as nonfunctional, and Spinoza concludes, "[W]e do not endeavor, will, seek, or desire something because we judge it good, but rather we judge it good because we endeavor, will, seek or desire it." To understand the affects one must determine their antecedent causes, not the imagined objects to which they tend.

Affectivity occurs when the organism undergoes a change of state that encompasses either increased vitality, or control of its environment, or decreased vitality. In the former case, "satisfaction" (*laetitia*, sometimes rendered "pleasure") results; in the latter case, "dissatisfaction" (*dolor*, sometimes rendered "pain") results. These are the two fundamental affects. Taking these as primitive, Spinoza defines love as "pleasure which is accompanied by the idea of an external cause" (*Amor est laetitia, concomitante idea causae externae*) and hate as "pain or dissatisfaction accompanied by the idea of an external cause" (scholium to prop. 13, *Ethics* 3). Both are derivative affects. Love occurs whether the idea is true or false, whether the imagined idea exists or not. If the pleasure is experienced under the modality of "bodily mixing," it is by definition sexual (see Matheron,

"Spinoza"). (At one point in *World as Will and Representation* [vol. 2, 533], Schopenhauer misquotes and ridicules Spinoza's definition: "[O]n account of its excessive naïveté, [it] deserves to be quoted for the sake of amusement: '*Amor est titillatio* [*sic*], *concomitante idea causae externae.*' ")

The account of affectivity is perhaps the least fully studied portion of the *Ethics* (but see Jung; Schrijvers), and there are many ambiguities and problems. "Bodily mixing" requires far more explanation and development than Spinoza provides. But in its steadfast rejection of mind-body dualism and functional explanation, it marks a revolutionary change from what went before and is wholly consistent with Spinoza's naturalism.

The roots of Spinoza's naturalism lie in his metaphysics: God and nature are one and the same infinite totality. The Cartesian dualism of body and thought is refigured by Spinoza as a duality of descriptions of this one infinite substance, for which Spinoza's preferred term is "nature." Science is capable of giving complete and "mechanical" descriptions of this nature, whether conceptualized as matter, in physics, or as thought, in psychology. The descriptions are isomorphic or parallel: "The order and connection of ideas is the same as the order and connection of things" (prop. 7, *Ethics* 2). That connection is one of mathematically expressed and exceptionless causal laws, that is, determinism. Understanding these causal chains constitutes the basis of the "therapy" that Spinoza develops in *Ethics* 4 and whose objective is not the extinction of the affective drives, as in Stoicism or Descartes, but their integration into a life that maximizes the power (*potentia*) of the organism in dealing with its environment. Much has been written about Spinoza's therapeutic principles and their relation to subsequent thinkers (Bernard; Gabhart; Rice, "Notes").

Spinoza does not provide examples of the therapeutic principles in relation to sexual behavior. Any attempt to do so would constitute what French scholars call "spinozéan," that is, attempts to extend his thought to problems not treated by him (for example, Rice ["Homosexualization"] on **homosexuality**), rather than "spinoziste," that is, textual or historical analysis.

Monistic naturalism and its rejection of a supernatural order are the basis of Spinoza's social and political thought. The central problem he attacked in the *Theologico-Political Treatise* was the fragmentation of civil authority by religious sects and dogmas; this problem is still very much with us. His resolution is a secularism combined with an eloquent plea for individual freedom. Religious dogma is restricted to the private domain, and its impact on civil society falls under the control of sovereign political power. The best state is one that maximizes human freedom and stresses diversity. **Marriage** is conceived neither as a religious nor sexual institution but as a rational social contrivance for the rearing of children (explanation 20, appendix, *Ethics* 4). Spinoza adds that marriage is best when "the love of both man and woman has for its cause not merely physical attractiveness but especially freedom of spirit," a refreshingly egalitarian remark in a century not usually regarded as amicable to feminist thought. Alexandre Matheron ("Femmes") offers a "spinozéan" development of Spinoza's ideas in connection with contemporary feminist themes. I suspect we will eventually see the development of Spinoza's suggestions in the area of "**queer theory**." While Spinoza wrote little about sexuality, the framework he provided for understanding affectivity in general and human sexuality in particular holds rich promise.

See also Descartes, René; Fichte, Johann Gottlieb; Freud, Sigmund; Leibniz, Gottfried; Schopenhauer, Arthur

REFERENCES

Aristotle. *De generatione et corruptione*. Trans. H. H. Joachim. In W. David Ross, ed., *The Works of Aristotle*, vol. 2. Oxford, U.K.: Clarendon Press, 1930; Barbone, Steven, and Lee Rice. "Spinoza and Human Sexuality." In Alan Soble, ed., *Sex, Love, and Friendship*. Amsterdam, Holland: Rodopi, 1997, 265–77; Bernard, Walter. "Psychotherapeutic Principles in Spinoza's *Ethics*." In Siegfried Hessing, ed., *Speculum Spinozanum: 1677–1977*. London: Routledge and Kegan Paul, 1977, 63–80; Bertrand, Michéle. "Spinoza et la psychanalyse." *Studia Spinozana* 8 (1992), 171–90; Bickel, Lothar. "On Relationships between Psychoanalysis and a Dynamic Psychology." In Siegfried Hessing, ed., *Speculum Spinozanum: 1677–1977*. London: Routledge and Kegan Paul, 1977, 81–89; Birnbacher, Dieter. "Freiheit durch Selbsterkenntnis: Spinoza–Schopenhauer–Freud." *Schopenhauer-Jahrbuch* 74:1 (1993), 87–102; Burbage, Frank, and Nathalie Chouchan. "Freud et Spinoza: la question de la transformation et le devenir actif du sujet." In Olivier Bloch, ed., *Spinoza au XXième siècle*. Paris: Presses Universitaires de France, 1993, 527–48; Descartes, René. (1641) *Meditations*. Trans. Donald Cress. Indianapolis, Ind.: Hackett, 1982; Fóti, Véronique M. "Thought, Affect, Drive, and Pathogenesis in Spinoza and Freud." *History of European Ideas* 3:2 (1982), 221–36; Gabhart, Mitchell. "Freedom, Understanding, and Therapy in Spinoza's Moral Psychology." *International Journal of Applied Philosophy* 9:1 (1994), 1–9; Hessing, Siegfried. "Freud's Relation with Spinoza." In Siegfried Hessing, ed., *Speculum Spinozanum: 1677–1977*. London: Routledge and Kegan Paul, 1977, 224–39; Jung, Gertrud. "Die Affektenlehre Spinozas." *Kant Studien* 32:1 (1927), 85–150; Kaplan, Alan. "Spinoza and Freud." *Spinoza Studies* (Haifa) (1978), 85–110; Matheron, Alexandre. "Femmes et serviteurs dans la démocratie spinoziste." In Siegfried Hessing, ed., *Speculum Spinozanum: 1677–1977*. London: Routledge and Kegan Paul, 1977, 368–86; Matheron, Alexandre. "Spinoza et la sexualité." In *Etudes sur Spinoza: Anthropologie et politique au xviiième siècle*. Paris: Vrin, 1986, 209–30; Mistura, S. "Verso una teoria dell'affetto. Spinoza e Freud." In Filippo Mignini, ed., *Dio, l'Uomo, la Libertà*. Rome, Italy: Japadre Editore, 1990, 349–74; Nails, Debra. "Conatus versus Eros/Thanatos: On the Principles of Spinoza and Freud." *Dialogue* (PST) 21:2–3 (1979), 33–40; Rice, Lee C. "Emotion, Appetition, and Conatus in Spinoza." *Revue Internationale de Philosophie* 31:1 (1977), 101–16; Rice, Lee C. "Freud, Sartre, Spinoza: The Problematic of the Unconscious." *Giornale di Metafisica* 17:1 (1995), 87–106; Rice, Lee C. "Homosexualization and Collectivism." *Philosophy and Theology* 12:2 (2000), 275–92; Rice, Lee C. "Notes on Spinozistic Therapy." In M. Czelinski, T. Kisser, R. Schnepf, M. Senn, and J. Stenzel, eds., *Transformation der Metaphysik in die Moderne*. Würzburg, Ger.: Königshausen and Neumann, 2003, 100–111; Rice, Lee C. "Spinoza's Account of Sexuality." *Philosophy Research Archives* 10 (1984), 19–34; Schopenhauer, Arthur. (1818, 1844, 1859) *The World as Will and Representation*, 2 vols. Trans. E.F.J. Payne. New York: Dover, 1966; Schrijvers, Michael. *Spinozas Affektenlehre*. Stuttgart, Ger.: Verlag Paul Haupt, 1989; Schulz, Ortrun. "Schopenhauers spinozistische Grundansicht." *Schopenhauer-Jahrbuch* 74:1 (1993), 51–72; Spinoza, Baruch. *Ethics and Selected Letters*. Trans. Samuel Shirley. Indianapolis, Ind.: Hackett, 1990; Spinoza, Baruch [Benedictus]. *Opera Omnia*, 2 vols. Ed. R. van Vloten and J.P.N. Land. The Hague: Martinus Nijhoff, 1914; Spinoza, Baruch. *Principles of Cartesian Philosophy, Metaphysical Thoughts*. Trans. Samuel Shirley. Introduction and notes by Steven Barbone and Lee C. Rice. Indianapolis, Ind.: Hackett, 1998; Spinoza, Baruch. *Theological-Political Treatise*, 2nd ed. Trans. Samuel Shirley. Indianapolis, Ind.: Hackett, 1998.

Lee C. Rice

ADDITIONAL READING

Barbone, Steven, and Lee Rice. "Coming Out, Being Out, and Acts of Virtue." In Timothy F. Murphy, ed., *Gay Ethics: Controversies in Outing, Civil Rights, and Sexual Science*. Binghamton, N.Y.: Harrington Park Press, 1994, 91–110; Ben-Ze'ev, Aaron. "Emotions and Change: A Spinozistic Account." In Yirmiyahu Yovel, ed., *Desire and Affect: Spinoza as Psychologist*. New York: Little Room

Press, 1999, 139–54; Beyssade, Jean-Marie. "De l'émotion intérieure chez Descartes et l'affect actif spinoziste." In Edwin Curley and Pierre-François Moreau, eds., *Spinoza: Issues and Directions*. Leiden, Holland: E. J. Brill, 1990, 176–90; Bicknell, Jeanette. "An Overlooked Aspect of Love in Spinoza's *Ethics*." *Iyyun* 47 (1988), 41–55; Damasio, Antonio. *Looking for Spinzoa: Joy, Sorrow, and the Feeling Brain*. Orlando, Fla.: Harcourt, 2003; Davidson, Donald. "Spinoza's Causal Theory of the Affects." In Yirmiyahu Yovel, ed., *Desire and Affect: Spinoza as Psychologist*. New York: Little Room Press, 1999, 95–112; Duroux, Françoise. "Puissance et utopie au péril de la différence sexuelle." In Myriam D'Allones and Hadi Rizk, eds., *Spinoza: Puissance et ontologie*. Paris: Editions Kimé, 1994, 127–38; Fóti, Véronique M. "Thought, Affect, Drive, and Pathogenesis in Spinoza and Freud." *History of European Ideas* 3:2 (1982), 221–36. Reprinted in Genevieve Lloyd, ed., *Spinoza: Critical Assessments*, vol. 4. London: Routledge, 2001, 289–305; Greenspan, Patricia S. "A Case of Mixed Feelings: Ambivalence and the Logic of Emotion." In Amélie Oksenberg Rorty, ed., *Explaining Emotions*. Berkeley: University of California Press, 1980, 223–50; Groen, J. J. "Spinoza's Theory of Affects and Modern Psychobiology." In Jon Wetlesen, ed., *Spinoza's Philosophy of Man*. Oslo, Nor.: Universitetsforlaget, 1978, 97–118; Hannan, Barbara. "Love and Human Bondage in Maugham, Spinoza, and Freud." In Roger E. Lamb, ed., *Love Analyzed*. Boulder, Colo.: Westview, 1997, 93–106; Neu, Jerome. *Emotion, Thought, and Therapy: A Study of Hume and Spinoza and the Relationship of Philosophical Theories of the Emotions to Psychological Theories of Therapy*. London: Routledge and Kegan Paul, 1977; Ogilvie, Bertrand. "Spinoza dans la psychanalyse." In Olivier Bloch, ed., *Spinoza au XXième siècle*. Paris: Presses Universitaires de France, 1993, 549–76; Ravven, Heidi M. "The Garden of Eden: Spinoza's Maimonidean Account of the Genealogy of Morals and the Origin of Society." *Philosophy and Theology* 13:1 (2001), 3–47; Schneider, Monique. "Spinoza et Freud: la problématique du savoir dans ses rapports avec l'étendue." In Renée Bouveresse, ed., *Spinoza: Science et Religion*. Paris: Vrin, 1988, 77–88; Schrijvers, Michael. "The *Conatus* and the Mutual Relationships between Active and Passive Affects in Spinoza." In Yirmiyahu Yovel, ed., *Desire and Affect: Spinoza as Psychologist*. New York: Little Room Press, 1999, 63–80; Yovel, Yirmiyahu, ed. *Desire and Affect: Spinoza as Psychologist*. New York: Little Room Press, 1999.

STDs. *See* Diseases, Sexually Transmitted

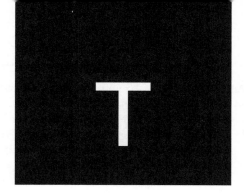

TANTRISM. The terms "tantra" and "tantrism" refer to a diverse range of religious traditions that arose in South Asia around the middle of the first millennium, apparently first in **Hinduism** and subsequently in **Buddhism**. In South Asia, tantric themes also developed in some traditions of **Jainism** and **Islam**, and in East Asia such themes were synthesized with amenable elements of Taoism. Since the nineteenth century, the West has generated numerous invectives against tantrism as well as popular efforts to appropriate it, both of which have influenced the self-understandings of the Asian traditions. While some popular appropriations of tantrism make a potentially defensible effort to combine the values of "liberated" sexual pleasure with universalist spirituality, many are merely gross distortions that reflect a long-standing and often pernicious exploitation of the exotic and erotic Orient. (On the history of the intertwined Western and Indian imaginations about Tantra in the colonial and postcolonial periods, see Urban.)

Scholarly interpretations of Tantrism are also beset with difficulties. No category in any premodern Asian religion actually agrees in its extension with contemporary Western and Asian academic usages of "tantra." In the Sanskritic context, an important usage identifies as tantras a group of scriptures of Hindu Śaivism, Hindu Śāktism, and Buddhist Vajrayāna. Tantrism and Tantra may likewise refer to the movements that adhere to those scriptures. However, other scriptures and movements with very similar characteristics do not describe themselves as tantric. According to another common South Asian usage, "tantra" refers to a variety of folk traditions of "sorcery" to attain worldly ends.

Despite this confusion, scholars have been converging toward an illuminating new meaning for "tantra" and "tantrism," treating them as terms that classify together certain religious movements that do have important historical commonalities, regardless of their self-definitions. Several characteristic themes of this group of religious movements are relevant to the philosophy of sex.

Most obvious is the traditions' prominent sexual (predominantly heterosexual) mythic symbolism and correlated rituals. The tantric traditions usually conceive the Deity or Ultimate Reality in sexed or gendered terms: as a male God, such as Śiva or Viṣṇu/Kṛṣṇa, or as the Buddha in his ultimate nature; or as the Goddess Śakti ("Power") in one of her forms—Kālī, Durgā, Lakṣmī. Even though identified in this way as male or female, Ultimate Reality is viewed at the same time as an androgynous totality of both male and female polarities: Kālī with Śiva, Viṣṇu with Lakṣmī, Kṛṣṇa with Rādhā, and the Buddhist Prajñā (Wisdom, female) with Upāya (Skillful Means, male). According to the most common tantric mythic pattern, Ultimate Reality fragments into its polarized gender principles and then through the sexual union of those male and female principles emanates (emits from itself) and controls the universe. In Hinduism, whether the Ultimate is conceived as God or Goddess, it is through its feminine "maternal" polarity, Śakti, that it emanates, controls, and is immanent in the universe.

Tantric religious practices recapitulate the mythic archetype in various ways. These practices include, occasionally, sexual intercourse in which the partners become God and Goddess. Far more common, especially in later tantrism, are "domesticized," internalized, rites, that is, the contemplation of sexual symbolism in circular diagrams of emanation (*maṇḍalas*), empowered speech formulas (*mantras*), and theosophical and metaphysical speculation.

The most generic goal of tantric practices is Power, understood in the Hindu tantric traditions as, in essence, Śakti, the Goddess herself. The adept might identify with the Goddess, or be ecstatically possessed by her, or become her possessor (Śaktiman) by identifying with her consort (for example, one of the forms of Śiva or Viṣṇu). Much of the variety within tantrism derives from the different expressions of power that are pursued. These expressions of power range from the relatively limited "magical proficiencies" (*siddhis* or *vibhūtis*) of local shamans, through the sovereignty of kings (traditionally great sponsors of Hindu and Buddhist tantric traditions), to the omnipotence of the person who has become liberated by completely identifying with the deity. (For a general definition of tantra in terms of the quest for power, see White, "Introduction," *Tantra in Practice*, 7–9.)

The tantric traditions' concepts of sexuality are framed directly by their emanationist metaphysics and not only by their explicitly sexual mythic symbolism. Emanation's entailment, the simultaneous transcendence and immanence of the Ultimate, was already an important theme in broader traditions of Hindu devotionalism (*bhakti*) and in the Mahāyāna equation of *saṁsāra* (the phenomenal world in which occurs the cycle of reincarnation) and *nirvāṇa* (the soteriological realization of Ultimate Reality); however, this dialectic is given special emphasis in tantrism. The tantric adept discovers divine Power as pervading all worldly experience. Tantric theosophies establish numerous homologies between higher and lower planes of emanation. A formula found in a number of tantric traditions advocates the synthesis of liberation (*mokṣa*) with enjoyment (*bhoga*). Enjoyment includes not only sex but also all other pleasures realized through power.

Related to the valuation of immanence is the recognition by virtually all the tantric traditions that *embodiment* is integral to personal and soteriological identity. However, these traditions do not accept the *status quo* experience of the body but endeavor to transform it. Power emanating as the universe is often conceived as the body of the supreme God, Goddess, or the Buddha. The adept endeavors to expand the sense of his or her fleshly body into the experience of the cosmic body of emanatory Śakti. This process sometimes also makes the fleshly body itself *immortal*, as in tantric traditions of alchemy, which teach the way to become a *siddha*, "accomplished being" (see White, *Alchemical*).

Closely related to the aforementioned themes is a concern in tantric traditions to transgress, deliberately, cultural norms of bodily purity (*śuddhi*), for example, in the spheres of caste, hygiene, death, as well as sexuality. Great psychic and magical power accrues to the adept through the subversion of these norms, which delimit ordinary human agency (see Sanderson, "Purity and Power"). Transgression is also justified on the basis of divine immanence. Because the deity is immanent in the world, no entity or behavior is more or less pure than another. Everything is in its true nature identical with the deity.

There is great variation in the kinds and degrees of tantric transgression. A late medieval formula identifies sexual transgression as the culmination of the five "M's" (*makāras*, things whose designations start with the phoneme M): *madya* (wine), *matsya* (fish), *māṁsa* (meat), *mudrā* (many different things, from mystical or sexual postures to aphrodisiac beans and cereals), and *maithuna* (sexual intercourse). The sexual ritual is frequently performed between an upper-caste man and a lower-caste woman. For this reason it is also commonly adulterous for one or both partners. A few texts advocate **incest**, conceiving the ideal coupling, for example, between a man and his grandmother, mother, sister, daughter, or granddaughter (see Sanderson, "Meaning," 83). Many of the original tantric rites were originally performed in cremation grounds, which are traditionally viewed in South Asia as extremely impure. There are also prescriptions for the transgressive ingestion of sexual fluids as well as urine, excrement, phlegm, and even, rarely, human flesh.

An adept may perform the sexual ritual only after having received a qualified guru's initiation ($d\bar{\imath}k\d{s}\bar{a}$) and guidance. There are elaborate ritual preparations that may involve mantras, meditation, and worship. Frequently the female genitals (*yoni*) are worshiped as the locus of divine Power. In some cases the woman should be menstruating. Ejaculation is important in some traditions: The semen is mixed with the menstrual fluid, forming the *kuṇḍagolaka*, which is offered to Śakti and consumed. David White has argued that the consumption of sexual fluids was the core of the original Kaula form of the tantric ritual (this is the main argument of his *Kiss*). Other traditions advocate intercourse without ejaculation. Sometimes the man is trained to use his penis to suck the powerful fluids from the vagina. White has described this procedure (*vajrolī mudrā*) as the "fountain pen technique" (*Alchemical*, 199).

A topic much debated by scholars is the role of women in the sexual ritual and in tantric traditions more broadly. Tantric traditions do ascribe a certain dignity to women, insofar as they are the incarnations of Śakti (or Wisdom). Likewise, women are sometimes given authority as gurus competent to perform initiations, and at times tantric traditions describe women's experiences in the ritual and the benefits women gain from it. However, tantric practices were largely created by men and for men within strongly patriarchal societies. Most often, the female partner is seen as merely an accessory to the sexual rites. (For a positive evaluation of the role of women in Tantrism, see Shaw; for a different perspective, see Caldwell.)

Actual sexual rituals and other ostensible acts of transgression are truly quite rare in Asian tantric traditions. In fact, for over a thousand years there has been a tendency to "domesticize" the tantric traditions into forms more acceptable to orthodox and upper-caste audiences. Thus the great monistic Kashmiri Śaiva philosophical theologian Abhinavagupta (ca. 950–1020) interpreted the sexual ritual as leading to self-recognition as Śiva, through universalizing and transfiguring *pleasure* into its essential nature as the bliss of Śiva in union with Śakti. And he drew an analogy between this process and the universalization of emotions in aesthetic experience. This philosophical interpretation opened the way for purely internalized, contemplative versions of the sexual ritual in later Hindu tantrism (see Sanderson, "Meaning" and "Purity"; White, *Kiss*, 219–57). A similar internalization predominates in Tibetan and East Asian esoteric Buddhism, where the baroque tantric symbolism and ritual are largely placed at the service of Mahāyāna metaphysics and soteriology. An adept usually engages in contemplative rites in the effort to realize his or her own innate Buddhahood conceived as emptiness (*śūnyatā*) or flux consciousness (*vijñāna*).

As may readily be gathered from the role of women in sexual rituals and from the more extreme forms of tantric transgression, the question arises whether tantrism provides any scope for ethics. This is a recurring problem in constructive academic reflection. Magical powers (*siddhis*, *vibhūtis*) may be pursued or employed, of course, for ethical or unethical purposes. Some forms of tantrism may perhaps be described as expressions of a "megalomaniacal" quest for omnipotence without any concern for the well-being of others. Other forms of tantrism, however, integrate ethical objectives within their varieties of monistic metaphysics. Thus Vajrayāna Buddhism pursues the Mahāyāna ideal of the *bodhisattva*, that is, one who is dedicated to leading all beings to salvation. Though perhaps thematizing this concern less strongly, Hindu tantric traditions also praise the universal guru who channels divine grace to humanity.

See also Bataille, Georges; Buddhism; Chinese Philosophy; Freud, Sigmund; Gnosticism; Hinduism; Incest; Jainism; Manichaeism; Sade, Marquis de; Westermarck, Edward

REFERENCES

Caldwell, Sarah. "The Heart of the Secret: A Personal and Scholarly Encounter with Shakta Tantrism in Siddha Yoga." In Elliot R. Wolfson and Jeffrey J. Kripal, eds., *The Unknown, Remembered Gate: Religious Experience and Hermeneutical Reflection*. New York: Seven Bridges Press, 2004. <www.leavingsiddhayoga.net/caldwell.sarah.pdf> [accessed 19 January 2005]; Lawrence, David Peter. *Rediscovering God with Transcendental Argument: A Contemporary Interpretation of Monistic Kashmiri Śaiva Philosophy*. Albany: State University of New York Press, 1999; Sanderson, Alexis. "Meaning in Tantric Ritual." In Anne-Marie Blondeau and Kristofer Schipper, eds., *Essais sur le Rituel, III* (Colloque du Centenaire de la Section des Sciences Religieuses de l'École Pratique des Hautes Études). Louvain, France: Peeters, 1995, 15–95; Sanderson, Alexis. "Purity and Power among the Brahmans of Kashmir." In Michael Carrithers, Steven Collins, and Steven Lukes, eds., *The Category of the Person: Anthropology, Philosophy, History*. Cambridge: Cambridge University Press, 1985, 190–216; Shaw, Miranda. *Passionate Enlightenment: Women in Tantric Buddhism*. Princeton, N.J.: Princeton University Press, 1994; Urban, Hugh B. *Tantra: Sex, Secrecy, Politics, and Power in the Study of Religion*. Berkeley: University of California Press, 2003; White, David Gordon. *The Alchemical Body: Siddha Traditions in Medieval India*. Chicago, Ill.: University of Chicago Press, 1996; White, David Gordon. *Kiss of the Yoginī: "Tantric Sex" in Its South Asian Contexts*. Chicago, Ill.: University of Chicago Press, 2003; White, David Gordon, ed. *Tantra in Practice*. Princeton, N.J.: Princeton University Press, 2000.

David Peter Lawrence

ADDITIONAL READING

Bharati, Agehananda. *The Tantric Tradition*. Garden City, N.Y.: Anchor Books, 1970; Broido, Michael. "Killing, Lying, Stealing, and Adultery: A Problem of Interpretation in the Tantras." In Donald S. Lopez, Jr., ed., *Buddhist Hermeneutics*. Honolulu: University of Hawai'i Press, 1988, 71–118; Brooks, Douglas Renfrew. *Auspicious Wisdom: The Texts and Traditions of Śrīvidyā Śākta Tantrism in South India*. Albany: State University of New York Press, 1992; Brooks, Douglas Renfrew. *The Secret of the Three Cities: An Introduction to Hindu Śākta Tantrism*. Chicago, Ill.: University of Chicago Press, 1990; Chalier-Visuvalingam, Elizabeth. "Union and Unity in Hindu Tantrism." <www.infinityfoundation.com/mandala/i_es/i_es_visuv_e_unity.htm> [accessed 19 January 2005]; Dasgupta, Shashibhusan. *An Introduction to Tantric Buddhism*. Calcutta, India: University of Calcutta Press, 1974; Dasgupta, Shashibhusan. *Obscure Religious Cults*. Calcutta, India: Firma K. L. Mukhopadhyay, 1969; Davidson, Ronald M. *Indian Esoteric Buddhism: A Social History of the Tantric Movement*. New York: Columbia University Press, 2002; Dimock, Edward C. *The Place of the Hidden Moon: Erotic Mysticism in the Vaiṣṇava-sahajīya Cult of Bengal*. Chicago, Ill.: University of Chicago Press, 1966; Doniger, Wendy. "Tantric Bodies." [Review of *Kiss of the Yoginī: "Tantric sex" in Its South Asian Contexts*, by David Gordon White] *Times Literary Supplement* (20 May 2004). <www.the-tls.co.uk/this_week/story.aspx?story_id=2107312> [accessed 9 September 2004]; Dupuche, John R. *Abhinavagupta: The Kula Ritual as Elaborated in Chapter 29 of the Tantrāloka*. Delhi, India: Motilal Banarsidass, 2003; Dyczkowski, Mark, S.G. *The Doctrine of Vibration: An Analysis of the Doctrines and Practices of Kashmir Shaivism*. Albany: State University of New York Press, 1987; Faure, Bernard. *The Red Thread: Buddhist Approaches to Sexuality*.

Princeton, N.J.: Princeton University Press, 1998; Guenther, Herbert V. *The Tantric View of Life*. London: Shambhala, 1976; Gupta, Senjukta, and Richard Gombrich. "Kings, Power and the Goddess." *South Asia Research* 6 (1986), 123–38; Gupta, Senjukta, Dirk Jans Hoens, and Teun Gourdriaan. *Hindu Tantrism*. Leiden, Holland: Brill, 1979; Hakeda, Yoshito S., trans. *Kūkai: Major Works*. New York: Columbia University Press, 1972; Harper, Katherine Ann, and Robert L. Brown. *Roots of Tantra*. Albany: State University of New York Press, 2002; Jackson, Roger R. "Ambiguous Sexuality: Imagery and Interpretation in Tantric Buddhism." *Religion* 22:1 (1992), 85–100; Kakar, Sudhir. *Shamans, Mystics, and Doctors: A Psychological Inquiry into India and Its Healing Traditions*. Boston, Mass.: Beacon Press, 1983; Kripal, Jeffrey J. (1995) *Kālī's Child: The Mystical and the Erotic in the Life and Teachings of Ramakrishna*, 2nd ed. Chicago, Ill.: University of Chicago Press, 1998; Lawrence, David Peter. "The Dialectic of Transcendence and Immanence in Contemporary Western and Indian Theories of God." In Liu Shu-hsien et al., eds., *Transcendence and Immanence: Comparative and Multi-Dimensional Perspectives*. Hong Kong: New Asia College, Chinese University of Hong Kong, 2001, 347–63; Marglin, Frédérique Apffel. *Wives of the God-King: The Rituals of the Devadasis of Puri*. Delhi, India: Oxford University Press, 1985; Sanderson, Alexis. "Śaivism and the Tantric Traditions." In Stewart Sutherland, Leslie Houlden, Peter Clarke, and Friedham Hards, eds., *The World's Religions*. London: Routledge, 1988, 660–704; Shipper, Kristofer. (1982) *The Taoist Body*. Trans. Karen C. Duval. Berkeley: University of California Press, 1994; Silburn, Lilian. (1983) *Kuṇḍalinī: The Energy of the Depths. A Comprehensive Study Based on the Scriptures of Nondualistic Kashmir Śaivism*. Trans. Jacques Gontier. Albany: State University of New York Press, 1988; Strickmann, Michel. *Mantras et mandarins: Le Bouddhisme tantrique en Chine*. Paris: Gallimard, 1996; Svoboda, Robert. *Aghora*, 3 vols. New Delhi, India: Rupa, 1986, 1993, 1998; Wayman, Alex. *The Buddhist Tantras: Light on Indo-Tibetan Esotericism*. New York: Samuel Weiser, 1973.

THOMAS AQUINAS (SAINT) (1224/25–1274). Mentioning Thomas Aquinas while discussing sexuality can invite a grimace. What could a thirteenth-century virginal priest, a Dominican friar, have to say in contemporary dialogue about sexuality? If anything, the spectres of Vatican rulings on **contraception** and the place of women loom (see, for example, Paul VI's [1897–1978] encyclical *Humanae vitae* [1968]), for Aquinas's teachings are regularly held up as the final word in such papal positioning.

In Aquinas's world, the Roman Catholic Church defined Christendom for Europeans, which definition was being challenged by the rediscovered writings of **Aristotle** (384–322 BCE). Thomas gained widespread respect for his theological synthesis of traditional Augustinian Christianity and Aristotle's philosophy (see Owens), which withstood the assaults of reactionary Augustinians as well as skeptical Aristotelians. Aquinas's was not the only such synthesis; his teacher Albertus Magnus (1206–1280) had already made an attempt. During the Counterreformation Thomas was named a "Doctor of the Church" by Pius V (1504–1572). After a period of obscurity, Leo XIII (1810–1903) elevated him, in *Aeterni patris* (1879), to the heights of doctrinal authority.

Thomas's understanding of sexuality begins with his conception of nature. "Nature" often refers to "how things are in the world," and our conception of "nature" derives from our scientific understanding of the world; the discoveries of cell biology, genetics, and chemistry comprise what we take to be "natural." Thomas's conception of "nature" is different. First, even though he links it to "how things are in the world," his idea of science drew not on Francis Bacon's (1561–1626) experimentalism (*Novum Organum*) but on Aristotle (e.g., *Metaphysics*). Second, in accepting the doctrine of Original Sin, Thomas believed that humans were created one way but are now by nature different. Third, while we construe "nature" as relative to the state of scientific knowledge (and various cultures might describe nature differently), for Aquinas "nature" is not relative. A statement is an objective truth of nature if it is a self-evident natural truth or if it is an accurate observation interpreted according to self-evident natural truths (*Summa theologiae* [*ST*], IaIIae, ques. 91, art. 3; ques. 94, art. 2). We share with animals inclinations to behave instinctually, as in sexual intercourse and the education of offspring, which Thomas describes as Natural Law (*ST*, IaIIae, ques. 94, art. 2). But, unlike animals, it is also natural for us to use reason to understand good and evil, the successful fruits of which are also Natural Law, our participation in God's Eternal Law (*ST*, IaIIae, ques. 91, art. 2). Thus Thomas's use of "natural" refers to two categories: behavior in accord with reason and behavior that is instinctive. For example, adulterous sex might be instinctively motivated, and hence natural in that sense, but it violates reason. For Aquinas, licit sex must satisfy both conditions, which on his view limits it to procreative marital coitus (*Summa contra gentiles* [*SCG*], III, ques. 122).

Social constructionism asserts that culture creates gender. Aquinas, by contrast, is an essentialist: People have a divinely created nature, an essence defining them as a species different from other animals. We are composites of material body and immaterial soul, each having an operation particular to itself, yet functioning together. Sight involves a physical eye and an action, seeing, that gives the eye form and fulfillment. Similarly, the soul gives the body both its human form and its highest purpose (*SCG*, II, ques. 57; *ST*, Ia, ques. 76; *Commentary on Aristotle's De Anima*, lectures 2, 6, 7). Aristotle believed our highest purpose was understanding the world, but Aquinas argues that Aristotle misses the higher purpose of understanding the goodness of divine perfection. The soul is "a spiritual being present in the body and in its several parts—the form of the whole body in such fashion as to be also the form of each part" (*SCG*, II, ques. 72; *Quaestiones de Anima*, ques. 1–3).

Aristotle and Aquinas differ about the soul's surviving the body, but they agree that it does not exist beforehand. (On the soul's immortality, see *Quaestiones de Anima*, ques. 14; *SCG*, II, ques. 79–81; *ST*, Ia, ques. 75, art. 6.) Nor is generation as simple as the soul's being contributed by the father, the body by the mother. For Aquinas, a father's semen contributes nutritive elements that organize the development of the fetus, but semen does not contain the intellectual soul. The generative power of the father provides the catalyst for the organizing nutritive elements, which during fetal development are transformed into the child's blood. The intellectual soul, by which we are human, is given at conception by a creative act of God. This does not mean that God intervenes directly in each act of conception (God does not act in time). Rather, our intellectual souls are created as potential in the seed generated by our fathers, which potential stretches back to the divinely enacted creation of the first human, Adam (*SCG*, II, ques. 87–89; *ST*, Ia, ques. 118–19).

Thomas's account apparently makes women secondary in generation. Having no knowledge of cell biology, Aquinas used the agricultural analogy of seeds, fertilization, and earth to grasp generation. Speculating about what Aquinas's notion of the ideal state of male-female relations would have been were he aware of cellular mitosis is interesting. He would not have denied this science, nor would he have kept it from influencing his views of sexuality. But he would have still adhered to Genesis's account of human beginnings, in which the creation of man and woman and their experience in Paradise resulted in introducing sin and death into the world. In Genesis 2, God creates the first man from the slime of the earth, breathing life into his face and bestowing the newborn soul into the newly formed body (see *ST*, Ia, ques. 90, art. 1, art. 4). Because it was not good for man to be alone, God created a helper, the woman, like in form to the man. Aquinas's term for helper is the Latin *adiutorium*, which connotes assistant, not servant or slave. Aristotle had said that women are misbegotten men. Aquinas understands Aristotle as meaning that while the semen's power tends to produce a male, some other circumstance (e.g., a moist, south wind) shifts generation from male to female. Thomas agrees but denies moral value to this shift, read too easily into "misbegotten": "as regards universal human nature, woman is not misbegotten, but is included in nature's intention as directed to the work of generation" (*ST*, Ia, ques. 91, art. 1, reply 1).

Women are by nature different from men, but not only in their reproductive role. Men of diminished reasoning capacity should be subject to men of higher capacity, even before the Fall, for some would have better senses of justice or knowledge (*ST*, Ia, ques. 96, art. 3). Similarly, in the family women should be subject to men in virtue of their lesser reason (*ST*, Ia, ques. 91, art. 1, reply 2). Men thus largely have the responsibility of educating children (*SCG*, III, ques. 122). Nevertheless, Aquinas thinks **marriage** involves natural **friendship** between man and woman (*SCG*, III, ques. 124). This is one basis for lifelong monogamy: Husband must not abandon wife. While other animals were created male and female, woman's creation from the man's rib created a deep bond between them (Gen. 2:21). Aquinas takes this, too, as a basis for lifelong monogamy. In this union, the woman must acknowledge her reliance on the man as symbolically prefigured in the first woman's creation and "neither use authority over the man . . . nor be subject to man's contempt as a slave" (*ST*, Ia, ques. 91, art. 3). Why does Aquinas not refer to Genesis 1:27 ("male and female created He them")? Some readers prefer this apparently separate creation story because it lacks male hegemony. For Aquinas, citing Ecclesiasticus 17:5 for support, the two passages describe the same event.

Original Sin—the reason all humans are by nature prone to sin—is inherited from Adam. Our natures are created differently than the natures of other created substances. Man was endowed with "original justice," the means by which the lower powers are subject to reason and which God intended to be passed from parent to child. On sinning by his own free choice, Adam deprived himself and his progeny of this original justice. The emphasis is on Adam, not Eve. Had only Eve sinned, sin would not have been transmitted to their offspring. Semen contains the active causality in generating the nutritive soul of the child, so this defect must be traced back to the father (*ST*, IaIIae, ques. 81, art. 5; see **Saint Paul** [5–64?], Rom. 5:12–14, 1 Cor. 15:21–23, 45–49). **Augustine** (354–430) argued that lust in coitus, not coitus itself, transmitted Original Sin (*On Marriage and Concupiscence*, bk. 1, chap. 27), while for Anselm of Canterbury (1033–1109), semen no more contained sin than does spittle or blood ("Virgin Conception," chap. 7). In disagreeing, Aquinas did not claim that semen is intrinsically evil. Semen is nutriment that contains the tendency to sin, which was transmitted from Adam. Just as our intellectual souls are created in potential in the seed of our father, which potential stretches back to Adam, so does seed contain sin in potential or, as Aquinas puts it, it contains sin virtually, not actually (*De Malo* [*DM*], ques. 4).

Aquinas embraces Augustine's definition of sin (*Contra Faustum*, bk. 22, chap. 27) as "a transgression in word, deed, or desire of the eternal law" (*ST*, IaIIae, ques. 71, art. 6). Sin is not a uniform phenomenon. Mortal sin deserves eternal punishment, for, like mortal disease, they kill us, they destroy "life principles." Venial sin affects the results of the life principles of the soul and can be overcome by these principles (*ST*, IaIIae, ques. 72, art. 5; *SCG*, III, ques. 143–44). These principles are the sources of our right actions, those by which we attain our final end, to behold God, and they compel us (mediately) to **love** our fellows and (ultimately) love God. The word Aquinas uses for these interrelated loves is *caritas*. A soul deprived of *caritas* by its own actions is no longer drawn to God, while one in which charitable tendencies are impeded by some force soluble by *caritas* is culpable, yet is still capable of being charitably motivated. The soul's vision of its end is clouded by sensual appetites, Aquinas argues, but they do not destroy it. Acts that destroy love for God, like blasphemy and devil worship, or that destroy the common life of society, like theft and homicide, are mortal sins (*DM*, ques. 7, art. 1).

Sins against man's spiritual nature are generally worse than sins against the body, which makes carnal sins, or sins of physical desire, less serious (*Commentary on Ephesians*, chap. 5, lec. 2). After all, they stem from wrong ordering of the satisfaction of bodily desires, a turn toward a lesser good, while spiritual sins turn the spirit away from God (*ST*, IaIIae, ques. 73, art. 5). But sins of the flesh are not uniformly less serious than spiritual sins. **Adultery** involves as much the sin of greed for another's spouse as of lust for that person; adultery is more than fornication alone, for it is the usurpation of that which belongs to another (*ST*, IaIIae, ques. 73, art. 7). Note that Aquinas's Latin is "*homo usurpat rem alterius*." That which is appropriated might be interpreted as the physical person of the spouse or the right of the absent spouse to that physical person. (The Blackfriars translation suggests the latter; the earlier English Dominican translation [Pegis] suggests the former.) What about **seduction** and **rape**? Destroying another person's innocence must be worse than consensual fornication. After all, "the man who seduces a woman thereby deprives her of the life of grace and leads her into mortal sin. If the seriousness of the sin were determined by the amount of harm done, it would follow that the seducer would be worse than a murderer." But the seducer's intention is not to destroy the victim's spiritual life, Aquinas says, but to satisfy lust. The victim's spiritual death depends on *her* free will, not the actions of another. (*ST*, IaIIae, ques. 73, art. 8. See Augustine, *City of God* [*COG*], bk. 1, chap. 18: "Tush, another's lust cannot pollute thee. . . . What man of wit will think he loseth his chastity, though his captivated body be forcedly prostitute unto another's bestiality?")

Lust is one of the seven "deadly" or capital sins, those having the power of acting as army generals, marshaling hosts of lesser sins to lead us to destruction. Paul wrote that covetousness—for Aquinas, the turning toward a perceived, passing good—lies at the root of all evils (1 Tim. 6:10). In Ecclesiasticus 10:15, pride is at every sin's beginning, "a turning away from God, whose command man refuses to obey" (*ST*, IaIIae, ques. 84, art. 2). These faults ground the seven capital sins, *viz.*, vainglory, envy, anger, sloth, avarice, gluttony, and lust (*ST*, IaIIae, ques. 84, art. 4). While "lust" is used for many hungers—for food, drink, gold—its venue is venery, the carnal delight associated with sexuality. Not every sexual act is sinful, except when lust lies at its base (*SCG*, III, ques. 126). Augustine had argued that coitus is not sinful, if motivated by "the health of the race" (*On the Good of Marriage*, 25). Aquinas follows suit. Reproduction is necessary to preserve the species, and because the need for an act's direction by reason is directly related to the act's importance, anything that clouds reason regarding sexual behavior is dangerous (*ST*, IIaIIae, ques. 153, art. 2, art. 3; Augustine notes the complication that sexuality itself clouds reason [*COG*, bk. 14, chap. 16]). Concupiscence that turns a pleasure like that accompanying coitus, which is for propagation, into an end in itself is cupidity. The agent is thereby put in jeopardy (*ST*, IaIIae, ques. 30, art. 3).

Thomas uses "fornication" to refer to illicit sex, explaining that the term comes from *fornice*, the arch under which prostitutes met their clients in antiquity (*DM*, ques. 15, art. 3). Spiritual fornication is delighting in things against God's order; simple fornication is "intercourse between two people who are not committed to one another" in marriage (*ST*, IIaIIae, ques. 151, art. 2; ques. 154, art. 2). In simple fornication, coitus apparently involves two people mutually sharing their bodies. But, despite its instinctiveness, it flouts Natural Law when it involves "souls wickedly loving pleasures" to the detriment of spiritual health (*SCG*, III, ques. 122). Thomas sometimes speaks of fornication as involving three people: the two engaged in coitus and the child that might result. Fornication is thus worse than theft, because it is disadvantageous not merely to property but to this child's good. Fornication, however, is not as bad as murder, which sins against an existing life (*ST*, IIaI-Iae, ques. 154, art. 2, art. 3). Fornication might not even involve coitus, for libidinous kisses and caresses can be as lasciviously enjoyed, as can fantasizing about sex (*ST*, IIaI-Iae, ques. 154, art. 4; see Matt. 5:28).

Regarding nonconsensual fornication, Thomas argues that the wrong done by the rapist is as much against the prospect of marriage as it is against the victim. A seducer violates both father and daughter or, if the daughter consents, only the father. If violence is involved, the crime is rape, not seduction, although Thomas thinks they usually amount to the same thing (*ST*, IIaIIae, ques. 154, art. 6, art. 7). **Incest**, too, is a sin, because it is disrespectful of our parents (Lev. 18) and prevents people from widening their circle of friends. Worse, it tends to lead to excessive desire between the persons involved (*ST*, IIaI-Iae, ques. 154, art. 9; *DM*, ques. 15, art. 3). Lust combines with sacrilege, Thomas says, when one seduces or rapes another whose life is dedicated to divine service (nun, priest, monk). This Aquinas calls "spiritual rape" (*ST*, IIaIIae, ques. 154, art. 10).

Adultery—from the Latin *ad alter* ("to another"), referring to invading a bed not one's own—is a special lechery. This sin wrongs not only the spouse(s) of the fornicating couple but also their offspring, in addition to damaging the souls of the adulterous individuals. The only licit **sexual activity** is between two people married to one another. Even then, lust haunts every sexual act. If the man behaves with abandon or too fiercely with his wife, the act is as much adulterous as if he were with another woman (*ST*, IIaIIae, ques. 154, art. 8, reply 2). If "it is not as a wife, but as a woman, that a man treats his wife, and if he is ready to use her in the same way if she were not his wife, it is a mortal sin. . . . If however he seeks pleasure within the bounds of marriage so that it would not be sought in another than his wife, it is a venial sin" (*ST*, Supplement, ques. 49, art. 6). The marriage debt (*annexis matrimonio*; see 1 Cor. 7:4–5) binds wife and husband mutually. But because the wife has periodic generative powers the husband lacks, the husband is more bound to have intercourse with her to beget children than she is bound to have sex with him when she knows conception is unlikely. Thus the wife has a duty to refrain from sex during menses, and the husband must not force himself on her (*ST*, Supp., ques. 64, art. 1; see art. 3, art. 4).

Contraception seems precluded by a central dimension of Aquinas's **sexual ethics**: "The end which nature intends in sexual union is the begetting and rearing of the offspring; and that this good might be sought after, it attached pleasure to the union. . . . [U]se of sexual intercourse on account of its inherent pleasure, without reference to the end for which nature intended it, is to act against nature" (*ST*, Supp., ques. 65, art. 3; *SCG*, III, ques. 122; for commentary, see Gudorf, 65). It does not follow, however, that sex in which conception is uncertain is wrong. In the case of the elderly, marriage and marital sex are permitted, despite their being unable to conceive, although Thomas does not think this preferable to **abstinence** (*ST*, Supp., ques. 58, art. 1, reply 3). If a married person is sterile, or if the wife is already pregnant (and does not know it), conception is impossible, yet sex is not against nature (*SCG*, III, ques. 122). Even if a couple's taking active measures to prevent pregnancy contraceptively makes their sex illicit, having sex under conditions that might be construed as avoiding pregnancy, while doing nothing actively to prevent conception, is not. (Such is one precursor of the "natural family planning" or "periodic continence" of twentieth-century Catholicism; see Anscombe.)

Because sex is both generative and a marital binding force, impotence and frigidity are matters of concern. Impotence can arise either from a natural, intrinsic cause or an artificial, extrinsic cause. If it is natural but temporary, it can be remedied, and the marriage will not suffer; but if it is permanent, the marriage is voided. The man will remain "forever without the hope of marriage," while the woman is free to marry someone else (*ST*, Supp., ques. 58, art. 1). The hallmark of permanence is three years, according to Church practice: Three years of honest effort without an erection renders the marriage void. But, Thomas warns, if afterwards the man regains his powers, the marriage is reinstated. The extrinsic cause of impotence Aquinas had in mind was witchcraft (not a figment of superstitious imaginations, for Scripture speaks of its reality). The Church, when dealing with impotence, must be alert to the possibility that someone is engaged in sorcery (*ST*, Supp., ques. 58, art. 2). Frigidity in women is a lesser impediment; it does not preclude intercourse. "Yet there may be a natural impediment from another cause, namely stricture, and then we must judge of stricture in the woman in the same way as of frigidity in the man" (*ST*, Supp., ques. 58, art. 1, reply 6). A tough hymen, Thomas comments, may be broken by a medical instrument.

While marriage is best for many people as a means whereby carnal sin may be defeated (1 Cor. 7:9), not everyone should marry. Celibacy is better for some, particularly some (but not all) who spend their lives studying theology. Celibacy is not unnatural, despite the disturbance it might cause, although celibacy without a spiritual reason suggests the vice of insensibility (*SCG*, III, ques. 137). At the resurrection, we will have bodies for enjoying Paradise in perfect beatitude, but the saved have no need of sustenance or reproduction, so the pleasures of eating and sex will be gone. These pleasures, for Thomas, are instrumental for the preservation of the individual and the species. But there will be no new people born, as it would be awkward to have one class born in sin and saved by Christ and another born without sin. Hence, there is no sexual activity after resurrection. Those who believe there would be, like Jews, Saracens, and millenarian heretics who envision a thousand-year earthly paradise, are wrong (*SCG*, IV, ques. 83).

In Eden, people were immortal, having bodies resistant to corruption, thanks to constant subjective connection to God (*ST*, Ia, ques. 97, art. 1). Woman was created to help man (Gen. 2:18). Since "another man would have proven a more effective help in anything else," generation must have been why she was created (*ST*, Ia, ques. 98, art. 2; Augustine, *Good of Marriage*, 1.1, 3.3; *Literal Reading of Genesis*, 9.3.5, 9.3.9). In natural generation, Thomas argues, there must be active and passive principles, one that acts by fertilizing, one that is fertilized. Given the mechanics of the procreative organs, the male acts, the female is acted on. So coitus has been part of our nature from creation. This does not mean that the sensual delights of sexuality would be pursued as if impelled by desire. Reason instead would determine when sex was appropriate, and since reason controlled lower human nature, the pleasure would be rich but not an end in itself (*ST*, Ia, ques. 98, art. 2). People did not have sex in Paradise for fun, even with physical pleasure possible. Concupiscence, which entices one to hunger for more pleasure, would have been wholly absent. Further, the virginal integrity of the woman would not have been compromised by sex, "for the semen could enter without the impairment of the genital organs, just as now the menstrual flow in a virgin does not impair her integrity" (*ST*, Ia, ques. 98, art. 2, reply 3, reply 4; see Augustine, *COG*, bk. 14, chap. 26). Sexual pleasure is not a consequence of the Fall, for the anticipation of sexual delight encourages reproduction even in Eden. Before the Fall, the sexual experience would have been intense, but we would not have been driven by its prospect, or addicted to it, as we are now. Indeed, "the pleasure of sense would have been all the greater, given the greater purity of man's nature and sensibility of his body. But the pleasure urge would not have squandered itself in so disorderly a fashion on this sort of pleasure when it was ruled by reason" (*ST*, Ia, ques. 98, art. 2, reply 3).

Of the unnatural sexual vices, **bestiality** is, for Aquinas, the worst, for it goes beyond the bounds of humanity (*ST*, IIaIIae, ques. 154, art. 12; he refers to Gen. 37:2). Following that is "the vice of sodomy," sexual activity between two men (or two women), then lechery that departs from the right mode of intercourse ("according to other rather beastly and monstrous techniques"), and finally, **masturbation** (*ST*, IIaIIae, ques. 154, art. 11). Masturbation, the least grave unnatural vice, is an "unchaste softness" that involves sin against the right order and use of one's body (*DM*, ques. 15, reply 4). Finding sexual release with another person of the opposite sex in ways other than coitus, that is, elsewhere than in the "right vessel" (the genitals of one's partner), is next in gravity. This is worse than if "the inordinateness concerns other modes of intimacy" (*ST*, IIaIIae, ques. 154, art. 12), by which Aquinas likely means coitus in some position other than the "missionary." Next in gravity are same-sex acts. Thomas reads Paul, whose authority he views as final, as condemning same-sex acts in Romans 1:26 and 2 Corinthians 12:21. "A practice opposed to the pattern set for us by nature" exceeds in wickedness the seduction of an innocent of the opposite sex, adultery, and rape (*ST*, IIaIIae, ques. 154, art. 12).

Some scholars have tried to ameliorate Aquinas's condemnation of **homosexuality**. John McNeill (97n.30) cites a passage in which Thomas lists pleasures that, while not strictly speaking natural, might be considered accompanying nature. "Consequently it happens that something which is not natural to man . . . becomes connatural to this individual man, on account of there being some corruption of nature within him" (*ST*, IaIIae, ques. 31, art. 7). Thomas's examples are sick people who perceive sweet as bitter, deranged people with a taste for dirt, and the disturbed who take pleasure in cannibalism or bestiality. Because same-sex acts are, for Aquinas, only marginally less grave than bestiality (*ST*, IIaIIae, ques. 154, art. 12), reading Thomas as open to more lenient views of homosexuality is difficult. **John Boswell** (1947–1994) suggests that Thomas's calling homosexuality unnatural is more a social than purely theological decision (303–22, 328). In the third objection of *ST* IaIIae, question 94, article 2, the argument is rehearsed that virtue is not common to all: Something might be virtuous for one person and vicious for another. Thomas responds that this applies to acts in themselves, which might be proportionate to some but disproportionate to others. Boswell interprets Aquinas here as perhaps permitting some social relativism about homosexuality. Had Aquinas viewed homosexuality as a natural variation of the norm, as something "we are born with" (as in Jung and Smith, 30–31), one might follow Boswell. But Thomas's earlier description of it as a disordered state of one's nature, akin to cannibalistic hunger or enjoying animals sexually, makes this implausible. However, for a theological analysis of homosexuality in a tradition open to Aquinas's thought, see Charles Hefling.

See also Abstinence; Adultery; Anscombe, G.E.M.; Aristotle; Augustine (Saint); Bestiality; Bible, Sex and the; Boswell, John; Casual Sex; Catholicism, History of; Catholicism, Twentieth- and Twenty-First-Century; Completeness, Sexual; Contraception; Homosexuality, Ethics of; Homosexuality and Science; Incest; Masturbation; Natural Law (New); Paul (Saint); Perversion, Sexual; Russell, Bertrand; Sherfey, Mary Jane; Social Constructionism; Wojtyła, Karol (Pope John Paul II)

REFERENCES

Anscombe, G.E.M. "Contraception and Chastity." *The Human World*, no. 7 (1972), 9–30; Anselm. (1099–1100) "On the Virgin Conception and Original Sin." In Brian Davies and Gillian Evans, eds., *The Major Works*. Oxford, U.K.: Oxford University Press, 1998, 357–89; Aristotle. (ca. 350 BCE?)

Metaphysics. Trans. David Ross. Oxford, U.K.: Oxford University Press, 1924. Reprinted, 1997; Augustine. (413–427) *The City of God* [*De civitate Dei*]. Trans. John Healey. Ed. R.V.G. Tasker. London: J. M. Dent, 1945; Augustine. (401–414) *The Literal Reading of Genesis* [*De genesi ad litteram*]. Trans. John Hammond Taylor. Mahwah, N.J.: Paulist Press, 1983; Augustine. (418?–421) *On Marriage and Concupiscence* [*De nuptiis et concupiscentiae*]. Trans. Peter Holmes and Robert Ernest Wallis. In Philip Schaff, ed., *Library of Nicene and Post-Nicene Fathers*, vol. 5. Grand Rapids, Mich.: Eerdmans, 1989, 263–308; Augustine. (401–402) *On the Good of Marriage* [*De bono coniugali*]. Ed. and trans. Patrick G. Walsh. Oxford, U.K.: Clarendon Press, 2001; Augustine. (400) *Reply to Faustus the Manichaean* [*Contra Faustum*]. Trans. R. Stothert. In Philip Schaff, ed., *Library of Nicene and Post-Nicene Fathers*, vol. 4. Grand Rapids, Mich.: Eerdmans, 1989, 155–345; Bacon, Francis. (1620) *The New Organon* [*Novum Organum*]. Ed. Lisa Jardine and Michael Silverthorne. Cambridge: Cambridge University Press, 2000; Boswell, John. *Christianity, Social Tolerance, and Homosexuality: Gay People in Western Europe from the Beginning of the Christian Era to the Fourteenth Century*. Chicago, Ill.: University of Chicago Press, 1980; Gudorf, Christine E. *Body, Sex, and Pleasure: Reconstructing Christian Sexual Ethics*. Cleveland, Ohio: Pilgrim Press, 1994; Hefling, Charles, ed. *Our Selves, Our Souls, and Bodies*. Boston, Mass.: Cowley Press, 1996; Jung, Patricia B., and Ralph Smith. *Heterosexism: An Ethical Challenge*. Albany: State University of New York Press, 1993; Leo XIII (Pope). "*Aeterni Patris*, Encyclical on the Restoration of Christian Philosophy, August 4, 1879." In Claudia Carlen, ed., *The Papal Encyclicals 1878–1903*. Raleigh, N.C.: Pierian Press, 1990, 17–27; McNeill, John J. *The Church and the Homosexual*, 4th ed. Boston, Mass.: Beacon Press, 1993; Owens, Joseph. "Aquinas as Aristotelian Commentator." In *St. Thomas Aquinas, 1274–1974: Commemorative Studies*. Toronto, Can.: Pontifical Institute of Medieval Studies, 1974, 213–38; Paul VI (Pope). "*Humanae Vitae*, Encyclical on the Regulation of Birth." In Claudia Carlen, ed., *The Papal Encyclicals 1958–1981*. Raleigh, N.C.: Pierian Press, 1990, 223–36; Thomas Aquinas. (1267–1268) *Commentary on Aristotle's De Anima*. Trans. Kenelm Foster and Silvester Humphries. New Haven, Conn.: Yale University Press, 1951. Reprinted, Notre Dame, Ind.: Dumb Ox Books, 1994; Thomas Aquinas. (1273?) *Commentary on Saint Paul's Epistle to the Ephesians*. Trans. Matthew Lamb. Albany, N.Y.: Magi Books, 1966; Thomas Aquinas. (1269) *De Malo* [*On Evil*]. Trans. Richard Regan. Oxford, U.K.: Oxford University Press, 2003; Thomas Acquinas. (1265–1266) *Quaestiones de Anima* [*Questions on the Soul*]. Trans. James H. Robb. Milwaukee, Wis.: Marquette University Press, 1984; Thomas Aquinas. (1258–1264) *Summa contra gentiles*, 5 vols. Trans. Anton Pegis. South Bend, Ind.: University of Notre Dame Press, 1975; Thomas Aquinas. (1265–1273) *Summa theologiae*, 60 vols. Trans. Blackfriars. Cambridge, U.K.: Blackfriars, 1964–1976; Thomas Aquinas. *Summa theologiae*. In *Basic Writings of St. Thomas Aquinas*. Ed. and trans. Anton Pegis. New York: Random House, 1945.

Stephen E. Lahey

ADDITIONAL READING

Anscombe, G.E.M. "Contraception and Chastity." *The Human World*, no. 7 (1972), 9–30. Reprinted in Michael Bayles, ed., *Ethics and Population*. Cambridge, Mass.: Schenkman, 1976, 134–53; HS (29–50); Anscombe, G.E.M., and Peter T. Geach. *Three Philosophers*. [Aristotle, Thomas Aquinas, Frege] Ithaca, N.Y.: Cornell University Press, 1961; Beis, Richard H. "Contraception and the Logical Structure of the Thomist Natural Law Theory." *Ethics* 75:4 (1965), 277–84; Brundage, James A. *Law, Sex, and Christian Society in Medieval Europe*. Chicago, Ill.: University of Chicago Press, 1987; Davies, Brian. *Aquinas*. London: Continuum, 2002; Davies, Brian. *The Thought of Thomas Aquinas*. Oxford, U.K.: Clarendon Press, 1992; Dougherty, Jude P. "Thomism." In Ruth Chadwick, ed., *Encyclopedia of Applied Ethics*, vol. 4. San Diego, Calif.: Academic Press, 1998, 365–72; Elliott, Dyan. *Fallen Bodies: Pollution, Sexuality, and Demonology in the Middle Ages*. Philadelphia: University of Pennsylvania Press, 1999; Finnis, John M. *Aquinas: Moral, Political, and Legal Theory*. Oxford, U.K.: Oxford University Press, 1998; Fuchs, Josef. "Natural Law." In Judith Dwyer, ed., *The New Dictionary of Catholic Social Thought*. Collegeville, Minn.: Liturgical Press, 1994,

669–75; Gilson, Étienne. *The Christian Philosophy of St. Thomas Aquinas*. Trans. L. K. Shook. New York: Random House, 1956; Gracia, Jorge, and Timothy Noone. *A Companion to Philosophy in the Middle Ages*. London: Blackwell, 2003; Haakonssen, Knud. "Natural Law." In Lawrence C. Becker and Charlotte B. Becker, eds., *Encyclopedia of Ethics*, 2nd ed., vol. 2. New York: Routledge, 2001, 1205–12; Jordan, Mark D. *The Invention of Sodomy in Christian Theology*. Chicago, Ill.: University of Chicago Press, 1997; Kenny, Anthony, ed. *Aquinas: A Collection of Critical Essays*. London: Macmillan, 1969; Kerr, Fergus. *After Aquinas: Versions of Thomism*. London: Blackwell, 2002; Kretzman, Norman, and Eleonore Stump, eds. *The Cambridge Companion to Aquinas*. Cambridge: Cambridge University Press, 1993; Lahey, Stephen E. "Saint Thomas Aquinas [on Love]." In Ellen K. Feder, Karmen MacKendrick, and Sybol S. Cook, eds., *A Passion for Wisdom: Readings in Western Philosophy on Love and Desire*. Englewood Cliffs, N.J.: Prentice Hall, 2004, 136–39; Levy, Donald. "Perversion and the Unnatural as Moral Categories." *Ethics* 90:2 (1980), 191–202. Reprinted (revised, expanded) in POS1 (169–89); Lonergan, Bernard. *Verbum: Word and Idea in Aquinas*. Ed. David Burrell. South Bend, Ind.: University of Notre Dame Press, 1967; Noonan, John T. (1965) *Contraception: A History of Its Treatment by the Catholic Theologians and Canonists*, enlarg. ed. Cambridge, Mass.: Harvard University Press, 1986; O'Connor, D[aniel] J[ohn]. *Aquinas and Natural Law*. London: Macmillan, 1967; O'Meara, Thomas. *Thomas Aquinas, Theologian*. South Bend. Ind.: University of Notre Dame Press, 1997; Pasnau, Robert. *Thomas Aquinas on Human Nature*. Cambridge: Cambridge University Press, 2002; Paul VI (Pope). "*Humanae Vitae*, Encyclical on the Regulation of Birth." In Claudia Carlen, ed., *The Papal Encyclicals 1958–1981*. Raleigh, N.C.: Pierian Press, 1990, 223–36. Reprinted in P&S1 (131–49); P&S2 (167–84); P&S3 (96–105); Payer, Pierre. *The Bridling of Desire: Views of Sex in the Later Middle* Ages. Toronto, Can.: University of Toronto Press, 1993; Pope, Stephen J. "Primate Sociality and Natural Law Theory." In Robert W. Sussman and Audrey R. Chapman, eds., *The Origins and Nature of Sociality*. New York: Aldine de Gruyter, 2004, 313–31; Principe, Walter. "Loving Friendship According to Thomas Aquinas." In David Goicoechea, ed., *The Nature and Pursuit of Love: The Philosophy of Irving Singer*. Amherst, N.Y.: Prometheus, 1995, 128–41; Schott, Robin May. (1988) "Aquinas's Views of Women and Sexuality." In *Cognition and Eros: A Critique of the Kantian Paradigm*. University Park: Pennsylvania State University Press, 1993, 59–71; Soble, Alan. "Kant and Sexual Perversion." *The Monist* 86:1 (2003), 57–92; Thomas Aquinas. *Commentum in quartum librum sententiarum magistri Petri Lombardi*. In *Opera omnia*, t. 7/2. Parmae, Italy: Typis Petri Fiaccadori, 1858, 872–1259; Thomas Aquinas. (1258) *Faith, Reason, and Theology* [*Commentary on the De Trinitate of Boethius*]. Trans. Armand Maurer. *Medieval Sources in Translation* 32. Toronto, Can: Pontifical Institute of Medieval Theology, 1987; Thomas Aquinas. *Summa theologiae: A Concise Translation*. Trans. Timothy McDermott. Allen, Tex.: Christian Classics, 1991; Torrell, Jean-Pierre. *Saint Thomas Aquinas*, vol. 1: *The Person and His Work*. Washington, D.C.: Catholic University of America, 1996; Westerman, Pauline C. *The Disintegration of Natural Law Theory: Aquinas to Finnis*. Leiden, Holland: Brill, 1998.

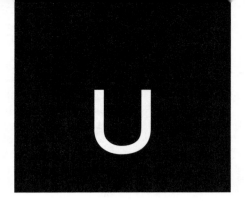

USE, SEXUAL. *See* Kant, Immanuel; Objectification, Sexual

UTILITARIANISM. *See* Consequentialism

UTOPIANISM. Sexual utopianism is essentially a modern phenomenon, beginning with writings in the late 1800s and early 1900s. **Plato**'s (427–347 BCE) *Republic* is not utopian, in the sense that this theoretical work describes the ideal state but makes no claims about its possibility. Similarly, in *Utopia* Thomas More (1477/78–1535) presents an ironic vision of communal society that the author did not really consider a possibility. Neither Plato nor More proposes a sexual utopia and not even a liberating conception of relations between the sexes. Plato's equality of male and female guardians is not based on individual rights or assumptions about the sameness of the sexes (see Buchan, *passim*). Instead, it was meant to avoid the evils of inheritance and familial preferences. Male and female guardians are, for eugenic reasons, mated at religious festivals by a rigged lottery, and personal ties among them are thereby eliminated. Men and women of this class exercise naked together, sexual relations are occasionally permitted as rewards, and children are raised communally. But Plato denies that men and women are in general equally capable (*Republic*, bk. 5). More's *Utopia* likewise upholds traditional values. It has strict rules for **marriage** and divorce and severe penalties for their infraction. Though prospective spouses are presented to each other in the nude, a chaperone is present; the sole purpose of this ritual is to increase the chance of long-term marital compatibility. More's *Utopia* is a vision of economic but not sexual liberation. In Plato and More sexual fulfillment is a mere side effect of reproductive requirements and is subordinated to "higher" social goals.

Sexual utopians typically diagnose personal unhappiness and social ills in terms of either sexual frustration caused by outdated or irrational social practices and institutions or the production of unhealthy sexuality by sociopolitical arrangements. Healthy, satisfying sexuality is presented as central to the good life and a stable and progressive social order. (**Margaret Mead**'s [1901–1978] influential but questionable studies of Polynesian sexuality might be seen as an attempt of this kind, perhaps more manifesto or science fiction than social science.) But some writers find fault in nature itself (see **Sigmund Freud** [1856–1939], "Universal Tendency," 188–89). Our biological or psychological limitations prevent us from attaining fulfillment; the ideal society would change us sexually and emotionally in ways that allow us to meet our moral and spiritual aspirations.

Both types of explanation of human misery, the social and the natural, appear in the work of **Jean-Jacques Rousseau** (1712–1778). In his philosophical essay "Discourse on the Origin and Foundations of Inequality" and novels *Emile* and *Julie, or the New Heloise*,

Rousseau presents physical **love** as a simple appetite, easily satisfied in the state of nature with a wide range of partners, but which is complicated through the social construct of moral love (the result of a sort of conspiracy among women to enslave men), just as self-love (*amour de soi*) is now complicated by egotism (*amour propre*). Moral love involves desire for a particular person of virtue or merit as determined by social standards. When it is unrequited or otherwise thwarted, **jealousy**, frustration, deception, coercion, and violence result. Romance is a temporary condition, often vitiated by barriers of social class and propriety, wealth and practicality, age and familiarity. Lovers fall out of love and go their separate ways or, if they are lucky, transform their relationship into the calm, comfortable partnership of conventional marriage (see **Roger Scruton**, 244). In either case, moral love ends. But that need not be entirely bad, for moral love is in tension with the need for self-identity and autonomy, an opposition that (in contrast to the conflict of individual rights with state sovereignty) cannot ever be fully reconciled under any social system, for it is metaphysical, rooted in human nature. Rousseau is a pessimist about sex and love, not a utopian (see Rapaport).

Elements of sexual utopianism first appear in Western thought in the writings of the **Marquis de Sade** (1740–1814; on his utopianism, see Heumakers, 116–20) and followers of the French socialists Henri de Saint-Simon (1760–1825) and Charles Fourier (1772–1837). Sade, as Aldous Huxley (1894–1963) tells us, "regarded himself as the apostle of the truly revolutionary revolution, beyond mere politics and economics—the revolution in individual men, women, and children, whose bodies were henceforward to become the common sexual property of all and whose minds were to be purged of all the natural decencies, all the laboriously acquired inhibitions of traditional civilization" ("Foreword" [1946] to *Brave New World*, xvi–xvii). Sade's credo of total abandonment to sexual impulses, including the most perverse, whatever the moral cost, was adumbrated in the seventeenth century, well before Sade, by the Sabbatean movement within **Judaism**, whose eccentric leader Sabbatai Zevi married a prostitute and preached in favor of vice in general, finding a divine aspect to even the most evil deeds (see Rothstein, 209–11).

Saint-Simon's utopian socialist vision was rooted in religious faith, as evidenced in his most important work, *New Christianity* (1825). Unlike his sometime friend Auguste Comte (1798–1857), an atheist who sought to adapt the motivations and trappings of orthodox Catholicism to his own secular-rationalistic purposes, Saint-Simon saw his program as truly Christian, restoring body or the physical to its proper place in relation to the spiritual (see Manuel, 348–63). His follower Barthèlemy Prosper Enfantin (1796–1864) applied this idea sexually by founding a marriage-optional commune in which "free love" was encouraged (see Bazard). The French government perceived the commune as a threat to conventional marriage and abolished it in 1832.

Fourier similarly held that human misery was a result of our deviating from the divine plan, specifically our repression of the thirteen passions implanted by God but at odds with civilization: the five senses; four social passions (ambition, love, **friendship**, and family feeling); three distributive passions (of intrigue, diversification, combining pleasures); and the synthesizing passion for harmony. Freeing these passions would lead to human happiness and unity, he believed. Fourier proposed organizing society into a network of communes or "phalanxes" of 1,600 to 1,800 people matched scientifically for their talents and interests. These voluntary structures would successfully compete against the institutions of civilization, spreading and eventually replacing them without violence. Repressed passions are the cause of evil, and people can look forward to lives of joyful harmony once they are released. Women will be emancipated and free love the norm (see Beecher and Bienvenu, secs. III, IV,

VII). Thus Fourier anticipated socialists such as Emma Goldman (1869–1940) as well as the New Age and radical environmentalist movements of the late twentieth century.

The most significant attempt to realize such utopian ambitions in the nineteenth century was the Oneida community (1848–1879) in upstate New York, which combined Christianity, socialism, and group marriage. This scheme of "Bible Communism" was created by John Humphrey Noyes (1811–1886), an itinerant preacher who accepted Perfectionism, a doctrine that implies that those who fully embrace God can be totally free of sin. The moral law is written in their hearts, so there is no need for the external constraints of conventional morality (Klaw, 29). Earlier Christian collectivists, such as the renegade Catholic Thomas Müntzer (1486/89–1525) had attempted communities in which, on the basis of their religious beliefs, private property was abolished. Social groups devoted to the principle of "free love," such as the Berlin Heights Society of Ohio, also existed (Klaw, 236). But Noyes's community associated Christianity, common property, and nonconventional sexual arrangements for perhaps the first time. His "complex marriage" differed from free love, which he rejected as much as he did monogamy and celibacy, because it was, he thought, anarchist and sensualist. Romantic love, prone to jealousy and possessiveness, and the preferential bonds of normal parental love, were "selfish" and "sickly" and hence to be shunned. Universal love, not "egotism," was the foundation of their ethic. Sexual love must not be the "false love" of the "pleasure-seeker" but should bring people closer to God (as in **Tantrism**). It is properly regarded as sacramental, Noyes maintained, as much an occasion for celebration as Thanksgiving or Christmas (Klaw, 157).

The Oneidan system, reminiscent of Plato's *Republic*, was centrally administered by Noyes and his designated female intermediaries, who granted or denied permission to those who wanted to engage in sexual relations, or "interviews." Permission was given or withheld on various grounds, including religious and genetic fitness, and as a reward or punishment. His principle of "ascending fellowship" increased the prospects of the older and less attractive members having desirable partners: Older women would initiate boys after puberty, and most of the girls would have their first sexual experiences with Noyes himself, as in the medieval practice of the *droit du Seigneur* and, closer to home, the Branch Davidian cult of David Koresh (born Vernon Howell; 1959–1993; see Reavis). Noyes's initiation of a young girl sometimes continued for a period of several months. This activity did not preclude his having incestuous relations with his niece. (Noyes's beliefs in sexual relations between siblings and public sex on stage were apparently never put into practice.) This initiation by the community's leader was avowedly for purposes of technical and religious instruction, so that females would consider him their lifelong authority on such matters. According to one ardent defender, Noyes did this "from a deep philosophical view and not from passion" (Klaw, 242). Indeed, when on account of age and physical state he could not adequately carry on these relationships, his authority over the community declined. Provided that sexual relations were permitted, accessibility was understood as a duty to the community, so that those, especially women, who refused **sexual activity** were subject to "mutual criticism" for being antisocial. Together with sexual denial and the threat of expulsion, this practice of public criticism for anything from perceived character flaws and lack of proper religious zeal to poor sexual technique (which has exemplars in twentieth-century totalitarianism and the People's Temple cult of Marxist minister Jim Jones [1931–1978]) was not only punishment but a method of remolding people into "new men" suited to the ideal society (in this case, Heaven on Earth). Cures for disease and immortality were promised by Noyes to those who submitted to this criticism and properly reformed.

Pregnancy was to be generally averted by the practice of male continence (as in Tantra), which had another advantage: increasing the likelihood of orgasm in the women. How a practice of nonorgasmic, nonejaculatory intercourse was satisfying or beneficial to the health of males, when even **masturbation** was forbidden, is unclear. A later program of eugenics implemented by Noyes encouraged designated couples to have spiritually advanced children so as to promote the community's religious and social goals. A "Stirpiculture Committee" under Noyes's control was established to determine who was suitable for such procreation. (For a defense of stirpiculture, see the early feminist Victoria Woodhull [1838–1927].) The progeny were raised in common in a Children's House administered by a surrogate father, as were the other children of the community. It is not obvious how supposedly superior children could be integrated with those of less favored unions in a purportedly egalitarian society that generally disapproved of individual excellence. (For a poignant example of the discouragement of the development of personal talents, see Klaw, 117–18, 294.) Since all children were thought to belong to the community conceived as one family, parents were allowed only limited time with their biological children, and that could be limited further as an antidote to an excessive degree "philoprogenitiveness" or as punishment for disobedience. Not only were parent-child sentiments and attachments discouraged, but emotional ties to the dead were as well. Children were taught not to grieve at funerals, which were simple and often perfunctory, sometimes even celebratory and joyful occasions. They were taught to sing songs expressing the doctrines of universal love and other tenets of the faith.

The status of women in the Oneida community was in some respects better than in the wider world but in others worse (Klaw, 130–38). Although Noyes viewed women as generally inferior to men, they had a measure of independence from particular men (other than Noyes), more sexual variety, less likelihood of unwanted pregnancy, financial security, others with whom to share burdensome domestic tasks, and a vote on community matters. What they lost were the right to have exclusive relationships with one man and their children. For Noyes, the gates of Heaven were closed to the monogamous by God's will: "You may say that you have no taste for anybody but your wife," Noyes said. "But . . . God will not have in his kingdom those who cannot love all that he loves" (Klaw, 168). As in many Christians from **Saint Paul** (5–64?) and **Saint Augustine** (354–430) to **Søren Kierkegaard** (1813–1855), Noyes condemned any particular love that was so passionate and exclusive as to turn the lovers from the demands of God (Klaw, 184). Girls were denied dolls (all were destroyed in a fire as ordered by Noyes), and women were discouraged from wearing long hair, long dresses, or jewelry. They were expected to be attractive to men, but without conventional methods of allure. Selfish, greedy sensualism was to be avoided; sex should be unselfish, even to the point of denying one's own tastes and inclinations (see Klaw, 188). Yet people should enjoy a variety of people sexually just as they enjoy eating various fruits (one of Noyes's comparisons; Klaw, 157). One thereby loves the way an undiscriminating God loves.

Opposition from other religious groups and opinion leaders (one of whom characterized Oneida as a "utopia of obscenity"), threats of criminal prosecution, internal dissent about the autocratic leadership of the aging Noyes, and dissatisfaction with the administration of business interests and the system of sexual assignments led to the dissolution of the Oneida commune after thirty-one years. It remains the most successful example in American history of a functioning religious communist society, at its height including hundreds of members. Influenced by Noyes's readings of the Bible and Fourier, it was similar in some respects to Israeli kibbutzim and likely influenced a number of twentieth-century authors.

Despite his differences with **Marxism**, Edward Bellamy's (1850–1898) *Looking Backward* is a blueprint for a nationalistic, militaristic socialist state in many aspects not much different from the Soviet Union. Written as a romantic **fantasy** novel so as to attract readers, especially women, the book and its sequel, *Equality*, advocate neither free love nor female emancipation. Indeed, though many prominent feminists, whom Bellamy actively courted, were among his followers, he had traditional views about women and sex roles (not to mention racial prejudices). He favored a weakening of emotional ties within the family (see Strauss); deep emotional bonds were not only a threat to the solidarity of the state but a source of human suffering. In "Reorganization of Society to Extirpate Sorrow" (not published) and *Dr. Heiderhoff's Process* (1880), he presents Kafkaesque schemes, including the erasure of memory, to eliminate personal feelings for the greater good of society (Strauss, 83–85).

The extinguishing of deep sexual and familial ties is central to the imagined society of Aldous Huxley's *Brave New World* (*BNW*). No woman conceives and gives birth, for babies are created, gestated, and "decanted" artificially in "hatcheries," laboratories of human mass production that tailor the genetic profiles of infants to order. After "hypnopaedic" and other forms of conditioning in governmental child-raising facilities, the end result is a human who likes his place (whatever it is) in the rigid social class structure, aspiring to nothing better, perfectly suited to his economic role. Lower-class humans are cloned in large numbers, while those who fill the upper classes are more genetically unique. Sexual relations are casual, recreational, and definitely not meant to be reproductive (see Marcus's notion "pornotopia," 271). Long-term, exclusive relationships are strongly discouraged. Viviparous procreation is considered disgusting, and family life—with its sexual tensions, dysfunctional dynamics, and neurotic outcomes—is nothing to be missed. Children are taught to explore their bodies in sexual play. Morality requires lack of sexual restraint. Huxley (as if a member of **the Freudian Left**) comments, "As political and economic freedom diminishes, sexual freedom tends compensatingly to increase" ("Foreword" to *BNW*, xx).

Powerful emotions are perceived as a grave threat to the stability of society, and drugs such as soma ("A gramme is better than a damn") and occasional clinical treatments are readily available to head them off. For the same reason, **pornography**, sports, and frivolous entertainment have replaced the appreciation of serious art and literature; only a few world controllers have access to the great works. Religious faith and worship exist only in the form of a neopagan or New Age cult that stages "community sings" in which drugged participants dance into the sexual frenzy of "orgy-porgy." In what is essentially a Benthamite utilitarian society, even death is no occasion for sadness or suffering, for young children are conditioned to feel indifferent or even good when another human life ends. The life is assumed to have been a happy one, and its remains contribute energy to a factory. Mass consumption of technically sophisticated consumer goods and pastimes (Centrifugal Bumble-Puppy, Electromagnetic Golf, and the feelies), the pleasures of promiscuity, soma holidays, unchallenging jobs, and quasi-religious ecstasy are the ingredients of the good life this Panopticon.

In *BNW*, Huxley contrasts this society with that of the "savage reservation," an American Indian society in which veneration of nature, religious awe, ancient rituals, and traditional sexual mores give meaning to life and death. The physical conditions of disease, filth, brutality, extreme poverty, and old age, which are absent from "civilized society," are the price paid for richer personal, social, and spiritual lives. Love is made possible by conservative sexual morality, the reality of procreation, raising one's children to adulthood, and passing on wisdom and values. But while this is a more "human" society, it suffers from its own irrationality. Huxley expresses regret that he did not present a third alternative, a sane society based on cooperative economics, philosophically respectable religious beliefs, a higher form of utilitarianism, and a resolve that technology should serve human interests and not become our master ("Foreword" to *BNW*, xv).

Brave New World Revisited (*BNWR*), Huxley's retrospective essay on his book and observations on how some of it was becoming true, was written after the other great "dystopian" novel of the twentieth century appeared in 1948, George Orwell's *1984*. Orwell's Stalinesque state, based on coercion, punishment, and negative reinforcement, struck Huxley as less likely a picture of the future than something similar to *BNW* or B. F. Skinner's *Walden Two* (meant as a utopian novel), in which more efficient positive reinforcement and the genetic and/or environmental molding of the population to like their socioeconomic lots creates social stability and contentment. Huxley acknowledged that, at the time of writing *BNWR*, fascism had only recently been defeated, while communism increasingly threatened the free world. Overpopulation, he argued, would undermine the West and help the spread of Soviet domination.

In *1984* sexual and romantic love are discouraged by the state as threats to its stability. Instead of "free and frequent access to the opposite sex" serving to release tension among the masses (as in *BNW*; Huxley, *BNWR*, 11), erotic impulses are controlled and redirected by the government, transformed into the more useful feelings of a patriotic, hateful, warlike character. The relationship between two lovers—Winston and Julia—must be broken up because, as individual, voluntary, and private, it represents a loyalty to something other than the state. The state, as personified by "Big Brother," is to be the object of all love; hence private eroticism is subversive, even quasi-adulterous, as sex would be among Catholics in a holy order wedded to God and bound by vows of celibacy. The totalitarian societies of *BNW* and *1984* attempt to destroy "normal" human love relationships; one by trivializing sex, divorcing it from personal love, the other by punishing and redirecting it for the sake of social unity. Yet in Orwell's novel we find both the "Junior Anti-Sex League" *and* secret governmental production of pornography: Sexual appetites must be both stimulated and frustrated to be manipulable for state purposes.

Wilhelm Reich's (1897–1957) Freudo-Marxist diagnosis of the fascist impulse is pertinent here. His *The Sexual Revolution* appeared in 1930, the same year as Sigmund Freud's *Civilization and Its Discontents*, and it was shortly followed by another major work, *Character Analysis*. Reich hypothesized that sexual frustration, arising from external sources for which the family serves as a conduit, causes an "armoring" in the individual's personality and a sublimating of natural instincts into authoritarian impulses. In a healthy individual only pregenital desires would be sublimated and "orgiastic potency" would be maximized. The concentration of what Reich called "orgone energy" and its release in an intense orgasmic experience (contrast Noyes's continence) was paramount. Reich's sexual utopianism developed as he progressed from Marxism to anarchism, and it influenced the sexual revolution of the 1960s, as did the writings of Herbert Marcuse (1898–1979) (see King, 51–52, 62–77).

Another important influence on the 1960s sexual revolution was Robert Heinlein's (1907–1988) *Stranger in a Strange Land*. Its protagonist, Valentine Michael Smith, is the child of human parents raised by Martians after a crash landing on Mars killed his mother and father. Following his return to Earth, it emerges that he has extraordinary mental powers resulting from his alien upbringing. But his innocence and goodwill prevent him from misusing his abilities as he tries to "grok" (understand) the weird beliefs, customs, and mores of his parents' culture. Smith's powers include being able to remove the clothing of others and even inducing orgasm without direct physical contact. He seeks to know everyone within his circle as intimately as possible, encouraging them to surmount the sexual and psychological barriers that normally exist between individuals to achieve a kind of merging in universal love. Smith is an erotic Christ-figure who finally sacrifices his life for the salvation of humanity.

Robert Rimmer's (1917–2001) *The Harrad Experiment* was also an important influence. Advertised as "The Sex Manifesto of the Free-Love Generation," the 1966 novel chronicles a coeducational rooming arrangement among students at "Harrad" College (derived from Harvard and Radcliffe). Part four-year seminar, part encounter group, and part sensitivity-training workshop, this "structured experimental premarital environment" (*Harrad Letters*, 41) aimed at promoting self-realization and self-discovery through close communication and intimate contact with the other sex, which mitigates the tendency to **sexual objectification**. Common bathing and mixed-sex exercise in the nude, as in Plato's *Republic*, was the rule. Changing sex partners was allowed, but it would not be "swinging" or "free love." Sexual experience has more to do with the brain than the genitals and should be "an adventure in non-duality" (*Letters*, 54), not an athletic event or mere physical gratification. In his introductory essay preceding the *Letters*, Rimmer claims that "sexual humanism," which includes "a new understanding of the importance of love," can be the basis for "a new system of education" that could provide the nation and humanity with "a sense of purpose and direction" that it needs to surmount future challenges (*Letters*, 144–45). Yet, despite these grandiose aims, Rimmer denies that his novels are utopian, if that implies aiming at a perfect, unchanging outcome. We can try only to get closer to the ideal, to approximate it, and our conception of what that ideal is will inevitably change (see *Letters*, 8, 19–20, 28–29, 38–39, 42–43, 45–47). Left-liberal Rimmer remarks that he read *Stranger in a Strange Land* after writing his major novels, but he does recommend Right-libertarian Heinlein's exploration of alternative forms of marriage (*Letters*, 51, 53).

The influence of Huxley is evident in Robert Silverberg's 1970 science fiction novel *The World Inside*, set in 2381. Most people live in 1,000-floor skyscrapers ("urban monads"); hundreds of thousands of people, crammed into tiny apartments, fill each, and few ever leave unless they are needed to start a new "urbmon." The rest of humanity populates primitive farm communes that provide sustenance to the urbmons in return for manufactured goods. The religion of the urbmon dwellers condemns **contraception** and exalts parenting: The more children, the more blessed. Most are married while teenagers, but sexual exclusivity and jealousy are considered antisocial, a cause for counseling or even treatment from the "moral engineers." Those who fail to conform are sent "down the chute" into trash compactors and the urbmon's giant furnaces. "Nightwalking," mandatory promiscuous forays into the beds of other couples, is typically confined within one's own socioeconomic level (corresponding to groups of floors) but need not be. Anyone may have anyone, regardless of class or sex, at least in principle. This totally "free love" (along with drugs and entertainments) supposedly compensates for the stress and limitations of urbmon life, yet the lives of the characters in *World Inside* appear as desperately empty as those of their counterparts in *BNW*. Complete sexual freedom does not liberate or provide meaning or fulfillment to human lives.

Perhaps, then, a truly utopian society would be *asexual*. The radical vision of feminist theorist Ti-Grace Atkinson assumes that sexual differences between men and women, apart from their reproductive systems, are wholly the creation of culture, specifically of male oppressors who millennia ago took advantage of female weakness and vulnerability in pregnancy to assign them lesser social roles. For Atkinson, masculinity and femininity (gender roles) are social constructs that can and must be eliminated to attain social justice; along with them, biological procreation and sexual intercourse will also be dispatched to the trashbin of patriarchal history ("Institution of Sexual Intercourse"). Given, as in *BNW*, the artificial production of future generations, "men" and "women" will be obsolete, and both the need and desire for sex will wither away (just as Chairman Mao declared, during the Chinese Cultural Revolution, "In our society the piano is no longer needed"). The loss of sexual love should not be bemoaned, for it is pathological, "the natural response of the victim to the rapist" ("Radical Feminism"). Destructive dependency relationships are the inevitable result of erotic relationships; we simply do not realize this in our unhealthy, inegalitarian social order. The nearest thing remaining to sex would be "cooperative sensual experiences," group strokings serving as vehicles for expressing social approval of their recipients.

While Atkinson writes prose essays, other feminists have explored these issues in novels. Joanna Russ (*The Female Man*) and Marge Piercy (*Woman on the Edge of Time*) used time travel to bring together women of the present with those of future utopian and dystopian worlds. Russ's protagonists are Jeannine, an engaged woman with conventional aspirations; Joanna, a 1970s feminist; Janet, a woman from a future feminist utopian society; and Jael, who lives in a less distant future world in which men and women are literally at war, though stalemated. Janet's home "Whileaway" is devoid of men, who (she believes) died out in a plague. Men are not missed, for women become "men" by learning to do typically male tasks, employing strength-amplifying "induction helmets" when needed. (This is reminiscent of Thomas Berger's earlier novel *Regiment of Women*, with its stereotyped male-female role reversals.) In Jael's possible world "Manlanders" (men) are the enemy; they buy their male children from "Womanlanders," with whom they have a cease-fire (rich men can custom-order using their own sperm). At age five these boys are sent to a Spartan-style camp; those who fail to become brutal Real Men are turned into transsexuals or transvestites for the pleasure of those who do. (Compare the corrupt patriarchal dictatorships of Margaret Atwood's *The Handmaid's Tale* and Suzy McKee Charnas's *Walk to the End of the World*.) Jael, a professional assassin with sharp metal teeth and retractable cat claws, kills men for a living; she enjoys her ideologically justified work. Although masculine in most respects, Jael has a sex slave, a computerized boy-toy, as an appliance in her ultramodern rural Vermont house. At the novel's end Jael reveals to Janet that the existence of Janet's women-only paradise resulted not from disease but from her military success.

Piercy's novel offers a more detailed picture of a feminist utopia: a land of small eco-villages, primarily agricultural collectives based on adopted cultures, and a mixing of races. Children are created in "brooders" with random genetic combinations, except for occasional clones that continue the genome of some honored departed. In any case, culture and nurture are thought more important than biology. (The sinister Shapers, however, want to introduce eugenics.) These nonborn offspring have three co-mothers, including nursing males, who give them temporary names that are later replaced by those they choose for themselves, including "Mao," "Marat," "Neruda," and "Sappho." Co-mothers are often not lovers, to decrease conflicts over children that might adversely affect their bisexual, nonexclusive sex lives. Families are a matter of choice, not of biological or socioeconomic necessity. "Per" replaces "him" and "her," and everyone is referred to as "person" or "comrade." Political decisions are made in a long series of meetings among those with a stake in the outcome; the democratic process, which includes designated Earth and Animal Advocates, is of paramount importance. Meat-eating still occurs, as does capital punishment (for reasons of convenience, though admittedly unjust). War with the remnants of white male technoculture (mostly androids and cyborgs) necessitates universal military service. If "utopia" implies perfection, Piercy's vision is not quite it, but much closer than many existent societies.

While these sexual utopias may seem either unfeasible or undesirable, efforts toward their implementation typically producing dystopian nightmares, they are valuable as an expression of humanity's perennial, nearly ubiquitous discontent with the sexual status quo and as attempts, in fantasy, to overcome the limits of nature and traditional society. Fictional utopias illustrate theories and reveal their underlying assumptions, and they sometimes motivate reforms that at least approximate the ideals they uphold. Utopian visions, even when not explicitly religious (as in the Mormon faith), are often religiously inspired, providing pictures of the kingdom of heaven on earth. But they need not be static, complete, or perfect; nor must they be egalitarian, though more often than not, they are, in important respects. Sexual utopias have libertarian aspects, too. Robert Nozick's (1938–2002) conception of a utopia of utopias, each utopia competing with the others within a framework of freedom (*Anarchy, State, and Utopia*, part 3), has interesting implications for sexuality. The goal would be to encourage many different sexual and familial arrangements (what John Stuart Mill [1806–1873] called "experiments" in living; *On Liberty*, chap. 3, 309) among which people could choose, the most satisfactory eventually predominating. The multiplication of alternatives is, however, not always what people want (see Delaney's *Triton*), and history has taught us about the temptation to force one's favored vision of the best arrangement on everyone.

See also Arts, Sex and the; Bisexuality; Casual Sex; Consequentialism; Cybersex; Dworkin, Andrea; Fantasy; Feminism, French; Feminism, History of; Firestone, Shulamith; Freudian Left, The; Gnosticism; Kierkegaard, Søren; Liberalism; Love; Marriage; Protestantism, History of; Reproductive Technology; Westermarck, Edward

REFERENCES

Atkinson, Ti-Grace. (1968) "The Institution of Sexual Intercourse" and "Radical Feminism." In *Amazon Odyssey*. New York: Links Books, 1974, 13–23, 46–63; Atwood, Margaret. *The Handmaid's Tale*. New York: Houghton Mifflin, 1986; Bazard, Saint-Amand, Barthèlemy Prosper Enfantin, and Émile Barrault. *The Doctrine of Saint-Simon: An Exposition, First Year, 1828–1829*. Trans. Georg G. Iggers. Boston, Mass.: Beacon Press, 1958; Beecher, Jonathan, and Richard Bienvenu. *The Utopian Vision of Charles Fourier: Selected Texts on Work, Love, and Passionate Attraction*. Boston, Mass.: Beacon Press, 1971; Bellamy, Edward. (1880) *Dr. Heiderhoff's Process*. London: William Reeves, n.d.; Bellamy, Edward. *Equality*. New York: Appleton, 1897; Bellamy, Edward. (1888) *Looking Backward: 2000–1887*. Foreword by Erich Fromm (v–xx). New York: New American Library, 1960; Berger, Thomas. *Regiment of Women*. New York: Little, Brown, 1973; Buchan, Morag. *Women in Plato's Political Theory*. New York: Routledge, 1999; Charnas, Suzy McKee. *Walk to the End of the World*. New York: Ballantine, 1974; Delany, Samuel R. *Triton*. New York: Bantam, 1976; Freud, Sigmund. (1930) *Civilization and Its Discontents*. In *The Standard Edition of the Complete Psychological Works of Sigmund Freud*, vol. 21. Trans. and ed. James Strachey. London: Hogarth Press, 1953–1974, 57–145; Freud, Sigmund. (1912) "On the Universal Tendency to Debasement in the Sphere of Love." In *The Standard Edition of the Complete Psychological Works of Sigmund Freud*, vol. 11. Trans. and ed. James Strachey. London: Hogarth Press, 1953–1974, 179–90; Goldman, Emma. (1910) *Anarchism and Other Essays*. New York: Dover, 1969; Heinlein, Robert A. *Stranger in a Strange Land*. New York: Putnam, 1961; Heumakers, Arnold. "De Sade, a Pessimistic Libertine." In Jan Bremmer, ed., *From Sappho to De Sade: Moments in the History of Sexuality*. London: Routledge, 1989, 108–22; Huxley, Aldous. *Brave New World* [1932] and *Brave New World Revisited*

[1958]. New York: Harper and Row, 1965. Includes "Foreward" (1946); King, Richard. *The Party of Eros*. Chapel Hill: University of North Carolina Press, 1971; Klaw, Spencer. *Without Sin: The Life and Death of the Oneida Community*. New York: Penguin, 1993; Manuel, Frank E. *The New World of Henri Saint-Simon*. Cambridge, Mass.: Harvard University Press, 1956; Marcus, Steven. (1966) *The Other Victorians: A Study of Sexuality and Pornography in Mid-Nineteenth-Century England*, 2nd ed. New York: Basic Books, 1975; Mead, Margaret. (1928) *Coming of Age in Samoa: A Psychological Study of Primitive Youth for Western Civilization*. New York: Morrow, 1968; Mill, John Stuart. (1859) *On Liberty*. In Bernard Wishy, ed., *Prefaces to Liberty: Selected Writings of John Stuart Mill*. Boston, Mass.: Beacon Press, 1959; More, Thomas. (1516) *Utopia*. Ed. George R. Logan and Robert M. Adams. Cambridge: Cambridge University Press, 1989; Nozick, Robert. *Anarchy, State, and Utopia*. New York: Basic Books, 1974; Orwell, George. (1948) *Nineteen Eighty-Four*. New York: New American Library–Dutton, 1950; Piercy, Marge. *Woman on the Edge of Time*. New York: Fawcett, 1974; Plato. (ca. 375–370 BCE) *The Republic*. Trans. Benjamin Jowett. Oxford, U.K.: Oxford University Press, 1945; Rapaport, Elizabeth. "On the Future of Love: Rousseau and the Radical Feminists." *Philosophical Forum* 5:1–2 (1973–1974), 185–205; Reavis, Dick J. *The Ashes of Waco*. New York: Simon and Schuster, 1995; Reich, Wilhelm. (1933) *Character Analysis*, 3rd ed., enlarged. New York: Farrar, Straus and Giroux, 1972; Reich, Wilhelm. (1930) *The Sexual Revolution*. New York: Farrar, Straus and Giroux, 1974; Rimmer, Robert. *The Harrad Experiment*. New York: New American Library, 1966; Rimmer, Robert, ed. *The Harrad Letters to Robert H. Rimmer*. New York: New American Library, 1969; Rothstein, Edward. "Utopia and Its Discontents." In Edward Rothstein, Herbert Muschamp, and Martin E. Marty, *Visions of Utopia*. New York: Oxford University Press, 2003, 1–28; Rousseau, Jean-Jacques. (1755) "Discourse on the Origin and Foundations of Inequality." In *The First and Second Discourses*. Trans. Roger D. Masters and Judith R. Masters. New York: St. Martin's Press, 1978, 76–248; Rousseau, Jean-Jacques. (1761) *Emile, or On Education*. Trans. Allan Bloom. New York: Basic Books, 1979; Rousseau, Jean-Jacques. (1761) *Julie, or the New Heloise: Letters of Two Lovers Who Live in a Small Town at the Foot of the Alps*. Trans. Philip Stewart and Jean Vaché. Hanover, N.H.: University Press of New England, 1997; Russ, Joanna. *The Female Man*. Boston, Mass.: Beacon Press, 1975; Saint-Simon, Henri de. (1825) *Nouvelle Christianisme* (*New Christianity*). Parts in Keith Taylor, ed., *Henri Saint-Simon 1760–1825: Selected Writings on Science, Industry, and Social Organization*. New York: Holmes and Meier, 1975, 289–304; and Ghita Ionescu, ed., *The Political Thought of Saint-Simon*. New York: Oxford University Press, 1976, 204–18; Scruton, Roger. *Sexual Desire: A Moral Philosophy of the Erotic*. New York: Free Press, 1986; Silverberg, Robert. *The World Inside*. New York: Doubleday, 1970; Skinner, B. F. *Walden Two*. New York: Macmillan, 1948; Strauss, Sylvia. "Gender, Class, and Race in Utopia." In Daphne Patai, ed., *Looking Backward, 1888–1988: Essays on Edward Bellamy*. Amherst: University of Massachusetts Press, 1988, 68–90; Woodhull, Victoria. (ca. 1875) *The Victoria Woodhull Reader*. Ed. Madeleine B. Stern. Weston, Mass.: M & S Press, 1974.

Robert M. Stewart

ADDITIONAL READING

Anderson, Harriet. *Utopian Feminism: Women's Movements in Fin-de-Siècle Vienna*. New Haven, Conn.: Yale University Press, 1992; Barthes, Roland. (1971) *Sade, Fourier, Loyola*. Trans. Richard Miller. New York: Hill and Wang, 1976; Bartkowski, Frances. *Feminist Utopias*. Lincoln: University of Nebraska Press, 1989; Bean, Orson. *Me and the Orgone*. New York: St. Martin's Press, 1961; Beecher, Jonathan, and Richard Bienvenu. *The Utopian Vision of Charles Fourier*. Boston, Mass.: Beacon Press, 1971; Bobonich, Christopher. (2002) "Plato on Utopia." In Edward N. Zalta, ed., *Stanford Encyclopedia of Philosophy*. <plato.stanford.edu/entries/plato-utopia/> [accessed 26 January 2005]; Bobonich, Christopher. *Plato's Utopia Recast: His Later Ethics and Politics*. Oxford, U.K.: Clarendon Press, 2002; Burroughs, William S. (1959) *Naked Lunch*. New York: Grove Press, 1992; Califia, Pat. "Whoring in Utopia." In *Public Sex: The Culture of Radical Sex*. Pittsburgh, Pa.: Cleis Press, 1994, 242–48. Reprinted in POS4 (475–81); Chauhan, M. Rafiq. "A Comparative Study of Plato's *Republic* and Huxley's *Brave New World*." *Pakistan Philosophy Journal* 13 (1974), 63–74; Dawson, Doyne. *Cities of the Gods: Communal Utopias in Greek Thought*. New York: Oxford University Press, 1992; Donawerth, Joan, and Carol Kolmerten, eds. *Utopian and Science-Fiction by Women: Worlds of Difference*. Syracuse, N.Y.: Syracuse University Press, 1994; Eckstein, Arthur. *Orwell, Masculinity, and Feminist Criticism*. Amherst: University of Massachusetts Press, 1984; Foster, Lawrence. "That All May Be One: John Humphrey Noyes and the Origins of the Oneida Community Complex Marriage." In *Religion and Sexuality: The Shakers, the Mormons, and the Oneida Community*. Urbana: University of Illinois Press, 1984, 72–122; Foster, Lawrence. *Women, Family, and Utopia: Communal Experiments of the Shakers, the Oneida Community, and the Mormons*. Syracuse, N.Y.: Syracuse University Press, 1991; Francoeur, Robert T. *Utopian Motherhood: New Trends in Human Reproduction*. Garden City, N.Y.: Doubleday, 1970; Freud, Sigmund. (1927) *Future of an Illusion*. In *The Standard Edition of the Complete Psychological Works of Sigmund Freud*, vol. 21. Trans. James Strachey. London: Hogarth Press, 1953–1974, 1–56; Hull, Richard T., ed. *Ethical Issues in the New Reproductive Technologies*. Belmont, Calif.: Wadsworth, 1990. 2nd ed., *Ethical Issues in the New Reproductive Technologies*. Amherst, N.Y.: Prometheus, 2005; Jacoby, Russell. *The End of Utopia: Politics and Culture in an Age of Apathy*. New York: Basic Books, 1999; Kern, Louis J. *An Ordered Love: Sex Roles and Sexuality in Victorian Utopias. The Shakers, the Mormons, and the Oneida Community*. Chapel Hill: University of North Carolina Press, 1981; Kesten, Seymour R. *Utopian Episodes: Daily Life in Experimental Colonies Dedicated to Changing the World*. Syracuse, N.Y.: Syracuse University Press, 1993; Kolmerten, Carol A. *Women in Utopia: The Ideology of Gender in the American Owenite Communities*. Bloomington: Indiana University Press, 1990; Kolnai, Aurel. *The Utopian Mind and Other Papers: A Critical Study in Moral and Political Philosophy*. Ed. Francis Dunlop. London: Athlone, 1995; LeGuin, Ursula. *The Left Hand of Darkness*. New York: Ace Books, 1969; Martin, Biddy. "Sexualities without Genders and Other Queer Utopias." In Mandy Merck, Naomi Segal, and Elizabeth Wright, eds., *Coming Out of Feminism?* Oxford, U.K.: Blackwell, 1998, 11–35; Masters, R.E.L. (1962) "The Homosexual Revolution." In Henry Anatole Grunwald, ed., *Sex in America*. New York: Bantam, 1964, 256–82; McClymond, Michael J. "John Humphrey Noyes, the Oneida Community, and Male Continence." In Colleen McDannell, ed., *Religions of the United States in Practice*, vol. 1. Princeton, N.J.: Princeton University Press, 2001, 218–33; McLellan, David. *Utopian Pessimist: The Life of Simone Weil*. New York: Poseidon Press, 1990; Nussbaum, Martha C., ed. *On Nineteen Eighty-Four: Orwell and Our Future*. Princeton, N.J.: Princeton University Press, 2005; Patai, Daphne. *Orwell: A Study in Male Ideology*. Amherst: University of Massachusetts Press, 1984; Patai, Daphne, ed. *Looking Backward, 1988–1888: Essays on Edward Bellamy*. Amherst: University of Massachusetts Press, 1988; Pippin, Robert, Andrew Feenberg, and Charles P. Webel, eds. *Marcuse: Critical Theory and the Promise of Utopia*. South Hadley, Mass.: Bergin and Harvey, 1988; Rapaport, Elizabeth. "On the Future of Love: Rousseau and the Radical Feminists." *Philosophical Forum* 5:1–2 (1973–1974), 185–205. Reprinted in POS1 (369–88); Robinson, Paul. *Sex, Opera, and Other Vital Matters*. Ithaca, N.Y.: Cornell University Press, 1995; Rosenblum, Nancy L. "Democratic Sex: Reynolds v. U.S., Sexual Relations, and Community." In David M. Estlund and Martha C. Nussbaum, eds., *Sex, Preference, and Family: Essays on Law and Nature*. New York: Oxford University Press, 1997, 63–85; Roth, Philip. *The Dying Animal*. Boston, Mass.: Houghton Mifflin, 2001; Rowbotham, Sheila, and Jeffrey Weeks. *Socialism and the New Life: The Personal and Sexual Politics of Edward Carpenter and Havelock Ellis*. London: Pluto Press, 1977. London: Longwood, 1980; Sargisson, Lucy. *Contemporary Feminist Utopianism*. London: Routledge, 1996; Sargisson, Lucy. "Contemporary Feminist Utopianism: Practising Utopia on Utopia." In John Horton and Andrea Baumiester, eds., *Literature and the Political Imagination*. London: Routledge, 1996, 238–55; Sisk, John P. (1960) "The Dream Girl as Queen of Utopia." In Henry Anatole Grunwald, ed., *Sex in America*. New York: Bantam, 1964, 284–90; Soble, Alan. *Pornography: Marxism, Feminism, and the Future of Sexuality*. New Haven, Conn.: Yale University Press, 1986; Spurlock, John C. *Free Love: Marriage and Middle-Class Radicalism in America, 1825–1860*. New York: New York University Press, 1988; Stokes, Walter R. (1962) "Sexual Utopia." In Henry Anatole Grunwald, ed., *Sex in America*. New York: Bantam, 1964, 152–60; Tucker, Scott.

"Gender, Fucking, and Utopia: An Essay in Response to John Stoltenberg's *Refusing to Be a Man*." *Social Text*, no. 27 (1990), 3–34; Vonnegut, Kurt, Jr. (1968) "Welcome to the Monkey House." In *Welcome to the Monkey House*. New York: Dell, 1970, 28–47; Webb, Randall, and Doug Raynor. "The Connubial Utopias of Robert Rimmer." *The Futurist* 2:5 (1968), 99–100; Zamiatin, Eugene. (1920) *We*. Trans. Gregory Zilboorg. New York: Dutton, 1924, 1952.

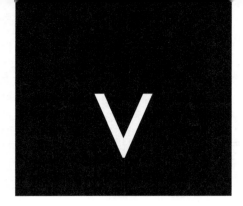

VIOLENCE, SEXUAL. Sexual violence takes many forms: violence in **sexual activity** (**rape**, sexual assault, **acquaintance rape**), violence that occurs within relationships (domestic abuse, wife-battering), and the violence threatened or suggested against subjects of sexual interest (**sexual harassment**). It might also include sexual activity that might not be violent were both partners consenting adults but is violence when one person is incompetent: a child, an underage adolescent, the intoxicated, the mentally handicapped. Sexual violence is often carried out physically but can also be done verbally, psychologically, or emotionally. Some might consider **sadomasochism** sexual violence, although the presence of **consent** among the parties might imply that these acts are not truly violent or that consensual sadomasochism is, *ceteris paribus*, an acceptable type of sexual violence. (It still might be a "manifestation of our society's eroticization of dominance"; Gudorf, 143, 148.)

Studies of victims of sexual violence (men, women, children) have demonstrated that it undermines or prevents the development or maintenance of important aspects of personhood: a sense of control and responsibility for one's body and life, self-esteem, and the inclination to self-preservation that depends on it (Draucker and Stern; Russell, 139–40). Sometimes the damage is temporary. Sexual violence that happens to someone at a young age, or for extended periods of time, or with considerable physical pain, or at the hands of trusted friends or family members causes more serious, long-term damage (Russell, 200–203). Studies also show that most sexual violence includes at least one or two of these aggravating factors. Over 50 percent of female rape victims are under eighteen at the time, and 21 percent are under twelve. Being raped before the age of eighteen enhances the likelihood that a woman will be raped again (Merrill et al.; Tjaden and Thoennes).

The U.S. Department of Justice estimated that 987,400 rapes occur annually: 876,100 male on female, 111,300 male on male. Women also experience significantly more partner violence than men. Twenty-five percent of surveyed women, versus 8 percent of surveyed men, said they had been raped or physically assaulted by a current or former spouse, cohabiting partner, or date in their lifetime; 1.5 percent of surveyed women, versus 0.9 percent of surveyed men, said they had been raped or physically assaulted by such a person in the previous twelve months (Tjaden and Thoennes). There are also cases in which men are the victims of sexual violence carried out by aggressive women, with sometimes equally damaging psychological effects (Anderson and Struckman-Johnson).

Most offenders in some categories of sexual violence are habitual, especially **pedophilia** and domestic abuse, and have high rates of recidivism. In the twenty-five years following conviction, 38 percent of rapists were charged again, 24 percent were tried, and 19 percent were convicted, while the respective rates for convicted child molesters were 75 percent, 58 percent, and 46 percent (Prentky et al., 645–50). Some who commit violence (e.g., spouse abusers) can be "retrained," since they often act consistently with what they perceive as accepted, and hence acceptable, social practices (Muehlenhard and Kimes;

Seabloom et al.). Studies of police responses to spousal abuse show that arrest deters more effectively than other responses (Goldman, 99–100).

Other than "retraining" those who commit sexual violence, what solutions are there? Some emphasize teaching women physical self-defense techniques and helping them recognize and avoid dangerous situations (Clay-Warner; DeWeld). Similarly, children can be taught the difference between "good touches" and "bad touches" and be encouraged to report strange or scary adult behavior to parents and teachers (DeYoung). Others, who reject polluting the "innocence" of girls and children with exaggerated fears and suspicions, emphasize legal changes that would treat sexual violence more seriously, such as the permanent incarceration of repeated sex offenders or their surgical or chemical castration ("Court Splits"; Mansnerus; Meisenkothen; Wright). This view finds support in the existence of many repeat offenders and in the pattern of escalation often (but not always) observed in those who commit sexual violence (Erchak). Many violent offenders begin their criminal careers with **masturbation** to violent **pornography** (or **fantasy**) or Peeping Tom (voyeuristic) activity (Abel et al.; Zolondek et al.). Yet many men who routinely engage in these activities never become violent. Social science research on the role of pornography in producing sexual violence is equivocal.

While some biologists (e.g., Thornhill and Palmer) argue that the tendency of men to coerce women sexually is genetic and heritable, because during human **evolution** it conveyed an adaptive advantage, others disagree, on the grounds that most men do not rape and the propensity to rape dramatically varies from culture to culture (see Sanday). Further, rapists impregnate their female victims only 2 percent of the time, and only 38 percent of that 2 percent results in live births. If so, rape confers unreliable evolutionary advantage (Stanford). Nevertheless, some writers argue that the **evolutionary psychology** approach to understanding sexual violence, including sexual harassment, yields a "feminist advantage" (Kenrick et al.) Much social science research on rape understands sexual violence as more a product of socialization than individual pathology. Peggy Sanday's study of rape in ninety-five societies concluded that women in the United States are much more likely to be raped than women in other societies. Abramson and Hayashi contrast the high level of sadistic pornography in Japan with that country's relatively low incidence of rape. The frequency of rape in a society seems most influenced by the nature of the relations between the sexes, the status of women, and the attitudes of boys during their developmental years.

Many feminists comprehend all sexual violence as proceeding from a social conception of sexuality that bases it on domination (a basis that many urge should be changed to mutuality; see Gudorf, 139–59). Sexuality is conceived as the "taking," by a bigger, stronger, usually male person, of a smaller, weaker, usually female, person. (For how we conceive sex as "possession," see **Andrea Dworkin** [1946–2005].) The use of violence in sexual interactions is an implicit aspect of this conception of sexuality. As **Catharine MacKinnon** makes the point, "Perhaps the wrong of rape has proved so difficult to define because the unquestionable starting point has been that rape is defined as distinct from intercourse, while for women it is difficult to distinguish the two under conditions of male dominance" (174). Much of our sexual **language**, particularly slang, expresses violence and domination and treats sex as something men want and obtain by possessing women (see Baker). Male domination and possession is socially presumed to be "natural" and exactly what women want, regardless of what they say. The thesis that rape is not primarily motivated by **sexual desire** but is meant to dominate women (Fortune, 177–80) seems not to be true for date and acquaintance rapists, who constitute the majority (Crooks and Baur, 551, 555; Hickman and Muehlenhard). Still, many feminists agree with Susan Brownmiller's claim (15, 209) that all men benefit from rape and other sexual violence committed by a few men, insofar as these acts intimidate women and thereby increase men's power over them. In what is called the "sexual revolution" of the late twentieth century, some women adopted a masculine approach to sex, seeing themselves as hunting for the commodity of sex from a male population. While considerably less likely to use physical force than men in their search for sexual satisfaction, some women are skillful at harassment and emotional sexual violence (Anderson and Struckman-Johnson). Whether we should applaud or bemoan this turning of the tables, or the sexual autonomy and assertiveness exhibited by these women, is unclear and cannot be resolved by facile and dogmatic philosophy, theology, or social analysis.

Many reforms have been instituted since the 1970s in the law, policing, health care, **sex education** programs, and counseling services. These have served to detect, protect, and treat the victims of sexual violence, to punish and, if possible, reform offenders, and to educate males and females about appropriate sexual behavior. The effects of these reforms have been uneven. The stigma of having been sexually victimized has abated little for women, children, and especially males and still inhibits the reporting of offenders. When child and women victims are financially or psychologically dependent on men, they often despair of rescue. But sexual attitudes have gradually shifted and continue to shift, however slowly. The ownership of and trading in women by men, as represented in sacred texts and past law, and the exclusion of women from education and political rights that supported such a status, are increasingly rejected in those areas where they persist. During the modern period, **marriage** became more companionate as men and women came to have more interests and training in common, motherhood was drastically abbreviated (by **contraception**, for example), and the life span was extended. While specific programs for ending sexual violence will be proposed, scrapped, and modified, the historical trajectory toward the equality of men and women seems destined to continue, in sexuality as well as in social, economic, and political arenas.

See also Coercion (by Sexually Aggressive Women); Consent; Dworkin, Andrea; Genital Mutilation; Harassment, Sexual; Incest; Language; MacKinnon, Catharine; Military, Sex and the; Objectification, Sexual; Paglia, Camille; Pedophilia; Pornography; Psychology, Evolutionary; Rape; Rape, Acquaintance and Date; Sade, Marquis de; Sadomasochism

REFERENCES

Abel, Gene G., Suzann S. Lawry, Elisabeth Karlstrom, Candice A. Osborn, and Charles F. Gillespie. "Screening Tests for Pedophilia." *Criminal Justice and Behavior* 21:1 (1994), 115–27; Abramson, Paul R., and Haruo Hayashi. "Pornography in Japan: Cross-Cultural and Theoretical Considerations." In Neil M. Malamuth and Edward Donnerstein, eds., *Pornography and Sexual Aggression*. Orlando, Fla.: Academic Press, 1984, 173–83; Anderson, Peter B., and Cindy Struckman-Johnson, eds. *Sexually Aggressive Women: Current Perspectives and Controversies*. New York: Guilford, 1998; Baker, Robert B. " 'Pricks' and 'Chicks': A Plea for 'Persons.' " In Robert B. Baker and Frederick A. Elliston, eds., *Philosophy and Sex*, 1st ed. Buffalo, N.Y.: Prometheus, 1975, 45–64; Brownmiller, Susan. *Against Our Will: Men, Women, and Rape*. New York: Simon and Schuster, 1975; Clay-Warner, Jody. "The Effect of Protective Actions and Situational Factors on Rape Outcomes." *Violence against Victims* 17:6 (2002), 691–705; "Court Splits on Use of Actuarial Instruments in Sex Offender Civil Commitment Hearings." *Criminal Law Reporter* 74:13 (2003), 207–12; Crooks, Robert, and Karla Baur. *Our Sexuality*, 8th ed. Belmont, Calif.: Wadsworth, 2002; DeWeld, Kristine. "Getting Physical: Subverting Gender Violence Through Self-Defense." *Journal of Contemporary Ethnography* 32:3 (2003), 247–78; DeYoung, Mary. "The Good Touch/Bad Touch Dilemma." *Child Welfare* 67:1 (1998), 60–68; Draucker, Claire Burke, and Phyllis Noerager Stern. "Women's Responses to Sexual

Violence by Males." *Western Journal of Nursing Research* 22:4 (2000), 385–402; Dworkin, Andrea. *Intercourse*. New York: Free Press, 1987; Erchak, Gerald M. "The Escalation and Maintenance of Spouse Abuse: A Cybernetic Model." *Victimology* 9:2 (1984), 247–53; Fortune, Marie. *Sexual Violence: The Unmentionable Sin*. New York: Pilgrim, 1983; Goldman, Jessica L. "Arresting Abusers Would Reduce Domestic Violence." In Karin Swisher, Carol Wekesser, and William Barbour, eds., *Violence against Women*. San Diego, Calif.: Greenhaven Press, 1994; Gudorf, Christine E. *Body, Sex, and Pleasure: Reconstructing Christian Sexual Ethics*. Cleveland, Ohio: Pilgrim, 1994; Hickman, Susan E., and Charlene L. Muehlenhard. "College Women's Fears and Precautionary Behaviors Related to Acquaintance Rape and Stranger Rape." *Psychology of Women Quarterly* 21:4 (1997), 527–47; Kenrick, Douglas T., Melanie R. Trost, and Virgil L. Sheets. "Power, Harassment, and Trophy Mates: The Feminist Advantages of an Evolutionary Perspective." In David M. Buss and Neil M. Malamuth, eds., *Sex, Power, Conflict: Evolutionary and Feminist Perspectives*. New York: Oxford University Press, 1996, 29–53; MacKinnon, Catharine A. "Rape: On Coercion and Consent." In *Toward a Feminist Theory of the State*. Cambridge, Mass.: Harvard University Press, 1989, 171–83; Mansnerus, Laura. "Questions Rise over Imprisoning Sex Offenders Past Their Terms." *New York Times* (17 November 2003), A1; Meisenkothen, Christopher. "Chemical Castration: Breaking the Cycle of Paraphiliac Recidivism." *Social Justice* 26:1 (1999), 139–55; Merrill, Lex L., Carol E. Newell, Cynthia J. Thomsen, Steven R. Gold, Joel S. Milner, Mary P. Moss, and Sandra G. Rosswork. "Childhood Abuse and Sexual Revictimization in a Female Navy Recruit Sample." *Journal of Traumatic Stress* 12:2 (1999), 211–25; Muehlenhard, Charlene L., and Leigh Ann Kimes. "The Social Construction of Sexual and Domestic Violence." *Personality and Social Psychology Review* 3:3 (1999), 234–45; Prentky, Robert A., Austin F. S. Lee, Raymond H. Knight, and David Cerce. "Recidivism Rates among Child Molesters and Rapists: A Methodological Analysis." *Law and Human Behavior* 21:6 (1997), 635–59; Russell, Diana E. H. *The Secret Trauma: Incest in the Lives of Girls and Women*. New York: Basic Books, 1986; Sanday, Peggy Reeves. "The Socio-Cultural Context of Rape: A Cross-Cultural Study." *Journal of Social Issues* 37:4 (1981), 5–27; Seabloom, William, Mary E. Seabloom, Eric Seabloom, Robert Baron, and Sharon Hendrickson. "A 14–24 Year Longitudinal Study of a Comprehensive Sexual Health Model Treatment Program for Adolescent Sex Offenders." *International Journal of Offender Therapy and Comparative Criminology* 47:4 (2003), 468–81; Stanford, Craig B. "Darwinians Look at Rape, Sex, and War." *American Scientist* 88:4 (2000), 360–68; Thornhill, Randy, and Craig Palmer. *A Natural History of Rape: Biological Bases of Sexual Coercion*. Cambridge, Mass.: MIT Press, 2000; Tjaden, Patricia, and Nancy Thoennes. *Prevalence, Incidence, and Consequences of Violence against Women: Findings of the National Violence against Women Survey*. Washington, D.C.: National Institute of Justice, 1998; Wright, Richard G. "Sex Offender Registration and Notification: Public Attention, Political Emphasis, and Fear." *Criminology and Public Policy* 3:1 (2003), 97–104; Zolondek, Stacey C., Gene G. Abel, William F. Northey, Jr., and Alan D. Jordan. "The Self-reported Behaviors of Juvenile Sexual Offenders." *Journal of Interpersonal Violence* 16:1 (2001), 73–86.

Christine E. Gudorf

ADDITIONAL READING

Baker, Robert B. " 'Pricks' and 'Chicks': A Plea for 'Persons.' " In Robert B. Baker and Frederick A. Elliston, eds., *Philosophy and Sex*, 1st ed. Buffalo, N.Y.: Prometheus, 1975, 45–64. Reprinted in P&S2 (249–67); P&S3 (281–97), with " 'Pricks' and 'Chicks': A Postscript after Twenty-Five Years" (297–305); Brison, Susan J. *Aftermath: Violence and the Remaking of a Self*. Princeton, N.J.: Princeton University Press, 2002; Brison, Susan J. (1993) "Surviving Sexual Violence: A Philosophical Perspective." In Robert B. Baker, Kathleen J. Wininger, and Frederick A. Elliston, eds., *Philosophy and Sex*, 3rd ed. Amherst, N.Y.: Prometheus, 1998, 567–82; Broadus, Loren. "Sex and Violence in the Family and Church." In Elizabeth Stuart and Adrian Thatcher, eds., *Christian Perspectives on Sexuality and Gender*. Grand Rapids, Mich.: Eerdmans, 1996, 400–409; Buss, David M., and Neil M. Malamuth, eds. *Sex, Power, Conflict: Evolutionary and Feminist Perspectives*. New York: Oxford

University Press, 1996, 231–68; Carlson, Eric S. "Sexual Assault on Men in War." *The Lancet* 349:9045 (11 January 1997), 129; Christensen, F[errel] M. "The Alleged Link between Pornography and Violence." In J. J. Krivacska and John Money, eds., *The Handbook of Forensic Sexology: Biomedical and Criminological Perspectives.* Amherst, N.Y.: Prometheus, 1994, 422–48; Comstock, Gary D. *Violence against Lesbians and Gay Men.* New York: Columbia University Press, 1991; Dershowitz, Alan M. "The Other Rape Epidemic." In *The Abuse Excuse and Other Cop-outs, Sob Stories, and Evasions of Responsibility.* Boston, Mass.: Little, Brown, 1994, 279–81; Douglas, Lawrence. "The Force of Words: Fish, Matsuda, MacKinnon, and the Theory of Discursive Violence." *Law and Society Review* 29:1 (1995), 169–90; Duggan, Lisa. *Sapphic Slashers: Sex, Violence, and American Modernity.* Durham, N.C.: Duke University Press, 2000; Dworkin, Andrea. *Pornography: Men Possessing Women.* New York: Penguin Books, 1989; Eccles, Anthony, William L. Marshall, and Howard E. Barbaree. "Differentiating Rapists and Non-rapists Using the Rape Index." *Behavior Research and Therapy* 32:5 (1994), 539–46; French, Stanley G., Wanda Teays, and Laura M. Purdy, eds. *Violence against Women: Philosophical Perspectives.* Ithaca, N.Y.: Cornell University Press, 1998; Girshick, Lori B. *Woman-to-Woman Sexual Violence: Does She Call It Rape?* Boston, Mass.: Northeastern University Press, 2002; Hall, Gordon C. Nagayama, and Christy Barongon. "Prevention of Sexual Aggression: Sociocultural Risk and Protective Factors." *American Psychologist* 52:1 (1997), 5–14; Hartsock, Nancy C. M. "Gender and Power: Masculinity, Violence, and Domination." In *Money, Sex, and Power: Toward a Feminist Historical Materialism.* New York: Longman, 1983, 155–85; Kennedy, Duncan. "Sexual Abuse, Sexy Dressing, and the Eroticization of Domination." In *Sexy Dressing Etc.* Cambridge, Mass.: Harvard University Press, 1993, 126–213; MacKinnon, Catharine A. (2000) "Disputing Male Sovereignty: On *United States v. Morrison.*" In *Women's Lives, Men's Laws.* Cambridge, Mass.: Harvard University Press, 2005, 206–39; MacKinnon, Catharine A. (1993) "From Silence to Silence: Violence against Women in America." In *Women's Lives, Men's Laws.* Cambridge, Mass.: Harvard University Press, 2005, 345–51; MacKinnon, Catharine A. "Rape: On Coercion and Consent." In *Toward a Feminist Theory of the State.* Cambridge, Mass.: Harvard University Press, 1989, 171–83. Reprinted in Katie Conboy, Nadia Medina, and Sarah Stanbury, eds., *Writing on the Body: Female Embodiment and Feminist Theory.* New York: Columbia University Press, 1997, 42–58; Murphy, Jeffrie G. "Some Ruminations on Women, Violence, and the Criminal Law." In Jules Coleman and Allen Buchanan, eds., *In Harm's Way: Essays in Honor of Joel Feinberg.* Cambridge: Cambridge University Press, 1994, 209–30; Rosenfeld, Diane L. *"Why Doesn't He Leave?* Restoring Liberty and Equality to Battered Women." In Catharine A. MacKinnon and Reva B. Siegel, eds., *Directions in Sexual Harassment Law.* New Haven, Conn.: Yale University Press, 2004, 535–57; Russell, Diana E. H. "Pornography and Rape: A Causal Model." *Political Psychology* 9:1 (1988), 41–73. Revised version in Diana E. H. Russell, ed., *Making Violence Sexy: Feminist Views on Pornography.* New York: Teachers College Press, 1993, 120–50; Russell, Diana E. H., ed. *Making Violence Sexy: Feminist Views on Pornography.* New York: Teachers College Press, 1993; Russell, Gordon W., ed. *Violence in Intimate Relationships.* New York: PMA Publishing, 1988; Sanday, Peggy Reeves. *A Woman Scorned: Acquaintance Rape on Trial.* New York: Doubleday, 1996; Smith, Abbe. "The 'Monster' in Us All: When Victims Become Perpetrators." *Suffolk University Law Review* 38:2 (2005), 367–94; Smuts, Barbara. "Male Aggression against Women: An Evolutionary Perspective." In David M. Buss and Neil M. Malamuth, eds., *Sex, Power, Conflict: Evolutionary and Feminist Perspectives.* New York: Oxford University Press, 1996, 231–68; Spiegel, Marcia Cohen. *Bibliography of Sexual and Domestic Violence in the Jewish Community* (2004). <www.mincava.umn.edu/documents/bibs/jewish/jewish.html> [accessed 1 January 2005]; Waldner, Lisa K. "Domestic Violence." In Timothy F. Murphy, ed., *Reader's Guide to Lesbian and Gay Studies.* Chicago, Ill.: Fitzroy Dearborn, 2000, 190–91; Weisberg, D. Kelly, ed. "Battered Women." In *Applications of Feminist Legal Theory to Women's Lives: Sex, Violence, Work, and Reproduction.* Philadelphia, Pa.: Temple University Press, 1996, 277–401.

VIRTUE ETHICS. *See* Ethics, Virtue

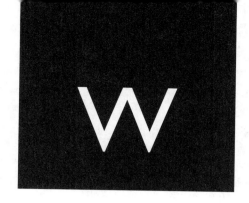

WESTERMARCK, EDWARD (1862–1939). The Swedish-speaking Finn Edward Alexander Westermarck was born and educated in Helsinki. As an undergraduate he developed an aversion to German philosophy, especially **Immanuel Kant**'s (1724–1804), and a predilection for British empiricism. A desire to visit the British Museum Library (then the world's best) prompted him in 1887 to travel to England, a country he subsequently considered his second home and intellectual fatherland (*Memories*, 30, 72, 263). In the course of a long career as philosopher and anthropologist, he wrote voluminously, and mainly in English, on three subjects: sex and **marriage**, morality, and Morocco. The first six chapters of *The History of Human Marriage* were submitted for his doctoral thesis in 1889, and the whole work (then only one volume) was published in 1891, with a short laudatory introduction written by Alfred Russel Wallace (1823–1913). Three further editions appeared before the work was rewritten and enlarged threefold for the fifth edition (1921). For twenty-three years (1907–1930), Westermarck held simultaneously two professorial chairs: one in Practical Philosophy (first at Helsinki, then from 1918 at Åbo Academy, of which he was a cofounder and the first rector) and one in sociology at the London School of Economics. He declined many generous invitations to other posts, including some in Sweden and one at Harvard. He died in Lappvik, Finland.

Although Westermarck never married and revealed in his autobiography that he had no practical interest in the subject (*Memories*, 69), the study of marriage engrossed his attention for much of his working life. The question that led him to examine human sexuality and to write *History*—one that also preoccupied **Saint Augustine** (354–430; *City of God*, bk. 14, chaps. 17, 18)—was the origin of sexual modesty. How can we explain the veil of discretion that is almost universally drawn over the sexual life? Surprisingly, his favored answer is intimated in just a few lines in the early editions of *History* (2nd ed., 211–12, 541) but is accorded the whole of chapter XII in the fifth. One explanation is that modesty is a mechanism of self-defense. Since animals are unable to defend themselves during intercourse, they seek seclusion to be less vulnerable. This explains the loss of the instinct in domesticated animals but is inconsistent with its intensification in the most polite and civilized people (*History*, 5th ed., vol. 1, 429–30). Westermarck believed that modesty has more than one root. The main one is a naturally selected aversion to **incest**, which is why sexual modesty is particularly strong among members of the same family and especially between those of opposite sex (see Wolf). The influence of sentiments and habits thus acquired early in life extends beyond the family circle (439–53).

History incorporates a vast compendium of ethnographic data but also includes discussion of particular contentious theories. Prominent in all editions (especially the last) are his criticisms of the hypothesis of promiscuity, *viz.*, that our prehistoric ancestors lived promiscuously and some primitive races continue to do so. This view had been common in the post-Darwinian world and one that Westermarck had at first accepted. He abandoned it because he found it incompatible with the evidence of natural history. The spirit of Darwinian theory underpins most of his work.

> [T]he institution of marriage . . . has developed out of a primeval habit. It was, I believe, even in primitive times, the habit for a man and a woman (or several women) to live together, to have sexual relations with one another, and to rear their offspring in common, the man being the protector and supporter of his family and the woman being his helpmate and the nurse of their children. This habit was sanctioned by custom, and afterwards by law, and was thus transformed into a social institution. (*History*, 5th ed., vol. 1, 27–28; see *Future of Marriage*, 5; *Three Essays*, 166)

This theory is expressed in his much quoted dictum that "marriage is rooted in the family, not the family in marriage" (*History*, 5th ed., vol. 1, 72; *Future*, 9; *Short History*, 30). Extending his discussion back to the anthropoid apes, he points out that they seem to be induced by an instinct acquired through natural selection to form lasting bonds that help preserve the next generation and therefore the species. Such an arrangement is indispensable in a species where there is prolonged infant dependency (*History*, 5th ed., vol. 1, 32–37; *Future*, 5). For this reason, the family probably existed among primitive man, just as it does, he believed, among many nonhuman primates (cf. Diamond, 7).

Chapter III of *History* (5th ed.) challenges the claims of ancient and modern writers that there were, or still are, promiscuous races. Westermarck rejects such reports as inherently unreliable or resulting from a failure to understand the data. Chapters IV–VIII consider and dismiss other attempts to interpret a wide range of sexual practices as vestigial evidence of a prehistoric state of widespread promiscuity. "The numerous facts put forward in support of the hypothesis do not entitle us to assume that promiscuity has ever been the prevailing form of sexual relations among a single people, far less that it has constituted a general stage in the social development of man, and least of all, that such a stage formed the starting-point of all human history" (*History*, 5th ed., vol. 1, 297–98; see *Future*, 15–16). Chapter IX presents the positive case for the implausibility of the promiscuity hypothesis: The prevalence of **jealousy** among our prehuman progenitors would have been a forceful deterrent. (Contrast more recent work on promiscuity: Barash and Lipton; Buss; Hrdy.)

Because Westermarck saw jealousy as a potent stabilizing influence in the psychodynamics of sexual relations, he rejected as impracticable and undesirable the proposals of contemporary authors to eradicate it (e.g., William Robinson [1867–1936], 386–88; **Bertrand Russell** [1872–1970], *Marriage and Morals*, 188, 114–15, 239, 249). Recognizing jealousy as a deeply rooted and serviceable instinct, Westermarck thought that this complex emotion should be respected. Russell may well have been right to maintain that **love** is generous, but when it is gratified in **adultery**, it is at someone else's expense and this leads to resentment (*Future*, 73–79).

According to Westermarck, the rules of exogamy (which forbid people to marry within their family, tribe, or clan) and prohibitions against incest are closely related, being derived from an almost universal aversion acquired by natural selection and founded on the biological fact that plant and animal species are harmed by self-fertilization and inbreeding (*History*, 5th ed., vol. 2, chap. XX; *Short History*, chap. IV). This thesis is central to *Three Essays on Sex and Marriage* (1934). While Westermarck believed that there is a natural aversion to incest, **Sigmund Freud** (1856–1939) maintained that everyone has incestuous desires that are subject to repression (*Totem and Taboo*; see Spain; Walter). In the first essay, "The Oedipus Complex" (1–123), Westermarck rejects this theory as a mass of unverifiable assumptions and fanciful speculation. The second essay, "Recent Theories of Exogamy" (125–59), is a rejoinder to criticisms of Westermarck's work that had appeared in the 1920s and early 1930s. In the third, "The Mothers" (161–335), he vigorously rebuts objections raised in a recently published book of that name by Dr. Robert Briffault (1876–1948). Briffault had attributed to Westermarck opinions he did not hold and impugned his integrity as a scholar.

The Future of Marriage in Western Civilization (1936), dedicated to **Havelock Ellis** (1859–1939), was Westermarck's penultimate book, published when he was seventy-three. It draws on a lifetime of learning and well-informed reflection. The first third of the twentieth century had seen an explosion of writing about sex, much of which asserted that amid the ongoing changes in human relations marriage was facing a crisis. Some even predicted the family's demise. Westermarck examined whether the causes that had brought the family into existence were likely to continue and to what extent family life would decline or undergo change (1–2). In this work he defines marriage as "a social institution sanctioned by custom or law" (5), but in early editions of *History* he had used a wider definition, including more or less durable relationships between other animals. He was convinced that pair bonding had been necessary for the survival of highly evolved species and therefore had deep biological foundations. In humans, habits became customs, which in turn became institutions.

> If . . . men are induced by instincts to remain with a woman with whom they have had sexual relations and to take care of her and of their common offspring, other members of the group, endowed with similar instincts, would feel moral resentment against a man who forsook his mate and children. As I have pointed out in another work [*Origin and Development of the Moral Ideas*, vol. 1, 118–22, 135–37, 139 ff.], public or moral resentment or disapproval is at the bottom of the rules of custom and of all duties and rights. That the functions of the husband and father are not merely of the sexual and procreative kind, but involve the duties of supporting and protecting the wife and children, is testified by an array of facts relating to peoples in all quarters of the world and in all stages of civilization. (8; see Thomas Aquinas [1224/25–1274], *Summa contra gentiles*, bk. 3, pt. 2, chap. 122)

Westermarck concludes the first chapter by claiming that marriage and the family stem from "deep-rooted instincts which will help to preserve them" (20).

While conceding that under the protection afforded by modern states women and children might survive without husbands or fathers to look after them (*Future*, 20), Westermarck was profoundly skeptical that alternative domestic or social arrangements would serve as well as traditional ones. He dismissed the suggestion that people might live more happily in communes and castigated the communism advocated by **Plato** (427–347 BCE) in *Republic* (bk. 5, 457c–d, 460b–62e)—men will share women; parents will not know who their children are—and that recently realized in Soviet Russia, both being founded on a dogmatic aversion to private property. Socialistic and collectivistic innovations would, he believed, prove unsatisfactory to all parties: parents, children, and the state. Recent experience in the United States, Russia, and elsewhere had indicated that normal family life is a prerequisite of personal development (156–64).

Marriage normally has three essential elements: sex, companionship, and children (*Future*, 21). Conjugal affection, as distinct from lust, was probably an early ingredient of sexual relations (29). Though he does not in this context mention **David Hume** (1711–1776; *Treatise*, bk. II, pt. ii, sec. 11), like him and in common with other writers on the psychology of sex, Westermarck maintains that there is a two-way transfusion between love and lust (31–32). Home-building, companionship, and the economic interdependence that these imply will probably remain powerful incentives to marriage (33–36). As he noted,

> [L]ike the sexual impulse, the other elements in marriage have a deep foundation in human and even pre-human instincts. Combined with that impulse, there must from the beginning have been some degree of attachment which kept the individuals of different sex together till after the birth of the offspring. This was the germ of that unity and intermingling of the spiritual and the sensual elements in sexual love which characterises the normal relations between husband and wife among ourselves. It has led to a more or less durable community of life in a common home, to which the promiscuous gratification of the sexual impulse affords no equivalent. (155–56)

"So far as I can see, then, there is every reason to believe that [these] . . . are factors which will remain lasting obstacles to the extinction of marriage and the collapse of the family, because they are too deeply rooted in human nature to fade away, and can find adequate satisfaction only in some form of marriage and the family founded upon it" (170).

Westermarck did realize, however, that change was in the wind. "It seems to me very likely . . . that [henceforth] in questions of sex people will be less tied by conventional rules and more willing to judge each case on its merits, and that they will recognise greater freedom for men and women to mould their own amatory lives" (*Future*, 201). Many of his predictions have come true. A champion of **feminism**, he welcomed the emancipation of women and anticipated further progress in this direction, realizing that this would affect relations between the sexes (92–93). By the 1930s the use of **contraception** had become more widespread, and some thinkers had already asserted that pleasure, not procreation, was the primary object of sex (25–26; cf. Wilson, 125–27). Westermarck was aware that this development had both good and bad implications. By facilitating safer intercourse, contraception diminished the incentive to hasty marriage (54) and encouraged premarital cohabitation or trial marriage of a kind that was practiced in primitive and rural communities, enjoyed some advocacy in early-twentieth-century America (104–7), and has now become common. He feared, however, that contraception would promote license outside marriage and would lower the quality of the population by being practiced more frequently by better educated and wealthier people, who were thought to be genetically superior, than by the lower classes (100–103). At this time the notion of eugenics was both scientifically and politically more acceptable than it is today.

Though Western society had long been almost exclusively monogamous, matrimonial legislation has varied widely from one country to another. By the mid-1930s divorce was becoming more easily available in Europe and the United States. Westermarck believed that this trend toward more liberal attitudes would continue as the influence of Christianity waned. A staunch agnostic, he was severely critical of orthodox Christian teachings on sex, which are largely negative and irrational. Christianity had introduced into Europe a rigid asceticism (*Christianity and Morals*, chap. 9) that maintained that **sexual activity** is unclean and defiling (128) and that intercourse within marriage is tolerable only as essential to procreation. All other forms of sexual activity were forbidden (*Future*, 23–24, 130, 228–31). "It is strange to think that such crude notions have for ages exercised a dominant influence upon the moral attitude towards sex behaviour in Western civilization" (*Future*,

232). Although he believed Christianity's anticarnal tradition to be firmly rooted in the writings of **Saint Paul** (5–64?), in *Christianity* he thoroughly discussed controversies about sexuality that raged in the church from the apostles to his own time.

Westermarck was homosexual, though he lived at a time when he could not be openly so. He knew at first hand that **homosexuality** was not deliberately chosen by willfully degenerate people but rather an orientation that develops spontaneously (see Sullivan, 3–9). His work as a scholar informed him that it is found in most human races and some animals and that most cultures do not display the extreme hostility to it of Judeo-Christianity (*Origin*, chap. XLIII). He was acquainted with research published in Europe and America that indicated a relatively high incidence of homosexuality. Westermarck believed that legal prohibitions are incapable of extinguishing homosexual desire and, judging from the frequencies of homosexual acts in countries with and without such laws, are ineffective in deterring this activity (*Christianity*, 374). By contrast, laws against incest are scarcely felt as restraining, since very few people experience incestuous desires (*History*, 5th ed., vol. 2, 192; see *Three Essays*, 69–72; *Future*, 249, 261). Westermarck rightly predicted that growth in understanding would lead to a decline in intolerance of homosexuality and expressed the hope that the demise of "antiquated religious ideas" would lead to a reappraisal on utilitarian grounds (*Future*, 251–55).

Early in his life Westermarck espoused the empiricist doctrine that morality is rooted in feeling, not reason (*Memories*, 101; *Origin*, chaps. I–V [first published in 1906]). He consistently maintained that ethics is not an autonomous or prescriptive discipline that reveals *sui generis* moral truths but a branch of descriptive anthropology and psychology. Late in his career he defended this position by making an onslaught on the views of his opponents in *Ethical Relativity* (1932) and *Christianity and Morals* (1939). This, his last book, makes uncomfortable reading for those who regard Christianity as the bedrock of exalted and immutable morality. Although Westermarck denied the existence of objective moral truth to a degree that made his own moral pronouncements seem as questionable as any other, he was by no means a moral nihilist, adopting a kind of nondogmatic utilitarianism. No feelings can be the basis of objective truth, but since the retributive sentiments on which morality is based are produced by **evolution**, they can be justified to some extent by their functional efficiency. A species as reflective as man can and should review its moral practices in the light of experience. Though he thought that many entrenched attitudes about sexual issues were ill-founded, and pleaded for more open-minded and critical appraisal, he was no advocate of reckless innovation: He was a critic of promiscuity and a staunch defender of stable marriage as the arrangement in which partners and dependent children are most likely to thrive. He therefore castigated the "uncritical spirit of revolt" (*Future*, 239) that rejected this institution without good reason.

See also Adultery; Animal Sexuality; Augustine (Saint); Bestiality; Casual Sex; Ellis, Havelock; Evolution; Feminism, Lesbian; Feminism, Liberal; Fichte, Johann Gottlieb; Freud, Sigmund; Homosexuality, Ethics of; Homosexuality and Science; Hume, David; Incest; Jealousy; Love; Marriage; Marxism; Paul (Saint); Plato; Psychology, Evolutionary; Russell, Bertrand; Sherfey, Mary Jane; Tantrism; Thomas Aquinas (Saint); Utopianism

REFERENCES

Augustine. (413–427) *The City of God*. Trans. Marcus Dods. New York: Modern Library, 1993; Barash, David P., and Judith Eve Lipton. *The Myth of Monogamy: Fidelity and Infidelity in Animals and People*. New York: Henry Holt, 2001; Briffault, Robert. *The Mothers*, 3 vols. London: George Allen and Unwin, 1927; Buss, David M. *The Evolution of Desire: Strategies of Human Mating*. New

York: Basic Books, 1994; Diamond, Jared. *Why Is Sex Fun? The Evolution of Human Sexuality*. New York: Basic Books, 1997; Freud, Sigmund. (1913) *Totem and Taboo*. In *The Standard Edition of the Complete Psychological Works of Sigmund Freud*, vol. 13. Trans. James Strachey. London: Hogarth Press, 1953–1974, ix–161; Hrdy, Sarah Blaffer. *The Woman That Never Evolved*. Cambridge, Mass.: Harvard University Press, 1981; Hume, David. (1739) *A Treatise of Human Nature*. Ed. David Fate Norton and Mary J. Norton. Oxford, U.K.: Oxford University Press, 2000; Plato. (ca. 380 BCE) *Republic*. Trans. G.M.A. Grube. Indianapolis, Ind.: Hackett, 1992; Robinson, William J. (1917) *Woman: Her Sex and Love Life*, 8th ed. New York: Critic and Guide, 1923; Russell, Bertrand. *Marriage and Morals*. London: George Allen and Unwin, 1929; Spain, David H. "The Westermarck-Freud Incest-Theory Debate: An Evaluation and Reformulation." *Current Anthropology* 28:5 (1987), 623–45; Sullivan, Andrew. *Virtually Normal: An Argument about Homosexuality*. New York: Knopf, 1995; Thomas Aquinas. (1258–1264) *On the Truth of the Catholic Faith. Summa contra gentiles. Book Three: Providence. Part II*. Trans. Vernon J. Bourke. Garden City, N.Y.: Image Books, 1956; Walter, Alex. "Putting Freud and Westermarck in Their Places: A Critique of Spain." *Ethos* 18:4 (1990), 439–46; Westermarck, Edward. *Christianity and Morals*. London: Kegan Paul, Trench, Trubner; New York: Macmillan, 1939; Westermarck, Edward. *Ethical Relativity*. London: Kegan Paul, Trench, Trubner; New York: Harcourt Brace, 1932; Westermarck, Edward. *The Future of Marriage in Western Civilization*. London and New York: Macmillan, 1936; Westermarck, Edward. (1891) *The History of Human Marriage*, 2nd ed. London: Macmillan, 1894. 5th ed., 3 vols. London: Macmillan, 1921; New York: Allerton Book Co., 1922; Westermarck, Edward. *Memories of My Life*. Trans. from the Swedish by Anna Barwell. London: George Allen and Unwin; New York: Macauley, 1929; Westermarck, Edward. (1906–1908) *The Origin and Development of the Moral Ideas*, 2nd ed., 2 vols. London: Macmillan, 1912–1917; Westermarck, Edward. *A Short History of Marriage*. London and New York: Macmillan, 1926; Westermarck, Edward. *Three Essays on Sex and Marriage*. London: Macmillan, 1934; Wilson, Edward O. *On Human Nature*. New York: Bantam, 1979; Wolf, Arthur P. *Sexual Attraction and Childhood Association: A Chinese Brief for Edward Westermarck*. Stanford, Calif.: Stanford University Press, 1995.

J. Martin Stafford

ADDITIONAL READING

Davis, Kingsley. "Jealousy and Sexual Property." *Social Forces* 14:3 (1936), 395–405; Malinowski, Bronislaw. Review of *The History of Human Marriage* [5th ed.], by Edward Westermarck. *Man* 24:5 (1924), 502–4; Shalit, Wendy. "Can Modesty Be Natural?" In *A Return to Modesty: Discovering the Lost Virtue*. New York: Free Press, 1999, 118–43; Small, Meredith. *What's Love Got to Do with It? The Evolution of Human Mating*. New York: Anchor, 1995; Stroup, Timothy. "Westermarck, Edvard Alexander." In Brian Harrison, ed., *New Oxford Dictionary of National Biography*, vol. 58. Oxford, U.K.: Oxford University Press, 2004, 265–69; Stroup, Timothy. "Westermarck, Edward [Alexander]." In Lawrence C. Becker and Charlotte B. Becker, eds., *Encyclopedia of Ethics*, 2nd ed., vol. 3. New York: Routledge, 2001, 1798–99; Stroup, Timothy. *Westermarck's Ethics*. Publications of the Research Institute of the Åbo Akademi Foundation, No. 76. Åbo, Fin.: Åbo Akademi, 1982; Stroup, Timothy, ed. *Edward Westermarck: Essays on His Life and Works. Acta Philosophica Fennica*, vol. 34. Helsinki, Fin.: Societas Philosophica Fennica, 1982; Symons, Donald. *The Evolution of Human Sexuality*. Oxford, U.K.: Oxford University Press, 1979.

WITTGENSTEIN, LUDWIG (1889–1951).

Ludwig Josef Johann Wittgenstein was born in Vienna, Austria, and died in Cambridge, England. Few philosophers have had greater impact on twentieth-century thought than Wittgenstein, through his *Tractatus Logico-Philosophicus* (completed in 1912), the later *Philosophical Investigations* (1940s), and a number of books and a multitude of lectures between them. His influence ranged over psychology, sociology, linguistics, as well as analytic and Continental philosophy; that some of his central ideas would find application to contemporary issues about human sexuality is therefore not surprising. Yet Wittgenstein wrote nothing about matters relevant to sexuality in itself, and he evinced only ambivalence toward, or anxious silence about, his own (homo)sexual identity (see Duffy; Levi; Monk, 117, 138, 369, 376–77). Regardless, at least three Wittgensteinian themes promise useful insight into human sexuality: his thought that the meaning of a word is its use; his view of embodiment; and the relationship of each to the contingencies of epistemic context.

Wittgenstein's work is commonly divided into two periods, an earlier one represented by *Tractatus* and a later period by *Philosophical Investigations* (*PI*). There are also many posthumously published works. What philosophical ideas connect these two periods or whether even such a distinction should be drawn has been the subject of much scholarly debate. One observation from this endeavor is important here: Much of what concerned Wittgenstein throughout his career had to do with the evolving and intimate relationship between what can be said and the constellation of intentions, beliefs, and activities that inform what (in his later works) he calls a "form of life":

> "So you are saying that human agreement decides what is true and what is false?"—It is what human beings *say* that is true and false; and they agree in the *language* that they use. That is not agreement in opinions but in form of life. (*PI*, §241)

What connects the two periods is not a concern for ethics or traditional philosophical ideas like "the good life." Rather, what drove a thinker so otherwise unsure about the practical value of philosophy was his conviction that the key to this value lay in a clear understanding not only of the relationship between belief, action, and **language** but of the epistemic contexts within which language has a use. As Wittgenstein makes the point, "to imagine a language means to imagine a form of life" (*PI*, §19).

The difference, then, between these two periods involves no abandonment, much less a repudiation, of his ideas but a shift of focus away from studying the representational link between words and states of affairs and toward a concentration on language use. This turn to context signals a transition from the *Tractatus*'s preoccupation with the syntactical structure of language to the specific epistemic conditions in which words are used:

> When philosophers use a word—"knowledge," "being," "object," "I," "proposition," "name"—and try to grasp the *essence* of the thing, one must always ask oneself: is the word ever actually used in this way in the language-game which is its original home?—What *we* do is to bring words back from their metaphysical to their everyday use. (*PI*, §116)

> A main source of our failure to understand is that we do not *command a clear view* of the use of our words.—Our grammar is lacking in this sort of perspicuity. A perspicuous representation produces just that understanding which consists in "seeing connections." (*PI*, §122)

The key to this more "perspicuous" understanding is discerning that the meaning of a word is its use: "For a *large* class of cases—though not for all—in which we employ the word 'meaning' it can be defined thus: the meaning of a word is its use in the language" (*PI*, §43). Language is not an object of investigation but the distinctive activity of a certain kind of creature, human beings. Usefulness thus signals the "life" of words and obsoleteness their "death":

> But how many kinds of sentences are there? Say assertion, question, and command?—There are *countless* kinds; countless different kinds of use of what we call "symbols," "words," "sentences." And this multiplicity is not something fixed, given once and for all; but new types of language, new language-games, as we may say, come into existence, and others become obsolete and get forgotten. . . . Here the term "language-*game*" is meant to bring into prominence the fact that the *speaking* of language is part of an activity, or a form of life. (*PI*, §23)

That a linguistically mediated exchange is like playing a game demonstrates that, for Wittgenstein, language use is a (loosely) rule-governed activity whose variable "strategies" fulfill a wide variety of purposes: stating claims, asking questions, giving orders, expressing pain, announcing beliefs, evincing desire, and so on. Such exchanges cannot be adequately characterized as those of, say, disembodied Cartesian minds but reflect the embodied individual and collective experiences of beings who are embedded psychologically, epistemically, and materially in a form of life (Orr, 322–43). In Wittgenstein's nondualist, non-Cartesian ontology, or philosophical anthropology, the human being is grounded in the body and lived experience, and these together encompass both "instinctive" or prelinguistic behaviors and social practices. The body and experience are "the weft into which language is woven" to create the patterns of our lives (Orr, 323). Wittgenstein puts this point eloquently: "The human body is the best picture of the human soul" (*PI*, p. 178e).

As the "weft into which language is woven," the human body grounds the meaning of linguistic exchanges as these take place within particular epistemic contexts that are themselves coded or "patterned" by factors of, for example, race, sex, gender, age, ability, and sexuality. What, indeed, constitutes racial, sex and/or gender identity, what it means to be old, or abled, or "normal" depends in large measure on one's embodied location within (or without) relevant, empowered, and evolving language games. If Wittgenstein is correct that the meaning of a word is its use, then significant insight into how race, sex, gender, age, and ability are inscribed upon the bodies and actions of human persons may be provided by careful examination of the ways in which we use words, whose words count or are empowered, and how particular uses identify and reinforce the social, economic, political, and cultural conditions of our forms of life.

Consider two examples relevant to human sexuality. One involves the birth of intersexed infants. Within what we might call the language game of gender identification, there are only two possible "moves," as it were, "boy" or "girl" (not and/or). To be born intersexed, with some or all of the reproductive organs of both biological sexes, is to be born not "fitting" the game. As this child matures, (s)he cannot be expected to be able to "play" in accord with the gender game's rules. Indeed, it seems we have no language within which to situate such infants as "normal" with respect to sexual identity. This is at least part of the reason doctors often advise the devastated parents, themselves similarly "at a loss for words" in trying to describe their child's "disabled" condition, to make use of sex-reassignment surgery.

The point is not merely that our language fails to include intersexed infants but that the way we conceive of the "normal" with respect to gender identification is largely determined by the language games we enter long before the birth of a child. That among the first things people want to know about a new baby is what sex it is indicates some measure of the importance we attach to this aspect of identification. The issue, though, is not merely one of, say, embarrassment. After all, one could respond to such a question candidly with "intersexed." The issue is that this response lacks an adequate epistemic context: The social expectations ordinarily met by playing the language game correctly are wanting in this case because they are unknowable. Such expectations, moreover, are not unknowable because intersexed children somehow fall outside of "human being" (clearly they do not) but because the existence of intersexed persons poses a serious challenge to the institutions, norms of behavior, and social practices that support cultural **heterosexism**. Surgery, then, reinforces the conditions for the forms of life determined by such institutions by engendering (literally and figuratively) the bodies on which social expectations can be encoded. Medicine creates the avenue for entrance into the language games deemed appropriate to the sexes and thereby helps to fix the epistemic, social, and political conditions of individual persons according to their sexed bodies.

We can take a similarly Wittgensteinian approach to the political debate over **same-sex marriage**. Each time a conservative proponent of traditional heterosexual **marriage** appeals to the dictionary to find the definition of "marriage" (and in doing so, treats human artifacts as if they were a guide to Platonic forms), he or she is playing a language game whose legitimacy depends not only on a rigid division of human beings into two sexes but also on the institutions, norms, and practices through which the game itself is reinforced as a representation of the "normal" and "natural." When these proponents insist that marriage is *by definition* exclusively heterosexual, they are, plausibly, saying: "This is how the game is played. These are its players, one man and one woman. And for other combinations, some other game, but not *marriage*, is being played." These proponents arguably commit the mistake Wittgenstein attributes to philosophers when he says that their error is to look for the essence of a word instead of its use in a language. But if so, then as new uses enter the language, others become obsolete. In some areas of the country the marriage game has undergone this sort of transformation, which is effected each time a same-sex couple is issued a *marriage* license. This does not necessarily mean that marriage can no longer be defined (used) as heterosexual. It does, though, illustrate a key theme of Wittgenstein's later philosophy, that the capacity for change is a condition of a language's survival, intimately tethered as it is to the evolving circumstances and conditions of human life and without which it has no meaningful application. This is why—to mention briefly one more example—the feminist expansion of the meaning of "**rape**" to include what the traditional definition considered only or, at most, **seduction** "can be a legitimate linguistic move in the language game of rape" (Reitan, 45).

See also Anscombe, G.E.M.; Bisexuality; Descartes, René; Genital Mutilation; Intersexuality; Language; Marriage, Same-Sex; Money, John; Queer Theory

REFERENCES

Duffy, Bruce. *The World as I Found It*. New York: Ticknor and Fields, 1987; Levi, Albert W. "The Biographical Sources of Wittgenstein's Ethics." *Telos*, no. 38 (Winter 1978–1979), 63–76; Monk, Ray. *Ludwig Wittgenstein: The Duty of Genius*. New York: Penguin, 1990; Orr, Deborah. "Developing Wittgenstein's Picture of the Soul: Toward a Feminist Spiritual Erotics." In Naomi Scheman and Peg O'Connor, ed., *Feminist Interpretations of Wittgenstein*. University Park: Pennsylvania State University Press, 2002, 322–43; Reitan, Eric. "Rape as an Essentially Contested Concept." *Hypatia* 16:2 (2001), 43–66; Wittgenstein, Ludwig. (1953) *Philosophical Investigations*, 3rd ed. Trans. G.E.M. Anscombe. New York: Macmillan, 1973; Wittgenstein, Ludwig. *Tractatus Logico-Philosophicus*. Trans. D. F. Pears and B. F. McGuinness. New York: Routledge, 1961.

Wendy Lynne Lee

ADDITIONAL READING

Burnyeat, M. F. "Wittgenstein and Augustine *De magistro*." In Gareth B. Matthews, ed., *The Augustinian Tradition*. Berkeley: University of California Press, 1999, 286–303; Cavell, Stanley. *Must We Mean What We Say? A Book of Essays*. Oxford, U.K.: Oxford University Press, 1976; Cerbone, David. "Don't Look But Think: Imaginary Scenarios in Wittgenstein's Later Philosophy." *Inquiry* 37:2 (1994), 159–83; Crary, Alice, and Rupert Reed. *The New Wittgenstein*. New York: Routledge, 2000; Diamond, Cora. *The Realistic Spirit: Wittgenstein, Philosophy, and the Mind*. Cambridge, Mass.: MIT Press, 1991; Feder, Ellen K. " 'Doctors' Orders': Parents and Intersexed Children." In Eva Feder Kittay and Ellen K. Feder, eds., *The Subject of Care: Feminist Perspectives on Dependency*. Lanham, Md.: Rowman and Littlefield, 2002, 294–320. <www.bodieslikeours.org/research-and-studies/feder-docsorders-2.html> and <www.bodieslikeours.org/respdf/Feder2002.pdf> [accessed 16 February 2005]; Genova, Judith. *Wittgenstein: A Way of Seeing*. New York: Routledge, 1995; Gier, Nicholas F. *Wittgenstein and Phenomenology: A Comparative Study of the Later Wittgenstein, Husserl, Heidegger, and Merleau-Ponty*. Albany: State University of New York Press, 1981; Hamilton, Christopher. "Sex." In *Living Philosophy: Reflections on Life, Meaning and Morality*. Edinburgh, Scot.: Edinburgh University Press, 2001, 125–41; Heyes, Cressida. *The Grammar of Politics: Wittgenstein and Political Philosophy*. Ithaca, N.Y.: Cornell University Press, 2003; Houston, Lynn Marie. "Wittgenstein, Ludwig." In Timothy F. Murphy, ed., *Reader's Guide to Lesbian and Gay Studies*. Chicago, Ill.: Fitzroy Dearborn, 2000, 640–42; Janik, Allen, and Stephen Toulmin. *Wittgenstein's Vienna*. New York: Simon and Schuster, 1973; Lee-Lampshire, Wendy. "The Sound of Little Hummingbird Wings: A Wittgensteinian Investigation of Forms of Life as Forms of Power." *Feminist Studies* 25:2 (1999), 409–26; Levi, Albert W. "Wittgenstein Once More: A Response to Critics." *Telos*, no. 40 (Summer 1979), 165–73; Lovibond, Sabina. *Realism and Imagination in Ethics*. Minneapolis: University of Minnesota Press, 1983; Mulhall, Stephen. *Inheritance and Originality: Wittgenstein, Heidegger, Kierkegaard*. Oxford, U.K.: Clarendon Press, 2001; O'Connor, Peg. *Oppression and Responsibility: A Wittgensteinian Approach to Social Practices and Moral Theory*. University Park: Pennsylvania State University Press, 2002; Pears, David. *The False Prison: A Study of the Development of Wittgenstein's Philosophy*. New York: Oxford University Press, 1988; Phillips, D. Z., and Peter Winch, eds. *Wittgenstein: Attention to Particulars*. New York: St. Martin's Press, 1989; Pitkin, Hanna Fenichel. *Wittgenstein and Justice: On the Significance of Ludwig Wittgenstein for Social and Political Thought*. Berkeley: University of California Press, 1972; Rudebush, Thomas, and William M. Berg. "On Wittgenstein and Ethics: A Reply to Levi." *Telos*, no. 40 (Summer 1979), 150–60; Schatzki, Theodore R. *Social Practices: A Wittgensteinian Approach to Human Activity and the Social*. Cambridge: Cambridge University Press, 1996; Scheman, Naomi. *Engenderings: Constructions of Knowledge, Authority and Privilege*. New York: Routledge, 1993; Scheman, Naomi, and Peg O'Connor, eds. *Feminist Interpretations of Wittgenstein*. University Park: Pennsylvania State University Press, 2002; Schulte, Joachim. *Experience and Expression: Wittgenstein's Philosophy of Psychology*. Oxford, U.K.: Oxford University Press, 1993; Schwarzschild, Steven S. "Wittgenstein as Alienated Jew." *Telos*, no. 40 (Summer 1979), 160–65; Sluga, Hans, and David Stern, eds. *The Cambridge Companion to Wittgenstein*. Cambridge: Cambridge University Press, 1996; Stern, David. *Wittgenstein on Mind and Language*. New York: Oxford University Press, 1995; Tanesini, Alessandra. *Wittgenstein: A Feminist Interpretation*. Malden, Mass.: Polity, 2004; Winch, Peter. *Studies in the Philosophy of Wittgenstein*. London: Routledge, 1969; Wittgenstein, Ludwig. *Culture and Value*. Ed. G. H. von Wright and Heikki Nyman. New York: Blackwell, 1980; Wittgenstein, Ludwig. *On Certainty*. Trans. Denis Paul and G.E.M. Anscombe. Ed. G.E.M. Anscombe and G. H. von Wright. New York: Harper and Row, 1969; Wittgenstein, Ludwig. *Philosophical Grammar*. Ed. Rush Rhees. New York: Blackwell, 1974; Wittgenstein, Ludwig. *Remarks on Colour*. Trans. Linda L. McAlister and Margarete Schattle. Ed. G.E.M. Anscombe. Berkeley: University of California Press, n.d.; Wittgenstein, Ludwig. *Remarks on the Foundation of Mathematics*. Trans. G.E.M. Anscombe. Ed. Rush Rhees, G. H. von Wright, and G.E.M. Anscombe. New York: Blackwell, 1967; Wittgenstein, Ludwig. *Remarks on the Philosophy of Psychology*. Vol. 1: Trans. G.E.M. Anscombe.

Ed. G.E.M. Anscombe and G. H. von Wright. Vol. 2: Trans. C. G. Luckhardt and M.A.U. Aue. Ed. G. H. von Wright and Heikki Nyman. Chicago, Ill.: University of Chicago Press, 1980; Wittgenstein, Ludwig. *Zettel*. Trans. G.E.M. Anscombe. Ed. G.E.M. Anscombe and G. H. von Wright. New York: Blackwell, 1981.

WOJTYŁA, KAROL (POPE JOHN PAUL II) (1920–2005). John Paul II was born Karol Józef Wojtyła in Wadowice, Poland. In 1938 he began his university studies intending to pursue philology, literature, and theater. His college years coincided with World War II. In 1942 he began study as a clandestine seminarian with the Archdiocese of Kraków. Ordained in 1946, he left Poland for Rome to pursue his doctoral degree in philosophy. He was later appointed Chair of Ethics at the Catholic University of Lublin, where he lectured on philosophical and theological questions related to ethics. Most memorable were his lectures in **sexual ethics**, which became the basis for *Love and Responsibility* (1960). In 1967, Paul VI (1897–1987; papacy, 1963–1978) elevated him to cardinal, and about a decade later, at age fifty-eight, he was elected pope (1978).

As the leader of the Roman Catholic Church, John Paul II guided it through a cultural environment at odds with the Church's teaching, especially regarding sexual morality. John Paul II's theology of human sexuality was deeply embedded in a vision of cataclysmic struggle between the forces of good (culture of life) and evil (culture of death). This belief that there is a vast divide between the values of Catholic Christianity and those of modern culture is a key to understanding his philosophy and theology. Catholic teachings about **marriage**, **homosexuality**, **contraception**, and **masturbation** are not matters of private morality. Adhering to these teachings is, in his view, a way to side with the forces of good as articulated in the "the gospel of life" and exemplified by Jesus Christ.

Interpreting "the gospel of life" is not easy, especially when it comes to specifying its principles into guides for action. Catholic tradition prides itself on immutable, consistent moral teachings. The role of any pontiff is to maintain that steady course even as he confronts seemingly new moral problems. He "is the perpetual and visible source and foundation of the unity both of the bishops and of the whole company of the faithful" (*Catechism*, par. 882). Catholics believe that guided by the holy spirit the pontiff speaks in a universal and timeless voice on issues regarding faith and morals. Although he interprets Catholic teachings anew to respond to developments in the world around him, his role is not to invent new truths. His task is to specify the objective moral truths that are known to all reasonable persons as a result of God's revelations of eternal law in the forms of natural and divine law.

The Catholic moral evaluation of human sexuality hinges on two elements. First, the two agents engaged in the act must be married and one must be male, the other female. Second, the act itself must always be open to procreation. The first of these points emerges from the theology of marriage, which insists that marriage is a sacrament, a sign of God's saving power on earth. It is through marriage that the human sexual act receives its full meaning as part of God's plan. The origin of the second is more complex, but most scholars of Catholic sexual ethics attribute it to the Natural Law approach that is central to Catholic ethics. More particularly, it is the teleological view that bodily organs have divinely ordained purposes. Using them in a way that deliberately frustrates those purposes is a violation of God's order. Sexual organs are ordained for the purpose of propagating the species, and using them solely for pleasure upsets the divine and natural order.

Attitudes about the first element have remained consistent in the history of Catholic teaching on sex. The second element has been debated more strongly. The notion of the ends of marriage was developed most fully by **Augustine** (354–430) and **Thomas Aquinas** (1224/25–1274). Both argued that marriage had several purposes, but procreation was by far the most important. The other purposes—unity, sacrament, companionship—could never substitute for procreation as an end. Beginning in the early twentieth century, this insistence on procreation as the sole or primary end of sexuality became less prominent. Most notably, at the Second Vatican Council in the 1960s, the bishops declared that "marriage . . . is not instituted solely for procreation" (*Gaudium et Spes*, par. 50). They did not intend to deny the fact that procreation remains the central purpose of the sexual act, but they wanted to emphasize that sexual acts served to bring couples closer together. The intimacy of the act strengthened the bond between spouses. In recent Catholic documents, the meaning of the sexual act is said to lie in the inseparability of the unitive and procreative meanings of marriage (see Paul VI's "Humanae vitae").

Views about the significance of this shift away from procreation as the sole or primary end of sexual acts vary among Catholic theologians. More liberal ("revisionist") moral theologians see this as a sign that Catholicism is adapting to modern understandings of sex and marriage. They argue that the logical conclusion of this shift should be more liberal attitudes about contraception and **reproductive technology**. Conservative theologians argue that this shift is merely linguistic. It does not signify a major change or development in Catholic teaching and does not affect the traditional norms of Catholic sexual morality. They claim that Catholic theology has always insisted on several purposes of sex.

John Paul II began his papacy at a moment in Catholic history when these questions about sexual morality were at the forefront of the collective Catholic psyche. Paul VI's "Humanae vitae" (1968), which articulated the Catholic opposition to contraception, caused much controversy. This resulted in a crisis in the teaching authority of the Church, as many Catholics looked to their own consciences to decide which moral norms were right. John Paul II's papacy was a response to this crisis, combining a strong authoritarian tone with a pastoral message of care and compassion. It is no exaggeration to say that John Paul II's papacy centered on sexual morality. Much of his theology is built around sexual and familial images. For example, he described the body as having a "nuptial meaning" and referred to the **love** that humans have for God as spousal love. He developed these bodily metaphors in a series of addresses compiled in *The Theology of the Body* (*TOB*), which fully articulates his ideas about sex, marriage, and theology. To understand his sexual ethics, however, one must begin with *Love and Responsibility* (*LAR*), written while he was Karol Wojtyła.

The human person is a central theme of this work. For Wojtyła, the norms of Catholic sexual morality must be founded on the most fundamental good—the person. "Sexual morality is within the domain of the person. It is impossible to understand anything about it without understanding what the person is, its mode of existence, its functioning, its powers. The personal order is the only proper plane for all debate on matters of sexual morality" (*LAR*, 18). Every person, for Wojtyła, is both object and subject (21). The visible world consists of all sorts of entities that can be called objects. Human persons are one such entity, but they differ from all other objects (including nonhuman animals) by virtue of their capacity for rationality and the existence in each person of an "inwardness" or "interior life" that is oriented around truth and goodness.

While Wojtyła acknowledges that physiological and psychological information about human sexual functions is vital, the morality of sexual acts is ultimately determined by respect for the person *as* a person. Wojtyła refers to this as the "personalistic norm" (drawn in opposition to utilitarianism), according to which one may not use another merely as a means to an end. Persons are not objects and must not be utilized, as is often the case in sex, merely as an object for one's pleasure. Wojtyła's formulation of the personalistic norm follows **Immanuel Kant**'s (1724–1804) Categorical Imperative, which prohibits treating a person who is the object of one's activity as only a means to an end. Ignoring this prohibition violates the subjectivity of the person and fails to acknowledge that each person has "distinct personal ends" (*LAR*, 28). Wojtyła was in most of his career a critic of Kant's formalistic ethic, yet here he embraces a similar theme of respect for the person. Nevertheless, Wojtyła's personalistic norm is based on a different anthropology of the person than Kant's. Wojtyła's anthropology derives from his understanding of the person as God's creature and the view that humans were created with "a very particular resemblance to God" (40). For Wojtyła, the personalistic norm can be stated as the Christian New Testament commandment to love the neighbor. He acknowledges that while the personalistic norm is not identical to the love commandment, it shares a similar axiology, one that always values the person over pleasure. The essence of the love commandment, formulated in personalistic language, is that "the person is a good towards which the only proper and adequate attitude is love" (41).

The problem of how to avoid using another person is especially pronounced in the sexual encounter. Wojtyła describes it as a struggle: "The sexual instinct wants above all to take over, to make use of another person, whereas love wants to give, to create a good, to bring happiness" (*LAR*, 138). Love is the antithesis of using the other person as a means; when you love the other, you desire his or her good. Wojtyła believes that love puts a couple on "a footing of equality" because they "are bound by the same aim or common good" (28). If love is present and a couple shares the same good, then the "possibility that one might be subordinated to the other" is diminished. Without abiding by the personalistic norm, and its implications for love, the sexual encounter can easily be governed by a utilitarian mentality. The kind of love that Wojtyła has in mind is not romantic or erotic. It is the New Testament's *agape* that urges Christians to love one another as God loves them. Wojtyła acknowledges that there is a problem of "introducing love into love" (*LAR*, 17). By this he means the classic problem in Christian ethics that emerges from the emphasis given to *agape* (disinterested neighbor love): how to transform erotic love, which is particularistic, into a neighbor love that sees the other as special not merely because of attraction or **sexual desire** but because the other is a creature of God.

Sexuality is a natural part of what it is to be human. Every human experiences the sexual urge, a natural drive or orientation. But unlike animals, in which the sexual urge cannot transcend mere physical instinct, humans can exercise free will and are capable of acting on the sexual urge in various ways. The urge is necessary for maintaining the species and in that sense is part of the natural order. Wojtyła refers to this aspect of the urge as its "existential significance" (*LAR*, 53). It is the human participation in God's creative activity. Even though this purpose of the sexual urge is predetermined, humans, by treating the sexual partner as an object of love, give the sexual act its specific character as an experience of the consciously taken decision to "participate in the whole natural order of existence to further the existence of the species *Homo*" (53). When the person enters into the natural order or "immerses himself so to speak in its elemental processes . . . he *must not forget he is a person*" (236). One way to remember one's personhood is to make sure that the sexual urge is directed to procreation. Directed that way, it becomes the occasion for love between spouses and for the love they will express for the fruit of their union. Procreation is the shared good that protects married couples from trying to attain their own selfish ends. The sexual encounter is driven by the desire for the other. If one views the other merely as an object, desire remains at the stage of concupiscence. The human will, "with its natural aspiration to the infinite good which is happiness," must start to want the good for the other person (137). Sexual morality, then, in Wojtyła's view, applies the personalistic norm to the fulfillment of the natural purpose of sex. Merely responding to the dictates of nature is not enough. That is precisely why the procreative and unitive ends must be inseparable. Without the unitive end, procreation can become a way to treat the other merely as a means to an end.

The nature of the love between the spouses includes a reciprocal gift of self. Wojtyła uses "self-giving" to describe this distinguishing character of betrothed love. "What might be called the law of *ekstasis* seems to operate here: the lover 'goes outside' the self to find a fuller existence in another. In no other form of love does this law operate so conspicuously as it does in betrothed love" (*LAR*, 126). "Going outside" oneself does not culminate only in the proximate good of the other, for "to desire 'unlimited' good for another person is really to desire God for that person" (138). The idea of reciprocal self-giving derives from Wojtyła's beliefs about the complementarity of male and female. On his interpretation of Genesis, Adam and Eve were both created in God's image. In that sense, male and female are unified in a shared humanity, and both are distinct from every nonhuman species. Yet they are separate and exist for one another's sake. Together they form a community of persons, especially in the sexual act where they become "one flesh." Wojtyła reads the Christian creation accounts as descriptions of the process of human self-consciousness. Humans are revealed to themselves through their bodies in the realization that they are different from other species. This realization leads to an experience of solitude, which is not remedied by God's other creations. Man, in Genesis's second creation account, was still alone, and he needed someone who would be bone of his bone, flesh of his flesh. God created Eve from Adam's rib to remedy this need. The original solitude of man, understood as having no sex or gender, is re-created into the unity of male and female. This unity is damaged by Adam and Eve's disobedience and its punishment by God (original sin), which leads to male domination over the female. But in sexual intercourse, man and woman become "one flesh" and in doing so relive that original unity and appreciate the value of the other as a person created in God's image. They also "submit their whole humanity to the blessings of fertility" (*LAR*, 44). Genesis describes every human experience of conjugal sex.

John Paul II derives another idea from Genesis: "original nakedness." Before the Fall, male and female were naked. Nakedness, in his view, signifies an original simplicity and integrity. By disobeying God, Adam and Eve shattered this original purity and introduced the experience of shame and lust. Nevertheless, their capacity to give themselves as gifts to one another persists. One can read this "nuptial attribute" of the body in the bodily distinction of male and female. They give to one another, and through sex, they experience a true reciprocity, the gift of themselves to the other. Yet for sex to have both a theological and personalistic (ethical) dimension, the human body must always be viewed as more than just sexual. It is the vehicle for expressing an interpersonal meaning through the personal communion of male and female. The body, in John Paul II's view, speaks the **language** of true personalism. "The human body is not merely an organism of sexual reactions." In addition, it is "the means of expressing the entire man, the person, which reveals itself by means of the language of the body" (*TOB*, 397). The body "speaks" this language, which John Paul II describes as mysterious, through "action and interaction." In the sexual act, man and woman continue the "dialogue" that "had its beginning on the day of creation" (398). The language of the body is authentic when persons express the whole truth of what it means to be a person through the actions of their bodies. Mastery over the body is a prerequisite for giving oneself freely to the other. Thus, the truth of personhood is the capacity to give oneself to the other. In the conjugal act, "man and woman reciprocally express themselves in the fullest and most profound way possible" (398).

Through marriage, humans strive to imitate God's love, and they participate in his creative activity through sexual intercourse. Nevertheless, sex is not the only way to achieve this good. In fact, the Church has always viewed consecrated celibacy as superior to marriage. This option is not available to everyone, but it is important because it plays a role in preparing certain people for eternal union with God. By choosing to remain celibate, they devote themselves in a special way to this task and point the way for others. Still, marriage is good and necessary. It serves the natural purposes of propagating the species and combines that with the love needed between humans. Any sex outside marriage (**adultery**, premarital sex) is immoral because the sexual partner will necessarily be degraded "to the status of an object of pleasure for another person" (*TOB*, 222). Marriage justifies the sexual act by directing it to its appropriate ends, the propagation and education of offspring and faithful self-giving love.

The prohibition of contraception is a central tenet of Catholic sexual ethics. Much of John Paul II's writing focused on this issue. He supported the prohibition of artificial contraception as stated definitively in "Humanae vitae": deliberately impeding the procreative process of the human sexual act is intrinsically evil. He did, however, develop and elaborate this position in several different directions. For example, he connected contraceptive acts with other contra-life acts such as **abortion**; both are motivated by the similar utilitarian mentality that views human life as something to be used. In "Evangelium vitae," he refers to the "contraceptive mentality" as based on a "conspiracy against life" (par. 12–13). His primary argument against the use of contraception is that any sexual act that is deliberately nonprocreative violates the order of the true communion of persons. It constitutes a withholding of self; a contraceptive act can never be a true gift of self.

This argument about "withholding of self" is distinct from Paul VI's Natural Law arguments and, some argue, distinct from Wojtyła's own writing in *Love and Responsibility*. For example, in his earlier book he appeals to the "order and the laws of nature" (235) to condemn artificial methods of birth regulation and to justify "periodic continence" to avoid pregnancy. It is possible to avoid procreation by "having intercourse during infertile periods, and abstaining during fertile periods. If [people do] this procreation is excluded in the natural way. . . . [The man and woman] are merely adapting themselves to the laws of nature. . . . The fertility cycle in woman is part of that order." By contrast, some "devices . . . are artificial [and so] they deprive conjugal relations of their 'naturalness,' which cannot be said when procreation is avoided by adaptation to the fertility cycle" (235). But having been trained as a philosopher, Wojtyła realizes the objections to the position he has just laid out and immediately asks: "But is it not all the same a total avoidance of procreation, and by definition morally bad? To answer this question we must examine . . . the ethics of periodic continence."

Wojtyła dislikes the term "rhythm method," preferring to call the practice "periodic continence" (*LAR*, 240). His point is that the regulation of birth for the proper reason(s) is not to be conceived as a "birth-control technique" or "method" in any sense but only as a method for regulating conception. The distinction as he sees it is "if periodic continence can be regarded as a 'method' at all, it is a method of regulating conception and not of avoiding family" (242). Further, "If continence is to be a virtue and not just a 'method' in the utilitarian sense, it must not serve to destroy readiness for parenthood in a husband and wife, since acceptance [of parenthood] is what justifies the marital relationship and puts it on a level of a true union of persons" (242). There is an apparent tension here; Wojtyła wants the intention of every sexual act to be procreative, but he acknowledges that couples can use periodic continence to regulate procreation.

In more recent works, John Paul II argued using different terms: A conjugal act that separates the procreative from the unitive ends cannot be an act of love because the persons engaged in the act are not "speaking" the language of the body in a way that "correspond[s] to the interior truth and to the dignity of personal communion" (*TOB*, 398). He still acknowledges that married couples can licitly avoid the birth of children by abstaining from sex during the woman's fertile period. The main difference between **abstinence** and artificial methods is that the latter violates the virtue of chastity, while the former is an expression of that virtue. There are several ways to understand the connection between chastity and contraception. First, the practice of abstaining from sex is a way to exhibit self-mastery, which enables the person to give himself or herself more fully to the other. Second, when couples engage in sex using artificial contraception, they are in danger of using each other only for the sake of pleasure. By precluding the possibility of conception, the shared good of sexual intercourse, the husband and wife turn their gaze toward another good, their own pleasure and satisfaction. All discussion of the rhythm method stresses that a couple should choose to limit births only for legitimate reasons. Thus, the morally relevant difference between "artificial" and "natural" contraception need not be intention. Rather, in the former case, the couple has sex for pleasure with no thought of procreation, whereas in the latter they abstain from sex and, in John Paul II's view, are less likely to treat each other as means.

This description of artificial contraception as a violation of chastity is different from his earlier view that abstinence was preferable because it is more in tune with the cycles of nature. For example, in *Theology of the Body* he writes that "the virtuous character of the attitude which is expressed in the natural regulation of fertility is determined not so much by fidelity to an impersonal natural law as to the Creator-Person, the Source and the Lord of the order which is manifested in such a law" (401).

On another important issue, Catholic teaching considers all homosexual acts intrinsically evil because they violate the order of God's creation. For John Paul II, the centrality of gender complementarity means that personal communion can never exist when the parties to a sexual act are not male and female. He considers a homosexual act, by its very nature, to be an instance where the dignity of the other cannot be upheld. The other is only being used for the purpose of satisfying a sexual urge. In the homosexual act, the language of the body is not being expressed in its integrated and authentic truthfulness.

John Paul II made sexual morality central to his Catholic message by reinforcing the traditional Catholic norms that govern licit sexual behavior. Yet some saw him as an innovator because he expanded on those teachings in several ways. First, his teachings had a stronger grounding in appeal to Scripture. Second, he elevated the discussion of sexual morality to the level of a most pressing concern for Catholic morality: Maintaining traditional sexual norms protects the culture of life from the forces of the culture of death. In "Evangelium Vitae" he wrote that "the loss of contact with God's wise design is the deepest root of modern man's confusion" (par. 22). For John Paul II, the properly ordered sex act is the most significant manifestation of this design. Third, he insisted that the body cannot be understood apart from the person, a change from the pre-Vatican II physicalist Natural

Law interpretation of the body and sex. Indeed, the body provides a language for understanding the dignity of the person. That language is the language of love as self-donation. Because each body is male or female, it exists in a state of readiness to give itself to its complementary other. This act of reciprocity (sex within marriage) reveals the full dignity of the person. This reminder that one ought to treat the other in such a way that values the other's dignity is, perhaps, John Paul II's greatest contribution to Catholic sexual ethics.

See also Abstinence; Anscombe, G.E.M.; Augustine (Saint); Catholicism, History of; Catholicism, Twentieth- and Twenty-First-Century; Consequentialism; Contraception; Homosexuality, Ethics of; Kierkegaard, Søren; Love; Marriage; Natural Law (New); Thomas Aquinas (Saint)

REFERENCES

Catechism of the Catholic Church, 2nd ed. Washington, D.C.: United States Catholic Conference, 2000; Paul VI (Pope). "Humanae Vitae." *Catholic Mind* 66 (September 1968), 35–48; Vatican Council II. "*Gaudium et Spes*: The Pastoral Constitution on the Church in the Modern World." *Acta Apostolicae Sedis* 58:15 (1966), 1025–1120. Vatican translation in David J. O'Brien and Thomas A. Shannon, eds., *Catholic Social Thought: The Documentary Heritage*. Maryknoll, N.Y.: Orbis Books, 1992, 164–237; Wojtyła, Karol (Pope John Paul II). "Evangelium Vitae." *Origins* 24:42 (6 April 1995), 689–727; Wojtyła, Karol. (1960) *Love and Responsibility*. Trans. H. T. Willetts. New York: Farrar, Straus, Giroux, 1981; Wojtyła, Karol. *The Theology of the Body: Human Love in the Divine Plan*. Boston, Mass.: Pauline Books, 1997.

Aline Kalbian

ADDITIONAL READING

Buttiglione, Rocco. *Karol Wojtyła: The Thought of the Man Who Became John Paul II*. Trans. Paolo Guietti and Francesca Murphy. Grand Rapids, Mich.: Eerdmans, 1997; Congregation for the Doctrine of Faith. *Homosexualitatis Problema: Letter to the Bishops of the Catholic Church on the Pastoral Care of Homosexual Persons* (1 October 1986). Boston, Mass.: Pauline Books, 1986. <www.vatican.va/roman_curia/congregations/cfaith/doc_doc_index.html> [accessed 21 September 2004]; Curran, Charles, and Richard McCormick, eds. *John Paul II and Moral Theology*. New York: Paulist Press, 1998; Dulles, Avery. *The Splendor of Faith: The Theological Vision of Pope John Paul II*. New York: Crossroad, 1999; Gudorf, Christine, E. "Encountering the Other: The Modern Papacy on Women." In Charles E. Curran, Margaret A. Farley, and Richard McCormick, eds., *Feminist Ethics and the Catholic Moral Tradition*. New York: Paulist Press, 1996, 66–89; Kalbian, Aline. *Sexing the Church: Gender, Power, and Contemporary Catholic Ethics*. Bloomington: Indiana University Press, 2005; Paul VI (Pope). "Humanae Vitae." *Catholic Mind* 66 (September 1968), 35–48. Reprinted in Claudia Carlen, ed., *The Papal Encyclicals 1958–1981*. Raleigh, N.C.: Pierian Press, 1990, 223–36; P&S1 (131–49); P&S2 (167–84); P&S3 (96–105); Pontifical Council for the Family. *The Truth and Meaning of Human Sexuality: Guidelines for Education within the Family* (8 December 1995). Boston, Mass.: Pauline Books, 1995. <www.vatican.va/roman_curia/pontifical_councils/family/index.htm> [accessed 21 September 2004]; Sacred Congregation for the Doctrine of Faith. *Persona Humana: Declaration on Certain Questions Concerning Sexual Ethics* (29 December 1975). Boston, Mass.: Pauline Books, 1975. <www.vatican.va/roman_curia/congregations/cfaith/doc_doc_index.html> [accessed 21 September 2004]; Simpson, Peter. "Love and Responsibility." In *On Karol Wojtyła*. Belmont, Calif.: Wadsworth, 2001, 46–67; Weigel, George. *Witness to Hope: The Biography of John Paul II*. New York: HarperCollins, 1999; West, Christopher. *Theology of the Body Explained: A Commentary on John Paul II's "Gospel of the Body."* Boston, Mass.: Pauline Books, 2003; Wojtyła, Karol (Pope John Paul II). *The Acting Person*. Trans. Andrzej Potocki. Dordrecht, Holland: Reidel, 1979; Wojtyła, Karol. "Authentic Concept of Conjugal Love." *Origins* 28:37 (1999), 654–56; Wojtyła, Karol. *Familiaris Consortio: The Role of the Christian Family in the Modern World.* (Apostolic Exhortation, 22 November 1981) Boston, Mass.: Pauline Books, 1981. <www.vatican.va/

holy_father/john_paul_ii/index.htm> [accessed 21 September 2004]; Wojtyła, Karol. *Mulieres Dignitatem: On the Dignity and Vocation of Women on the Occasion of the Marian Year*. (Apostolic Letter, 15 August 1988) Boston, Mass.: Pauline Books, 1988. <www.vatican.va/holy_father/john_paul_ii/index.htm> [accessed 21 September 2004]; Wojtyła, Karol. *Ordinatio Sacerdotalis: On Reserving Priestly Ordination to Men Alone*. (Apostolic Letter, 22 May 1994) Boston, Mass.: Pauline Books, 1994. <www.vatican.va/holy_father/john_paul_ii/index.htm> [accessed 21 September 2004]; Wojtyła, Karol. *The Papal Encyclicals of John Paul II*. Ed. J. Michael Miller. Huntington, Ind.: Our Sunday Visitor, 1996; Wojtyła, Karol. *Person and Community: Selected Essays*. (*Catholic Thought from Lublin*, vol. 4) Trans. Theresa Sandok. Frankfurt, Ger.: Peter Lang, 1994; Wojtyła, Karol. *Redemptoris Mater: Mother of the Redeemer*. (Encyclical, 27 March 1987) Boston, Mass.: Pauline Books, 1987. <www.vatican.va/holy_father/john_paul_ii/index.htm> [accessed 21 March 2004]; Wojtyła, Karol. *Veritatis Splendor: The Splendor of Truth*. (Encyclical, 6 August 1993) Boston, Mass.: Pauline Books, 1993. <www.vatican.va/holy_father/john_paul_ii/index.htm> [accessed 21 September 2004].

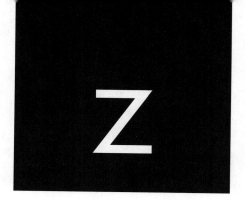

ZOOPHILIA. *See* Bestiality

SELECTED GENERAL BIBLIOGRAPHY

Readers, students, teachers, and scholars investigating the philosophy of sex will find the following works interesting and helpful. This list includes, beyond the central texts listed in the "Abbreviations," several more philosophy (or theology) of sex anthologies, textbooks, monographs, and works in general philosophy (marked with an asterisk) but also collections and treatises from other fields.

Abelove, Henry, Michèle Aina Barale, and David M. Halperin, eds. *The Lesbian and Gay Studies Reader*. New York: Routledge, 1993.

Bell, Alan P., and Martin S. Weinberg. *Homosexualities: A Study of Diversity among Men and Women*. New York: Simon and Schuster, 1978.

Bullough, Vern L., and Bonnie Bullough, eds. *Human Sexuality: An Encyclopedia*. New York: Garland, 1994.

*The Catholic Encyclopedia. <newadvent.org/cathen> [accessed 11 January 2005].

*Chadwick, Ruth, ed. *Encyclopedia of Applied Ethics*, vols. 1–4. San Diego, Calif.: Academic Press, 1998.

Coleman, Julie. *Love, Sex, and Marriage: A Historical Thesaurus*. Amsterdam, Holland: Rodopi, 1999.

*Corvino, John, ed. *Same Sex: Debating the Ethics, Science, and Culture of Homosexuality*. Lanham, Md.: Rowman and Littlefield, 1997.

*Devine, Philip E., and Celia Wolf-Devine, eds. *Sex and Gender: A Spectrum of Views*. Belmont, Calif.: Wadsworth, 2003.

*Dixon, Nicolas, ed. *The Philosophy of Love and Sex*. *Essays in Philosophy* 2:2 (June 2001). <www.humboldt.edu/~essays/archives.html> [accessed 20 April 2005].

Dynes, Wayne R., ed. *The Encyclopedia of Homosexuality*, 2 vols. New York: Garland, 1990.

Eadie, Jo, ed. *Sexuality: The Essential Glossary*. London: Arnold, 2004.

Ellis, Albert, and Albert Abarbanel, eds. *The Encyclopedia of Sexual Behavior*, 2 vols. New York: Hawthorne Books, 1961. New and revised 2nd ed., 1967. New 2nd ed. (1 vol.), Jason Aronson, 1973.

*Feder, Ellen K., Karmen MacKendrick, and Sybol S. Cook, eds. *A Passion for Wisdom: Readings in Western Philosophy on Love and Desire*. Upper Saddle River, N.J.: Prentice Hall, 2004.

Flood, Michael. (1992) *The Men's Bibliography*, 13th ed. (20 September 2004). <mensbiblio.xyonline.net/> [accessed 25 May 2005].

Francoeur, Robert T., Timothy Perper, Norman A. Scherzer, George P. Sellmer, and Martha Cornog. *A Descriptive Dictionary and Atlas of Sexology*. Westport, Conn.: Greenwood, 1991.

*Hanson, Anthony, Jennifer Campbell Koella, and Michael Keene. "Philosophy on the Internet." In *The Mayfield Quick View Guide to the Internet*. Mountain View, Calif.: Mayfield, 2001, 47–82.

*The Internet Classics Archive. MIT Web site. <classics.mit.edu> [accessed 18 January 2005].

*The Internet Encyclopedia of Philosophy. <www.utm.edu/research/iep> [accessed 18 January 2005].

Jackson, Stevi, and Sue Scott, eds. *Feminism and Sexuality: A Reader*. New York: Columbia University Press, 1996.

*Jung, Patricia Beattie, Mary E. Hunt, and Radhika Balakrishnan, eds. *Good Sex: Feminist Perspectives from the World's Religions*. New Brunswick, N.J.: Rutgers University Press, 2001.

Katz, Jonathan, ed. *Homosexuality: Lesbians and Gay Men in Society, History, and Literature*. New York: Arno Press, 1975.

Laumann, Edward O., John H. Gagnon, Robert T. Michael, and Stuart Michaels. *The Social Organization of Sexuality: Sexual Practices in the United States*. Chicago, Ill.: University of Chicago Press, 1994.

Laumann, Edward O., and Robert T. Michael, eds. *Sex, Love, and Health in America: Private Choices and Public Policies*. Chicago, Ill.: University of Chicago Press, 2001.

*Lebacqz, Karen, with David Sinacore-Guinn, eds. *Sexuality: A Reader*. Cleveland, Ohio: Pilgrim Press, 1999.

Magnus Hirschfeld Archive for Sexology, Humboldt University of Berlin. (Web site) <www2.rz.hu-berlin.de/sexology> [accessed 10 February 2005].

*Murphy, Timothy F., ed. *Gay Ethics: Controversies in Outing, Civil Rights, and Sexual Science*. Binghamton, N.Y.: Harrington Park Press, 1994.

————. *Reader's Guide to Lesbian and Gay Studies*. Chicago, Ill.: Fitzroy Dearborn, 2000.

Nye, Robert A., ed. *Sexuality*. Oxford, U.K.: Oxford University Press, 1999.

*The Perseus Digital Library. Tufts University Web site. <www.perseus.tufts.edu> [accessed 18 January 2005].

*Priest, Graham, ed. *Perversion. The Monist* 86:1 (January 2003).

*Reich, Warren T., ed. *Encyclopedia of Bioethics*, rev. ed., 5 vols. New York: Simon and Schuster; Macmillan, 1995. (1st ed., New York: Free Press, 1978.)

*————. *The Ethics of Sex and Genetics*, rev. ed. New York: Macmillan, 1998.

"Researching Sex: A Resource Guide to Sexology." <www.pages.drexel.edu/~jlc42/sexology.html> [accessed 16 February 2005].

*Rogers, Eugene F., Jr., ed. *Theology and Sexuality: Classic and Contemporary Readings*. Oxford, U.K.: Blackwell, 2002.

*Shelp, Earl E., ed. *Sexuality and Medicine*. Vol. 1: *Conceptual Roots*. Vol. 2: *Ethical Viewpoints in Transition*. Dordrecht, Holland: Reidel, 1987.

*Singer, Irving. *The Nature of Love*. Vol. 1: *Plato to Luther* [1st ed., 1966], 2nd ed. Chicago, Ill.: University of Chicago Press, 1984. Vol. 2: *Courtly and Romantic*, 1984. Vol. 3: *The Modern World*, 1987.

*Soble, Alan. "The Fundamentals of the Philosophy of Sex." In Alan Soble, ed., *The Philosophy of Sex: Contemporary Readings*, 4th ed. Lanham, Md.: Rowman and Littlefield, 2002, xvii–xlii.

*————. *The Philosophy of Sex and Love: An Introduction*. St. Paul, Minn.: Paragon House, 1998.

*————. "Philosophy of Sexuality." In James Fieser, ed., *The Internet Encyclopedia of Philosophy* (2000). <www.iep.utm.edu/s/sexualit.htm> [accessed 18 January 2005].

*————. "Sexuality, Philosophy of." In Edward Craig, ed., *Routledge Encyclopedia of Philosophy*, vol. 8. London: Routledge, 1998, 717–30.

*————. "Sexuality and Sexual Ethics." In Lawrence C. Becker and Charlotte B. Becker, eds., *Encyclopedia of Ethics*, 1st ed., vol. 2. New York: Garland, 1141–47. Reprinted, revised, in Lawrence C. Becker and Charlotte B. Becker, eds., *Encyclopedia of Ethics*, 2nd ed., vol. 3. New York: Routledge, 2001, 1570–77.

*————. (Web site) <www.uno.edu/~asoble> [accessed 2 January 2005].

*————, ed. *Eros, Agape, and Philia: Readings in the Philosophy of Love*, 1st printing. New York: Paragon House, 1989. 2nd printing, corrected, St. Paul, Minn.: Paragon House, 1999.

*Solomon, Robert C., and Kathleen M. Higgins, eds. *The Philosophy of (Erotic) Love*. Lawrence: University Press of Kansas, 1991.

Stanford Encyclopedia of Philosophy. <plato.stanford.edu/contents.html> [accessed 18 January 2005].

Stimpson, Catharine R., and Ethel Spector Person, eds. *Women: Sex and Sexuality*. Chicago, Ill.: University of Chicago Press, 1980.

*Stuart, Elizabeth, and Adrian Thatcher, eds. *Christian Perspectives on Sexuality and Gender*. Grand Rapids, Mich.: Eerdmans, 1996.

*Swidler, Arlene, ed. *Homosexuality and World Religions*. Valley Forge, Pa.: Trinity Press, 1993.

*"Symposium on Consent and Sexual Relations." *Legal Theory* 2:2–3 (1996), 87–264.

*Trevas, Robert, Arthur Zucker, and Donald Borchert, eds. *Philosophy of Sex and Love: A Reader*. Upper Saddle River, N.J.: Prentice-Hall, 1997.

*Verene, Donald, ed. *Sexual Love and Western Morality: A Philosophical Anthology*, 1st ed. New York: Harper and Row, 1972. 2nd ed., Boston, Mass.: Jones and Bartlett, 1995.

*Vitek, William. "Bibliography." In Robert B. Baker and Frederick A. Elliston, eds., *Philosophy and Sex*, 2nd ed. Buffalo, N.Y.: Prometheus, 1984, 471–521.

Ward, Sally K., Jennifer Dziuba-Leatherman, Jane Gerard Stapleton, and Carrie L. Yodanis, eds. *Acquaintance and Date Rape: An Annotated Bibliography*. Westport, Conn.: Greenwood Press, 1994.

Williams, Christine L., and Arlene Stein, eds. *Sexuality and Gender*. Malden, Mass.: Blackwell, 2002.

*Williams, Clifford, ed. *On Love and Friendship: Philosophical Readings*. Boston, Mass.: Jones and Bartlett, 1995.

*Wilson, John. *Love, Sex, and Feminism: A Philosophical Essay*. New York: Praeger, 1980.

JOURNALS (All accessed 24 June 2005)

AllPsych Journal. <allpsych.com/journal>

Annual Review of Sex Research. <www.sexscience.org/publications/index.php?category_id=437>

Archives of Sexual Behavior. <www.ingentaconnect.com/content/klu/aseb>

Canadian Journal of Human Sexuality. <www.sieccan.org/cjhs.html>

Electronic Journal of Human Sexuality. <www.ejhs.org>

GLQ: A Journal of Lesbian and Gay Studies. <www.ingentaconnect.com/content/dup/glq>

International Journal of Sexuality and Gender Studies. <www.ingentaconnect.com/content/klu/jlbi>

J. Paul Leonard Library: Sexuality Journals. <online.sfsu.edu/~chrism/journals.html>

Journal of Bisexuality. <www.haworthpress.com/web/JB>

Journal of Homosexuality. <www.haworthpress.com/web/JH>

Journal of Human Sexuality. <www.leaderu.com/jhs>

Journal of Lesbian Studies. <www.haworthpress.com/web/JLS>

Journal of Psychology and Human Sexuality. <www.haworthpress.com/web/JPHS>

Journal of Sex Research. <www.sexscience.org/publications/index.php?category_id=439>

Journal of the History of Sexuality. <www.utexas.edu/utpress/journals/jhs.html>

Law and Sexuality: A Review of Lesbian, Gay, Bisexual, and Transgender Legal Issues. <www.law.tulane.edu/tuexp/journals/law_sex/default.htm>

Maledicta: The International Journal of Verbal Aggression. <www.sonic.net/maledicta/journal.html>

Sex Education: Sexuality, Society and Learning. <www.tandf.co.uk/journals/titles/14681811.asp>

Sexualities, Evolution and Gender: An International Journal of Feminist and Evolutionary Standpoints. <www.tandf.co.uk/journals/titles/14792508.asp>

Sexualities: Studies in Culture and Society. <sexualities.sagepub.com>

Sexuality and Culture. <www.csulb.edu/~asc/journal.html>

Sexuality Research and Social Policy: Journal of the National Sexuality Resource Center. <www.ucpress.edu/journals/srsp/>

Society for Human Sexuality: Scholarly Sexuality Journals. <www.sexuality.org/l/sex/sexjrn.html>

Studies in Gender and Sexuality. <www.analyticpress.com/sgs.html>

Theology and Sexuality. <tse.sagepub.com>

EDITORS AND CONTRIBUTORS

The biographical sketches are followed by the entry or entries written by that contributor or editorial board member.

VOLUME EDITOR

Alan Soble is professor of philosophy and University Research Professor at the University of New Orleans. He has been writing about and teaching the philosophy of sex and love since 1977. He has also published in feminist epistemology, the philosophy of science, and the history of philosophy (Augustine, Francis Bacon, Immanuel Kant, John Stuart Mill). Some of his essays have been translated into Chinese, French, German, Hungarian, Italian, and Portuguese. He has two daughters, Rebecca Jill (b. 1969) and Rachel Emőke (b. 1993).

Activity, Sexual; Completeness, Sexual; Ethics, Sexual; Hobbes, Thomas; Masturbation; Personification, Sexual; Philosophy of Sex, Overview of; Singer, Irving

ADVISORY BOARD

David Archard is professor of philosophy and public policy and director of the Institute for Environment, Philosophy and Public Policy at the University of Lancaster. He has published on social, political, legal, and applied moral philosophy. Among his books are *Sexual Consent* (1998) and *Children, Family and State* (2003). He is currently working on *Rape: An Essay in Moral and Legal Philosophy*.

Flirting; Rape

Martha Cornog, M.A., M.L.S., authored *The Big Book of Masturbation* (2003), which won a Benjamin Franklin Award from the Publishers Marketing Association, and coauthored *For Sex Education: See Librarian* (with Timothy Perper, 1996). Her anthology *Libraries, Erotica, and Pornography* (1991) won the American Library Association's Oboler Award. She has written on sexuality research and sexual language and is collaborating with her husband Timothy Perper on romantic/erotic Japanese comics (manga). She was book review editor for the *Journal of Sex Education and Therapy* and was named *Library Journal* Book Reviewer of the Year/Nonfiction in 2001.

Bullough, Vern L.; Ellis, Albert; Rimmer, Robert

John Corvino is assistant professor of philosophy at Wayne State University in Detroit. He is the editor of *Same Sex: Debating the Ethics, Science, and Culture of Homosexuality* (1997) and is a contributor to the Independent Gay Forum <www.indegayforum.org/authors/corvino>. His other research interests include business ethics and Hume's metaethics.

Homosexuality, Ethics of; Orientation, Sexual; Social Constructionism

Joseph A. Diorio is dean of the Division of Postgraduate Studies at Unitec, New Zealand. Born on Staten Island, he received his Ph.D. in philosophy and education from Columbia University. He has published articles on educational theory and sexuality education in *Educational Theory, Curriculum Inquiry, Gender and Education, Educational Philosophy and Theory, Journal of Social Philosophy*, and *Sex Education*.

Dysfunction, Sexual; MacKinnon, Catharine; Money, John; Sex Education

Ann Garry is professor and chair of the Philosophy Department and former director of the Center for the Study of Genders and Sexualities at California State University, Los Angeles. She specializes in feminist philosophy and also writes and teaches about sexuality and contemporary moral issues more generally. She edited, with Marilyn Pearsall, *Women, Knowledge, and Reality: Explorations in Feminist Philosophy* (1989; 2nd ed., 1996) and is an associate editor of *Hypatia: A Journal of Feminist Philosophy*.

Christine E. Gudorf is professor of religious studies and chair of her department at Florida International University. She publishes in the area of social and religious ethics, especially regarding gender and sexuality, and has written *Body, Sex, and Pleasure: Reconstructing Christian Sexual Ethics* (1994) and, with James Huchingson, *Boundaries: A Casebook in Environmental Ethics* (2003).

Catholicism, Twentieth- and Twenty-First-Century; Genital Mutilation; Herdt, Gilbert; Violence, Sexual

Sarah Hoffman earned her Ph.D. at the University of Alberta and is associate professor of philosophy at the University of Saskatchewan. In addition to the philosophy of sex, her research interests center on topics in the philosophy of science and mathematics, especially those related to existence and fictionalism.

Dworkin, Andrea; Perversion, Sexual

Richard T. Hull is professor emeritus of philosophy, State University of New York at Buffalo. During the 2003 fall term, he was Visiting Distinguished Professor in the Institute of Medicine and Humanities, University of Montana, Missoula. He edited *Ethical Issues in the New Reproductive Technologies* (1990; e-book edition, <www.richard-t-hull.com>, 2003) and contributed several entries to Annette Burfoot, ed., *Encyclopedia of Reproductive Technologies* (1999). He also edits the series *Presidential Addresses of the American Philosophical Association* (Kluwer, 1999–2001; Prometheus, 2003–   ) and the series *Histories and Addresses of Philosophical Societies* (Rodopi, 1994–   ).

Reproductive Technology

Edward Johnson is professor and chair of the Philosophy Department, University of New Orleans, where he has taught since receiving his Ph.D. from Princeton University in 1976. He is the author of essays in applied ethics, including "Inscrutable Desires" (*Philosophy of* *the Social Sciences*; 1990), "Beauty's Punishment: How Feminists Look at Pornography" (D. Bushnell, ed., *Nagging Questions: Feminist Ethics in Everyday Life*; 1995), and "Loves-expressed" (A. Soble, ed., *Sex, Love, and Friendship*; 1997).

Bestiality; Ellis, Havelock; Humor; Language

John Kleinig is director of the Institute for Criminal Justice Ethics and professor of philosophy at John Jay College of Criminal Justice in New York. He also holds the Charles Sturt University Chair of Policing Ethics in the Centre for Applied Philosophy and Professional Ethics (Canberra, Australia). Among his books are *Paternalism* (1984), *Ethical Issues in Psychosurgery* (1985), and *The Ethics of Policing* (1996). He is the editor of *Teaching Criminal Justice Ethics: Strategic Issues* (1997; with Margaret Leland Smith); *From Social Justice to Criminal Justice: Poverty and the Administration of Criminal Law* (2000; with William C. Heffernan); and *Private and Public Corruption* (2004; with William C. Heffernan).

Bible, Sex and the

Timothy F. Murphy holds a Ph.D. from Boston College and is professor of philosophy in the Biomedical Sciences at the University of Illinois College of Medicine at Chicago. He is the author of *Gay Science: The Ethics of Sexual Orientation Research* (1997) and *Case Studies in Biomedical Research Ethics* (2004). He has been a visiting scholar at the American Medical Association Institute for Ethics.

Homosexuality and Science

James Lindemann Nelson is professor of philosophy and faculty associate, Center for Ethics and Humanities in the Life Sciences, at Michigan State University, and a fellow of the Hastings Center. The coauthor (with Hilde Lindemann Nelson) of *The Patient in the Family* (1995), he has also written *Hippocrates' Maze: Ethical Explorations of the Medical Labyrinth* (2003) and edited *Rationing Sanity: Ethical Issues in Managed Mental Health Care* (2003).

Nagel, Thomas

Igor Primoratz is professor of philosophy at the Hebrew University, Jerusalem, and principal research fellow in the Centre for Applied Philosophy and Public Ethics at the University of Melbourne. His publications include *Ethics and Sex* (1999) and *Human Sexuality* (editor, 1997) and articles on prostitution, sexual perversion, and pedophilia.

Pedophilia; Prostitution

J. Martin Stafford was born in Hyde, N.W. England, in 1948 and educated at Manchester and Sheffield Universities. He has never held an academic post but has written several articles on sexuality and the history of ethics and one short book, *Homosexuality and Education* (1988). In 1997, he published an acclaimed collection of the contemporary responses to Bernard Mandeville. He has also produced CDs, including the first complete recordings of E. J. Moeran's piano music (1994) and William Croft's harpsichord works (1999). (Inquiries about the books and CDs may be sent to Ismeron99@aol.com.) He has finished an account of the life and work of Alec Baldwin, which he began while writing for this encyclopedia.

Hume, David; Mandeville, Bernard; Scruton, Roger; Spencer, Herbert; Westermarck, Edward

Robert M. Stewart received his Ph.D. from the University of Michigan in 1981 and is professor of philosophy at California State University, Chico. His areas of interest include ethics, social and political philosophy, and the philosophy of sex and love. With Brooke Moore, he wrote *Moral Philosophy: A Comprehensive Introduction* (1994), and he edited *Philosophical Perspectives on Sex and Love* (1995) and *Readings in Social and Political Philosophy* (2nd ed., 1996).

Paglia, Camille; Sex Work; Utopianism

Edward Collins Vacek, S.J., has a license in sacred theology from Loyola University of Chicago and a Ph.D. (philosophy) from Northwestern University. He came to Weston Jesuit School of Theology in 1981, where he is professor of Christian ethics. He has contributed over fifty articles to various journals and books and is the author of *Love, Human and Divine* (1994).

Posner, Richard; Sexuality, Dimensions of

Alan Wertheimer is John G. McCullough Professor of political science at the University of Vermont. He is the author of *Coercion* (1987), *Exploitation* (1996), and *Consent to Sexual Relations* (2003). He has also taught at the John F. Kennedy School of Government at Harvard University.

Consent

CONTRIBUTORS

Douglas Adeney, M.A. (Monash), Ph.D. (St Andrews), lectures in philosophy at the University of Melbourne. The coauthor, with John Weckert, of *Computer and Information Ethics* (1997), his main interests and publications are in moral and political philosophy.

Liberalism

Timo Airaksinen, Ph.D. (Turku), has been professor of philosophy at the University of Helsinki since 1983. He has published on the philosophy of literature (Marquis de Sade, H. P. Lovecraft) and the history of philosophy (Thomas Hobbes, George Berkeley, G.W.F. Hegel). He is a life member of Clare Hall College, Cambridge, England, and a former fellow of the Pittsburgh Center for the Philosophy of Science.

Bataille, Georges; Sade, Marquis de

Peter B. Anderson is professor in the department of Human Performance and Health Promotion, University of New Orleans. He received his Ph.D. from New York University in human sexuality and has published two edited books, ten book chapters, and over thirty articles in professional journals on AIDS, women's sexual aggression, and sexual violence.

Coercion (by Sexually Aggressive Women)

David Archard. *See* Advisory Board, above.

Neera K. Badhwar is associate professor of philosophy at the University of Oklahoma. Her articles on friendship, love, unity of virtue, happiness, and liberalism have appeared in

Ethics, Noûs, American Philosophical Quarterly, Philosophy and Phenomenological Research, and *Social Philosophy and Policy*. She edited *Friendship: A Philosophical Reader* (1993).

Friendship

Alison Bailey is associate professor of philosophy and a member of the Women's Studies Program at Illinois State University. She is the author of *Posterity and Strategic Policy: A Moral Assessment of Nuclear Policy Options* (1989) and coeditor (with Paula Smithka) of *Community, Diversity, and Difference: Implications for Peace* (2002). Her research on race privilege and resistance has appeared in *Hypatia* and the *Journal of Social Philosophy*.

Firestone, Shulamith

Robert Baker is professor of philosophy at Union College, director of the Center for Bioethics of the Graduate College of Union University, and a continuing visiting fellow at the University of Pennsylvania's Center for Bioethics.

Ethics, Professional Codes of

David L. Balch, who teaches at Brite Divinity School in Fort Worth, Texas, earned a B.A. from Abilene Christian University, a Master of Divinity from Union Theological Seminary in New York, and a Ph.D. in New Testament from Yale University, where he studied with Abraham Malherbe. He has had two Fulbrights to Tübingen, the first with Ernst Käsemann, and has been ordained by the Evangelical Lutheran Church in America.

Paul (Saint)

Elizabeth Brake, B.A. (Oxford), M. Litt. and Ph.D. (St Andrews), is assistant professor of philosophy at the University of Calgary. She has published articles on Immanuel Kant's and G.W.F. Hegel's accounts of marriage, Henry James, and Catharine MacKinnon. Her research interests also include feminist ethics, philosophy and literature, and paternity.

Hegel, G.W.F.; Kant, Immanuel

Marla Brettschneider is associate professor of political philosophy and feminist theory in Women's Studies and Political Science at the University of New Hampshire (UNH), where she also coordinates UNH's Queer Studies program.

Judaism, Twentieth- and Twenty-First-Century

Keith Burgess-Jackson, J.D., Ph.D., is associate professor of philosophy at the University of Texas, Arlington. He wrote his Ph.D. dissertation on constitutional interpretation under Joel Feinberg at the University of Arizona. He is coauthor (with Irving M. Copi [1917–2002]) of *Informal Logic* (2nd ed., 1992; 3rd ed., 1996), author of *Rape: A Philosophical Investigation* (1996), and editor of *A Most Detestable Crime: New Philosophical Essays on Rape* (1999).

Anscombe, G.E.M.

Cheshire Calhoun is Charles A. Dana Professor of Philosophy at Colby College (Maine). She is the author of *Feminism, the Family, and the Politics of the Closet: Lesbian and Gay Displacement* (2000). She has served on the American Philosophical Association's Committee on the Status of Gay, Lesbian, Bisexual, and Transgendered Persons in the Profession and was an expert witness in *Halpern et al. v. the Attorney General of Canada et al.*, the case that resulted in same-sex couples acquiring the legal right to marry in Ontario.

Marriage, Same-Sex

David Carr is professor of philosophy of education in the University of Edinburgh School of Education. He is author of *Educating the Virtues* (1991), *Professionalism and Ethics in Teaching* (2000), and *Making Sense of Education* (2003). He has edited *Education, Knowledge, and Truth* (1998) and coedited (with Jan Steutel) *Virtue Ethics and Moral Education* (1999) and (with John Haldane) *Spirituality, Philosophy, and Education* (2003).

Abstinence

Eric M. Cave is associate professor of philosophy at Arkansas State University in Jonesboro. He has published a book on rationality and the sense of justice, *Preferring Justice* (1998), as well as articles on rationality, justice, pluralism, marriage, and cohabitation.

Seduction

Elizabeth A. Clark is John Carlisle Kilgo Professor of Religion at Duke University and has authored or edited twelve books on early Christianity and the study of religion, including *Ascetic Piety and Women's Faith* (1986), *St. Augustine on Marriage and Sexuality* (1996), and *History, Theory, Text: Historians and the Linguistic Turn* (2004). She is a fellow of the American Academy of Arts and Sciences and founding editor of the *Journal of Early Christian Studies*, as well as past president of the American Academy of Religion, the American Society of Church History, and the North American Patristics Society.

Augustine (Saint)

Louise Collins is associate professor and chair of the Philosophy Department at Indiana University, South Bend. Her areas of interest are feminist theory, ethics, and social philosophy, and she has published on gossip, human cloning, cybersex, and teaching philosophy.

Cybersex

Martha Cornog. *See* Advisory Board, above.

John Corvino. *See* Advisory Board, above.

I. L. Coulter has studied at the Universities of Nevada, Alaska, and Houston. She read Mary Jane Sherfey's book in 1973, and it was, for her, a "eureka" moment. In her worldview (Coulter is now a great-grandmother), it is vital to create a cultural milieu in which the ancient riddle of the nature and evolution of the human female will be unraveled. Now living in northern Arizona, she does volunteer work in her local community.

Sherfey, Mary Jane

Charles M. Culver, M.D., Ph.D., is professor of medical education and associate director of the Physician Assistant Program at Barry University in Miami Shores, Florida. A fellow of the Hastings Center, he has authored articles and books in bioethics, including, with Bernard Gert, *Philosophy in Medicine: Conceptual and Ethical Issues in Medicine and Psychiatry* (1982) and *Bioethics: A Systematic Approach* (2005).

Paraphilia

Joseph A. Diorio. *See* Advisory Board, above.

Francis Dunlop has taught at a variety of educational institutions, both in England and abroad, including the University of East Anglia, where he is now honorary lecturer. His books include *The Education of Feeling and Emotion* (1984), *Scheler* (1991), and *The Life and Thought of Aurel Kolnai* (2002).

Kolnai, Aurel

Marvin M. Ellison completed doctoral studies at Union Theological Seminary in New York and teaches Christian social ethics at Bangor Theological Seminary. An ordained minister in the Presbyterian Church (U.S.A.), he was principal author of that denomination's study "Keeping Body and Soul Together: Sexuality, Spirituality, and Social Justice," reprinted as *Presbyterians and Human Sexuality* (1991). His other publications include *Body and Soul: Rethinking Sexuality as Justice-Love* (2003) and *Same-Sex Marriage? A Christian Ethical Analysis* (2004).

Protestantism, Twentieth- and Twenty-First-Century

Daniel M. Farrell is professor of philosophy at Ohio State University. His interests include ethical theory, applied ethics, aesthetics, social and political philosophy, the philosophy of law, the history of philosophy, and moral psychology. He has published in all these areas.

Jealousy

Leslie P. Francis, Ph.D. (philosophy, Michigan, 1974), J.D. (Utah, 1981), is Alfred C. Emery Professor of Law at the University of Utah and professor and chair of the Philosophy Department. She has written *Land Wars: The Politics of Property and Community* (with John G. Francis; 2003) and *Sexual Harassment as an Ethical Issue in Academic Life* (2001). She has edited, with Anita Silvers, *Americans with Disabilities: Implications of the Law for Individuals and Institutions* (2000).

Rape, Acquaintance and Date

Cynthia Freeland is chair and professor of philosophy at the University of Houston. She writes on issues in aesthetics, ancient philosophy, and feminist philosophy. Her books include *But Is It Art?* (2001) and *The Naked and the Undead: Evil and the Appeal of Horror* (2000). She has edited *Feminist Interpretations of Aristotle* (1998) and, with Thomas Wartenberg, *Philosophy and Film* (1995).

Beauty

Bernard Gert is Stone Professor of Intellectual and Moral Philosophy, Dartmouth College, and adjunct professor of psychiatry, Dartmouth Medical School. He has received Fulbright Awards (Israel, 1985–1986; Argentina, Fall 1995) and a National Humanities Center Fellowship (2001–2002). He is the author of *Common Morality: Deciding What to Do* (2004), *Morality: Its Nature and Justification* (2005), and, with Charles M. Culver, *Philosophy in Medicine* (1982) and *Bioethics: A Systematic Approach* (2005).

Paraphilia

James Giles was born in Vancouver and educated at the University of British Columbia and the University of Edinburgh. He is associate professor of philosophy at the University of Guam. Among his writings are *The Nature of Sexual Desire* (2004) and *No Self to Be Found: The Search for Personal Identity* (1997).

Hinduism; Indian Erotology

Carol Steinberg Gould is professor of philosophy at Florida Atlantic University. After receiving her Ph.D. from the State University of New York at Buffalo, she taught at Colgate University and Union College. She has published widely in Greek philosophy, especially Plato, philosophy of/in literature, and contemporary aesthetics.

Plato

Anthony J. Graybosch received a B.A. in philosophy from Fordham University and a Ph.D. from the City University of New York Graduate Center. At California State University, Chico, he teaches American philosophy and moral issues in parenting. He has one spouse, three sons, and two dogs.

Marriage

Lori Gruen is associate professor of philosophy and in the Program in Feminist, Gender, and Sexuality Studies at Wesleyan University. She is coeditor (with George Panichas) of *Sex, Morality, and the Law* (1997) and has published in practical ethics.

Law, Sex and the; Pornography

Christine E. Gudorf. *See* Advisory Board, above.

Mane Hajdin has taught at universities in Canada, Papua New Guinea, New Zealand, and the United States. His research is in the analytic tradition and covers topics in metaethics, applied ethics, philosophy of law, and social and political philosophy. He has written *The Boundaries of Moral Discourse* (1994), *Sexual Harassment: A Debate* (1997, with Linda LeMoncheck), and *The Law of Sexual Harassment: A Critique* (2004) and has edited *The Notion of Equality* (2001).

Harassment, Sexual; Privacy

Kim Q. Hall is associate professor of philosophy and a member of the Women's Studies faculty at Appalachian State University (North Carolina). She is the editor of the *NWSA Journal* special issue on feminist disability studies (2002) and coeditor, with Chris Cuomo, of *Whiteness: Feminist Philosophical Reflections* (1999).

Feminism, Lesbian; Queer Theory

Raja Halwani received his B.A. in economics from the American University of Beirut and his Ph.D. in philosophy from Syracuse University. He is associate professor of philosophy in the Department of Liberal Arts at the School of the Art Institute of Chicago. The author of *Virtuous Liaisons: Care, Love, Sex, and Virtue Ethics* (2003), he specializes in ethics, aesthetics, political philosophy, philosophy of sex and love, and gay studies.

Casual Sex; Ethics, Virtue

Sara Heinämaa is senior lecturer in theoretical philosophy at the University of Helsinki. She is also professor II in humanist women's studies at the University of Oslo. She has published several books on phenomenology and existentialism, including *Toward a Phenomenology of Sexual Difference: Husserl, Merleau-Ponty, Beauvoir* (2003).

Phenomenology

Jeffrey Hershfield is associate professor of philosophy at Wichita State University. His research interests are in the philosophy of mind, philosophy of language, and philosophy of sex. In the philosophy of sex, he has written on social constructionism and acquaintance rape.

Animal Sexuality; Military, Sex and the

Darryl B. Hill received his Ph.D. from the University of Windsor in 1997 and is assistant professor of psychology at the College of Staten Island, City University of New York. He is the editor, with Michael Kral, of *About Psychology: Essays at the Crossroads of History, Theory, and Philosophy* (2003).

Psychology, Twentieth- and Twenty-First-Century

Sarah Hoffman. *See* Advisory Board, above.

Richard T. Hull. *See* Advisory Board, above.

Manyul Im has a B.A. in philosophy from the University of California, Berkeley, and a Ph.D. in philosophy from the University of Michigan, Ann Arbor. He is assistant professor of philosophy at California State University, Los Angeles. His research specialization is ancient Chinese philosophy, focused around the early Confucian figure Mencius (Mengzi).

Chinese Philosophy

Janice M. Irvine is professor of sociology at the University of Massachusetts and the author of *Talk about Sex: The Battles over Sex Education in the United States* (2002) and *Disorders of Desire: Sex and Gender in Modern American Sexology* (1990).

Sexology

Rockney Jacobsen is associate professor of philosophy at Wilfrid Laurier University in Waterloo, Ontario. He does research on the philosophy of mind and language, Wittgenstein, and metaethics. His photographs of life among the contemporary Ju/hoansi peoples in the Kalahari have been published in anthropology journals and textbooks.

Desire, Sexual

Edward Johnson. *See* Advisory Board, above.

Troy Jollimore is assistant professor of philosophy at California State University, Chico. He earned his B.A. from the University of Kings College and Dalhousie University in Halifax, Nova Scotia, Canada, and his Ph.D. from Princeton University. He is the author of *Friendship and Agent-Relative Morality* (2001).

Love

Patricia Beattie Jung is associate professor of theology, Loyola University, Chicago. With her husband of thirty years, L. Shannon Jung, she raised three sons. Together they edited the seventh edition of *Moral Issues and Christian Responses* (2003). She also edited *Good Sex: Feminist Perspectives from the World's Religions* (2001), with Mary Hunt and Radhika Balakrishnan, and *Abortion and Catholicism: The American Debate* (1988), with Thomas Shannon. In 1993, she wrote *Heterosexism: An Ethical Challenge* with the late Ralph Smith.

Heterosexism

Aline Kalbian, Ph.D. (University of Virginia, 1996), is assistant professor in the Religion Department, Florida State University. She has published articles on Catholic moral theology, sexual ethics, reproductive technology, and prenatal genetic testing and is the author of *Sexing the Church: Gender, Power, and Contemporary Catholic Ethics* (2005).

Wojtyła, Karol (Pope John Paul II)

Richard Kamber is professor of philosophy at the College of New Jersey. He holds a B.A. from Johns Hopkins University and a Ph.D. from Claremont Graduate University. He has written books and articles on existentialism, aesthetics, metaphilosophy, film, higher education, and the Holocaust. He thanks Teresa Rivas for her able assistance in collecting research materials for his entry.

Existentialism

James F. Keenan, S.J., is professor of moral theology at Weston Jesuit School of Theology. He writes on the history of Christian ethics and moral virtue. In the area of sexuality, he has worked as a group leader of the Surgeon General's Task Force on Responsible Sexual Conduct (2000–2002) and has authored "The Open Debate: Moral Theology and the Lives of Gay and Lesbian Persons" (*Theological Studies* 64:1 [2003], 127–50).

Catholicism, History of

Stephen Kershnar, an attorney and associate professor of philosophy at the State University of New York College at Fredonia, has published articles on adult-child sex and violent pornography and is the author of *Desert, Retribution, and Torture* (2001) and *Justice for the Past* (2004).

Fantasy

John Kleinig. *See* Advisory Board, above.

Andrew Koppelman is professor of law and political science at Northwestern University. He is the author of *Antidiscrimination Law and Social Equality* (1996) and *The Gay Rights Question in Contemporary American Law* (2002).

Natural Law (New)

Mathew Kuefler is associate professor of history at San Diego State University and the editor of the *Journal of the History of Sexuality*. He received his Ph.D. from Yale (1995), where he studied with John Boswell. The author of *The Manly Eunuch: Masculinity, Gender Ambiguity, and Christian Ideology in Late Antiquity* (2001) and "Male Friendship and the Suspicion of Sodomy in Twelfth-Century France" (in *Difference and Genders in the Middle Ages*, C. Pasternack and S. Farmer, eds., 2003), he has edited an anthology on the impact of Boswell's *Christianity, Social Tolerance, and Homosexuality*, titled *The Boswell Thesis* (2005).

Boswell, John

Stephen E. Lahey is lecturer in classics and religious studies at the University of Nebraska. He received his Ph.D. from the University of Connecticut in 1997; his dissertation was published as *Philosophy and Politics in the Thought of John Wyclif* (2003). An ordained Episcopal minister, he is interested in applying premodern theological approaches to the needs of contemporary society.

Thomas Aquinas (Saint)

Erik W. Larson is associate professor of religious studies at Florida International University. He is a member of the team of scholars editing the Dead Sea Scrolls and has contributed to several volumes of the series *Discoveries in the Judaean Desert*.

Gnosticism; Manichaeism

David Peter Lawrence earned his Ph.D. in the history of religions from the University of Chicago Divinity School in 1992. He has taught at the Hong Kong University of Science and Technology, Concordia University, Montreal, and the University of Manitoba. He now teaches at the University of North Dakota. His publications include *Rediscovering God with Transcendental Argument: A Contemporary Interpretation of Monistic Kashmiri Śaiva Philosophy* (1999).

Tantrism

Wendy Lynne Lee is professor of philosophy at Bloomsburg University of Pennsylvania and is the author of *On Marx* (2002). Her articles have appeared in *Hypatia, Feminist Studies, Journal of Mind and Behavior, Ethics and the Environment*, and the anthologies *The Grammar of Politics* (C. Heyes, ed., 2003) and *Feminist Interpretations of Wittgenstein* (N. Scheman and P. O'Connor, eds., 2002).

Marxism; Wittgenstein, Ludwig

Juhana Lemetti is a research student in the National Graduate School of Philosophy and lectures at Helsinki Open University and the University of Helsinki (Department of Moral and Social Philosophy). His research areas are political philosophy, early modern philosophy, Leopold von Sacher-Masoch, and Thomas Hobbes. His philosophical hobbies include Icelandic saga literature and the philosophy of sea monkeys.

Sacher-Masoch, Leopold von

Berel Dov Lerner was born in Washington, D.C., and is a member of Kibbutz Sheluhot in Israel's Beit Shean Valley, where he resides with his wife Batsheva and their five children. He studied philosophy and the social sciences at Johns Hopkins University and the University of Chicago, and Judaism at Yeshivat Ha-Kibbutz Ha-Dati in Israel. He received his Ph.D. in philosophy from Tel Aviv University and teaches at the Western Galilee Academic College. He is the author of *Rules, Magic, and Instrumental Reason: A Critical Interpretation of Peter Winch's Philosophy of the Social Sciences* (2002).

Judaism, History of

Michael P. Levine is professor of philosophy at the University of Western Australia. He edited *The Analytic Freud: Philosophy and Psychoanalysis* (2000) and, with Kristine Miller and William Taylor, the "Ethics and Architecture" issue of *Philosophical Forum* (35:2 [2004]). He has written articles on moral psychology, metaphysics, film, and Buffy (the vampire slayer).

Arts, Sex and the

Margaret Olivia Little is associate professor of philosophy and senior research scholar in the Kennedy Institute of Ethics at Georgetown University. Her research interests cluster around issues in ethics, from its metaphysics and epistemology to its applied side.

Abortion

Mike W. Martin is professor of philosophy at Chapman University (California). His degrees are from the University of Utah (B.S., M.A.) and the University of California, Irvine (Ph.D., 1977). His books include *Virtuous Giving: Philanthropy, Voluntary Service, and Caring* (1994), *Love's Virtues* (1996), *Meaningful Work: Rethinking Professional Ethics* (2000), and *Everyday Morality: An Introduction to Applied Ethics* (1989, 1995, 2001).

Adultery

Vincent A. McCarthy, M.A., Ph.D. (Stanford University), is professor of philosophy at Saint Joseph's University (Philadelphia) and a fellow of the Alexander von Humboldt Foundation (Bonn) and the American Council of Learned Societies. The author of *The Phenomenology of Moods in Kierkegaard* (1978) and *Quest for a Philosophical Jesus: Philosophy and Religion in Rousseau, Kant, Hegel, and Schelling* (1986), he has also published articles in *Kant-Studien, Kierkegaardiana*, and *International Kierkegaard Commentary*.

Kierkegaard, Søren

Laurence B. McCullough, Ph.D., is professor of medicine and medical ethics in the Center for Medical Ethics and Health Policy at the Baylor College of Medicine. He is also adjunct professor of ethics in obstetrics and gynecology and of public health at Weill Medical College of Cornell University and adjunct professor of philosophy at Rice University. With Frank A. Chervenak, he coauthored *Ethics in Obstetrics and Gynecology* (1994).

Contraception; Intersexuality

Jørgen Mejer has been professor of classics at the University of Copenhagen since 1974. In 2001–2003 he was director of the Danish Institute at Athens. He has written four books on Greek philosophy and Greek and Roman literature and has translated the Presocratics, Greek drama, Plato, and Cicero into Danish.

Greek Sexuality and Philosophy, Ancient; Roman Sexuality and Philosophy, Ancient

Timothy F. Murphy. *See* Advisory Board, above.

JoAnne Myers, Ph.D. (Rensselaer Polytechnic Institute), is codirector of Women's Studies and teaches political science at Marist College, Poughkeepsie, New York. She authored *The Historical Dictionary of the Lesbian Liberation Movement: Still the Rage* (2003) and articles on feminism, citizenship, and environmental policies.

Feminism, History of

James Lindemann Nelson. *See* Advisory Board, above.

Nkiru Nzegwu is associate professor in the Department of Africana Studies and the graduate program in Philosophy, Interpretation, and Culture at Binghamton University. The author of *Family Matters: Feminist Concepts in African Philosophy of Culture* (2005), she has published on African women and culture and on African and African diaspora arts.

African Philosophy

S. Jack Odell received his M.A. and Ph.D. (1967) from the University of Illinois (Urbana) and has been professor of philosophy at the University of Maryland since 1966. He is the author of *On Russell* (2000), *On Moore* (2001), *On Consequentialist Ethics* (2003), and *On the Philosophy of Language* (2004). With Charles Bontempo, he edited *The Owl of Minerva: Philosophers on Philosophy* (1975).

Consequentialism; Russell, Bertrand

Len O'Neill holds doctorates from Melbourne and Cambridge. He is senior research fellow in the Philosophy Department at the University of Melbourne. He has published in the areas of causation, probability, and induction and has focused on Buddhism since 1993.

Buddhism

Ed Pluth is assistant professor of philosophy at California State University, Chico. He specializes in psychoanalytic theory and contemporary continental philosophy and has published essays on Lacanian theory and Alain Badiou.

Freud, Sigmund; Lacan, Jacques

Nicholas P. Power is associate professor of philosophy at the University of West Florida. He received the Ph.D. at Temple University in 1996. He publishes in the areas of epistemology, philosophy of mind, and the philosophy of education.

Freudian Left, The; Psychology, Evolutionary

Igor Primoratz. *See* Advisory Board, above.

Carol V. Quinn, formerly assistant professor of philosophy, University of North Carolina at Charlotte, was also faculty associate for the University's Center for Professional and Applied Ethics. Her areas of interest include the philosophy of trauma, philosophical autobiography, medical ethics, feminism, queer philosophy, and philosophy of sex.

Addiction, Sexual; Diseases, Sexually Transmitted; Objectification, Sexual; Sadomasochism

Lee C. Rice is associate professor of philosophy at Marquette University. He was a Fulbright scholar at the University of Paris and completed his doctoral work as a Woodrow Wilson and Kent Fellow at St. Louis University. He is the author of over 100 articles on Baruch Spinoza and is one of the editors of the Samuel Shirley translations of Spinoza. He has also published articles on gay studies, psychometrics, and software design.

Spinoza, Baruch

Lance Byron Richey is associate professor of religious studies at Cardinal Stritch University in Milwaukee. He earned a Ph.D. in philosophy from Marquette University in 1995, with an emphasis in nineteenth-century German philosophy, and a Ph.D. in theology from Marquette in 2004, with an emphasis on the New Testament. His publications include an annotated edition of Anton Pannekoek's *Lenin as Philosopher*.

Fichte, Johann Gottlieb; Schopenhauer, Arthur

Stephen David Ross is professor of philosophy and comparative literature at Binghamton University (State University of New York), where he directs the program in Philosophy, Interpretation, and Culture. He is the author of *The Gift of Beauty: The Good as Art* (1996), *The Gift of Truth: Gathering the Good* (1997), *The Gift of Touch: Embodying the Good* (1998), *The Gift of Kinds: The Good in Abundance* (1999), and *The Gift of Property: Having the Good* (2001).

Feminism, French; Levinas, Emmanuel; Poststructuralism

Elisa Ruhl is the George F. Hourani Fellow in Ethics at the University at Buffalo (State University of New York). She is interested in the intersection of action theory and moral philosophy—the social and personal motivations that prompt reasoning, emotional response, and action. She has written articles on fetal homicide and pragmatic bioethics.

Islam

Michael Ruse was born in Birmingham, England, in 1940. From 1965 to 2000, he taught at the University of Guelph in Ontario, Canada. He moved to Florida State University in Tallahassee, where he is the Lucyle T. Werkmeister Professor of Philosophy. The author of books on the history and philosophy of biology, especially Darwinian evolution, Ruse has spent much time fighting Creationism. A former Guggenheim fellow, Ruse is a fellow of the Royal Society of Canada.

Evolution

Ruth Sample, Ph.D. (University of Pittsburgh, 1995), is associate professor of philosophy at the University of New Hampshire. The author of *Exploitation: What It Is and Why It's*

Wrong (2003) and editor, with Charles Mills and James Sterba, of *Philosophy: The Big Questions* (2004), she has written articles on John Locke, libertarianism, social contract theory, feminism, prostitution, and welfare rights.

Feminism, Liberal

Jana Sawicki is W. Van Alan Clark '41 Third Century Professor at Williams College, where she teaches philosophy and women's and gender studies. She is the author of *Disciplining Foucault: Feminism, Power, and the Body* (1991) and other pieces on Michel Foucault and feminist theory.

Foucault, Michel

Frank Schalow is associate professor of philosophy at the University of New Orleans. He has written *Heidegger and the Quest for the Sacred* (2001), *Language and Deed: Rediscovering Politics through Heidegger's Encounter with German Idealism* (1998), *The Renewal of the Heidegger-Kant Dialogue* (1992), *Imagination and Existence: Heidegger's Retrieval of the Kantian Ethic* (1986), and, with Patrick Bourgeois, *Traces of Understanding: A Profile of Heidegger's and Ricoeur's Hermeneutics* (1990).

Heidegger, Martin

Joel Schwartz is an adjunct senior fellow at the Hudson Institute in Washington, D.C. He has taught political philosophy and public policy at the University of Michigan, the University of Toronto, and the University of Virginia. He is the author of *The Sexual Politics of Jean-Jacques Rousseau* (1984).

Rousseau, Jean-Jacques

Juha Sihvola is director of the Helsinki Collegium for Advanced Studies (Finland), professor of history at the University of Jyväskylä, and vice-director of the Academy of Finland Centre of Excellence "History of Mind" <www.helsinki.fi/teol/steol/mind>. He has published articles on ancient philosophy and has edited *The Emotions in Hellenistic Philosophy* (with Troels Engberg-Pedersen, 1998), *Ancient Scepticism and the Sceptical Tradition* (2000), and *The Sleep of Reason* (with Martha Nussbaum, 2002).

Aristotle

Kim Skoog is professor of Asian and comparative philosophy at the University of Guam. He was the guest editor of a special issue of *Philosophy East and West* on Jainism (50:3 [2000]) and has contributed chapters to *Ahiṃsā, Anekānta, and Jainism* (T. Sethia, ed., 2004) and to *Jainism and Early Buddhism* (O. Qvarnström, ed., 2003).

Jainism

Alan Soble. *See* Volume Editor, above.

Ben Spiecker is professor of philosophy and history of education at Vrije University, Amsterdam. His publications in English include "Sex between Persons with 'Mental Retardation': An Ethical Evaluation" (*Journal of Moral Education* 31:2 [2002], 155–69) and "Is a

Traumatic Childhood Just Another Abuse Excuse?" (*Educational Philosophy and Theory* 35:4 [2003], 441–50), both coauthored with Jan Steutel.

Disability; Incest

J. Martin Stafford. *See* Advisory Board, above.

Jan Steutel is reader in philosophy of education at Vrije University, Amsterdam. With David Carr, he edited *Virtue Ethics and Moral Education* (1999), and with Ben Spiecker he wrote "Sex Education, State Policy, and the Principle of Mutual Consent" (*Sex Education* 4:1 [2004], 49–62).

Disability; Incest

Robert M. Stewart. *See* Advisory Board, above.

Mark Storey studied philosophy at the University of California, Santa Barbara (B.A.) and the University of Washington (M.A., 1988). He teaches logic, aesthetics, and Eastern philosophy at Bellevue Community College (Washington). He is the author of *Cinema Au Naturel: A History of Nudist Film* (2003) and is on the editorial staff of *Nude & Natural* magazine.

Nudism

James S. Stramel, Ph.D. (University of Southern California), has taught at Santa Monica College since 1992, specializing in ethics, applied ethics, gay and lesbian studies, the philosophy of sex, and epistemology.

Philosophy of Sex, Teaching the

Robert A. Strikwerda, Ph.D. (University of Notre Dame), is associate professor of philosophy and director of the Honors Program at Indiana University, Kokomo. With Larry May and Patrick D. Hopkins, he edited *Rethinking Masculinity: Philosophical Explorations in Light of Feminism* (2nd ed., 1996), which contains pieces, written with May, on male friendship and fatherhood.

Feminism, Men's; Mead, Margaret

Cindy Struckman-Johnson, Ph.D., is professor of psychology at the University of South Dakota, Vermillion. She and her spouse David have collaborated on research for over twenty years. Her primary research area is the sexual coercion of men and women. She has received a congressional appointment to serve on a national commission for legislation intended to eliminate prison rape.

Coercion (by Sexually Aggressive Women)

Garrett Thomson, D.Phil. (Oxford), is the author of *Needs* (1987), *Bacon to Kant* (2001), *On Leibniz* (2001), *On Locke* (2000), *On Kant* (1999), and *On the Meaning of Life* (2002). He is Compton Chair of Philosophy at the College of Wooster.

Leibniz, Gottfried

Edward Collins Vacek. *See* Advisory Board, above.

Kayley Vernallis, Ph.D. (University of California, Berkeley), is professor of philosophy at California State University, Los Angeles. She works in ethics and aesthetics and has been studying gender in seventeenth-century still-life painting and sexuality/gender in contemporary queer portraiture.

Bisexuality

Alan Wertheimer. *See* Advisory Board, above.

Hugh Wilder teaches philosophy at the College of Charleston (South Carolina). He received his Ph.D. from the University of Western Ontario. His essays have appeared in *Metaphilosophy*, *Canadian Journal of Philosophy*, *Australasian Journal of Philosophy*, *Philosophical Studies*, *Social Epistemology*, and *Philosophy and Literature*. With Judith de Luce, he edited *Language in Primates* (1983).

Communication Model

Kathleen J. Wininger, Ph.D. (Temple University), is associate professor of philosophy at the University of Southern Maine. She has written *Friedrich Nietzsche's Reclamation of Philosophy* (1997) and has edited, with Robert Baker and Frederick Elliston, *Philosophy and Sex* (3rd ed., 1998). She has taught at the University of Nairobi and lectured in other parts of Africa.

Nietzsche, Friedrich

Celia Wolf-Devine is associate professor of philosophy at Stonehill College. She holds a B.A. from Smith College and a Ph.D. from the University of Wisconsin, Madison. She has written *Descartes on Seeing: Epistemology and Visual Perception* (1993) and *Diversity and Community in the Academy: Affirmative Action in Faculty Appointments* (1997) and has edited, with Philip Devine, *Sex and Gender: A Spectrum of Views* (2003). She is also the author of "Abortion and the Feminine Voice" (*Public Affairs Quarterly* 3:3 [1989], 81–97).

Descartes, René

Joel Zimbelman, Ph.D., is professor and chair of the Department of Religious Studies at California State University (CSU), Chico. He is also coordinator for the Program in Humanities and a fellow in CSU/Chico's Center for Applied and Professional Ethics.

Protestantism, History of

NAME INDEX

The entries in this index are the names of persons (real or fictional; deceased or living; divine, human, animal, or a mixture) and places. If a name corresponds to an entry in the encyclopedia, the entry is indicated by **bold** numerals. Names in "References" and "Additional Readings" are not indexed. Alphabetization is by word. Cross-references (*See* and *See also*) are to both this index and to the Subject Index (pp. 1149–1176). Pages 1–620 are in volume 1; 621–1089 are in volume 2.

Ellison, Marvin M.: on progressive Protestantism, 872, 874. *See also* Protestantism, twentieth- and twenty-first-century

Elliston, Frederick A., 794, 795; on Johann Gottlieb Fichte, 349, 351; on marriage as union in Immanuel Kant, 646; on Martin Heidegger, 437; on promiscuity, 137, 437

Elshtain, Jean Bethke: problems in liberal feminism, 338

Emerson, Ralph Waldo, 259, 646

Empedocles: Love a driving force, 414

Engels, Friedrich, 383; prostitution, 832, 852; prostitution, marriage as, 274, 342; women's sexuality, commodification of, 661–62, 667; as Young Hegelian, 432. Works: *The Origin of the Family, Private Property, and the State*, 661, 667. *See also* Marx, Karl; Marxism

Epictetus (*Enchiridion*), 936; on marriage as distraction, 751; people disturbed only by their view of things, 259

Epicurus: abstinence ideal, 748; egoistic hedonist, 195; harmfulness of sexual activity, 414. *See also* Epicureans

Epiphanius of Salamis: on Gnosticism, 403, 409

Epstein, Louis M., 534; masturbation as seed-wasting in Judaism, 672

Epstein, Robert: on Albert Ellis, 259

Ericsson, Lars O.: defends prostitution, 853, 855

Ertman, Martha M.: androcentrism of Richard Posner, 826

Eskridge, William N.: defense of same-sex marriage, 652–54 passim; variety in forms of marriage, 651, 654

Estes, Yolanda: Kantian view of prostitution, 549

Estrich, Susan: acquaintance rape is real rape, 911, 912; resistance requirement in rape law, 912; whether women lie about rape, 916

Euripides, 711; dangers of *eros*, 411

Evans, Edward Payson: sex with a Jew seen as bestiality, 97

Eve, 161, 477, 511, 980; "Eve before Adam" (John Money), 1018; in Gnosticism, 406, 407; in Judaism, 521, 523; Søren Kierkegaard on, 555; in Manichaeism, 637–38; in Protestantism, 862, 863; Thomas Aquinas on, 1046–47; Karol Wojtyła on, 1084. *See also* Adam; Augustine (Saint)

Farrell, Daniel M.: definition of "jealous," 515–16; irrationality of jealousy, 517; jealousy contrasted with envy, 516. *See also* Jealousy

Fausto-Sterling, Anne: critic of John Money, 693; variation in human anatomical sex, 497

Feder, Ellen K., 793; called John Money's "John/Joan" case a "sham," 693; surgery on intersexed infants, 399

Feinberg, Joel, 784, 849; fraud in the factum contrasted with fraud in the inducement (in rape), 189; harm and the harm principle, 586, 719; legal moralism, 199, 586; offensiveness and the offense principle, 98, 199, 600, 718–21 passim; paternalism, 236

Ferenczi, Sándor: Hungarian colleague of Sigmund Freud, 563

Ferguson, Ann, 662

Ferguson, Frances: on Sadeian pornography, 455, 964

Ferree, Marnie: sexual addiction in women, 27

Feuerbach, Ludwig: influence on Karl Marx, 432, 660

Fichte, Johann Gottlieb, **347–53**, 795; adultery of men excused, 351; Aristophanes's myth (Plato's *Symposium*), 351; Aristotelean view of sexual generation, 349, 351; Kantianism of, 347–48, 350; law versus sexual morality, 350; on love, 348, 349, 351; marriage as school of virtue, 349–50; Karl Marx influenced by, 660; non-Kantianism of, 348–49; on prostitution, 350

Finkelhor, David: on pedophilia and incestuous abuse, 489, 490, 760

Finkelstein, Naomi: on disabled lesbian sexuality, 328

Finnis, John, 51, 283, 549; basic goods, 54, 702–4, 772; homosexual acts violate basic goods, 463–64, 704–5; infertile couples, sex permitted for, but not same-sex couples, 100, 160, 445, 656, 707; on masturbation, 676; New Natural Law theorist, 463–64, 655–56, 702–8 passim; (sexual) pleasure not a basic good, 703, 706. *See also* Anscombe, G.E.M., Catholicism, twentieth- and twenty-first-century; Grisez, Germain; Homosexuality, ethics of; Wojtyła, Karol

Firestone, Shulamith, **353–57**; on communal marriage, 644; extrauterine gestation needed for the liberation of women, 355; Freudian penis envy reinterpreted, 354; heterosexual love, corruption of, 354; incest taboo, 354,

Kantian grounds, 548–49; rape violates sexual bodily integrity, 906

Haraway, Donna, 209, 830

Hare, Richard M.: utilitarianism of, 231

Haring, Bernard, 158: stressed law of love for Catholicism, 154

Harlan, John (Justice): on privacy, 840, 841

Harlot, Scarlot. *See* Scarlot Harlot

Harrison, Beverly Wildung: sexuality and Christianity, 868–73 passim

Hart, Gary: adultery with Donna Rice, 35

Hart, H.L.A., 784; morality and the law, 199, 584, 587, 602–3

Hartley, Nina: satisfying life as pornographic performer, 818

Hartman, William, and Marilyn Fithian: benefits of nudism, 720; humanistic sexology, 1004–5

Hartmann, Heidi: patriarchy preceded capitalism, 667

Hartsock, Nancy C. M., 662; feminist standpoint theory, 256

Hartwig, Michael: on Saint Paul and homosexuality, 144

Haslanger, Sally: objectivity and objectification, 338, 549

Haynes, James: guilt from masturbating, 677

Hefling, Charles: Thomas Aquinas and homosexuality, 1051

Hegel, G.W.F., 4, 387, **429–35**, 790, 795, 829, 1022; Aristophanes's myth (Plato's *Symposium*), 351, 430; Georges Bataille influenced by, 84, 85; Simone de Beauvoir on, 433; biology of reproduction, 430; the dialectic, 85, 382, 430, 557, 558, 660, 663; existentialism, precursor of, 292; feminism and, 433; Johann Gottlieb Fichte influenced by, 348; homosexuality as logically incoherent, 433; on incest, 432; intersubjectivity, 174, 180, 385, 430, 663; Immanuel Kant's contractual marriage as "disgraceful," 432, 546; Søren Kierkegaard influenced by, 432; Søren Kierkegaard's spoof of the dialectic, 557, 558; love and/as union, 220, 431, 609–10; love, erotic, and self-fulfillment, 431, 976; Herbert Marcuse influenced by, 385; on marriage, 430–32 passim; Karl Marx influenced by, 660; Karl Marx, philosophy rejected by, 432, 660, 663; master-slave parable, 430, 433; Thomas Nagel influenced by, 180; Owl of Minerva, 430; Leopold von Sacher-Masoch influenced

by, 952; Jean-Paul Sartre influenced by, 174, 433; Friedrich von Schlegel (*Lucinde*), critique of, 431; Roger Scruton influenced by, 433, 976, 977; the state, 432, 977; Young Hegelians and, 432, 660

Heidegger, Martin, 313, **435–39**, 831; care (*Sorge*) and sexuality, 436, 437; concealing/revealing in erotic play, 436–37; *Dasein* as "asexual" (Jean-Paul Sartre), 297, 435; *Dasein* as gender-neutral, 435–36; Jacques Derrida on, 836; Albert Ellis influenced by, 259; as existentialist, 292, 435; existentialist label denied, 293; feminism and, 437; Heideggerian promiscuity, Frederick Elliston on, 437; Edmund Husserl and phenomenology, 435, 777, 778; Luce Irigaray on, 832; Søren Kierkegaard and anxiety, 436; Emmanuel Levinas influenced by, 593, 594; Herbert Marcuse influenced by, 385, 436; Nazi party, member of, 293; poststructuralism, influence on, 831; promiscuity and sexual experimentation, 436, 437; science of sexuality, critique of, 436, 830; "thrownness" of sexuality, 436, 831

Heim, Michael: computer technology and *eros*, 209

Heinämaa, Sara: Simone de Beauvoir's philosophy rooted in Edmund Husserl, 780. *See also* Phenomenology

Held, Virginia: fathers can mother, 335

Helen, 87, 221, 406, 411; abducted and sodomized by Theseus, 7. *See also* Lucretia

Helena: Gnostic mother, 406

Hellegers, André: founded Kennedy Institute of Ethics, 204

Helminiak, Daniel: on the crime of Sodom, 465

Helms, Jesse: blocked funding for sex research, 1005; opposition to artists of sexuality, 70

Hera: dispute with Zeus about sexuality of men and women, 413; seduces Zeus, 411

Heraclitus, 259

Herbert, Maria von: relationship with Immanuel Kant, 548

Herdt, Gilbert, **439–42**; dangers of coitus and vagina to men, 41, 439; fellatio insemination, 439; fellatio insemination not sexual, 225, 998; fellatio insemination as nutritive, 225; fellatio insemination required for boys to achieve manhood, 399, 439; orientation, sexual, implications of fellatio insemination for genesis and concept, 439–40, 471; Robert Stoller, collaboration with (*Intimate*

O'Carroll, Tom: on pedophilia, 757, 759

Odell, S. Jack: egoism not a moral theory, 195; hedonistic contrasted with nonhedonistic consequentialism, 199; G. E. Moore's utilitarianism, 195; practice consequentialism, 196, 200; Bertrand Russell's utilitarianism, 195, 946. *See also* Consequentialism; Russell, Bertrand

Oedipus (Sophocles, *Oedipus rex*): sexually desired his mother (opaquely), 227, 375

Okin, Susan Moller: on the feminism of John Stuart Mill, 342; sexual equality in marriage required, 335–36; traditional family unjust, 335–36

Olsen, Regine. *See* Kierkegaard, Søren

Onan (Genesis 38:8–10), 110; committed *coitus interruptus* (Saint Augustine, Pius XI), 76

O'Neill, Eileen: agency in lesbian sadomasochism, 962

O'Neill, Len. *See* Buddhism

O'Neill, Onora: Kantian ethics, 543, 544, 548

Ono, Yoko, 343

Origen: on Gnosticism, 405, 406

Orpheus: represents polymorphous perversity, 386

Orr, Deborah: Ludwig Wittgenstein's "weft," 1078

Ortega y Gasset, José, 1022; as existentialist, 293

Orwell, George: sex and love in *1984*, 1059

Osborne, Catherine: on Plato's *eros*, 608

Othello: sexual jealousy, 516, 519

Outka, Gene: on Christian love and Søren Kierkegaard, 557

Overall, Christine: compulsory heterosexuality, 326, 904; on prostitution, 854

Ovid, 936, 1022; art of seduction, 934; on flirting, 358

Padgug, Robert: ancient Greek and modern sexual categories different, 121; invention of homosexuality, 1028–29

Paglia, Camille, 576, **735–40**; casual sex, benefits of, 1000; beauty (of women) as a drug or trick, 87, 91, 736; bodies (reproductive) of women gross, disgusting, 91, 736; erotic dancing, "stripping," as art form, 736, 999; "orthodox" feminism on date rape and harassment criticized by, 737–78; Millian (liberal) feminism in, 736, 737, 999; Friedrich Nietzsche and, 91, 735; nudist colony not erotic, 718, 736; penis worship in,

70; Marquis de Sade and, 735, 737, 954; sadomasochism as sacred cult, 735, 964; Arthur Schopenhauer and, 91, 92, 735, 736; on sex work, 738, 999; sexuality as consumption, 16. Works: *Sex, Art, and American Culture*, 576, 735–38 passim, 964, 1000; *Sexual Personae: Art and Decadence from Nefertiti to Emily Dickinson*, 91, 735–38 passim, 999

Pakaluk, Michael, 390

Parent, W. A.: on privacy, 844

Paris (city): Natalie Barney, 316; Georges Bataille, 84; Havelock Ellis, 97; Michel Foucault, 362; Sigmund Freud, 371; Jacques Lacan, 567; Wanda Hulda Meister, 949; Jean-Jacques Rousseau, 940; Marquis de Sade, 953

Paris (Helen's lover), 221, 411

Parsons, Talcott: on incest prohibition, 488

Patai, Daphne: on sexual harassment, 424, 797

Pateman, Carole, 795; "consensual" intercourse as rape, 904; marriage and family in G.W.F. Hegel's political philosophy, 431, 432, 546; rejects prostitution, 336, 853; sex work contrasted with other work, 853, 998

Patterson, Charlotte: on children of homosexual parents, 470

Paul (Saint), 161, 548, 556, **748–54**, 861, 1048, 1075; "against nature" as "inordinate," 752; on homosexual acts, 109, 144, 1051; marital sex as *remedium ad concupiscentiae*, 144, 677, 750; marriage debt, 5, 156, 546, 677, 706, 750, 863, 913; marriage neither best (vs. celibacy) nor necessary (vs. childlessness), 77, 144, 145, 557, 612, 751, 859; marriage and sexuality as interfering with spirituality, 12, 750–51; 642–43, 1057; marry so as not to burn, 11, 612, 750; meaning of *arsenokoitai* in, 109, 465, 749; meaning of *malakoi* in, 109, 749; sin arises through "one man," 80; *soma* ("body") and *sarx* ("flesh") contrasted, 144; subjection of wife to husband (is like subjection of Church to God), 106, 161; veiling (covering) women, 504. Works: 1 Corinthians, 5, 11, 12, 77, 144, 156, 465, 504, 546, 557, 612, 642, 643, 677, 706, 748–52 passim, 859, 913; Ephesians, 161, 196; Romans, 12, 80, 109, 144, 752, 1051. *See also*: Catholicism, history of

Paul VI (Pope), 52, 156, 161, 1045, 1081; controversy over anti-contraception position of *Humanae vitae*, 157, 204, 1082; moral inseparability of procreation and union in

225; Thomas Nagel influenced by, 174–75, 180, 699; poststructuralism and, 830, 831; reciprocal incarnation, 223, 297, 699, 770; on seduction, 360, 981; sexual perversion and, 223, 770; sexuality and love attempt to curtail the freedom of the other, 174, 180, 223, 296–97, 771, 831, 963–64, 981. Works: *Being and Nothingness*, 180, 223, 296–98; 360, 435, 455–56, 571, 699, 770, 831, 963–64, 981. *See also* Beauvoir, Simone de; Existentialism

Saussure, Ferdinand de, 567, 737

Sawicki, Jana. *See* Foucault, Michel

Scalia, Antonin (Justice): legal moralism, 587

Scarlot Harlot: created term "sex work," 997

Schaeffer, Denise: on Catharine MacKinnon, 626, 628

Schalow, Frank. *See* Heidegger, Martin

Schalow, Paul Gordon: Japanese military pederasty, 685

Scheler, Max: phenomenology influenced Aurel Kolnai, 563

Schlafly, Phyllis: men improved by women, 445

Schlegel, Friedrich von: G.W.F. Hegel's critique of *Lucinde*, 431

Schmitt, David: males less sexually discriminating than females, 879

Schmitt, Richard: race and sexuality, 344

Schneider, Joseph W. *See* Conrad, Peter, and Joseph W. Schneider

Schopenhauer, Arthur, 63, 559, 795, **967–73**, 1022; anticipations of Sigmund Freud, 612, 968, 972; evolutionary biology in, 90, 92, 970–71; homosexuality and evolution, 971; on humor, 480; "I have no predecessors," 969; Immanuel Kant's influence on, 968–69; love reduced to sex, 612, 969; masturbation a medical, not ethical, problem, 676–77, 971; Friedrich Nietzsche influenced by, 711, 712, 714, 968, 972; Camille Paglia and, 91, 735; polygamy, advocacy of, 644–45, 971; on romantic love, 612; sexual desire contains illusions, 223, 644, 735, 788–89, 970, 972; Baruch Spinoza and, 969, 970, 1036, 1038; women trap men with beauty, 89, 736

Schott, Robin May: practical contrasted with pathological love in Immanuel Kant, 643

Schroeder, Jeanne L.: on marriage debt, 913; women deformed (says Catharine MacKinnon), 628

Schulhofer, Stephen, 184; consent to sex need not be verbal, 186, 902; "no" means no, 916;

rape contrasted with sexual assault, 912–13, 915; rape statutes and force, 185, 212; rape and violations of autonomy, 911, 913–15 passim; on "utmost resistance," 911–12

Schultz, Debra L., 538; Jewish women and the black civil rights movement, 537

Schulz, Ortrun: Arthur Schopenhauer and Baruch Spinoza, 969, 1036

Schwartz, Joel. *See* Rousseau, Jean-Jacques

Schwartz, Pepper. *See* Blumstein, Philip, and Pepper Schwartz (*American Couples*)

Schwarzenbach, Sibyl: on prostitution as selling a service, 854

Scruton, Roger, 283, 391, 433, 487, 724, 780, 788, 790, 795, 950, **973–80**; bestiality "a paradigm of perversion," 100; on casual sex, 140, 852; childhood sexuality, 757–58; criticism of sexology, 974–75; on David Hume on beauty, 88; death of sexual desire in marriage, 394, 1055; defense of heterosexism, 445, 978; embraces Nagelian completeness, 182; on incest, 488, 490; jealousy shows replace ability, 518; Kantian liberal feminism rejected, 591; on Richard Posner, 825, 827; sexual desire is interpersonal/intentional nature, 225, 770, 852, 975; sexual desire not transferable, 226, 975; on sexual perversion, 756, 770, 976; student of G.E.M. Anscombe, 51; union view of love, 607, 609. Works: *Sexual Desire: A Moral Philosophy of the Erotic*, 100, 140, 226, 394, 488, 518, 591, 607, 756, 758, 770, 780, 974–78 passim, 1055

Sedgwick, Eve Kosofsky: significance of queer theory, 895

Seidler, Victor: men's feminist, 343, 344

Seifert, Ruth: rape and war, 686, 687

Seneca, 259; temperate marital sexuality, 936

Shafer, Carolyn: on the harm of rape, 906

Shaffer, Jerome, 790; defining feature of sexual desire, 226–27; eating contrasted with sexual activity, 41

Shalit, Wendy: on nudism, 718

Shattuck, Roger, 580; value of implicit language, 579

Shaw, George Bernard, 1022

Sherfey, Mary Jane, **1016–22**; connection between reproductive function and sexual pleasure in male and female anatomy, 1017–18; criticism of Sigmund Freud on female sexuality, 1016–17; one-type-of-orgasm model of female sexuality, 1017;

Socrates, 195, 714, 802; criticized by Friedrich Nietzsche as antierotic, 711, 712; death/execution of, 640, 802, 805; instructed about love by Diotima, 222, 556, 672, 807, 1023; loved by Alcibiades, 89, 412, 807; marriage and, 639, 640; robust sexuality of in Plato's portrait, 804–5; teacher of Plato, 87. *See also* Plato

Sodom, 108–9, 149, 197, 235, 465, 522, 953

Solomon, Lewis: benefit of masturbation, 677

Solomon, Robert C., 213, 306, 790, 795, 1014; and Aristotle on pleasure, 175, 224–25; criticism of the pleasure model, 175; on love, 390, 391, 609, 610; love and sex, relationship between, 611; on masturbation, 175, 176, 225–26, 671, 678; on sexual perversion, 176, 213, 770; on Thomas Nagel's view of sexuality, 174–75, 182, 223, 698, 700, 770. *See also* Communication model

Solovyov, Vladimir: union view of love, 609–10

Sontag, Susan: on AIDS, 235; the "eschatology of immanence" of Norman O. Brown, 384

Sophia (wisdom), 405, 638; emanation of Christ in Gnosticism, 404

Soranus: abstinence healthy, 748

Søren Whiteley, C. H., and Winifred N. Whiteley, harm of masturbation, 677

Sparta, 939, 1061; *erastes-eromenos* relationship in, 685; sexuality in, 404, 803

Spears, Britney: as sex object, 671

Spelman, Elizabeth: Shulamith Firestone is too patriarchal, 355; "somatophobia," 355

Spencer, Herbert, **1033–36**; on chastity, 477, 1034; evolution and sexuality, 47, 1034–35; "survival of the fittest," 1035

Sperber, Hans: sexual origin of speech, 574–75, 578

Sperling, Susan: primate studies and human sexuality, 46

Spiecker, Ben: pederast has self-regarding motive, 757; on pedophilia, 755, 760; sexual decisions made by surrogates for the mentally disabled, 233. *See also* Disability; Incest

Spinoza, Baruch, 259, **1036–40**; Aristotelian teleology, rejection of, 970; and Johann Gottlieb Fichte 348; Sigmund Freud influenced by, 1036, 1037; Luce Irigaray on, 313; on jealousy, 516; Emmanuel Levinas influenced by, 594; on love, 1037–38; monistic naturalism opposed to dualism of

René Descartes, 1036–38 passim; queer theory and, 1038; Arthur Schopenhauer and, 969, 970, 1036, 1038

Sprinkle, Annie, 790; benefits and uses of sex, 277, 1013

Stafford, J. Martin: David Hume on love and lust, 477; Roger Scruton on homosexuality, 977–78. *See also* Hume, David; Mandeville, Bernard; Scruton, Roger; Spencer, Herbert; Westermarck, Edward

Stein, Edith: phenomenologist, 777

Stein, Edward: on definition of sexual orientation, 114, 729–30; essentialism–social constructionism debate, 46, 731, 834, 1029, 1030; the "Zomnian" analogy, 1030

Steinbock, Bonnie: on adultery, 33

Steinem, Gloria: on Linda Lovelace (*Deep Throat*), 337; *Ms.* magazine, co-founder of (with Betty Friedan), 335

Steiner, George: critic of pornography, 579–80; sexuality and language compared, 176

Stephen, James Fitzjames: critic of John Stuart Mill on liberty and women, 198, 334, 342; legal moralism, 199, 586, 601

Sternberg, Robert: triangular theory of love, 890

Steutel, Jan: pederast has self-regarding motive, 757; on pedophilia, 755, 760; sexual decisions made by surrogates for the mentally disabled, 233. *See also* Disability; Incest

Stewart, Robert M., 795. *See also* Paglia, Camille; Sex work; Utopianism

Stiglmayer, Alexandra: rape in war, 686, 905

Stoller, Robert J.: on bestiality, 76, 79; collaboration with Gilbert Herdt (*Intimate Communications*), 440–41

Stoltenberg, John: Andrea Dworkin, relationship with, 241; on pornography, 244, 343; sexual fantasies use other people, 305

Stone, Sandy [Allucquère Rosanne], 209; deception in cybersex, 213; telephone/cybersex works through fantasy and lack of cues, 211

Stopes, Marie Carmichael: early feminist promotion of heterosexuality, 320; family planning educator, 133; marriage annulled, 133

Storey, Mark: frequency of skinny-dipping, 719; on legal moralism, 718. *See also* Nudism

Storms, Michael: intensity factors in sexual orientation judgments, 114, 730, 890

SUBJECT INDEX

Entries in this encyclopedia on a concept, thing, or topic listed below are indicated by **bold** numerals. Alphabetization is by word. Court decisions are grouped under "Legal cases," passages from the Bible are grouped under "Scriptural passages," and encyclicals are grouped under "Encyclicals, papal." Cross-references (*See* and *See also*) are to both this index and to the Name Index (pp. 1113–1148). Pages 1–620 are in volume 1; 621–1089 are in volume 2.

Abortion, **1–7**, 51, 71, 81, 154, 205, 206, 538, 870, 926; in the Bible, 110; as contraception, 202, 203, 206; contraception, distinguished from by Pope Pius XII, 156; contraception, linked to by Karol Wojtyła (Pope John Paul II), 1085; couples who practice it are not really married, 78; effects, availability influences sexual activity, 826, 870; effects, reduces number of adoptable children, 921; in Hippocratic Oath, 268; the law and, 584, 656, 842; liberal feminist defense of, 1–2, 338; in Manichaeism, 637; minors consenting to, 190; in multiple pregnancies, 925; Phibionitic Gnostics eat fetal result of, 409; prohibiting premarital sex as a way to reduce, 199; reasons for, rape pregnancy, 686; reasons for, anatomical sex and sexual orientation selection, 473, 925; relevance of voluntariness and intention of sexual activity to moral permissibility of, 1–7; results from sexual addiction, 26; safer through medical technology, 154. *See also Planned Parenthood v. Casey*; *Roe v. Wade*

Abstinence, **7–14**, 74, 190, 226, 271; compulsory heterosexuality supported by derogation of, 904; contraception, a method of (rhythm), 156, 1085–86; contraception as an alternative to, 199; some cybersexual activity violates, 211; in Gnosticism, 11, 12, 403; health and other secular reasons for, 8, 9, 646, 748; in Manichaeism and among its Elect, 11, 12, 75, 638; masturbation, oral sex, and other noncoital sex acts may not negate, 8, 15, 16; masturbation assists in achieving,

677; one moral argument against same-sex acts is also an argument against, 197, 200, 461; morally or legally required of those with sexually transmitted diseases, 238; promotion of by (sex) education, 258, 931, 991–93; Protestant doubts about attainability of, 869; religious days on which one should be, 155; Saint Augustine and Saint Jerome debated requirement of, 77–78; Saint Augustine thought preferable to marriage and procreation, 12, 77, 632; Saint Jerome encouraged for all, 76–77, 642–43; Saint Paul recommended (1 Corinthians 7), 11, 145, 156, 612, 642, 749–50; Thomas Aquinas on, 1049; as a type of chastity but different from it, 7, 9–10, 51, 316, 1086. *See also* Anscombe, G.E.M.; Celibacy; Chastity; Rhythm method; Virginity

Abstinence, periodic. *See* Periodic continence; Rhythm method

Acquaintance rape. *See* Rape, acquaintance and date

Acquired Immunodeficiency Syndrome (AIDS), 154, 439, 441, 988, 1005; Africans blamed for, 38; bisexuals blamed for transmitting HIV to heterosexuals, 116, 236; caused by sexual addiction, 26; caused by tattooing, piercing, surgery, 399; in drug users and addicts, 235; fitting punishment for sexual immorality, 109; hazard of prostitution, 850; in New York Haitians, 235; occurs in "innocent" populations, 236; physicians refuse to treat infected persons, 270; provides reasons against premarital and other sexual

Continence. *See* Abstinence; Celibacy; Chastity; Periodic continence; Virginity

Contraception, 132, 133, 154, 186, 199, **202–9**, 213, 251, 258, 355, 445, 488, 536, 643, 784, 795, 826, 870, 988, 1012, 1060, 1068, 1074; abortion and, 1–3 passim, 81, 156, 656, 844, 921; Saint Augustine on, 74–76, 642, 676; in the Bible, 105, 110; cause of arguments within Catholicism, 158, 204, 1082; *coitus interruptus* a method of, 75, 204; contrary to freedom or well-being of women, 244, 319; and definition of sexual act, 18; George Drysdale, early defender of, 264; emergency, 206–7; the law and, 584, 656, 841, 842, 844, 921; not forbidden in Judaism, 538; not forbidden in Protestantism, 871; relationship between anal/oral sex and, 100; relationship between sex by infertile or homosexual couple and, 100, 445, 464, 465, 506, 656, 703, 707, 1049, 1085–86; rhythm method (periodic continence, abstinence) as a type of, or contrasted with use of, 52–54, 156, 871, 1085–86; rhythm method in Manichaeism, 75, 76; Margaret Sanger, proponent of, 263, 266, 319, 871; use of is contrary to nature, 150, 204, 702, 871, 1049; use of violates "inseparability," 157, 204, 1082, 1084; in Karol Wojtyła (Pope John Paul II), 1085–86. *See* Encyclicals, papal (*Humanae vitae*); Rhythm method

Coolidge effect (after President Calvin Coolidge): communication model explains, 176; familiarity attenuates sexual interest, 33, 34, 232, 394, 489, 1055; novel sex partner increases male performance, 90; a version of in Sigmund Freud's "On the Universal Tendency to Debasement in the Sphere of Love," 65, 140, 376, 786

Coprophilia, 70, 85, 767

Coprophagia: in Marquis de Sade, 85, 957, 958, 1043

Council of Trent: the goods of marriage, 150–51

Crossdressing. *See* Transvestism

Cultural views of sexuality. *See* African philosophy; Chinese philosophy; Greek sexuality and philosophy, ancient; Indian erotology; Roman sexuality and philosophy, ancient

Cybersex, **209–18**, 795; addiction to, 26, 213; as adultery, 16, 18, 30, 211, 213; anonymity allowed by, 26, 214; as casual sex, 136; deception in, 213–14; definition of, 209; fantasy in, 26, 999; involves sexual activities without physical contact, 210: e-mails, 16, 26, 213; instant messages, 16, 26; internet chatting, 15, 18–26 passim, 136; internet pornography, 26, 213, 585, 671, 813, 997; telephone sex, 15–21 passim, 211, 849, 997, 999; women cybersexuals, 26. *See also* Activity, sexual; Flirting; Masturbation, dual

Date rape. *See* Rape, acquaintance and date

Desire, sexual, **222–29**; abnormal, deviant, disordered, or unnatural, 27, 28, 99, 140, 151, 181, 276, 282, 283, 363, 460, 517, 519, 744–45, 752, 772, 813; as itself adultery, 3, 642, 704–5; analogy/disanalogy with desire for food or drink, 59, 226–27, 391, 494, 545, 611, 752, 787, 975, 1057; asymmetrical, unreciprocated, 23, 184, 191–92; Christian antipathy toward, 11–12, 143, 145–46, 150–51; conceptually linked with sexual activity, 23, 182, 211, 222; conceptually linked with sexual pleasure, 224–25, 456–57, 771; cultivation of, 9, 495; death of, 143, 158, 297, 316, 394, 487, 643, 646, 770; definition of, 224, 226–27, 678–79, 768, 771, 785, 794, 1012, 1014; disgust, repulsiveness, and, 98–99, 128, 310, 586–87, 768, 772; fantasy and, 225–26, 306, 327, 391, 547, 770, 961, 999; friendship incompatible with, 87, 392–93, 642; Gnostic contempt for, 12, 407, 637; hypoactive, 27, 250, 251; innateness contrasted with social construction of, 90–91, 115, 160, 222, 224, 225, 250, 326, 439–40, 988, 1010, 1011, 1027; (in)ordinate or (in)temperate, 281, 393, 494, 527, 752; as insatiable, 129, 558, 752, 1018; intersubjectivity of, 174–75, 181, 223, 225–26, 297–98, 752, 769, 780–81, 975–76; loveless casual sex and, 136, 137, 140, 765; marriage domesticates, tames, or is remedy (*remedium*) for, 144, 154, 158, 349–50, 431, 432, 445, 548, 642, 750, 859, 860, 863, 869; mastery, or struggle between will or reason, over, 75, 78, 127, 157, 168, 221, 282, 366, 407, 495, 545, 657, 787, 802, 804–5, 808, 859, 936, 968, 1050; morality of, 12, 53, 66, 107, 127, 274, 276–77, 319, 851; objectification or possession of the object or target of, 88, 139–40, 174, 223, 296–97, 328, 392, 393, 457, 518, 544–45, 613, 645–46, 699, 713, 724, 764, 853, 1083–84; pernicious because distracts from spiritual concerns, 12, 143, 525, 748; pleasure at being the target of, 170, 456–57; pornography's effect on, 305, 813; power and, 327–28, 455–58 passim, 622, 771, 889, 1067; relationship between love and, 87, 88, 136, 140, 220, 476–77, 607, 609–10, 611–12; repressed or unconscious elements in, 64, 66, 71, 327, 363, 364, 366, 1072; reproduction is the moral, natural, or ultimate goal of, 90, 146–47, 157, 181, 223, 251, 463, 664, 769, 787, 788–89, 970; sexual orientation and, 113, 115, 147, 612, 685, 729–30, 886, 890, 1011; for sexual variety, 33, 34, 646; union and, 220, 298, 390, 391, 392, 408, 430, 443, 468, 557, 609–12, 641, 646, 699, 807, 865, 871, 1014; women as denying, lacking, free of, or having mastery over, 41, 168, 354, 715; women as "the privileged objects of desire" (Georges Bataille), 86; women's perspectives on, 148, 446, 628. *See also* Arts, sex and the; Completeness, sexual; Communication model; Dysfunction, sexual; Ethics, sexual; Ethics, virtue; Freud, Sigmund; Freudian Left, the; Jealousy; Levinas, Emmanuel; Lust; Matthew 5:27–30; Nagel, Thomas; Paraphilia; Perversion, sexual; Plato; Rape; Sadomasochism; Scruton, Roger

Deviance, sexual, 213, 363, 514, 656, 768, 770, 861, 863, 963; African sexuality as, 38; bisexuality as, 115, 116; heterosexual variants as, 146; homosexuality as, 12, 27, 28, 115, 146, 769, 773, 803; immorality and, 174; incest as, 806; masturbation as, 12, 176; medicalization of, 28, 133, 362, 472, 676–77, 768–69, 874, 886–87, 896, 971, 1002–3, 1005, 1006; as mental disorder, 740–45 passim, 769; nymphomania as, 27; rape as not, 246. *See also* Paraphilia; Perversion, sexual; Psychology, in twentieth and twenty-first century

Diagnostic and Statistical Manual of Mental Disorders (American Psychiatric Association): homosexuality *per se* eliminated from, 28, 769

Diagnostic and Statistical Manual of Mental Disorders (American Psychiatric Association), I: homosexuality as mental disorder in, 769; issued in 1952, 27

Diagnostic and Statistical Manual of Mental Disorders (American Psychiatric Association), III: homosexuality eliminated, 769; Kantian psychological view of promiscuity, 27–28; mental disorder, definition of, 742–43; paraphilia, definition of, 742; transvestic fetishism, 742; zoophilia as paraphilia, 96

Diagnostic and Statistical Manual of Mental Disorders (American Psychiatric Association), III-R: included sexual addiction as sexual disorder, 27; paraphilia, definition of, 742–44; transvestic fetishism, 742

Diagnostic and Statistical Manual of Mental Disorders (American Psychiatric Association), IV: eliminated sexual addiction, 27; hypoactive sexual desire in, 9, 27, 250; Kantian psychological view of promiscuity in, 27–28; mental distress required for sexual dysfunction, 250; paraphilia, definition of, 742–45, 769–70; sadomasochism in, 962; sexual aversion disorder, 22; sexual dysfunctions in, 248–52 passim; transvestic fetishism, 742; voyeurism, 118; zoophilia, 96

Diagnostic and Statistical Manual of Mental Disorders (American Psychiatric Association), IV-TR: ego-dystonic sexual orientation as sexual disorder, 115; Kantian psychological view of promiscuity, 28; mental disorder, definition of, 740, 741–42; paraphilia, definition of, 742–45, 769–70; transvestic fetishism, 743

Disability, 71, 139, **229–34**, 251, 853, 895; consent and, 184, 232–33; deceptive cybersex and, 214; definition of, 239–40; intersexuality as, 1078; lesbian sexuality and, 328; in paraphilia, 740–41; queer theory and, 897; sexiness and, 244; welfare rights to sex and, 230–31. *See also* Dysfunction, sexual

Diseases, sexually transmitted, 38, 197, **235–41**, 646, 794, 870, 896; Africa and, 38, 235, 239; avoided by abstinence, 9, 988, 992; avoided by cybersex, 213; cause of infertility, 921; controlling depends on studying sexual activity, 22; deception about having, 189, 236, 585, 914; medical treatment of those with, 272, 988; result of adultery, 32; result of casual sex, 138, 461; result of premarital sex, 199; result of prostitution, 586, 634, 850, 987, 992; result of sexual addiction, 26; taking precautions against transmitting, 199, 233, 258, 275, 282, 441; testing for, morality and legality of, 237–39, 585. *See also* Sex education

peccadilloes of one's, 30, 31, 196, 743; animals as, 101; casual sex with, 136, 139; of love, marriage is the, 294; online, 214

Friendship, **390–97**, 592, 644, 802, 804, 836, 1055; a basic good for New Natural Law, 463, 703; between women, erotic or romantic, 116, 318, 325, 391; cannot be bought or sold, 851; damaged by sexuality, 26, 258, 305, 794; erotic love an excess of, 60; homosexuality and same-sex, 377, 391, 444; as love (*philia*) in Aristotle, 59, 528, 641, 801; marriage and, 60, 123, 295, 393, 478, 523, 529, 547–48, 613, 642, 643, 646, 704, 750, 860, 862, 1047; no better than erotic love, 557; not the same as love, 390–91, 596, 609, 611; nonsexual, 87, 123, 832; polluted by lust or sexuality, 87; required for the good life, 139; resulting from erotic love, 390, 414, 750. *See also* Love

Genital mutilation, 12, 38, 60, **398–402**, 957; castration, 11, 76, 108, 297, 316, 320, 450, 672, 712, 714, 833, 957, 1067; circumcision, 496, 505, 528, 643, 693; clitoridectomy, 505, 506; infibulation, 506

Gnosticism, 144, 146, **402–10**, 637, 639, 766, 788; Carpocratians, 403, 408–9; contempt for sexuality in, 11, 12, 403, 407; extreme sexual license in, 12, 403, 406, 408–9, 639; Manichaeism as, 637, 638; sex-negative influence on Christianity of, 12. *See also* Simonians; Valentinians

Good sex. *See* Ethics, sexual; Nonmoral evaluations

Gospel of Thomas. *See* Thomas, Gnostic Gospel of

Greek sexuality and philosophy, ancient, 145, 294, 403, **410–18**, 436, 556, 712, 749, 752, 946; antipathy to the flesh in, 12, 414, 528; bestiality in, 97; conception of masculinity in, 343; homosexuality in, 97, 121, 366, 367, 410, 412, 414, 465, 506, 684–85, 714, 757, 803, 934–35, 1027, 1030; homosexuality, passive male, in, 60, 147, 366, 412–13, 713, 803, 935; marriage in, 60, 123, 412, 413, 414, 640–41; medicine in, 133, 268–71, 366, 971; modesty in, 266; myths in, 7, 97; unnatural sexual acts in, 365, 465, 698. *See also* Aristotle; Athens; Plato; Roman sexuality and philosophy, ancient

Harassment, sexual, **419–29**, 622, 672, 784, 786, 795, 980, 1066, 1068; catcalling as, 723; convinced by others that one is a victim of, 171; cybersexual, 213; definition of, 419; evolutionary biology and, 91, 878, 1067; flirting can become, 359; language and, 425, 579, 785, 797; men's feminism and, 343, 538; in the military, 687–88; Camille Paglia on, 737–38; pornography and, 242, 623, 815; *quid pro quo*, 188, 419, 422, 425, 723; role of Catharine MacKinnon in developing the law of, 420–21, 579, 621; sexual humor as, 481–82, 797; treatment of, by professional codes of ethics, 270; violates Kantian morality, 549; in the workplace, 419, 535

Harm principle. *See* Utilitarianism

Hebrew philosophy. *See* Judaism, history of; Judaism, in twentieth and twenty-first century

Hedonism, 199, 880; of Jeremy Bentham's utilitarianism (pleasure as the good), 195, 196, 197, 462, 788; compatible with love, 592; egoism and, 195, 592; in (occasionally) John Stuart Mill's utilitarianism, 601; justifies necrophilia, 197; opposed to personalism, 564; pansexualism and, 175; responsible hedonism in Albert Ellis, 259

Heterosexism, 115, 117, 250, 320, **442–47**, 604, 652–53, 1079; adverse effects on women, 327, 962; defended by Roger Scruton, 445, 977–78; definition of, 442–43, 445; fought by queer theory, 115; homophobia and, 443, 874, 977, 989; homosexual groups fight, 116; purportedly in David Hume, 479; of Wilhelm Reich, 387

Heterosexual intercourse, 185, 210, 251, 297, 319, 940, 1017; creates obligation to possible fetus, 4–5, 1049; dangers and harmful effects of, 8, 10, 575–76, 922, 1048; dominance, rape, pornography, prostitution, sadomasochism, or violence are the models for, 245, 246, 274, 328, 339, 622, 724, 904; done in public, 600; foreplay and other precursors to, 19, 165, 211, 357, 575, 785, 787, 991, 1011; in marriage for procreation, 12, 45, 150, 157, 204, 213, 463–64, 521, 651, 655, 664, 768, 784, 868, 870–71, 923, 986, 1046; as necrophilia, 672, 675; pleasure and, 8, 21, 23, 146, 223, 988, 1018–19; the standard meaning of the word "coitus," 575; terminates virginity, 10; transmits original sin, 80, 146, 281, 642, 1047; vagina the dominant organ in, 40, 904; with

862; sexual desire, different from, 226, 611; transmits original sin, 1047; unnatural types of, 99, 109, 752; unsatisfiable, 87; of Kenneth Williams, 9. *See also* Desire, sexual

Manichaeism, **636–39**, 975; antipathy to the flesh in, 11, 12, 75, 638; Saint Augustine's relationship to, 75–76, 79–81 passim, 146, 638; promotion of rhythm method and contraception by, 75–76; vows of the Elect, 75, 510, 638. *See also* Mani

Marriage, 8, 45, 53, 55, 154–59, 281, 612–13, **639–50**, 704–5; annulment of, 133, 156, 1050; in Aristotle, 59–60, 641; in the Bible, 105–8 passim; "Boston," 116, 325, 391, 654; false promise of, 138, 904, 914; the goods of (in Saint Augustine), 12, 77–78, 81, 146, 642, 859, 1082; the goods of (according to Council of Trent), 150–51; the goods of (in G.W.F. Hegel), 431–32; group or communal, 640, 644, 864–65, 930–32 passim, 1056; Josephite, 12, 80, 155, 407–8, 530; in Immanuel Kant, 89, 139, 349, 393, 546, 613, 645–66, 764, 768; levirate, 76, 110; morganatic, 546; "open," 31, 33, 34, 258, 646, 944, 947; as prostitution, 274, 317, 342, 826, 827, 849, 945; sexual activity in as remedy against lust (*ad remedium concupiscentiae*), 144, 154, 158, 349–50, 431, 432, 445, 548, 642, 750, 859, 860, 863, 869; three stages of, in Richard Posner, 827; union view of, 155, 174, 351, 393, 546, 548, 613, 646. *See also* Adultery; Concubinage; Divorce; Westermarck, Edward

Marriage, polygamous (polygynous, polyandrous), 45, 90, 289, 408, 644–46, 1019; in Africa, 38, 39; among African Americans, 655; among Amerindians, 655; criticized by David Hume, 478, 644; criticized by Immanuel Kant, 546, 646; favored by Arthur Schopenhauer, 644–45, 971; implied by bisexuality, 117; implied by same-sex marriage, 650, 931; inconsistent with New Natural Law, 656; in Islam, 478, 506–7, 645; in Judaism, 506, 523, 655; the law and, 587, 650, 652; among Mormons, 645, 655, 864–65, 931; in Old Testament, 76, 105, 106–7, 655; unobjectionable if consensual, 198

Marriage, same-sex, 63, 351, 433, 470, **650–59**, 825, 859, 868, 897, 1023; in Africa, 40; bisexuality and, 116, 117; "Boston"

marriages a form of, 116, 325, 391, 654; definitional argument over, 603, 650–51, 702, 1079; Kantian defense of, 547; the law and, 117, 124, 443; leads to polygamy, 650, 931; sexually transmitted diseases and, 237; unofficial, 123, 538–39, 874

Marriage debt (conjugal debt; *annexis matrimonio*), 151, 155 277, 677; in Saint Augustine, 146; egalitarian in Saint Paul, 750, 913; polygamy removes drudgery from, 645; in Thomas Aquinas, 1049

Marxism, **660–71**, 1056; critique of biology in, 880; existentialism and, 293; joined with feminism, 353–54, 666–68; Catharine MacKinnon on, 621; poststructuralism and, 832, 834, 835; prostitution and, 660–61, 667, 832, 835, 852; utopianism of, 1058, 1059. *See also* Freudian Left, the; Marx, Karl

Masochism, 611; constitutional contrasted with elective, 700; contracts in, 951, 961; feminist critique of, 773, 964, 1066; Sigmund Freud on, 950, 962, 963; of Søren Kierkegaard, 555; as pathological, 69, 767, 950, 960, 962; reasons for, 963; of Jean-Jacques Rousseau, 939; in Jean-Paul Sartre, 296–98 passim, 455–56, 963–64; as scripted and staged, 950–51, 962; socialized in women, 241, 244, 246. *See also* Sacher-Masoch, Leopold von; Sade, Marquis de; Sadism; Sadomasochism

Masturbation, **671–82**. *See also* Autoerotism; Masturbation, dual; Masturbation, mutual; Masturbation, psychic; Masturbation, solitary; Narcissism; Onanism

Masturbation, dual (touch only the self, not each other), 674; cybersexual forms of, 20, 26, 209; cybersexual forms of as adultery, 30, 211; homosexual sex as, 704; whether a sexual activity, 15–20 passim, 210

Masturbation, mutual (one/each touches the other), 139, 445; benefits of, 251; in Buddhism, 129; conjoined with bestiality, 100, 137; in consequentialist ethics, 197; definition of, 673–76; as safe sex, 991; whether a sexual activity, 18–20 passim, 575; wrong in Catholicism and New Natural Law, 149, 706

Masturbation, psychic (fantasy alone), 495, 674

Masturbation, solitary (self-touch), 17, 96, 133, 96, 258, 350, 644, 743, 769, 784, 795, 825, 888, 939, 1003, 1013, 1057; adultery is really only, 675; benefits of, 251, 677, 788; in the Bible, 110; condemned as "wasting seed,"

524, 672; in consequentialist ethics, 197, 200; consistency with abstinence, celibacy, and chastity, 8, 9, 211; cured by clitoridectomy, 399; definition of, 673–76, 786; done in public, 411, 489, 673; as dual or mutual masturbation, 675, 679; as harmful, 257, 305, 547, 634–35, 676–77, 767, 770, 813, 886, 971, 992, 1003; in Havelock Ellis, 265, 494; with fantasies, as adultery, 30, 108, 110, 306, 672; fantasies accompany, 225–26, 547, 671–79 passim; Sigmund Freud on, 375, 677, 971; as a same-sex sexual act, 761; as incestuous, 149, 671; in Immanuel Kant, 544, 547, 676; lacks interpersonality or psychological completeness, 100, 176–77, 180, 182, 213, 214, 678, 770, 1014; liberal defenses of, 257, 945; *malakoi* as meaning those who engage in, 109, 110; morally objectionable or unnatural for same reason as bestiality, homosexuality, and oral sex acts (none procreative), 55, 99, 100, 160, 180, 213, 445, 463–64, 547, 643, 676, 703–7 passim, 768; as the paradigm case of sexuality, 175, 679; philosophy as, 775, 788, 791; pornography and, 1012, 1067; preference for, 9, 160, 770; pregnancy avoided by, 409; prostitution/sex work and, relationship between, 634–35, 998; in sexual addiction, 26; sexual sin in Catholicism and New Natural Law, 8, 12, 147, 148, 149, 159–60, 213, 702–6 passim, 860, 868, 1081; stigmatized, 132, 672; substitute for coupled sexual relations, 96, 177, 678, 771; in Thomas Aquinas, unnatural and mortally sinful, 99, 150, 160, 179, 463, 487, 643, 676, 768, 1051; whether a sexual act, 19, 20, 771

Medicine, 382, 443, 758, 1011, 1078–79; abortion and, 206–7; codes of ethics in, 268–71; confidentiality in, 235, 238, 269, 271, 472, 840, 843; control of women's bodies and sexuality by, 320, 355, 367, 748; genital mutilation and, 399, 400; history of, 132–33, 317, 318, 525, 748, 971, 1050; infertility, sterility, and, 154, 355, 691, 707, 708, 921, 925; informed consent in, 184, 189, 191, 206, 207, 230, 237–38, 399, 472, 500, 759, 913, 914, 922, 983; medical acts contrasted with sexual acts, 20, 225, 269–70, 1012; sexual activity as medical therapy, 42, 189, 903; prostitution and, 586, 850, 987, 998. *See also* Contraception; Deviance, sexual; *Diagnostic and Statistical Manual of*

Mental Disorders; Diseases, sexually transmitted; Dysfunction, sexual; Hippocratic oath; Homosexuality, science and; Intersexuality; Money, John; Paraphilia; Reproductive technology; Sexology

Men's feminism. *See* Feminism, men's

Men's liberation, 258, 765. *See also* Feminism, men's

Menstruation, 57, 58, 167, 736, 740, 1018, 1050; female inferiority and, 318, 512; female sexual desire and, 265; genital mutilation and, 398, 400; intercourse during, 100, 106, 464, 524, 1049; men's, 398; produces waste material, 85, 316; in spiritual ceremonies, 409, 450, 638–39, 1043

Military, the, 123, 537, 897, 934, 955, 1013, 1058, 1061; adultery and, 31, 35; rape and, 686–87, 905, 911, 1034; homosexuality and, 115–16, 160, 237, 443, 472, 684–86; sex and, **684–90**; sexual harassment and, 687–88

Misogyny, 244, 247, 304, 359, 443; in Buddhism, 128; in India, 511; in Islam, 505; in Judaism, 528, 529; in Friedrich Nietzsche, 295, 559; in Arthur Schopenhauer, 89, 972. *See also* Sexism

Modesty, 594, 953; Havelock Ellis's five factors in, 265–66; flirting and, 359; higher civilizations move beyond, 266; David Hume on, 476–78; in Islam, 503–4; in Judaism, 525; rape incited by lack of, 512, 576; required for love, 266; as response to disgust, 265, 266; as social or natural, 266, 477–78, 633, 940–41

Morality, sexual. *See* Ethics, sexual

Morality and the law. *See* Consequentialism; Law, sex and the; Liberalism

Mormons, 864–65; polygamy among, 645, 655, 865, 931

Muslim. *See* Islam

Mutilation. *See* Genital mutilation

Narcissism, 64, 66, 309, 387, 808; adultery and, 34; autoerotism and, 264, 374, 678; masturbation and, 671, 678

Natural Law, 157, 654, 771, 789, 794, 825, 863, 1081, 1086; adultery violates, 32, 860, 1048, 1049; contraception violates, 53, 203, 204, 463, 656, 1049, 1085–86; goods of marriage in, 860; in Christine Gudorf, 46; homosexuality violates, 463, 487, 643, 802, 860, 977, 1051; incest violates, 491, 860; masturbation violates, 463, 487, 643, 860;

monogamy required by, 45, 48, 643, 1047, 1049; in Plato (*Laws*), 806; in Marquis de Sade, 956; unnatural sex violates, 180, 203–4, 768, 977; in Thomas Aquinas, 203, 305, 463, 487, 795, **1045–53**. *See also* Catholicism: history of; Catholicism: in twentieth and twenty-first centuries; Natural Law (New)

Natural Law (New), 651, 654, **702–11**; on homosexuality, 463–64, 702–8 passim; on infertility, 656, 707–8; married pair as organic unit in, 655, 704, 707, 708; on masturbation, 676, 702–7 passim; on same-sex marriage, 655–56, 708. *See also* Catholicism: history of; Catholicism: in twentieth and twenty-first centuries; Natural Law

Necrophilia, 281; as casual sex, 136; consequentialism on, 197; incestuous, 85; legal moralism and, 587; as masturbation, 672, 675; as paired sex, 197, 672, 678; as a perversion, 767, 770, 772

Naturism. *See* Nudism

Nonmoral evaluations: adultery as good sex, 32, 34, 275; anal intercourse as good sex, 955; bad sex as boring, dull, tedious, unpleasurable, 21–22, 275, 770, 789; bad sex better than none at all, 700; bad and good sex in marriage, 21, 275, 293, 676, 677, 743; bad sex in prostitution, 23; better sex for women a sociopolitical goal, 67, 319, 335; casual sex can be good or bad, 140, 999; civilized sex better than state-of-nature sex, 940–41; cybersex can be better than "real" sex, 213; familiarity helps and hinders good sex, 140, 176; good sex as exciting, pleasurable, satisfying, 22, 275, 609, 784, 789, 1012; homosexual relations not good sex, 462; incompleteness in good sex, 181, 182, 700; morally bad sex better than none, 461; passionate and sensual sexuality compared, 1023–24; perversion as good sex, 700, 743, 769; pornography and good sex for women, 818; promiscuity as good sex, 677; sex of prelapsarian Adam and Eve as bad and good, 223; utopias promise good sex, 1054; whether sex is good or bad for a man depends on the woman, 41–42

Nudism, 133, **718–22**

Objectification, sexual, 71, 186, 297, 318, 337, 505, **723–28**, 768, 784, 786, 1060; acquiescing to, 337, 725; casual sex, promiscuity, as involving, 139, 141, 245, 726; in fantasy, 305–6, 671; focuses on body parts, 139, 646, 723, 726, 765; harassment, pornography, prostitution, and rape as involving, 139–40, 242, 243, 328, 549, 575, 623, 723, 724, 738, 816, 853, 905, 975; marriage and, 546, 646, 764; personification as attenuating, 764–66; personification as opposite of, 764–65; sexuality essentially involves, 245, 393, 454, 545, 546, 549, 645–46, 724, 738, 764, 765, 795. *See also* Kant, Immanuel; Personification; Sex object; Sexual use

Oedipal and Electra complexes, 70, 101, 354, 375, 383, 567, 569, 572, 735, 806

Onanism: *coitus interruptus*, a contraceptive method, 76, 110; understood as masturbation, 676

Orgasm, simultaneous, 17; as sign of union, 610

Orgasm, women's, 317, 525, 1013; challenge to men, 458; dysfunctions in, 250, 251; Sigmund Freud on, 375, 887, 1016–17, 1019; Shere Hite's survey of, 672; Sarah Blaffer Hrdy on mystery of, 772, 1017–18; William Masters and Virginia Johnson's clitoral (single) orgasm thesis, 41, 257, 1017, 1023, 1024; Sappho on, 414; Irving Singer's rejection of single-orgasm theory, 1018, 1019, 1024–25; Donald Symons on, 1018, 1019. *See also* Sherfey, Mary Jane

Orientation, sexual, 160, 176, 250, 251, 437, 506, **728–34**, 786, 793, 872, 1083; anatomical sex and gender do not always correlate with, 114, 729, 891; in ancient Greece, 121, 413, 730–31, 1026–27; in ancient Rome, 121; behaviors, importance of in, 109, 114, 160, 282, 460–61, 471, 729, 769, 1004, 1011; bestiality as a, 95, 96, 99; in the Bible, 109; continuum versus discrete types view of, 114, 730, 890, 1004; definition of, 113, 114, 728–29; difficulties of explaining or understanding, 64, 90–91, 115, 116, 160, 289–90, 439–40, 460, 463, 468, 471–72, 499, 500, 692, 731, 780, 890–91, 1075; dispositions in, 114, 460, 514, 729–30, 1011; fantasies in, 114; heterosexist discrimination and, 442, 874, 989, 1011; liberalism and, 334, 337, 604; marriage and, 653; non-behavioral morality of, 160, 282, 460, 470, 524, 873; pansexualism as a, 115; preferences in, 114, 117, 337, 440, 472, 497,